HANDBOOK OF COSMETIC DERMATOLOGY

VOLUME 2

ADVANCED AESTHETIC PROCEDURES AND EMERGING THERAPIES

Dr. Shreya Das

ALLIED
HEALTH
PRESS

Handbook of Cosmetic Dermatology Volume 2

Advanced Aesthetic Procedures and Emerging Therapies

Author: **Dr. Shreya Das**

Allied Health Press
4164 Lakeshore Road
Burlington ON L7L 1A4
Canada
www.alliedhealthpress.com
Email: orders@arclereducation.com

ISBN: 978-1-77956-829-8

ABOUT THE AUTHOR

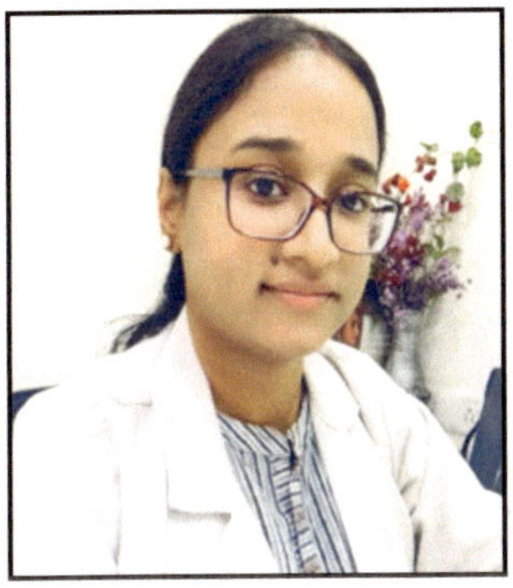

Dr. Shreya Das is an Oral and Maxillofacial Surgeon with specialized training and clinical experience in facial cosmetic surgery and aesthetic medicine. A university gold medalist, she completed her MDS in Oral and Maxillofacial Surgery and has since worked across reputed hospitals and wellness organizations. With a strong interest in facial aesthetics, her work bridges surgical precision and minimally invasive cosmetic procedures. She is passionate about advancing evidence-based practices in facial cosmetic and reconstructive surgery and contributing to the education of clinicians in this evolving field.

Brief Table of Contents

Getting Started with This Book

Chapter Openers

A list of Chapter Outline is presented providing a brief Introduction to what will be covered in the chapter.

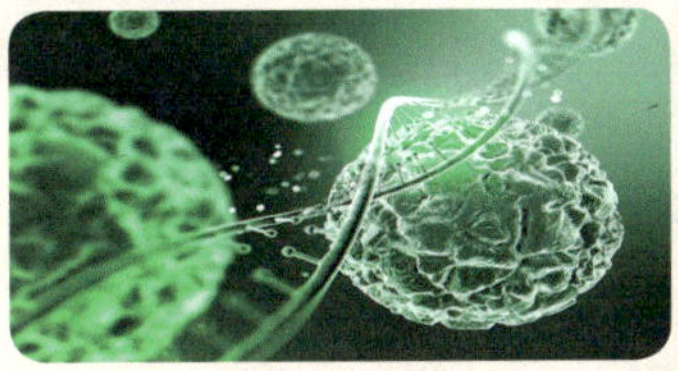

Introduction

Often referred to as the science of life, biology is a broad field of study aimed at comprehending the several kinds of life on Earth, from tiny creatures to sophisticated multicellular entities. Comprising several subfields, including molecular biology, ecology, and evolutionary biology, each of which advances our knowledge of living systems, this field clarifies the mechanisms controlling life events, including development, reproduction, and interaction with the surroundings, which is the central goal of biology. Moreover, biology fills in the void between the natural sciences and medicine by offering a necessary understanding of health, illness, and the interactions between organisms and their environments. Dealing with urgent global issues such as climate change, biodiversity loss, and new diseases depends on an awareness of these complex biological interactions, therefore highlighting the critical part biology plays in modern civilization. Fundamentally, biology explores and tests ideas about the living world using the scientific method. Through methodical observation and experimentation,

LEARNING OBJECTIVES

After studying this chapter, you will be able to:

1. Discuss the scientific method in biology;
2. Explain the cell theory;
3. Discuss the genetics and heredity;
4. Evolution and natural selection;
5. Focus on ecology and ecosystems;
6. Learn about human biology;
7. Evaluate the plant biology;
8. Explain the microbiology;
9. Focus on current trends in biology.

1.1. The Scientific Method in Biology

Learning Outcome

1. Describe the steps of the scientific method;
2. Focus on hypothesis formation;
3. Learn about experimental design.

Learning Outcomes

The beginning of each section of every chapter contains a set of Learning Outcomes that inform students of concepts they should understand. These outcomes help students understand what they should be able to do if they have mastered the material in that section.

Test Your Knowledge

Throughout each chapter, Test Your Knowledge cues you to note which topics have been covered and to self-test your understanding of the material presented.

Test Your Knowledge

1. Explain why correlation does not imply causation in scientific experiments.
2. How does the scientific method help reduce the influence of personal opinions in research?

Chapter Summary

The Summary Section appear at the end of each chapter and summarize main concepts covered throughout the chapter. These points provide key concepts in an engaging and meaningful way.

Summary

The investigation of biological principles highlights the importance of a comprehensive view of life by reflecting the intricate interactions that occur within living systems. The complexity of biology goes beyond individual species or systems, as this essay highlights; it also includes the interactions that mold ecosystems and affect biodiversity. Researchers can conduct in-depth analyses of metabolomic data using sophisticated technologies like MetaboAnalyst, which offer insights into the molecular mechanisms underlying these interactions. As demonstrated by the developments in MetaboAnalyst, for example, the integration of diverse omics data promotes a thorough understanding of metabolic pathways and helps identify important biological markers necessary for research on development and disease (Chong et al., 2018). Additionally, the phenomenon of ecological invasions is a key component of biological research and a vital field of study. The introduction of non-native species into unfamiliar habitats has significant ramifications and calls for multidisciplinary management strategies. Examining the origins and effects of these biological incursions, invasion science has become a crucial field that highlights the need to comprehend ecological dynamics and community interactions. As interest in biological invasions increases, new findings are emerging that put conventional ecological theories and practices to the test. The importance of incorporating various scientific viewpoints is shown by this developing discipline, which also highlights how invasive species shape ecosystems and advances our knowledge of ecological resilience (David et al., 2013). When taken as a whole, these discoveries from invasion science and metabolomics highlight the value of multidisciplinary biology research. Fostering cross-disciplinary collaboration and utilizing technological breakthroughs to improve our comprehension of intricate biological interactions are crucial as we look to the future of biological research. In addition to deepening our understanding of the complexities of life, this method lays the groundwork for tackling urgent environmental issues. Future studies can ensure the continued relevance of biology in a world that is constantly changing by acknowledging the interconnection of biological systems and opening the door to creative solutions that support sustainability and biodiversity conservation. We might imagine a thorough comprehension of life that serves both academia and society at large through ongoing investigation and integration of scientific knowledge.

Knowledge Assessment

The chapter includes material designed to review and reinforce each content. It includes Critical Thinking Questions to help test of your understanding of information presented in the chapter and Short answer Questions to review your understanding of the key concepts presented in the chapter.

Critical Thinking Questions

1. **Who is known as the "Father of Modern Biology"?**
   a. Aristotle
   b. Charles Darwin
   c. Gregor Mendel
   d. Louis Pasteur
2. **What is the basic unit of life?**
   a. Atom
   b. Molecule
   c. Cell
   d. Organism
3. **Which branch of biology studies the interaction of organisms with their environment?**
   a. Genetics
   b. Ecology
   c. Physiology
   d. Botany
4. **Which macromolecule is the main source of energy for living organisms?**
   a. Proteins
   b. Lipids
   c. Carbohydrates
   d. Nucleic acids
5. **DNA is primarily responsible for which function in living organisms?**
   a. Energy production
   b. Protein synthesis
   c. Storing genetic information
   d. Regulating body temperature

Short Answer Questions

1. What is biology, and why is it important to study biology?
2. What are the three main domains of life, and how are they different from one another?
3. Define homeostasis and give an example of how it works in living organisms.
4. What is the cell theory, and why is it fundamental to biology?
5. How do autotrophs and heterotrophs differ in the way they obtain energy?
6. What is the scientific method, and how is it applied in biological research?
7. Discuss how biology helps address global challenges such as climate change, disease, and food security.
8. Explain the levels of biological organization from the smallest unit to the largest. Provide examples at each level.
9. Describe the relationship between structure and function in biology, giving specific examples from cells or organs.
10. How has the discovery of genetics shaped our understanding of inheritance and variation among organisms?

Supplementary Materials

Key Terms: A list of key terms is given for quick reference

KEY TERMS FROM THIS CHAPTER

Annotation enrichment analysis
Cell theory
Ecosystems
Microbiology
Plant biology
Biological structure
Cellular structure
Genetics
Natural selection
Cell
Ecology
Human biology
Organism

Further Resources: Recommendations for additional readings, websites, and multimedia resources.

References

1. Argelaguet, R., Velten, B., Arnol, D., Dietrich, S., Zenz, T., Marioni, J. C., Buettner, F., et al. (2018). Multi-omics factor analysis—A framework for unsupervised integration of multi-omics data sets. *Molecular Systems Biology, 14*. https://doi.org/10.15252/msb.20178124.
2. Bacher, S., Blackburn, T. M., Essl, F., & Genovesi, P. (2017). *Socio-Economic Impact Classification of Alien Taxa (SEICAT)*. https://core.ac.uk/download/286567949.pdf (accessed on 8th March 2025).
3. Barnett, R., Brace, S., Cucchi, T., & Dobney, K. (2013). *Divergent Evolutionary Processes Associated with Colonization of Offshore Islands*. https://core.ac.uk/download/20664364.pdf (accessed on 8th March 2025).

Detailed Table of Contents

CHAPTER 5

Nail Aesthetic Conditions and Treatments 135

CHAPTER 6

Thread Lifting and Skin Tightening Techniques 169

CHAPTER 7

Liposuction Techniques 203

CHAPTER 10

Psychodermatology and Body Dysmorphic Disorder 301

CHAPTER 11

Tattoo Removal and Scar Management 335

CHAPTER 12

Cosmetic Sclerotherapy 365

LIST OF FIGURES

PREFACE

Cosmetic dermatology has experienced the most vigorous development over the past few decades, evolving from a specialism within dermatology to a distinct discipline addressing both cosmetic and functional concerns of the skin, hair, and nails. Influenced by advances in cellular biology, immunology, and materials science, practitioners today have a range of minimally invasive and noninvasive techniques at their disposal with which to achieve results formerly deemed feasible only through lengthy surgery. Patients today expect more than mere correction; they want therapies that enhance their natural appearance, restore self-confidence, and harmonize with their active lifestyles. This evolution has been fueled by an increased understanding of the interaction between photodamage, skin aging, and genetic susceptibility, as well as improvements in delivery systems that ensure therapeutic agents reach their target sites optimally and safely.

At the same time, the interaction between patient psychology and dermatologic therapy has come to be increasingly understood as a critical element of effective treatment. Beauty beliefs and self-image are profoundly personal and shaped by a combination of cultural, social, and individual factors. Practitioners, therefore, need to balance technical skill with insight, modifying treatment plans to address both the physical attributes and the psychosocial needs of individual patients. Such an integrative approach is also adopted in pre- and posttreatment management, with patient education, proper setting of expectations, and longitudinal follow-up being important in maintaining long-term satisfaction. By integrating evidence-based treatment practices with customization, modern cosmetic dermatology creates effects that result in a synthesis of physical and emotional impact.

The aim of this book, *Handbook of Cosmetic Dermatology: Volume 2*, is to provide a comprehensive resource for clinicians, researchers, and students seeking to expand their knowledge of the most current therapeutic regimens. Based on fundamental understanding, this book presents cutting-edge methods and protocols, highlights pragmatic concerns in patient selection and management, and reviews the results of current clinical trials. It contains detailed procedural descriptions, example cases, and summaries of consensus guidelines that document the safe and effective use of these treatments in practice.

Chapter 1 provides a comprehensive overview of platelet-rich plasma (PRP) applications, outlining the principles of autologous blood processing, techniques for optimizing growth factor concentration, injection and topical application protocols, and procedures for assessing tissue rejuvenation and regeneration. Safety protocols, contraindications, and comparisons of PRP with adjunct treatments are emphasized. Chapter 2 discusses the multifaceted problem of hair loss, reviewing diagnostic models for androgenetic and non-androgenetic alopecias, trichoscopy-directed treatment, evidence-based drug treatments, microneedling and low-level laser therapy (LLLT) devices, surgical transplantation techniques, and patient counseling methodologies for setting reasonable goals. Chapter 3 explores treatment options for hyperpigmentation and melasma, including descriptions of pigmentary pathways, chemical peeling, laser and light treatments, topical treatments with tranexamic acid (TXA) and hydroquinone alternatives, and combination treatments that are maximally effective and minimally hazardous. Chapter 4 discusses treatments for vitiligo, including cosmetic camouflage approaches, narrowband UVB phototherapy, autologous melanocyte transplantation techniques, and newer molecular agents that induce repigmentation in both stable and active disease.

Chapter 5 describes nail cosmetic disorders, ranging from brittle nail syndrome to onycholysis and pitting disease, by examining diagnostic characteristics, systemic and topical treatments, including biotin supplementation and novel peptidomimetic drugs, as well as procedural treatments such as nail matrix micrografting. Chapter 6 addresses thread lifting and skin tightening procedures, comparing suture materials, insertion technique by facial zone, mechanisms of collagen induction, management of potential complications, and patient satisfaction measures. Chapter 7 provides a comprehensive overview of liposuction methods, ranging from traditional tumescent to power-assisted, ultrasound-assisted, and laser-assisted modalities, along with recommendations on fluid management, contouring techniques, and post-treatment compression regimens. Chapter 8 covers vascular lesions, demonstrating classification techniques for hemangiomas and telangiectasias, the selection of pulsed dye and Nd:YAG lasers, sclerotherapy solutions, and adjunctive pharmacologic agents, as well as management of purpura and scarring, including risk prevention and monitoring strategies.

Chapter 9 discusses cellulite and stretch mark management, covering current theories behind dermal-adipose interactions, mechanical massage devices, subcision techniques, fractionated resurfacing lasers, and topical retinoids, with comparative patient-reported outcome data. Chapter 10 considers psychodermatology and body dysmorphic disorder (BDD) by outlining screening protocols, collaborative care models with mental health professionals, behavioral therapy strategies, and considerations for ethical treatment boundaries.

Chapter 11 collates tattoo removal and scar treatment modalities, including Q-switched laser parameters, picosecond pulse technologies, adjunctive chemical and mechanical methods, and second-generation silicone-based and growth factor-enhanced scar therapies. Chapter 12 concludes with a discussion of cosmetic sclerotherapy, including foam versus liquid sclerosants, duplex ultrasound guidance, dosing algorithms, and strategies for preventing pigmentation and recanalization, supported by the results of long-term follow-up.

This guidebook is addressed to practicing dermatologists, plastic surgeons, aesthetic physicians, nurse practitioners, physician assistants, and residents seeking a broad, clinically applicable text. Researchers and industry experts will also find utility in the detailed protocol descriptions and discussions of new technologies. As a reference for routine clinical use or as an introduction to further advanced study, this book presents a methodical, practical route to mastering the diverse array of treatments typical of contemporary cosmetic dermatology.

PLATELET-RICH PLASMA: APPLICATIONS IN COSMETIC DERMATOLOGY

1

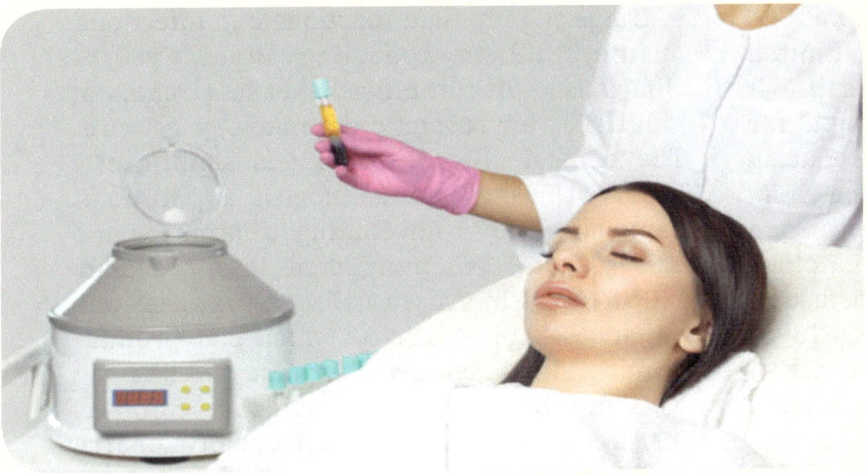

LEARNING OBJECTIVES

After studying this chapter, you will be able to:

1. Understand the mechanism of platelet-rich plasma (PRP) in cosmetic dermatology
2. Describe common applications of PRP in cosmetic dermatology
3. Explain benefits of PRP procedures
4. Define risks and considerations for PRP procedures
5. Compare other cosmetic treatments
6. Highlight current research and future direction

Introduction

The field of cosmetic dermatology has made huge strides in the recent past, and many new therapies have emerged to provide added aesthetic advantages. Platelet-rich plasma (PRP) therapy is one such therapy that has gained immense prominence because it purports to harness the body's own healing mechanism. It is a therapy in which a patient's blood is taken and subsequently prepared to load the platelets and the growth factors that stimulate tissue growth. With growing demands for minimally invasive interventions, PRP therapy presents a lucrative option for individuals choosing to undergo cosmetic treatments without the necessity for surgical interventions. It has now been apparent that researchers have begun exploring the multifaceted applications of PRP in various cosmetic procedures, such as in facial rejuvenation, scar revision, and hair restoration, thus outlining its significance in modern dermatological interventions. Various studies have indicated the positive outcomes of PRP therapy on healing and skin quality. For instance, PRP is increasingly regarded as effective in addressing challenging dermatological conditions such as scarring from acne and alopecia. A research study on white Wistar mice described the wound healing properties of the PRP and revealed that PRP significantly increases the tissue regeneration process compared to other therapies like salmon DNA serum dermapen (Chiuman et al., 2023). This directs towards the particular growth factors within the PRP, which act crucially in tissue remodeling and proliferation. The regenerative potential of PRP is not limited to purely cosmetic beautification because it accesses the body's biological reaction for healing and re-vitalization, ultimately producing a heightened aesthetic beauty of the skin. Beyond its medical benefits, the application of PRP therapy within cosmetic dermatology raises significant safety and patient satisfaction concerns that must be addressed. As PRP is drawn from the patient themselves, the risk of side effects that would otherwise be associated with foreign substances is significantly decreased. That being said, the efficacy of PRP is largely determined by standards of collection and processing, making it even more essential to adhere to the procedure when using it (Suruchi et al., 2018). In addition, continued scientific investigation further improves our knowledge of the capabilities of PRP, alongside its limitations in the treatment of skin disorders. As science keeps unfolding, practitioners are prompted to employ evidence-based protocols in order to maximize treatment efficacy as well as patient safety, and thus PRP therapy remains a paradigm of regenerative medicine's transformative power on cosmetic dermatology.

Definition of Platelet-Rich Plasma (PRP)

The concept of PRP emerged out of a desire to harness the body's own natural healing processes for therapeutic gain. PRP is harvested from a patient's blood using a process of centrifugation, which separates out the plasma, a pale yellow liquid made up of platelets, from the red and white blood cells. The concentrated plasma is loaded with platelets, growth factors, and cytokines, all of which play an important role in wound healing and tissue regeneration. On injection, PRP induces various cellular activities, including collagen synthesis, angiogenesis, and cell growth, with the result of stimulating repair and regeneration of damaged tissues. Its autologous nature precludes the possibility of triggering immune reactions and infections, making PRP an appealing alternative for clinicians to provide efficient yet safe treatment modalities for cosmetic dermatology patients. The clinical efficacy of PRP is significantly observed in most dermatological applications, particularly for rejuvenating treatments and hair growth. When injected into the skin, PRP triggers increased collagen synthesis and enhances skin elasticity, which can produce remarkable reductions in wrinkle and fine line visibility. Besides, clinical evidence confirms its effectiveness in the treatment of alopecia, where the growth factors contained in PRP are intended to stimulate hair follicles and increase hair density by a minimally invasive method. However, the clinical effectiveness of PRP may vary on the basis of different parameters, such as platelet concentration, application mode, and the characteristics of the patient. These parameters direct the importance of employing standardized protocols to optimize their therapeutic applicability in different dermatological scenarios, thus paving the way for more uniform results in practice (Rizvi, 2021). Moreover, the convergence of PRP therapy and regenerative medicine offers an interesting insight into its future scope in cosmetic dermatology. Through its ability to enhance tissue repair and cellular regeneration, PRP is also said to be beneficial for cosmetic use, but even for medical use such as scar revision and healing of wounds. New research also shows the efficacy of PRP when mixed with other regenerative agents such as polydeoxyribonucleotide (PDRN), which would further advance the advantage in the instance of acne scars and skin rejuvenation (Akaberi et al., 2025). The growing evidence suggests that the flexibility may render it a keystone in the future of cosmetic procedures. Nonetheless, ongoing research is paramount to ascertain its efficacy, shed off existing contradictions, and improve methodologies, thereby solidifying PRP as a mainstream option within the ever-evolving field of cosmetic dermatology (Figure 1.1).

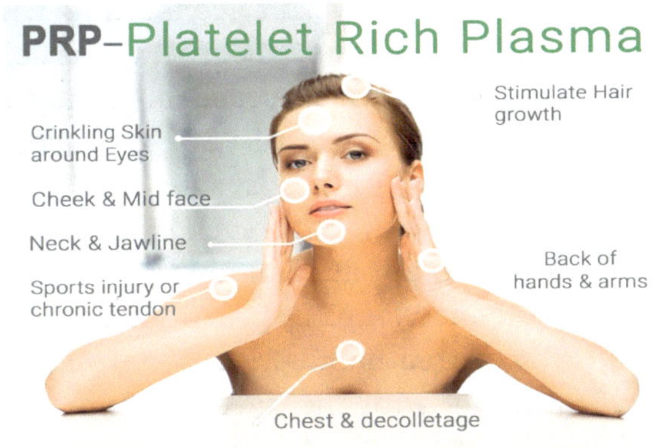

Figure 1.1. Platelet-rich plasma (PRP).

Source: https://dermnurse.ca/wp-content/uploads/2023/11/cd29f1ac158b7f18c7305c0d01fc56d3b5fda090_s2_n1.jpg.

Historical Background of PRP in Medicine

The concept of using PRP in medical therapy originated in surgery in the late 20th century. Initially, PRP was developed as a means to enhance healing in orthopedic and dental operations. The density of growth factors contained within platelets rendered them theoretically capable of substantially enhancing the repair and regeneration of tissue. This encouraged researchers to examine the effectiveness of PRPs in other medical fields, including sports medicine and reconstructive surgery. With its advantages being realized, the application of PRP grew, with numerous studies reporting its effectiveness in quick healing and improving surgical results. Specifically, among the most crucial milestones in its history was its application in dermatology, where it began to be considered a new form of treating skin pathology and optimizing cosmetic outcomes, eventually leading to its transition into cosmetic dermatology and cosmetic treatments. The development of PRP as a cosmetic treatment indicates a significant shift in the mindset of medical treatments to aesthetics. Dermatologists began investigating the potential for treating overall skin conditions, such as acne scars and overall rejuvenation, with PRP. Saeed et al. (2016) demonstrate this development by describing techniques such as fractional microneedling radiofrequency (RF) with PRP, demonstrating a three-dimensional method of improving facial scars and texture of the skin. This union of cosmetic dermatology and regenerative medicine laid the basis for numerous clinical research studies examining its efficacy in aesthetic applications. The positive outcomes noted in these aforementioned studies spurred patient interest and acceptance of PRP as a valid treatment modality for anti-aging resistance and beauty enhancement, solidifying its position in cosmetic dermatology. Refining the functions of PRPs in dermatology, several studies have also elucidated the mechanisms through which PRP contributes to the rejuvenation and healing of the skin. Oh et al. (2014) note that the concentration of growth factors in PRP, such as platelet-derived growth factor (PDGF), enhances tissue remodeling and production of collagen, which is imperative for the restoration of skin integrity. This biological foundation explains the success of PRP in conditions like depressed acne scarring, in which traditional treatments have met with restrictions. The inclusion of LED phototherapy with PRP also illustrates combination therapies that are pioneering in cosmetic dermatology. As practitioners more and more critically investigate and affirm PRP's clinical efficacy through intense research, its history is a foundation for ongoing advances that enable it to mature as an option for treatment of a vast variety of dermatological conditions.

Overview of PRP's Rise in Cosmetic Dermatology

The entry of PRP into cosmetic dermatology is a significant departure from conventional aesthetic treatments, driven by an increasing demand for minimally invasive interventions whose outcome is natural. The application of traditional aesthetic interventions, fillers, and injectables has given way to innovative, regenerative therapies. PRP is distinguished for its autologous nature; it is implemented utilizing the patient's components of blood, removing side effects and enhancing biocompatibility. Improved recent years in knowledge of growth factors and their use in tissue regeneration have prompted the utilization of PRP as a highly sought-after treatment among patients who want rejuvenation of facial appearance without undergoing surgery. Greater consumer awareness and exposure to natural treatments are also accelerating the trend, which solidifies PRP's position as a leader in the latest cosmetic dermatology.

With greater popularity for a broad array of dermatological applications, PRP's utility for hair restoration and facial rejuvenation has been in the spotlight. Research confirms that the growth factors in PRP strongly stimulate hair follicles, triggering hair growth in patients with androgenetic alopecia and other types of hair loss. Moreover, its application extends to treating skin laxity, fine lines, and overall skin texture, showcasing its versatility. Clinicians increasingly integrate PRP into comprehensive treatment regimens, often combining it with procedures such as microneedling to enhance results. This synergistic approach not only amplifies the therapeutic effects but also appeals to patients seeking holistic solutions to aesthetic concerns. The favorable outcomes shown in clinical trials contribute to the proven efficacy of PRP in cosmetic dermatology and thus encourage increased research and utilization of this new treatment. The use of PRP in cosmetic dermatology is supported by a strong evidence base demonstrating its safety and efficacy, but practitioners need to be aware of potential contraindications. Emerging studies enhance our understanding of the interaction between cosmetic procedures and autoimmune disorders, where some procedures can harm patients with underlying conditions, rendering patient care a tailored process. For instance, while PRP is generally safe, consulting with patients with autoimmune disorders is crucial as their response to such procedures may be unpredictable (Górska et al., 2024). Further, the understanding of PRP's role in healing chronic wounds supports its regenerative power beyond cosmetic application, and thus, there should be full knowledge by practitioners when adding PRP to treatment protocols (Everts et al., 2018). Along with the development of the topic, ongoing research and clinical experience will be important in maximizing protocols and utilizing PRP most safely and effectively within cosmetic dermatology (Figure 1.2).

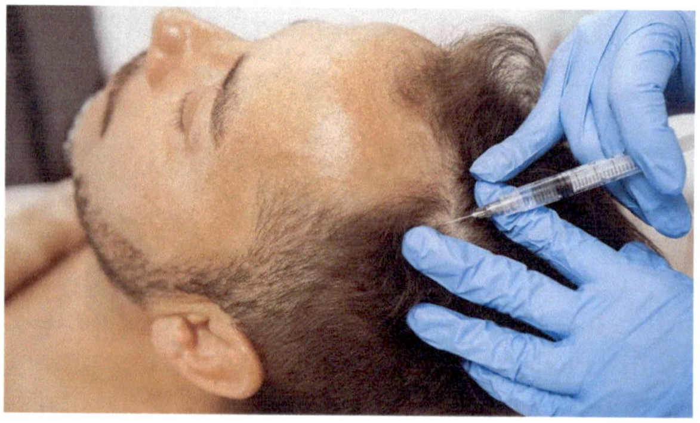

Figure 1.2. Platelet-rich plasma (PRP) therapy being administered for hair restoration.

Source: https://sa1s3optim.patientpop.com/filters:format(webp)/assets/production/practices/7c07f9409168f5d49e2231d3b69d75ff1f8b14a2/images/2532110.png.

1.1. Mechanism of Action

Learning Outcome

1. Understand the composition of platelet-rich plasma
2. Discuss growth factors and their role in skin rejuvenation
3. Explain the process of PRP extraction and preparation

The mechanism of action of PRP in cosmetic dermatology involves primarily the release of an array of growth factors and cytokines that facilitate tissue repair and regeneration. On injection into the epidermis or the dermis, PRP significantly enhances wound healing by triggering many cellular activities. Release of the significant growth factors such as PDGF, vascular endothelial growth factor (VEGF), and transforming growth factor-beta (TGF-β) that play a role in collagen synthesis, angiogenesis, and control of inflammatory processes takes place, and all together lead to increased tissue remodeling and rejuvenation, which renders PRP a promising therapeutic agent for improving skin texture and appearance in cosmetic therapy (Thanh et al., 2021). Apart from the delivery of growth factors, PRP's success also comes from its capacity to enhance the skin's regenerative power. Because PRP is autologous, it ensures that the patient's own biological substance is applied, lessening the risk of allergic reactions or other adverse effects. Evidence suggests that PRP triggers the proliferation of dermal fibroblasts and keratinocytes, both of which are crucial to skin integrity and function. By fostering a dynamic environment for cellular growth and differentiation, PRP treatment revitalizes skin vitality, targeting in particular problems such as wrinkles, scars, and other signs of aging. Synergistic interaction of these growth factors renders PRP capable of employing a multipronged approach towards revitalizing the skin not so readily achieved through conventional therapy (Oh et al., 2014). In the domain of specific applications, PRP action has demonstrated great promise in the treatment of depressed facial scars as well as overall skin quality. As clinical evidence has hinted, PRP enhances wound healing facilitated by therapy like laser therapy since it stimulates the healing potential of the skin by upregulating such processes critical in tissue remodeling. The application of PRP, coupled with adjunct therapies, including LED phototherapy, even strengthens its effect, where the phototherapy assists in alleviating inflammation and simultaneously enhances regeneration processes stimulated by PRP. Together, these effects accentuate its healing potential in aesthetic dermatology, optimizing the recovery process and minimizing undesirable side effects, thereby increasing its application in aesthetic treatments (Thmanh et al., 2021).

1.1.1. Composition of Platelet-Rich Plasma

PRP content is what makes PRP useful in cosmetic dermatology and has been of interest because of its regenerative capacity. PRP is derived from autologous blood, wherein blood is treated to harvest platelets and condense them into a minimal volume of plasma. This procedure collects key growth factors and cytokines that are involved in regeneration and repair of tissues. Among the components, platelets discharge substantial proteins like fibrin, fibronectin, and vitronectin that support healing. PRP can enhance the structural integrity of dermal tissues with this very composition and triggers an intense healing reaction, making it a valuable commodity in cosmetic applications. With the use of the natural regenerative powers of the body's own platelets, PRP is a procedure that aligns with the ethics of minimally invasive cosmetic treatments. With regard to cosmetic dermatology, the presence of growth factors in PRP makes it pertinent to the demand for repair and rejuvenation of tissue. These growth factors, which reside within the alpha-granules of the platelets, are accountable for the stimulation of cellular functions such as proliferation, migration, and differentiation. Clinical studies have established that PRP can hasten the process of wound healing, enhance skin texture, reduce wrinkles, and cause hair regrowth in alopecia. Such factors are not only limited to repair in tissues but also stimulation of collagen synthesis, which is responsible for retaining the elasticity and youthful appearance of the skin. Thus, the understanding of the subtle interaction of constituents in PRP allows practitioners to formulate treatment protocols effectively and yield maximum effect in enhancing skin quality and patient satisfaction (Unal et al., 2017). Moreover, preparation of PRP also influences not only its composition but the efficacy of PRP in cosmetic procedures. Numerous methods are employed to prepare PRP, including differential centrifugation and filtration, which influence the concentration of platelets and growth factors. Variability in preparation protocol can lead to variation in platelet-to-plasma ratio and leukocyte content, influencing the therapeutic efficacy of PRP. More concentrated platelets have been reported to correlate with greater clinical benefit in studies on PRP evaluation for hair growth and skin rejuvenation. Therefore, optimizing the production of PRP optimizes not only the treatment's therapeutic profile but also underscores the need for standardization among clinical procedures. Such advances minimize variability and enable improved understanding of the relationship between PRP content and its clinical effect in cosmetic dermatology (Cyran et al., 2024) (Figure 1.3).

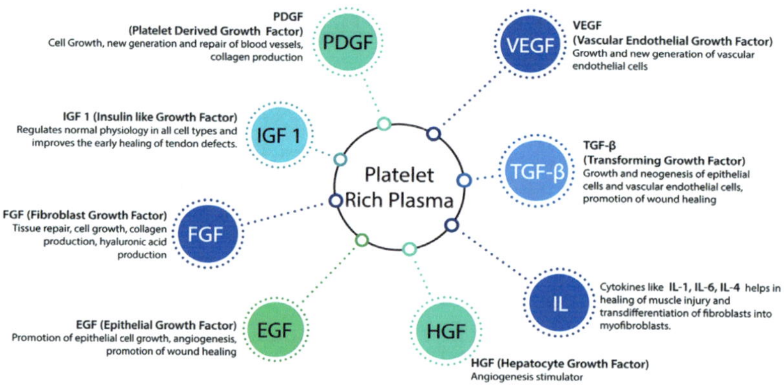

Figure 1.3. The components of platelet-rich plasma and their functions.

Source: https://www.researchgate.net/publication/330453033/figure/fig1/AS:957660107137024@1605335370728/The-components-of-platelet-rich-plasma-and-their-functions.png.

1.1.2. Growth Factors and Their Role in Skin Rejuvenation

The pursuit of youthful, radiant-looking skin has led to phenomenal expansion in cosmetic dermatology, primarily through the application of growth factors. These protein molecules play a vital role in dermal rejuvenation, allowing proliferative, migratory, and differentiating cellular activity. In the instance of PRP, growth factors are concentrated and derived from the patient's own platelets. This autologous preparation not only has a decreased risk of adverse effects but also functions to enhance the body's intrinsic healing mechanisms of the skin. PRP has been demonstrated to improve collagen production and elasticity of the skin by injecting it into damaged or aging tissues, which effectively reverses the signs of aging and improves the overall texture of the skin. Thus, growth factors have deep impact on the rejuvenation of skin is the cornerstone of contemporary aesthetic treatments, particularly when utilized through the might of contemporary methods such as PRP therapy (Wang et al., 2025). In this vein, recent research has confirmed that specific PRP origins possess differential potentials for stimulation of skin regeneration, with some factors playing crucial roles to enhance therapeutic efficacies. For instance, PRP from animal sources, particularly from deer, has delivered highly satisfactory outcomes in comparative research examining wound healing and skin rejuvenation properties (Wang et al., 2025). The synergistic effect of a combination of various growth factors in PRP, such as PDGF and TGF-β, creates a complex biological niche that highly promotes skin healing and rejuvenation. By stimulating fibroblast activity and angiogenesis, these growth factors not only repair the young skin but also reverse such conditions as atrophic scarring and pigmentary disorders. The subtle application of these findings can bring the promise of individualized therapeutic interventions in aesthetic dermatology (Wang et al., 2025). Moreover, the application of PRP with other modalities such as microneedling or laser therapy enhances the effectiveness of generalized skin rejuvenation therapy. This is due to the improved delivery and penetration of growth factors into the dermal tissues, which result in better effects. There is evidence supporting the hypothesis that multi-modal approaches leveraging the regenerative properties of growth factors are more effective in addressing the texture, tone, and elasticity of the skin. With advancements in aesthetic medicine, understanding how these growth factors function will provide practitioners with the power to further customize treatment protocols. Hence, further research into growth factors and their broader connotations within dermatology must be undertaken to design standard practices with optimal patient benefit for cosmetic procedures (Łukasz et al., 2024) (Figure 1.4).

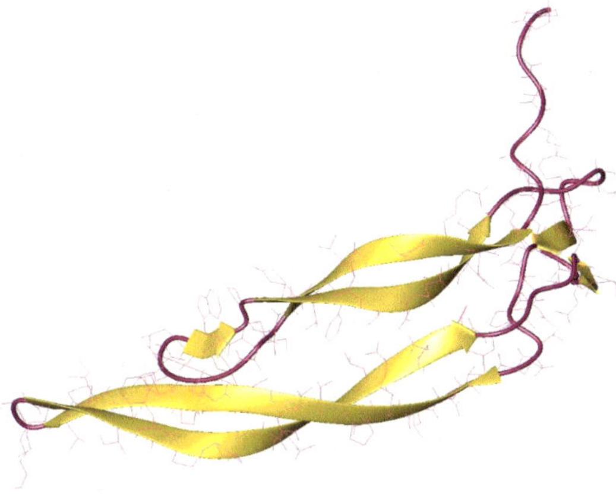

Figure 1.4. Platelet-derived growth factor BB monomer, human.

Source: https://upload.wikimedia.org/wikipedia/commons/e/ee/1pdg.jpg.

1.1.3. The Process of PRP Extraction and Preparation

Preparation and harvesting of PRP is an attentive process, beginning with the taking of the patient's blood. A standard 10 to 60 milliliter blood draw typically occurs, and the blood is then transferred to a sterile tube that is filled with an anticoagulant to prevent clotting. Following blood draw, the blood is centrifuged, a process vital to the separation of the components of the blood based on their densities. There are often two spins of centrifugation: one separating the red blood cells and the plasma, and another pelleting the platelets into the plasma's top layer. This double centrifugation process ensures a platelet-rich dense plasma layer required for the therapeutic application in cosmetic dermatology, including tissue remodeling and skin rejuvenation. Once the centrifugation process is completed, preparation of the PRP involves extracting the uppermost platelet-rich layer, which is also referred to as platelet-rich plasma, while leaving behind the bottom layers of red blood cells and white blood cells in minimal quantity. This is typically achieved by the employment of a pipette or other suitable equipment to softly aspirate the plasma without disturbing the sedimented components at the bottom. The ideal PRP should be concentrated with a significantly higher degree of platelets than regular blood, typically a five- to ten-fold concentration. As noted in the literature, the success of PRP is dependent on factors such as dosage and method of preparation, so practitioners must adhere to standard protocols to achieve optimal results (Rizvi, 2021). This is scrupulous handling and precise extraction, which play critical roles in maximizing the therapeutic value of PRP for various cosmetic procedures. At the time of extraction, the PRP can be activated depending on the intended use. Activation of PRP is often performed with agents such as thrombin or calcium chloride, which cause platelets to release healing and regeneration-activating growth factors and cytokines. These growth factors induce a variety of biological activities, including angiogenesis, collagen synthesis, and keratinocyte proliferation, enhancing the overall efficacy of treatment in correcting abnormalities such as wrinkles, acne scars, and alopecia. Recent developments, including the development of activated PRP products with topical application, have enhanced the application of PRP in cosmetic dermatology (Roge et al., 2022). With these improvements in extraction and preparation techniques, PRP has proven itself to be a viable option for practitioners who wish to give patients valuable aesthetic improvements while utilizing the body's own potential for healing (Figure 1.5).

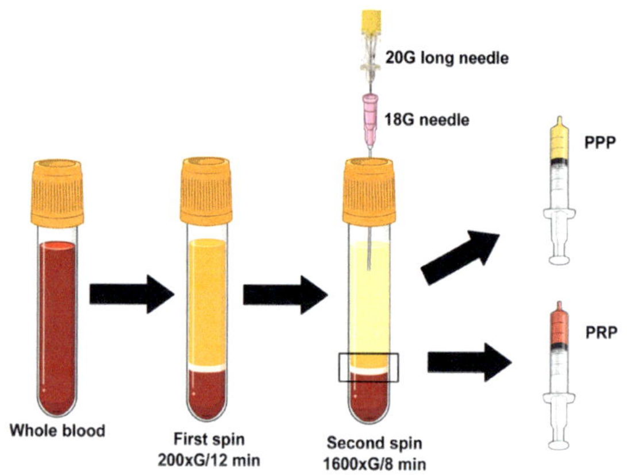

Figure 1.5. Method for preparing platelet-rich plasma (PRP).

Source: Machado E S, Soares F P, Yamaguchi R S, et al. (January 03, 2022) A Simple Double-Spin Closed Method for Preparing Platelet-Rich Plasma. Cureus 14(1): e20899. doi:10.7759/cureus.20899

Test Your Knowledge

1. What is the composition of PRP, and how is it different from whole blood?
2. What growth factors are present in PRP, and how do they contribute to skin rejuvenation in cosmetic dermatology?
3. What is the standard process for PRP extraction and preparation used in aesthetic dermatology?

1.2. Common Applications in Cosmetic Dermatology

Learning Outcome

1. Describe PRP for facial rejuvenation
2. Explain the role of PRP in hair restoration treatments
3. Define PRP for scar treatment and improvement

In aesthetic dermatology, PRP is now a multi-faceted tool with numerous applications. Most commonly applied to facial rejuvenation, PRP has been discovered to tighten the texture, tone, and look of skin. From the growth factors of the plasma for regenerative purposes, the extracted plasma is employed by professionals to induce collagen development, thereby increasing the elasticity of the skin and lessening the prominence of fine lines. Such therapies are of significant interest in an era where non-surgical cosmetic therapies are becoming more widespread, promising significant benefits with minimal downtime. The safety and efficacy profile of PRP also contributes to its popularity, particularly when applied to the treatment of conditions like acne scars and fine wrinkles, and further solidifies its established position in modern dermatologic treatment (Basily et al., 2024). Another important application of PRP in cosmetic dermatology is its use in hair restoration. Androgenetic alopecia is a common condition of hair loss, and many individuals are afflicted by it, so there is a demand for effective treatments. PRP is applied to stimulate hair follicles so that hair will regrow by establishing a healthier state for the scalp. With PRP injected into the scalp, growth factors induce the body's natural healing mechanism and increase blood circulation, both critical to the health of the hair. Scientific evidence attests to an increased thickness and density of the hair, thus making PRP an effective choice for those in search of non-invasive ways to treat hair loss. The ability of PRP to address this issue aesthetically with few side effects further establishes its status as a revolutionary procedure in cosmetic dermatology (Fareez et al., 2023). In addition, the combination of PRP with microneedling has also been emphasized due to its additive effects, particularly for the management of striae distensae, or stretch marks. Studies have indicated that a difference can be measured in skin texture and overall visual appearance with this combination. For instance, patients undergoing treatment of microneedling combined with PRP have better outcomes than patients treated with microneedling alone. This is because of the synergistic effect where microneedles cause micro-injuries that facilitate a greater rate of absorption of the PRP, and the latter delivers much-needed growth factors to the dermis. Although both procedures are well tolerated, note that neither treatment is completely devoid of side effects, which can vary depending on the individual. Still, the future of PRP in esthetics is bright and represents a significant paradigm shift towards regenerative therapy for the treatment of many cosmetic problems (Basily et al., 2024).

1.2.1. PRP for Facial Rejuvenation

In recent years, PRP has been a dominant subject in cosmetic dermatology, which reflects the shifting profile of aesthetic medicine. This new therapy employs the patient's own blood constituents to stimulate tissue regeneration and repair, drawing on the body's natural healing potential of platelets. On injecting PRP into the skin, it releases bioactive molecules that act as growth factors and thus stimulate cellular proliferation and accelerate the process of healing. It is particularly helpful in treating instances of fine lines, wrinkles, and even severe acne scars, as substantiated by recent research indicating the efficacy of PRP over other interventions like salmon DNA serum-based treatments, which were determined by study to produce the same results but at slower healing rates (Chiuman et al., 2023). The concepts of regenerative medicine set the stage for grasping its position within facial renewal. As skin ages and becomes subject to extensive structural alterations, such as a decline in elasticity and volume, the use of regenerative approaches further addresses not just returning the youthful complexion but also fostering skin health at a cellular level. By injecting PRP strategically, dermatologists can treat targeted areas of concern and permit the formation of collagen and elastin, which are crucial components in maintaining skin integrity. The growing trend of minimally invasive aesthetic treatments against aging occurs simultaneously with patients' demands for functional procedures that do not end with long recovery times, further establishing PRP as part of modern-day cosmetic clinics (Trovato et al., 2024).

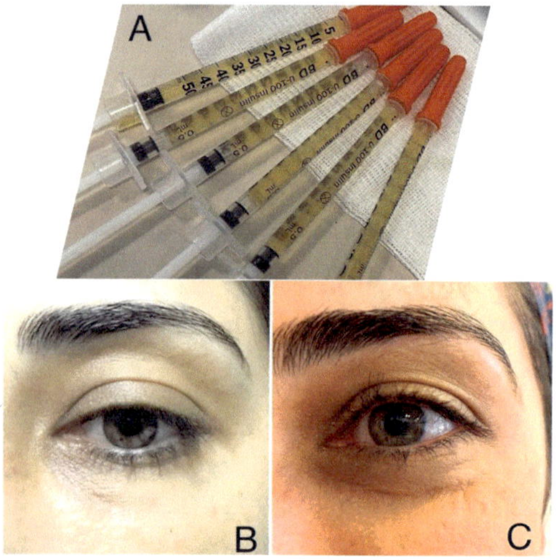

Figure 1.6. Platelet-rich plasma for facial rejuvenation. (A) Platelet-rich plasma in syringes; (B) Three months after the platelet-rich plasma applying; and (C) Before the platelet-rich plasma applying.

Source: https://www.researchgate.net/publication/390920895/figure/fig4/AS:11431281385772442@1745027451835/Platelet-rich-plasma-for-facial-rejuvenation-A-Platelet-rich-plasma-in-syringes-B-Three.jpg.

While the virtues of PRP therapy in facial rejuvenation are increasingly being valued, it becomes a matter of necessity to embrace its utilization with a focus on standardization and evidence-based practice. With the evolution of the branch of regenerative dermatology, more study is needed to evolve consensus for treatment protocols so that maximum patient safety and outcomes are achieved. There is a necessary need for well-designed *in vivo* trials that will be capable of verifying the efficacy of PRP relative to traditional dermatological treatment. Through such research, practitioners can refine methods, adapt therapy for individual patient needs, and confirm the long-term ramifications of PRP therapy, ensuring that this promising treatment remains a viable choice in the widening range of cosmetic dermatology (Trovato et al., 2024) (Figure 1.6).

1.2.2. PRP in Hair Restoration Treatments

The use of PRP therapy in hair rejuvenation procedures has been of significant interest to dermatologists and patients due to its potential benefits. This novel treatment takes advantage of the regenerative properties of platelets, which are abundant with growth factors necessary for the repair of tissues and the stimulation of hair follicles. By taking a patient's blood, spinning it to densify the platelets, and injecting this PRP into the scalp, physicians are hoping to promote the growth of hair and make hair thicker. Having an understanding of the deep influence of biological variables on hair loss, researchers have begun to look into the way PRP can promote healthier hair follicles and subsequently, turn balding around. Growing evidence demonstrates the promise of PRP for the treatment of androgenetic alopecia and other forms of alopecia, portending a rosy future for its use in aesthetic dermatology (Cyran et al., 2024). Clinical studies evaluating the efficacy of PRP for hair restoration have shown encouraging results, reliably reporting hair density improvements and overall hair growth. Outcomes from systematic reviews indicate that PRP therapy is favorable to the hair growth cycle by increasing the anagen phase and lowering shedding. Pleased patients usually report an acceptable enhancement in satisfaction rates in addition to noticeable results after treatment, maintaining the therapeutic significance of PRP in the management of baldness. More significantly, the customized aspect of PRP therapy lends itself to tailoring according to patient needs, promoting a personalized approach to cosmetic dermatology. However, there should still be a critical assessment of the various protocols employed between studies because PRP concentration and number of treatments are some of the factors that significantly influence outcomes (Cyran et al., 2024).

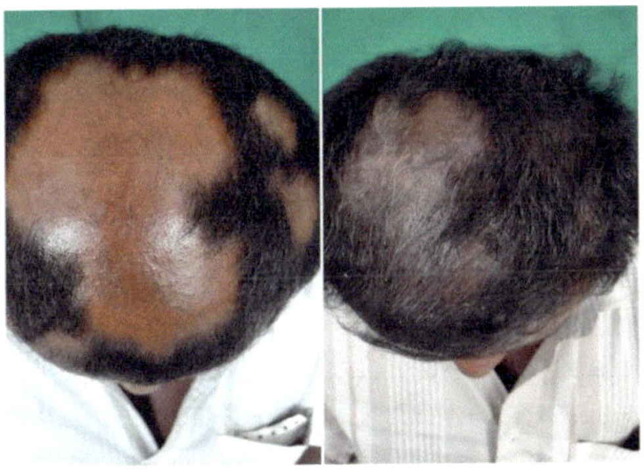

Figure 1.7. Before and after 6 sittings of PRP.

Source: https://www.researchgate.net/publication/333099702/figure/fig4/AS:758652210253827@1557888190825/Before-and-after-6-sittings-of-PRP.jpg.

As much as the promising evidence regarding PRP therapy is referenced, there are substantial concerns regarding safety and efficacy. Although patients normally experience few side effects, variability of response to treatment can lead to inconsistencies in outcome. In addition, the need for research on treatment protocol and method of preparation remains the paramount issue. Controlled trials comparing PRP with established treatments, such as topical minoxidil or hair transplant surgery, are needed to establish PRP's role in an extended therapeutic treatment plan. Additionally, the resolution of possible clinical evidence limitations will increase credibility of PRP in hair restoration clinics. As procedures are optimized and standardized by practitioners, further studies into their mechanisms of action will continue to increase understanding of the therapeutic value of PRP in the struggle against baldness (Figure 1.7).

1.2.3. PRP for Scar Treatment and Improvement

The fast-evolving arena of PRP therapy has gained wider and wider usage in cosmetic dermatology for the treatment of scars and for their improvement. The new treatment exploits the patient's own natural bodily elements, where the body's own healing processes are stimulated. PRP therapy involves taking a small quantity of the patient's blood, processing it to concentrate platelets, and then injecting it into the desired area. This technique may be highly effective for various types of scars, including acne scars, due to the potential of stimulating collagenesis and tissue remodeling. It has been demonstrated that PRP can be useful in improving homeostasis of treated tissues, and therefore it is an interesting therapeutic strategy for scar revision when combined with modern dermatology methodologies (Suruchi et al., 2018). In one of the largest and most important studies to evaluate the effectiveness of PRP in conjunction with fractional CO2 laser therapy, outstanding outcomes occurred in the condition of post-acne scars. The study comprised the administration of ablative fractional CO2 laser treatment and autologous PRP treatment on half of the face of each of the patients, where the control half received regular saline. The results were a substantial reduction in scarring on the PRP-treated side compared to the saline-treated side, which supports the adjunctive role of the procedure. The participants also had greater levels of satisfaction, and side effect incidence appeared to be lower with PRP, demonstrating not just its efficacy but also safety as an office-based treatment modality for scar management (Aswani et al., 2017).

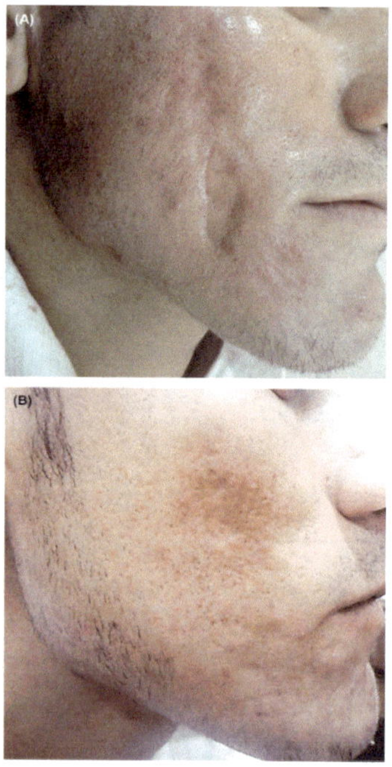

Figure 1.8. A male patient with Grade 4 acne scars and traumatic scars in Group C (combined skin needling and PRP). (A) Before treatment; and (B) Excellent response 2 months after the last session.

Source: https://www.researchgate.net/profile/Mohamed-Nasr-34/publication/263776594/figure/fig2/AS:296482981859328@1447698459072/A-male-patient-with-Grade-4-acne-scars-and-traumatic-scars-in-Group-C-combined-skin.png.

The advantages of incorporating PRP therapy into scar treatment plans extend beyond superficial enhancement; it also provides a way to improve patient comfort and satisfaction. By using a product derived from the patient themselves, PRP minimizes the risk of allergic reaction or complications from foreign products. In addition, the reduction in side effects, such as persistent erythema and edema, makes PRP an appealing option for individuals seeking effective and tolerable treatment for scars. With continuous research developments, the combination of PRP and traditional methods like laser therapy may transform what is regarded as best practice in dermatology, leaving practitioners with a robust tool to enhance patient outcomes and quality of care in scar revision therapy (Suruchi et al., 2018) (Figure 1.8).

Test Your Knowledge

1. How is PRP used for facial rejuvenation, and what are its clinical benefits?
2. What is the role of PRP in hair restoration treatments, especially for androgenetic alopecia?

1.3. Benefits of PRP Treatments

Learning Outcome

1. Describe minimally invasive nature of PRP procedures
2. Understand natural healing properties and biocompatibility of PRP
3. Discuss long-lasting results compared to other treatments

The application of PRP treatments in cosmetic dermatology has witnessed phenomenal returns in addressing numerous skin conditions and cosmetic concerns. One of the greatest advantages is that PRP can trigger skin rejuvenation on its own through innate growth factors that promote cellular turnover and healing. By utilizing the body's own bioelements, PRP stimulates collagen production, leading to greater skin quality and elasticity. This is a more authentic solution that reduces the application of artificial fillers or surgery, hence giving a more rounded solution for aging and skin damage. Furthermore, with less downtime and less exposure to side effects, patients are more likely to be satisfied than with traditional cosmetic procedures that can be invasive through surgery and have long recovery periods. PRP has also shown immense capability to treat pigmentation-related disorders like melasma, which affect many people and are difficult to treat with conventional methods. The regenerative capacity of PRP can reverse hyperpigmentation, thereby providing a more uniform complexion. As outlined in recent studies, PRP is now not only recognized as an adjunctive therapy for treating melasma, but even as an autonomous therapeutic measure. The unique composition of PRP, rich in platelets, serves the important role of attaining such therapeutic success through the repair and regeneration of skin tissue. This is particularly essential for patients who may risk experiencing psychological distress from noticeable skin imperfections, highlighting the significance of PRP treatments for physical presentation and the quality of life (Valentina et al., 2025). Another important benefit of PRP therapy is that they are applicable to curing a variety of cosmetic dermatologic problems aside from pigment-related issues. The applications of PRP can be broadened to include hair growth, acne scars, and overall skin rejuvenation. Since they are autologous, there is minimal risk of rejection, making it a relatively safe procedure for most patients. As noted in recent research, PRP may improve outcomes in such regions by its ability to induce angiogenesis and improve wound healing (Prokurat et al., 2024). Additionally, study shows that since it possesses a regenerative quality, PRP not only addresses superficially the skin but also corrects the underlying issues, thus guaranteeing a complete aesthetic improvement. The application of PRP treatments to cosmetic dermatology ultimately represents a step towards more patient-centered care, as it emphasizes the effectiveness of leveraging the body's natural repair processes to deliver cosmetic improvements (Figure 1.9).

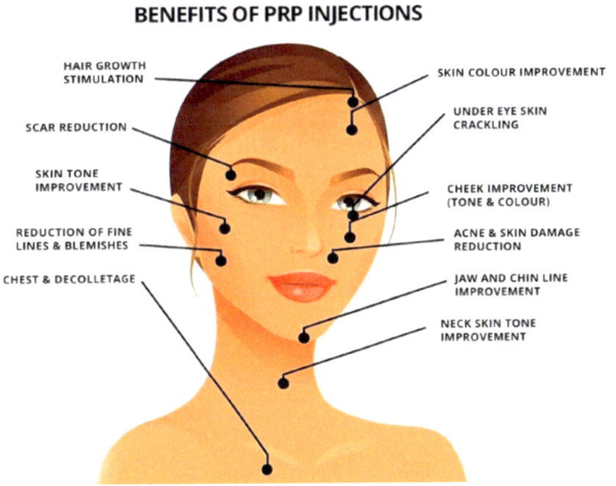

Figure 1.9. Benefits of PRP injections.

Source: https://drterrymadsen.com/assets/images/benefits-of-prp-injections.jpg.

1.3.1. Minimally Invasive Nature of PRP Procedures

The minimally invasive treatment of PRP is a revolutionary advancement in cosmetic dermatology. Unlike traditional surgery, PRP is a treatment that entails the extraction and re-injection of a small quantity of a patient's own blood to achieve a relatively simple treatment with less recovery time. The treatment involves venipuncture for the extraction of the blood, centrifugation for platelet concentration, and injection of the solution into the target areas of skin. This technique is designed to stimulate collagen production and growth of tissue, stimulating natural healing without the need for extensive cuts or stitches. As it includes the autologous factor, there is a much-reduced risk of harmful reactions, which has helped make it more sought after with patients seeking favorable cosmetic enhancements at the expense of less invasive treatments (Hidayat et al., 2024). Furthermore, increased patient satisfaction from minimally invasive PRP procedures is, in the most part, attributed to their rapid recovery periods and decreased amounts of pain. As patients are becoming more aware of their cosmetic treatments, demand for those treatments that involve a non-surgical technique continues to rise. Research demonstrates that patients who receive microneedling with PRP experience dramatic improvements in skin texture and appearance within a comparatively brief duration of time. This convergence not only enhances the efficacy of treatment but also aligns with patients' desires for perceptible results with zero extended time off (Pawlik et al., 2024). This rising trend represents a milestone towards less invasive, patient-catering treatments in cosmetic dermatology. In addition, the minimally invasive character of PRP expands its scope to other dermatological conditions, including alopecia and skin rejuvenation. In hair restoration, for example, PRP therapy has proved to be a successful treatment for conditions such as androgenetic alopecia. Through stimulating hair follicle regeneration, it provides a less invasive option compared to procedures such as hair transplants, which typically involve significant preparation and recovery time. The therapeutic efficacy of PRP in promoting hair growth has established it as the frontline non-surgical hair loss treatment among a broad patient population. With improving methods and increasing awareness, the application of PRP procedures to revamp practices in cosmetic dermatology only expands, and there is a strong argument for their wider acceptance into routine practices (Pawlik et al., 2024).

1.3.2. Natural Healing Properties and Biocompatibility

The intrinsic healing properties of PRP make it a revolutionary ingredient in cosmetic dermatology. PRP employs the body's own mechanism of healing through the separation of platelets and growth factors from the patients' own blood. Its autologous nature not only reduces the risk of rejection but also optimizes biocompatibility, making it an appealing treatment for facial rejuvenation and repair of the skin. As the demand for cosmetic procedures with minimal invasiveness has been rising, it is crucial to learn about the regenerative potential of PRP. The treatment causes a cascade of biological responses, promoting collagen production, angiogenesis, and tissue remodeling, all of which are critical for achieving young skin. Recent studies emphasize the synergy of PRP with skin health, demonstrating that off-the-shelf PRP use has the potential to significantly enhance wound healing with reassuring promise for patients seeking good and natural cosmetic therapies (Trovato et al., 2024). Beyond its healing aspect, PRP's biocompatibility is of extreme significance in its application in cosmetic therapies. The minimally invasive nature of PRP is because it utilizes the patient's biological materials, thus establishing compatibility and reducing potential side effects. Because PRP utilizes naturally occurring components, it eliminates the likelihood of inflammatory reactions or immune rejections that occur with foreign bodies. As elucidated in recent research, the addition of bioactive molecules, such as platelet-degrading growth factors, into scaffold material has been intensely researched, upholding the topic of biocompatibility in tissue engineering (Muchová et al., 2016). Not only are recovery times hastened by such compatibility, but there is also increased patient satisfaction, allowing treatments to occur in synchrony with the body's own recovery processes. With impending advancements in PRP therapy, its biocompatibility will be the most critical parameter in deciding optimal outcomes in aesthetic dermatology.

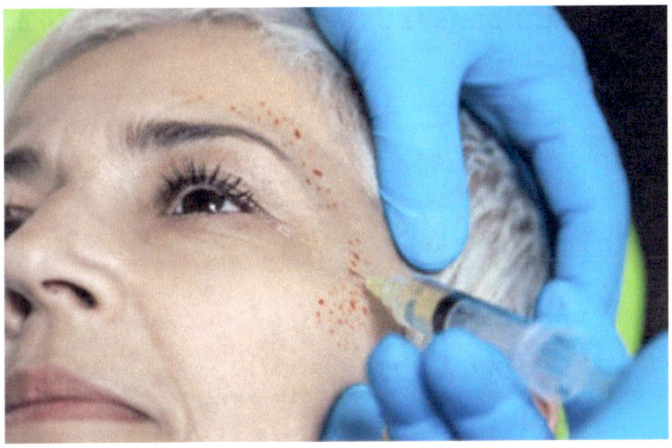

Figure 1.10. Platelet-rich plasma (PRP) therapy for facial rejuvenation.

Source: https://www.cumberlandskin.com/getmedia/d60c5833-27c0-4a7d-a936-efac7318f15e/PRP-6.jpg.

Wherever natural healing processes meet biocompatibility, PRP's role as a cornerstone for regenerative dermatology is reconfirmed. Practitioners need to realize that while the efficacy of PRP has been amply documented, there remains a need to standardize procedures and techniques. The current situation indicates a very good prospect for the utilization of PRP beyond the traditional use, such as in association with advanced collagen scaffolds that can be developed to optimize therapeutic effect. It is important in creating superior treatment regimens to consider carefully the mode of action of PRP at the cell level and optimize its biocompatibility and meet the needs of a large number of patients. Emphasizing these characteristics not only underscores the importance of PRP in cosmetic dermatology but also leaves room for new therapy that plays on the body's natural healing potential (Trovato et al., 2024) (Figure 1.10).

1.3.3. Long-Lasting Results Compared to Other Treatments

The effectiveness of PRP treatment in aesthetic dermatology is highlighted by its ability to produce enduring results, especially when compared with traditional forms of treatment. In the scenario of androgenetic alopecia, classical treatments such as minoxidil and finasteride have exhibited varying success, but generally are not sustainable in their outcomes. Research has shown that PRP not only increases the overall hair density but also significantly enhances the outcome when used in conjunction with these classic forms of treatment. Notably, combination therapy of PRP with minoxidil has been more effective than monotherapy with either agent, demonstrating a synergistic effect producing more robust and long-lasting results in hair growth. This suggests that PRP treatment presents a promising choice for patients seeking long-term results in hair loss therapy, addressing the limitations of standard treatment regimens (Marcinkiewicz et al., 2024). Therefore, PRP has also been found to be a good option for treating melasma, a condition famously hard to treat since it tends to easily recur. In comparative analysis between intradermal PRP and Qs Nd-YAG laser therapy, results proved that PRP not only provided significant improvement of pigmentation but also posed lower relapse risks within a three-month follow-up. While both treatment modalities were initially effective, the side treated with PRP was more resistant to the recurrence of melasma. This highlights PRP's role as not just an effective treatment for refractory forms of melasma but also as a possible leading candidate for maintenance therapy, eventually producing longer-lasting effects compared to traditional laser treatments (Rout et al., 2023). The consequences of the discoveries are that PRP therapy is advantageous in two respects: immediate enhancement of aesthetic state, and enduring outcomes. Since patients are progressively seeking long-lasting treatments, it becomes progressively sensible to bring PRP into cosmetic dermatology clinics. With the inclusion of enhancing effects of treatment in addition to the reduction of multiple procedures, PRP therapy is a leader in aesthetic medicine. The ongoing realization of the PRP's potential in various dermatological procedures opens new avenues for practitioners and patients alike, ultimately directing the way to sustained outcomes and patient satisfaction with cosmetic dermatology treatments. This shift is an extraordinary step toward successful and long-lasting cosmetic treatments (Figure 1.11).

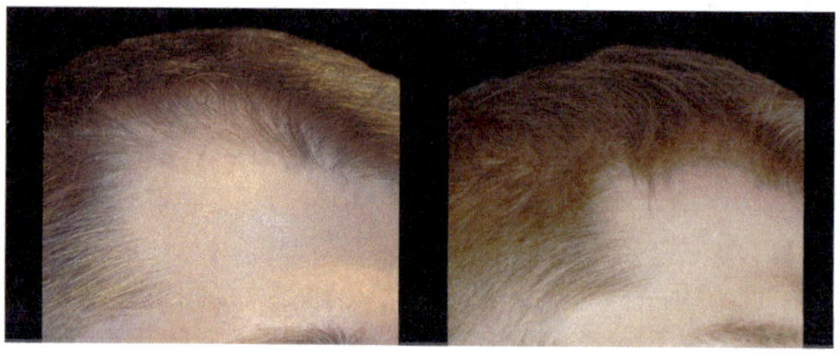

Figure 1.11. Significant increase in hair density and color with six monthly injections of PRP.

Source: https://www.skintherapyletter.com/wp-content/uploads/2019/09/img97-1024x422.jpg.

Test Your Knowledge

1. Why is PRP considered a minimally invasive cosmetic procedure, and what advantages does this offer to patients?
2. What makes PRP biocompatible, and how do its natural healing properties enhance cosmetic outcomes?
3. How do the results of PRP treatments compare in longevity to other aesthetic procedures?

1.4. Risks and Considerations

Learning Outcome

1. Discuss potential side effects and complications related to PRP
2. Deal with contraindications for PRP therapy
3. Explain the importance of professional administration in the context of PRP treatments

With regard to the cosmetic dermatology use of PRP, one consideration regarding the potential risks of the procedure is raised. Although PRP is a somewhat safe procedure since it utilizes the patient's own blood, issues can occur. These include local infection, allergy, and trauma to the injection site, all leading to additional psychological distress for patients trying to enhance their looks. Furthermore, the lack of unified protocols for PRP preparation and delivery may cause heterogeneous results, influencing patient satisfaction and the efficacy of procedures. One recent article highlights the prevalence of medical malpractice claims related to dermatological aesthetic procedures, reflecting on the need to understand the bigger picture surrounding such risks in conjunction with patient expectations and practitioner liability (Dereli et al., 2025). Ethical considerations are essential to any discussion of PRP therapy in the field of cosmetic dermatology. Providers should ensure that they properly educate their patients regarding the potential outcomes and limitations of PRP therapy. Inflammatory descriptions may increase expectations for unrealistic outcomes, particularly among those patients who can be affected by body dysmorphic disorders (BDD). The current social media phenomenon heightens such concern, driving an increasing demand for aesthetic procedures while concurrently driving the occurrence of body image-related mental health issues. As dermatologists are forced to work on these complex psychological landscapes, ethical transparency is crucial in assisting patients in making highly informed choices about their options for treatment (Keskinbora et al., 2023). Thus, professionals must balance technical competence with ethical sensitivity in order to put patient care first. There are also regulatory concerns involved in the type of materials that are used in the preparation and injection of PRP, making industry standards a must. Clinicians have to employ only Class 3 medical device materials for the procedure in order to minimize the risk of complications and ensure patient safety. Non-adherence to these guidelines may result in complications, such as necrosis of the tissue or severe inflammatory response, especially in dermal filler or mesotherapy with PRP treatments. Patients undergoing cosmetic treatment should be properly informed regarding the materials and methods used, promoting a culture of safety and responsibility in practice. Lastly, the confluence of efficacy, ethics, and regulation highlights heterogeneity of risks underlying platelet-rich plasma interventions in cosmetic dermatology (Keskinbora et al., 2023).

1.4.1. Potential Side Effects and Complications

PRP therapy has been heavily marketed in cosmetic dermatology for its regenerative properties. However, complications and side effects must be carefully evaluated to enable patient safety and optimal efficacy. The most common adverse effects seen are local pain, swelling, and bleeding at the site of injection, and these are typically mild and transient. These side effects are usually attributed to the invasive character of the procedure rather than the PRP itself. Yet, practitioners must still take precautions from patients' pre-existing conditions because certain factors such as concurrent medication or blood clotting disorder may enhance these side effects. Hence, a thorough patient assessment is required before treatment since it facilitates the minimization of risks of PRP treatments applied in cosmetic procedures (Suruchi et al., 2018). In addition to the short-term side effects, there are long-term complications that may be triggered by PRP therapy. These include the potential occurrence of infection, scarring, or thrombosis. While infections are fairly rare with the employment of autologous material, there remains no way to eliminate the risk entirely. The handling of the blood sample and the cleanliness of the equipment used in the procedure directly influence the probability of such complications arising. Furthermore, the indeterminate nature of the healing response within individuals who must undergo the procedure represents another level of risk that can result in less than desired aesthetic results. Though professionals aim to optimize the result of PRP therapy, they must also balance the benefits against the potential complications, pointing to the importance of protocol-based procedures and patient education regarding potential side effects (Dhillon et al., 2024). Due to the limitations of PRP therapy, it is essential to adopt an integrated clinical practice of managing side effects and complications. This can include pre-treatment screening, follow-up after the procedure, and customized aftercare instructions. Multidisciplinary management can also enhance safety outcomes and correct complications as they arise. Patient involvement in discussions about potential harm and realistic results enables better understanding and compliance. Lastly, although PRP therapy has great promise for cosmetic applications, more research is needed to determine long-term efficacy and safety. As new developments in the practice of cosmetic dermatology emerge, practitioners must keep abreast of new information on complications in order to continue refining treatment protocols (Suruchi et al., 2018) (Figure 1.12).

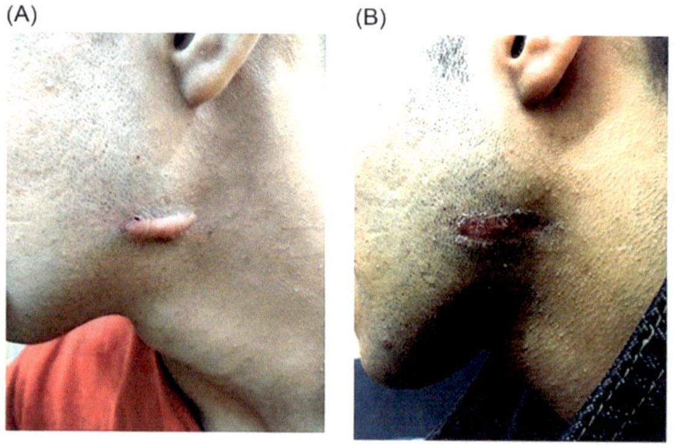

Figure 1.12. (A) Patient with keloid before treatment; and (B) and same patient after treatment with platelet rich plasma.

Source: https://www.researchgate.net/profile/Waleed-Albalat/publication/350887688/figure/fig2/AS:1143128119795722 7@1697145321536/A-Patient-with-keloid-before-treatment-B-and-same-patient-after-treatment-with.ppm.

1.4.2. Contraindications for PRP Therapy

PRP therapy is a rapidly growing area in the field of cosmetic dermatology owing to the potential it holds in the rejuvenation of the skin, healing of wounds, and regeneration of hair. Notwithstanding this, the application of PRP therapy is not contraindicated, mostly patient-related factors that would exclude or render the therapy unsafe or ineffective. Active infections, cutaneous conditions, or a history of some malignancies are a few such conditions that require caution. For instance, patients with infections of the skin can jeopardize worsening in case of PRP treatment since the introduction of the plasma can even activate inflammatory mechanisms. Therefore, careful assessment of the patient's medical history is required to prevent the unwanted outcomes arising from these contraindications, which is also aligned with general clinical standards that dictate safe procedures in cosmetic treatments (Rodriguez et al., 2024).

Moreover, concurrent medical conditions such as autoimmune diseases or blood dyscrasias are also absolute contraindications to PRP therapy. People with autoimmune diseases can exhibit erratic responses because they already possess compromised immune systems and can further exacerbate their situations. Similarly, platelet function or count disorders can ruin the desired therapeutic benefit of PRP therapies because competent platelet activity is required for successful treatments. The clinicians must ensure that patients undergo thorough examinations to determine the presence of any underlying blood disorders before they approve PRP injections. This failure can lead to not only ineffective management but also severe complications (Raquel et al., 2024). In addition, the success of the procedures is greatly dependent on the careful selection of candidates who are risk-free. However, certain factors like some medications, such as anticoagulants or immunosuppressants, may hinder the effect of PRP to a great extent. Further, patients with a history of adverse reactions to previous aesthetic treatments need to be handled with care. Hygiene is a very important factor too; poor sterile conditions at the time of application may increase the infection risk, as seen in the cases where complications were observed after PRP injections due to inadequate measures against hygiene. Thus, the use of rigorous pre-treatment procedures like patient education and informed consent is imperative not only for maximizing the effectiveness of PRP therapy but also for ensuring the general safety of all procedures (Rodriguez et al., 2024) (Figure 1.13).

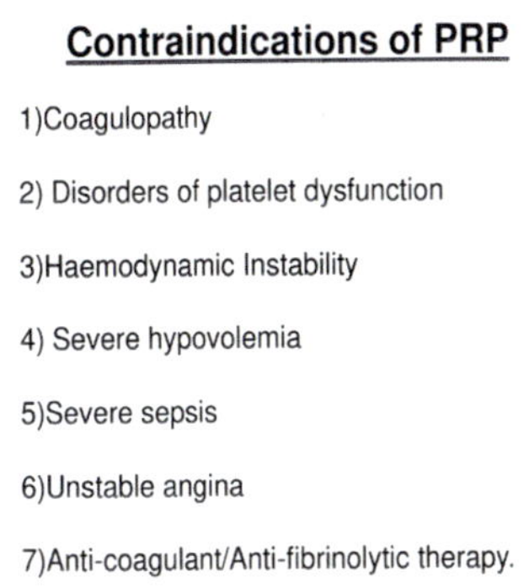

Figure 1.13. Contraindications of PRP.

Source: https://slideplayer.com/slide/12928787/78/images/37/Contraindications+of+PRP.jpg.

1.4.3. Importance of Professional Administration

The importance of professional application of PRP therapy extends beyond procedural application alone but encompasses an in-depth understanding of individual patient needs and sophisticated tissue repair mechanisms. Enhanced training enables practitioners to use PRP in a manner that maximizes its regenerative potential while minimizing risk derived from improper application. The technique, borrowed from sciences such as sports medicine and dentistry, requires scrupulous observance of the extraction and injection of the plasma.

The development of PRP use across medical specialties so far has eclipsed the accompanying scientific evidence of its efficacy, demanding strict professional regulation in its use for cosmetic purposes. By adherence to standardized protocols, professional practitioners can guarantee therapeutic claims associated with PRP, thereby ensuring patient safety and effectiveness of the treatment (López et al., 2018). Moreover, professional application is also essential in handling the ethical considerations of cosmetic procedures like PRP. Given that patients are likely to seek such interventions as a way of addressing pressures of societal appearance demands, it would be essential for practitioners to adopt a patient-centered approach. This involves not only the administration of the treatment but also a full consultation that assesses the psychological readiness and expectations of the patient. As reported in some research, such as case studies with atrophic acne scarring and chronic ulcers, the cosmetic applications of PRP have become more popular (Bendel et al., 2018). An expert clinician, with the capability to address realistic outcomes of PRP therapies, can remove potential dissatisfaction and enable an environment in which informed consent is paramount. This ethical responsibility further stresses professional administration in boosting the overall efficacy and safety of PRP procedures in dermatology. Finally, the economic factor of professional administration cannot be overlooked when discussing these applications in cosmetic dermatology. Proper training and certification can be a big game-changer in the success of a medical clinic offering PRP therapies. Investing in professionals not only raises the stature of the clinic but also patient retention as well as word-of-mouth recommendations. With increased demands for PRP treatments, professional guidelines and protocols become essential in practice compliance and competitiveness. The increasing interest in regenerative medicine has highlighted the need for practitioners to update themselves with the new developments, thereby enabling them to contribute meaningfully in the new scenario of cosmetic dermatology. With professional administration, clinics are able to shield their practice from potential liability while delivering treatments at the optimal level of care, ultimately being good for patients and providers alike (López et al., 2018).

Test Your Knowledge

1. What are the potential side effects and complications of PRP treatments in cosmetic dermatology?
2. What are the contraindications for PRP therapy in cosmetic procedures?

1.5. Comparison with Other Cosmetic Treatments

Learning Outcome

1. Differentiate between PRP and dermal fillers
2. Distinguish between PRP and laser treatments
3. Compare PRP and chemical peels

In cosmetic dermatology, treatments vie with one another on the basis of how much greater aesthetic value they can provide. PRP therapy stands out in its mechanism of using the body's own healing factor to rejuvenate young skin and stimulate hair growth. Compared to other well-liked treatments such as minoxidil and finasteride for androgenetic alopecia, PRP enjoys a big advantage. Studies have shown that treatment with PRP and these traditional therapies together produces greater improvements in hair density than with the individual therapy alone, thus demonstrating its value as a synergistic therapy in treating baldness (Marcinkiewicz et al., 2024). Consequently, patients desperate for solutions tend to seek PRP as an all-encompassing measure that could prove superior. Yet another intriguing comparison presents itself when one compares the outcome of PRP versus injectable platelet-rich fibrin (PRF) in facial skin rejuvenation. To be sure, both procedures involve utilization of the patient's own growth factors, yet some studies suggest that PRF may generate slightly better results on selected cosmetic parameters, i.e., canthal smoothness and wrinkle reduction, at a three-month postoperative time point. However, both total satisfaction and side effects were comparable between PRF and PRP treatment, which makes clinicians evaluate both as choices in aesthetic practice (Atsu et al., 2023). The slightly superior outcome associated with PRF can be appealing to practitioners and patients looking for more effects without using anticoagulants, choosing of the best treatment regimens in cosmetic dermatology even more complicated. Finally, awareness of the subtleties of PRP compared to other aesthetic treatments is the basis for making enlightened decisions in aesthetic medicine. The increased popularity of PRP can largely be attributed to the dual effect of reviving skin and stimulating hair growth, which makes it different from traditional treatments. Furthermore, the advantage of using PRP with existing therapies indicates the potential to design individual therapy regimens with optimal efficacy. With the advancement of cosmetic dermatology, future research and trials will continue to be essential in further delineating our understanding of these therapies and their relative effectiveness. The use of PRP as an augmentation to current protocols is an indicator of its use as a central figure in today's cosmetic therapies and firmly establishes it as an option in the pursuit of aesthetic enhancement.

1.5.1. PRP vs. Dermal Fillers

With the ever-increasing popularity of cosmetic procedures, PRP injections and dermal fillers have become two of the most prominent options in dermatology. PRP treatments involve the use of the patient's blood to extract growth factors and proteins, which naturally trigger healing and renewal of the skin. This autologous technique induces the formation of collagen and enhances skin texture and is now a popular choice for people who want non-surgical treatment. But with fillers, they typically need to use hyaluronic acid or other synthetic products that induce instant volume and moisture to the skin. While fillers can be used immediately, their effects are only temporary, and repeat sessions might be required to maintain desired outcomes. The decision between PRP and dermal fillers is ultimately dependent on patient goals, desired outcome, as well as patient tolerance to each. Between the safety profile of dermal fillers and that of PRP, there should be consideration of the fact that they greatly differ. Since PRP is derived from a patient's own body tissue, it reduces the potential for allergic reactions, something that is common with dermal fillers due to the synthetic production of the latter. Additionally, PRP can also improve the overall quality of the skin, rather than specifically address certain wrinkles or volume loss, and as such, is a very useful treatment for patients seeking to enhance skin health as a whole. Complications, however, still do occur with PRP injections, including minor swelling or bruising at the site of injection. In comparison, dermal fillers, although relatively safe, carry a higher risk for side effects like lumpiness, migration, and vascular occlusion if not applied correctly. Knowing about these risks is important for practitioners to guide their patients towards the optimum choice. The effect duration is another significant factor in the PRP vs dermal fillers debate. Dermal fillers usually give results immediately that last anywhere from six months to two years, depending on the filler and area treated. The instantaneous results are frequently very appealing to patients who desire quick fixes. Conversely, the impact of PRP treatment does not manifest immediately due to the natural healing process of the body, but can add to longer-term improvement in skin texture and quality in the future. Maintenance sessions are required to sustain PRP as well as filler effects; however, patients have to weigh the long-term improvement of better skin that PRP can provide against fillers' immediacy of augmentation. This thought highlights the necessity of customized treatment protocols, depending on patient preference and desired length of aesthetic gain (Table 1.1).

Table 1.1. PRP vs Dermal Filler: Pros and Cons

Pros of PRP	Cons of PRP
It utilizes the growth factors found in your blood, so your body won't reject the substance.	Aside from being expensive, it is not usually covered by most insurance plans.
This procedure can be performed with other facial treatments.	It may produce unsatisfactory results compared to Botox and surgeries.
It also heals skin allergies, existing wounds, and burnt skin.	Minor side effects include redness in the treated area that might last for days.

Pros of Dermal Fillers	Cons of Dermal Fillers
Dermal fillers reduce the noticeable signs of skin aging such as wrinkles, fine lines, and sunken cheeks.	They are not permanent; it can only last between 8–18 months.
The procedure is non-surgical, so there are fewer risks.	You may experience minor side effects such as itching, bruising, and swelling, as well as a mild infection.
The treatment has a quick recovery time.	In rare cases, you might encounter blood vessel blockage or develop lumps under your skin.

Source: https://myethosspa.com/prp-vs-dermal-filler/.

1.5.2. PRP vs. Laser Treatments

Use of PRP in cosmetic dermatology has come under a lot of attention, particularly compared to laser treatment. The treatment employs the body's natural power for wound healing by using a concentration of platelets in the form of blood from the patient. The innovative method is believed to enhance skin repair and regeneration compared to laser treatment, which typically depends on thermal damage to stimulate collagen synthesis. While lasers can be effective for conditions of the surface skin and scarring of other kinds, PRP is purported to penetrate deeper into the dermal tissues, provoking cell growth and tissue repair. Such a difference in mechanism is necessary because PRP is then more apt to effectively treat a wide variety of skin conditions, including those that are caused by aging and by scars due to acne, in which deeper action is needed to heal. Research comparing PRP to more traditional modalities like laser therapy also yields promising outcomes for each. For example, research highlighted the effectiveness of PRP in the wound healing process and demonstrated its better outcomes against salmon DNA serum treatments in a controlled environment using white Wistar mice. The significance of this finding lies in the fact that PRP encourages healing to happen faster, possibly due to the high content of growth factors and bioactive molecules that facilitate tissue regrowth and vasculogenesis (Chiuman et al., 2023). Compared to laser treatment, which is as valuable as it is regarding its immediate effects through skin tightening and resurfacing, it is perhaps not as capable of delivering the same form of healing that PRP delivers. This less obvious comparison indicates the importance of selecting the proper treatment for specific skin conditions and results. Further, deliberation about the full treatment possibilities for such diseases as alopecia, for which PRP and laser treatment are both standard practice, is essential. Research on the degree to which the look of alopecia can be improved also illustrates the variability of outcome with these treatments. Even though laser therapy has been efficient in stimulating the hair follicles, PRP is becoming more acknowledged for its ability to optimize the scalp's biological environment, an element that is crucial for hair growth in a majority of noncicatricial alopecias (Altunel et al., 2017). Each approach has its specific merits; therefore, the choice between PRP and laser treatments should be based on individual assessments of the patient's needs, skin, and specific dermatological conditions to achieve optimal cosmetic results (Figure 1.14).

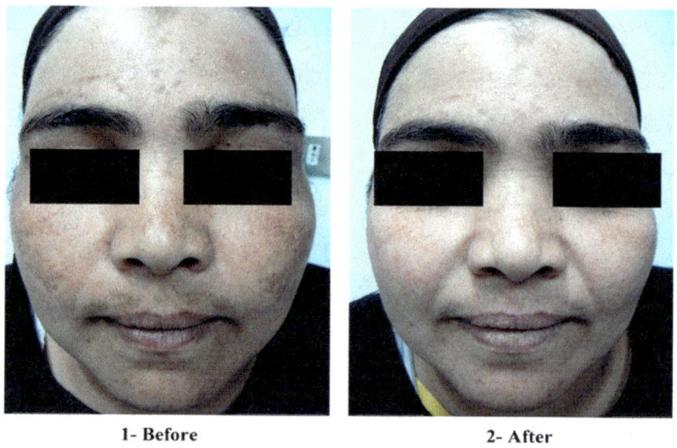

Figure 1.14. A case of fair improvement of both sides (Rt PRP-IPL and Lt PRP only), 1: before treatment, 2: after treatment. IPL, intense pulsed light; PRP, platelet-rich-plasma.

Source: https://www.researchgate.net/publication/351911946/figure/fig1/AS:11431281173844756@1689056677364/A-case-of-fair-improvement-of-both-sides-Rt-PRP-IPL-and-Lt-PRP-only-1-before.png.

1.5.3. PRP vs. Chemical Peels

In the last ten years, cosmetic dermatology has seen an increase in the application of various modalities of treatment to enhance skin texture and against the aging process. Two of the most used among these are PRP therapy and chemical peels, both having their own mode of action and therapeutic advantage. PRP therapy consists of applying platelets derived from autologous blood containing growth factors that promote regeneration and healing. This method has been increasingly popular for its capacity to trigger collagen production and augment the tone of skin, particularly in areas that are beset by scarring or uneven pigmentation.

Chemical peels, on the other hand, use acidic chemicals to strip off the outer layers of the skin, basically shedding away damaged tissue in the process of acquiring a fresh appearance. It is critical to appreciate these differences to optimize treatment options according to individual patient needs. The effectiveness of PRP therapy versus chemical peels largely depends on the specific skin concerns being addressed. PRP has shown significant promise in treating conditions like acne scars, where its regenerative properties facilitate healing by accelerating skin repair mechanisms. Another recent study highlighted increased outcomes in healing pockmarks with PRP as used with microneedling, showing a dramatic superiority to microneedling at elevated plasma levels (Edison et al., 2024). Chemical peels, on the other hand, are optimally effective for photoaging and epidermal pigmentation. Treatments involving chemical peels in conjunction with adjunct therapies such as carboxytherapy have also proved to have a significant effect on vascular circles and pigmentation in sensitive regions, including beneath the eyes, highlighting the customized nature required for aesthetic perfection (Kołodziejczak et al., 2024). On comparing the safety profiles and recovery periods of each technique, variations also emerge that affect patient preference. PRP therapy is generally considered a minimally invasive treatment with fewer side effects, given its autologous character. In the patient, bruising and swelling at injection sites may occur, necessitating a short recovery period. Chemical peels, however, have potential redness and peeling, especially with deeper peels, with possible prolonged downtime. This difference also complicates the decision-making process and highlights the importance of customized skincare regimens. Overall, both PRP therapy and chemical peels share certain advantages and disadvantages, which highlight the need for a holistic determination of individual patient goals and skin types in dermatologic cosmetics.

Test Your Knowledge

1. How does PRP compare to dermal fillers in facial rejuvenation?
2. How does PRP therapy differ from laser treatments in improving skin texture and tone?
3. What are the differences between PRP and chemical peels in cosmetic dermatology?

1.6. Current Research and Future Directions

Learning Outcome

1. Focus on recent studies on PRP efficacy
2. Understand the innovations in PRP technology
3. Deal with potential new applications in dermatology

Recent advances in PRP application in cosmetic dermatology have generated immense interest, with a particular emphasis on its efficacy in the management of cicatricial alopecia. As PRP's regenerative properties are increasingly unveiled through more research studies, studies indicate a viable role in improving hair density among these affected patients. The study shows that PRP not only stimulates hair growth but also improves the overall cosmetic outcome in patients with the disconcerting aftermath of hair loss. The multifaceted complexity of cicatricial alopecia, with its multicontoured clinical presentations, necessitates new treatment modalities. Based on a literature review made up of clinical trials and case reports, researchers highlight the necessity of standardized methods in an effort to evaluate its effectiveness in this arena ahead of firmer clinical guidelines and protocols that can significantly enhance patient outcomes in dermatologic therapy (Edaes & de Souza, 2023). The research on the use of PRPs in cosmetic dermatology extends beyond alopecia to cover numerous other conditions, highlighting its value as an intervention. New evidence shows extensive applications ranging from facial rejuvenation therapy to scar revision, illustrating the versatility of its benefits. However, the current evidence base illustrates significant heterogeneity in outcomes that is shaped by preparation protocol and injection method. This difference implies a call for more research aimed at formulating stringent guidelines that define best practices for the use of PRP in cosmetic procedures. This standardization is necessary because it will not only make treatment more effective but also safer and more satisfying for the patient, establishing PRP as a contender in the field of cosmetic dermatology (Altunel et al., 2017). Future directions for PRP research in cosmetic dermatology are promising but require intense study. To unlock its therapeutic potential, a partnership among researchers, dermatologists, and industry experts is important. Facilitating partnerships may result in the development of new therapies with a synergistic blend of PRP with other technologies such as stem cell therapy or low-level light therapy, thereby improving outcomes. Prospective longitudinal studies are needed to obtain further extensive data about the long-term consequences and overall patient satisfaction following PRP treatments. With continued advances in the science of cosmetic dermatology, constant exploration into the action mechanism of PRP not only expands our understanding of its applications but also opens the door to the establishment of specific and tailored treatment protocols to respond to the particular needs of patients (Edaes & de Souza, 2023).

1.6.1. Recent Studies on PRP Efficacy

PRP effectiveness in aesthetic dermatology has been of high interest in recent years, primarily on the basis of its regenerative potential because of growth factors released from platelets. Current studies highlight PRP's potential in various applications, particularly skin rejuvenation and hair loss treatment. PRP has been proven to cause collagen production and improve tissue healing, making it an excellent candidate for both medical and cosmetic treatment. For instance, synergistic application of PRP in conjunction with microneedling has been shown to have adequate improvements in the appearance of the skin and elasticity. Furthermore, while the dermatological community is more and more debating the extensive applications of PRP, the need for standardized guidelines and protocols becomes self-apparent to optimize patient outcomes in a variety of treatments and procedures, further solidifying its place in cosmetic dermatology. In hair restoration, recent studies have shown that PRP significantly increases hair density and thickness in androgenetic alopecia patients. The use of PRP in this area is believed to be an effective method of stimulating the hair follicles and prolonging the anagen phase of the hair cycle. Combined therapies, particularly microneedling with PRP, have yielded better outcomes than PRP alone, with some research demonstrating synergistic effects that maximize hair regrowth. These findings are significant because they address the growing demand for non-surgical methods of hair restoration so that patients can enjoy the benefits with minimal downtime. With growing utilization of such modalities, there is a critical need for more studies to ascertain the best treatment regimens and establish long-term benefits, thus ensuring consistent and reproducible results for patients suffering from hair loss. Another significant role of PRP efficacy is its use for the treatment of skin diseases such as acne scars, fine lines, and overall skin rejuvenation. Recent studies indicate that patients who are treated with PRP therapy combined with advanced techniques like laser therapy or chemical peeling show remarkable improvement in skin texture as well as facial volume. This synergy increases the healing potential of PRP and, at the same time, addresses familiar skin imperfections more comprehensively. Interestingly, research finds that PRP used along with microneedling can produce better results in the case of melasma, demonstrating its potential in curing various dermal conditions. Despite these developments, the dermatology industry is finding it difficult to formulate standard protocols and adequate preclinical evidence of PRP's efficacy in other treatments, emphasizing the necessity of strong clinical trials to determine its position in cosmetic dermatology and alleviate any liability issues in esthetic procedures, according to recent court reviews (Dereli et al., 2025) (Figure 1.15).

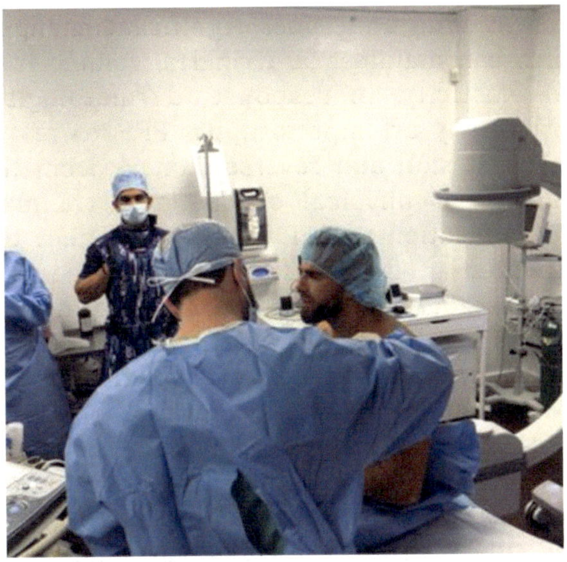

Figure 1.15. Clinical setting for platelet-rich plasma (PRP) therapy administration.

Source: https://s3-media0.fl.yelpcdn.com/bphoto/Y7pGC6aISYVVv4jJ8h3e4Q/348s.jpg.

1.6.2. Innovations in PRP Technology

The advent of new methods in the extraction and utilization of PRP technology is a new trend in cosmetic dermatology. New innovations are focused on optimizing platelet and growth factor concentration to enhance their therapeutic efficacy for skin rejuvenation. Automated devices for concentrating platelets from whole blood efficiently have made it easier, lowering the risk of contamination and guaranteeing uniform outcomes. These developments not only enhance the therapeutic efficacy of PRP treatments but also respond to the increasing demand for non-surgical aesthetic treatments. In particular, these advanced formulations enable practitioners to tailor PRP protocols to the individual patient's requirements and thus deliver optimal therapeutic effect. These developments demonstrate a commitment to an integration of science and aesthetic application and thus promote greater patient satisfaction and improved clinical outcomes. Moreover, awareness of the biological mechanisms underlying the effectiveness in the dermal layer has predisposed it to more targeted applications in addressing certain cosmetic problems. With the rich repertoire of growth factors found in PRP, tissue repair and regeneration have been promoted by dermatologists, particularly in dermal conditions that involve skin aging and alopecia. For example, PRP's function to induce differentiation of epithelial cells and orient collagen bundles is critical when regenerating older skin and healthier hair follicles. As advanced research by experts continues to determine PRP's regenerative factor, the window of opportunity for this technology to enhance treatment protocol widens. The new evidence on PRP applications, such as its established impact on cicatricial alopecia, indicates a potential all-purpose tool in cosmetic dermatology that guides practitioners in developing their therapeutic strategies and interventions (Edaes & de Souza, 2023). Parallel to these developments, ongoing studies on optimizing PRP formulation highlight the demand for standardization of treatment protocols. Variability in technique in the acquisition and utilization of PRP can result in uneven outcomes, complicating a demonstration of the acceptance of PRP as an effective treatment modality among cosmetic dermatologists. Consequently, industry stakeholders are demanding standards that outline best practices in the processing and injection of PRP. Furthermore, interdisciplinary collaboration is increasingly becoming a cornerstone, bridging the gaps between dermatology, regenerative medicine, and the life sciences. This collaborative effort ensures that new techniques are based on good scientific evidence and can address clinical needs effectively. As the industry continues to expand, integration of innovations into practice will be at the forefront of enhancing the safety, effectiveness, and popularity of PRP treatments in cosmetic dermatology (Unal et al., 2017) (Figure 1.16).

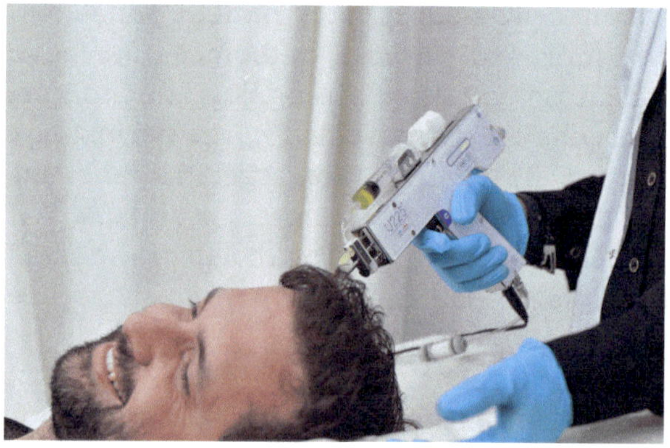

Figure 1.16. PRP treatments for hair.

Source: https://www.prpclinic.co.il/wp-content/uploads/2023/06/prp-%D7%9C%D7%92%D7%91%D7%A8-2-1024x683-1.png.

1.6.3. Potential New Applications in Dermatology

The investigation of new uses of PRP in dermatology is prompted by continuous developments in regenerative medicine. Among new promising developments, plasma gel can be identified as a major breakthrough over conventional PRP treatments. This plasma gel, formed through the controlled reduction of platelet-poor plasma to a more dense gel-like state, has the double benefit of not only exploiting the regenerative potential inherent in PRP but also offering supportive structure akin to cosmetic fillers. Such applications are particularly intriguing within facial rejuvenation, wherein plasma gel can increase elasticity, texture, and volume of the skin. Thus, the clinical efficacy and patient response associated with plasma gel is a notable research area in the search for newer dermatological treatments, as per Cheng et al (2025). The integration of this biomaterial in treatment protocols could potentially enhance overall patient satisfaction and aesthetic results. Moreover, physiological decline because of aging requires efficient regenerative therapies to reverse skin deterioration. As Manole et al. (2023) points out, the skin itself, especially after trauma, undergoes significant changes, which can manifest as wrinkles, volume loss, and elasticity. In response, dermatologists increasingly attempt to apply PRP to revive senescent skin and reverse damage from the majority of physical or chemical traumas. The application of PRP therapy to induce the activation of fibroblasts has been used for years, although its overall purposes for dermal repair are not as well-researched. Of particular interest in the study of long-term effects is the newly forming role of telocytes (TCs), recently identified cells in the dermis, with properties conducive to tissue repair and regeneration. Investigation of their interaction with PRP may hold future promise for new mechanisms of enhancing therapeutic outcomes, eventually maximizing treatment protocols in cosmetic dermatology. Future dermatological uses of PRP would involve synergistic treatment where PRP is used in concert with other regenerative therapies. A combination of PRP with growth factors, cellular treatments, or hyaluronic acid fillers may optimally exploit the advantages of each and present a lucrative field for innovation. Such approaches could potentially yield superior results in aesthetics, particularly for complex cases such as advanced skin laxity or extensive scarring. A study of how the combinations influence healing processes, patient satisfaction, and long-term results may reveal breakthrough treatment paradigms in dermatology. It is essential to demonstrate these new combinations with suitably designed clinical trials in a way to demonstrates them as effective and safe. In that manner, dermatology can move forward beyond the conventional approaches to cover high-level regenerative therapies, eventually resulting in improved care for deserving patients.

Test Your Knowledge

1. What do recent studies say about the efficacy of PRP in cosmetic dermatology?
2. What are some recent innovations in PRP technology that are enhancing its cosmetic use?

SUMMARY

The study in PRP in cosmetic dermatology reveals its vast potential for enhancing skin rejuvenation and healing procedures. As indicated through several studies, PRP therapy, including the new use of dermapens, has the potential to become an innovative treatment to mend skin blemishes like acne scars and more. The success of PRP lies in the fact that it contains a high concentration of growth factors and bioactive molecules, which trigger tissue regeneration and healing at the cellular level. The notable results from experimental studies attest to the fact that PRP not only induces rapid healing but is superior compared to other treatments. Therefore, the use of PRPs in cosmetic dermatology is a remarkable progress that signifies the potential for improvement in its application in aesthetic treatments in the future. Moreover, the comparative investigation between PRP and other plasma therapies, such as salmon DNA serum, makes the unique advantages of PRP in wound healing and rejuvenation of skin more strong. Research has established that PRP treatments have a greater healing efficacy than most other forms of treatment. Especially with ideal concentrations, PRP is extremely effective in accelerating the healing rate for pockmarks, as established in controlled lab studies using animal models. The ability of PRP to inhibit microorganisms and stimulate regenerative processes is a sign of its multi-faceted function in dermatology, which also makes it a pet among practitioners. This growing evidence attests to the role of PRP as a powerful tool for practitioners committed to innovating patient care in cosmetic and therapeutic dermatology. In conclusion, the present scientific and clinical application of Platelet-Rich Plasma is an evolution in cosmetic dermatology, driven by scientific interest and clinical evidence. With practitioners adopting PRP as a part of their treatment protocol, the ultimate outcome for patients cannot help but improve overall, further encouraging increased satisfaction and healthy skin. By the natural healing power of platelets, dermatologists can offer new options that are not only pleasing to the eyes but also healthy for the skin as a whole. As the present studies, including the comparisons with other treatments, have demonstrated, PRP is an effective method of addressing problematic skin conditions. The future of PRP in cosmetic dermatology appears promising, with future studies aimed at furthering research that may further enhance techniques and broaden its uses (Chiuman et al., 2023; Edison et al., 2024).

PRP application in cosmetic dermatology represents a significant leap forward in how dermatologists approach skin rejuvenation and hair growth. PRP treatment involves the application of the patient's own blood, which is then isolated to a high concentration of platelets with growth factors and cytokines. The autologous source not only minimizes the risk of allergic reaction but also promotes natural healing and cellular regeneration. In dermatology skin aesthetics, PRP has been applied in facial rejuvenation, acne scar remodeling, and overall skin texture improvement. With the growing demand for regenerative medicine procedures among dermatological experts, the introduction of PRP therapy has been very successful in improving patient satisfaction due to being a safe and minimally invasive method for maximizing cosmetic outcomes. Moreover, PRP therapy has also drawn interest in its application to treating baldness, including disorders like androgenetic alopecia and alopecia areata (AA). The rich content of growth factors in PRP is reported to cause hair follicle growth stimulation, therefore promoting new hair growth and hair density. Recent evidence indicates that the combination of PRP with microneedling might enhance these effects since microneedling is employed to facilitate growth factor penetration and uptake in the scalp. Clinical studies on the efficacy of PRP in treating baldness are still continuing, yet preliminary findings indicate significant potential, which is making it more and more popular amongst dermatologists as a treatment of choice for those experiencing thinning of hair. To this end is the recognition of the need for vigorous clinical trials for enhanced understanding of its long-term outcomes and effectiveness, adding to the body of knowledge in cosmetic dermatology. In addition to its application in skin rejuvenation and hair growth, the role of PRP therapy in cosmetic dermatology can also extend to other newer modalities, such as recovery following procedures and optimization of results of more invasive procedures. For instance, combined therapy of PRP with traditional treatments like dermal fillers and chemical peels could enhance tissue healing and overall aesthetic results. Combined therapy is in sync with a wider trend in medicine favoring individualized and holistic treatment protocols. But most importantly, it must be stressed that despite the promise of PRP, established procedures like hair transplantation and medical treatments like minoxidil are still mandatory in the management of hair loss and cosmetic enhancement. While cosmetic dermatology treads along the thin rope between tradition and innovation, ongoing evaluation of the effects of PRPs will affect future practice and inform optimal practices of care (Cholewa et al., 2025; Pawlik et al., 2024).

KEY TERMS FROM THIS CHAPTER

- Aesthetic dermatology
- Angiogenesis
- Autoimmune disorders
- Biological reaction
- Body dysmorphic disorders (BDD)
- Collagen synthesis
- Cosmetic fillers
- Cytokines
- Dermatological interventions
- Hair restoration
- Alopecia
- Anti-aging resistance
- Bioactive molecules
- Blood cells
- Cell growth
- Cosmetic dermatology
- Cosmetic procedures
- Dermatological conditions
- Facial rejuvenation
- Healing mechanism

CRITICAL THINKING QUESTIONS

1. **What is the primary component of Platelet-Rich Plasma (PRP)?**
   a. Red blood cells
   b. Platelets and growth factors
   c. Plasma proteins only
   d. Leukocytes
2. **Which of the following cosmetic conditions is PRP commonly used to treat?**
   a. Psoriasis
   b. Vitiligo
   c. Androgenetic alopecia
   d. Melasma
3. **What is the primary mechanism by which PRP exerts its effects in skin rejuvenation?**
   a. Immune modulation
   b. Bacterial inhibition
   c. Collagen stimulation and tissue regeneration
   d. Melanin suppression
4. **How is PRP typically prepared for cosmetic use?**
   a. Centrifugation of the patient's blood
   b. Bone marrow aspiration
   c. Synthetic chemical preparation
   d. Biopsy of skin tissue
5. **Which of the following is a potential side effect of PRP treatment?**
   a. Severe anaphylactic reaction
   b. Hyperpigmentation
   c. Autoimmune flare
   d. Infection at injection site

Short Answer Questions

1. What is PRP and how is it prepared for cosmetic dermatologic use?
2. Describe the proposed mechanisms of action for PRP in skin rejuvenation.
3. What are the most common cosmetic dermatologic indications for PRP therapy?
4. Compare and contrast the use of PRP as a monotherapy versus in combination with other treatments (e.g., microneedling, laser, fillers).
5. What are the key differences between leukocyte-rich and leukocyte-poor PRP, and how might these differences influence clinical outcomes in aesthetic applications?
6. What are the common side effects and potential complications of PRP in cosmetic dermatology?
7. Discuss the current evidence regarding the efficacy of PRP in the treatment of androgenetic alopecia. How does it compare to other treatment modalities?
8. What are the challenges and limitations in standardizing PRP protocols for cosmetic use, and how do they affect study comparisons and clinical outcomes?

Answer to Critical Thinking Questions

1. (b); 2. (c); 3. (c); 4. (a); 5. (d)

REFERENCES

1. Akaberi, S. M., Sharma, K., Ahmadi-Ashtiani, H. R., & Hedayati, M. (2025). Polydeoxyribonucleotide in skincare and cosmetics: Mechanisms, therapeutic applications, and advancements beyond wound healing and anti-aging. *Journal of Skin and Stem Cell.* https://www.semanticscholar.org/paper/a21b4f2b2588166c4ffe1ef558963c16674a9c1e (accessed on 11th June 2025).
2. Altunel, C., Gencler, B., & Kartal, S. P. (2017). *Cosmetic Procedures in The Treatment of Alopecia.* https://core.ac.uk/download/322430037.pdf (accessed on 11th June 2025).
3. Amici, J. M., Cogrel, O., Jourdan, M., Raimbault, C., Canchy, L., Kérob, D., Madfes, D., et al. (2023). Expert recommendations on supportive skin care for non-surgical and surgical procedures. *Journal of the European Academy of Dermatology and Venereology, 37*, 16–33. https://doi.org/10.1111/jdv.18855 (accessed on 11th June 2025).
4. Amir Adel Anis Basily, A. A. H. I., & Saleh, H. M. A. (2024). Comparative clinical trial of Dermapen microneedling and platelet-rich plasma versus Dermapen microneedling alone in the treatment of stretch marks in Egyptian adults. *QJM: An International Journal of Medicine.* https://www.semanticscholar.org/paper/3834d4900ed8c1923d93197a120f50f34852caaf (accessed on 11th June 2025).
5. Aswani, R. C., Borkar, M. A., Mehta, B. D., et al. (2017). Study of safety and efficacy of autologous platelet rich plasma combined with fractional CO_2 laser in the treatment of post acne scars: A comparative simultaneous split-face study. https://core.ac.uk/download/539914217.pdf (accessed on 11th June 2025).
6. Atsu, N., Ekinci-Aslanoglu, C., Kantarci-Demirkiran, B., Caf, N., & Nuhoğlu, F. (2023). The comparison of platelet-rich plasma versus injectable platelet rich fibrin in facial skin rejuvenation. *Dermatologic Therapy.* https://www.semanticscholar.org/paper/d00dfa512244463a054722cf96fb624500de0ed6 (accessed on 11th June 2025).
7. Avila, R. M., Camacho-Leon, G., Faytong-Haro, M., Merino-Alado, R., Pineda Carrillo, J., Mautong, H., Simancas-Racines, D., et al. (2024). Case report: Primary cutaneous histoplasmosis in an immunocompetent patient after cosmetic injection of platelet-rich plasma treated with trimethoprim-sulfamethoxazole. *The American Journal of Case Reports, 25*, e942660-1–e942660-7. https://www.semanticscholar.org/paper/9065f1658e83747c8adbc5b6cd19b746d1939025 (accessed on 11th June 2025).
8. Bagherani, N., Smoller, B. R., Tavoosidana, G., Ghanadan, A., Wollina, U., & Lotti, T. (2023). An overview of the role of carboxytherapy in dermatology. *Journal of Cosmetic Dermatology, 22*, 2399–2407. https://doi.org/10.1111/jocd.15741 (accessed on 11th June 2025).
9. Bendel, E. M. (2018). *Platelet Rich Plasma Treatment Application for Multiple Purposes.* https://core.ac.uk/download/232684123.pdf (accessed on 11th June 2025).
10. Pawlik, W., Nowotarska, A., Błaszczyński, G., Nojek, P., Zimonczyk, M., & Zawół, M. (2024). Hair loss therapies: a review and comparison of traditional and modern treatment methods. *Journal of Education, Health and Sport, 75*, 56191. https://doi.org/10.12775/JEHS.2024.75.56191(accessed on 11th June 2025).
11. Trovato, F., Ceccarelli, S., Michelini, S., Vespasiani, G., Guida, S., Galadari, H. I., Nisticò, S. P., Colonna, L., & Pellacani, G. (2024). Advancements in Regenerative Medicine for Aesthetic Dermatology: A Comprehensive Review and Future Trends. *Cosmetics, 11*(2), 49. https://doi.org/10.3390/cosmetics11020049(accessed on 11th June 2025).

12. Suruchi, G., Shweta, M., & Chandi, G. (2018). The Wonder Tool Platelet Rich Plasma in Cosmetic Dermatology, Trichology and Hair Transplant. InTech. doi: 10.5772/intechopen.70287(accessed on 11th June 2025).

13. Cheng, H., Li, J., Zhao, Y., Xia, X., & Li, Y. (2025). *In vivo* assessment of plasma gel: Regenerative potential and limitations as a filler. *Journal of Cosmetic Dermatology, 24*. https://www.semanticscholar.org/paper/b4e16826e793654f4b25d6c8649f256669acb463 (accessed on 11th June 2025).

14. Chiuman, L., Hestina, O., Xavier, N., & Tarigan, S. B. (2023). Dermapen treatments for healing pockmarked skin in male Wistar rats (*Rattus norvegicus*): A study comparing platelet-rich plasma with salmon DNA serum. https://core.ac.uk/download/599384510.pdf (accessed on 11th June 2025).

15. Cholewa, M., Jaglarz, K., Jasiewicz, M., et al. (2025). Non-pharmacological therapies in the treatment of chemotherapy-induced alopecia–A literature review. https://core.ac.uk/download/636386140.pdf (accessed on 11th June 2025).

16. Cyran, P., Jaroszyńska, A., Jaroszyński, F., et al. (2024). Platelet-rich plasma (PRP) in hair restoration treatments: A comprehensive review of existing literature. https://core.ac.uk/download/620863922.pdf (accessed on 11th June 2025).

17. Felipe Sanches Edaes, Cleide Barbieri de Souza (2023). PRP in cicatricial alopecia: Unraveling mechanistic insights, assessing clinical efficacy, and paving future directions. http://revista.lusiada.br/index.php/ruep/article/view/1773(accessed on 11th June 2025).

18. Dereli, A. K., İzci, A., Cenk, H., Şanlı, B., & Acar, K. (2025). Evaluation of medical malpractice claims arising from minimally invasive cosmetic procedures in the context of supreme court decisions. *TURKDERM*. https://www.semanticscholar.org/paper/d629cc666684f191a8b8642785afab0e16ca317e (accessed on 11th June 2025).

19. Dhillon, J., & Jusuf, N. K. (2024). Non–invasive vulvovaginal rejuvenation: A review. https://core.ac.uk/download/639389933.pdf (accessed on 11th June 2025).

20. Edison, R. E., Nila, E. D. W. R., & Wijaya, J. F. (2024). Comparison of the effectiveness of Dermapen using plasma from platelets with Dermapen on pockmarked skin surface of female Wistar rats (*Rattus norvegicus*). https://core.ac.uk/download/618209160.pdf (accessed on 11th June 2025).

21. Everts, P. A. (2018). *Autologous Platelet-Rich Plasma and Mesenchymal Stem Cells for The Treatment of Chronic Wounds*. https://core.ac.uk/download/322439011.pdf (accessed on 11th June 2025).

22. Fareez, I. M., Liew, F., Widera, D., Mayeen, N. F., Mawya, J., Abu Kasim, N. H., & Haque, M. N. (2023). Application of platelet-rich plasma as a stem cell treatment–An attempt to clarify a common public misconception. *Current Molecular Medicine*. https://www.semanticscholar.org/paper/680e2a0ac32f25fdcfb4f6fe4dd070e78a777ee9 (accessed on 11th June 2025).

23. Górska, M., Kmak, B., & Szot, A. (2024). Autoimmune disease and aesthetic medicine: A holistic approach. https://core.ac.uk/download/620863172.pdf (accessed on 11th June 2025).

24. Hidayat, A., Aswat, H. H., & Putri, L. D. (2024). Compare the effectiveness of a peel-off mask and sheet-mask with green tea extract on Dermapen-treated wounds on the back surface of female Wistar rats. https://core.ac.uk/download/599582055.pdf (accessed on 11th June 2025).

25. Keskinbora, K., & Kumbasar, E. (2023). Ethical concerns in dermatology and cosmetic applications. *Medical Research Archives.* https://www.semanticscholar.org/paper/888f1ad9b5a0c236c51f83cb5213b5e1b2859908 (accessed on 11th June 2025).

26. Kołodziejczak, A., & Rotsztejn, H. (2024). The impact of carboxytherapy and treatments combining carboxytherapy and selected chemical peels on vascular and pigmentary components of the dark circles. https://core.ac.uk/download/628489367.pdf (accessed on 11th June 2025).

27. López, J. M. S., & Rubio, J. A. (2018). *Clinical Applications of Plasma Growth Factors.* https://core.ac.uk/download/322436223.pdf (accessed on 11th June 2025).

28. Manole, C. G., Soare, C., Ceafalan, L. C., & Voiculescu, V. M. (2023). Platelet-Rich Plasma in Dermatology: New Insights on the Cellular Mechanism of Skin Repair and Regeneration. *Life (Basel, Switzerland), 14*(1), 40. https://doi.org/10.3390/life14010040(accessed on 11th June 2025).

29. Marcinkiewicz, A., Ochotnicka, A., Zatyka, P., Olczyk, M., Pawłowska, A., Rabenda, M., & Janik, P. (2024). The use of platelet-rich plasma in the treatment of alopecia–A review of the literature. *Archive Euromedica.* https://www.semanticscholar.org/paper/b57c75f8c50518957bfc23548f41fc63e16eac16 (accessed on 11th June 2025).

30. Muchová, J. (2016). *The Effect of Biologically Active Substances on The Structure and Properties of Collagenous Substrates.* https://core.ac.uk/download/44397957.pdf (accessed on 11th June 2025)

31. Navarro, R. M., Pino, A., Martínez, A., Garrigós, E., Grau, M., Gallego, E., Carme, A., et al. (2022). Combined therapy with laser and autologous topical serum for facial rejuvenation: A multiple case series report. *Journal of Cutaneous and Aesthetic Surgery, 15*, 363–370. https://www.semanticscholar.org/paper/3f8179881affcd85b1594740e7f3b0251d0f796e (accessed on 11th June 2025).

32. Ochyra, Ł., & Łopuszyńska, A. (2024). Platelet-rich plasma in dermatology and aesthetic medicine. *Quality in Sport.* https://www.semanticscholar.org/paper/c439f15d1ccc81d507195e6615b2ca9c5a1f2daf (accessed on 11th June 2025).

33. Oh, I. Y., Kim, B., & Kim, M. (2014). Depressed facial scars successfully treated with autologous platelet-rich plasma and light-emitting diode phototherapy at 830 nm. *Annals of Dermatology, 26*, 417–418. https://www.semanticscholar.org/paper/3633352ebb4584099c6a92eb234a00ea3dd7d178 (accessed on 11th June 2025).

34. Pham, T. T., Nguyen, T. M., Nguyen, T. N. H., Mai, T. H., & Nguyen, D. T. (2021). Platelet-rich plasma and its application in clinical trial. *VNU Journal of Science: Medical and Pharmaceutical Sciences.* https://www.semanticscholar.org/paper/669f9409c518102b795937833c1bc5c03fe0167a (accessed on 11th June 2025).

35. Prokurat, M., Grudnik, K., Niemczyk, W., Niemczyk, S., Migas, M., Wągrowska, K., Lau, K., et al. (2024). Platelet-rich plasma–A remedy present in every human being. History, functioning, and the benefits of therapy using it. *Polski Merkuriusz Lekarski: Organ Polskiego Towarzystwa Lekarskiego, 52*(2), 240–245. https://www.semanticscholar.org/paper/a48c6e814c5d89b14aa107db044614fa684e6fdc (accessed on 11th June 2025).

36. Ramadan, F. (2025). Microneedling: Monotherapy or adjuvant treatment? *Journal of Aesthetic Nursing.* https://www.semanticscholar.org/paper/abd366ccf0730d976364b39c7c3d5660b329503d (accessed on 11th June 2025).

37. Rizvi, S. A. (2021). Platelet-rich plasma in the treatment of alopecia. *International Journal of Research in Dermatology*. https://www.semanticscholar.org/paper/1dfd23e2e46f5c84c7fabd3948afd439ad005091 (accessed on 11th June 2025).

38. Rodriguez, M., & Mayrovitz, H. N. (2024). The history and current status of platelet-rich plasma therapy in dermatology. *Cureus, 16*. https://www.semanticscholar.org/paper/dadc23da41094fee24dbbf4522a431e85a2cfb86 (accessed on 11th June 2025).

39. Rout, A., Mani, S., & Pandey, A. (2023). Intradermal platelet-rich plasma vs. 1064 nm Q switched Nd-YAG laser (Qs Nd-YAG) in the treatment of resistant melasma–A split face comparative study in Indian subjects. *Pigment International, 10*, 158–164. https://www.semanticscholar.org/paper/d77f2bde21d0f4493818e693bfe417f9985eebc2 (accessed on 11th June 2025).

40. Saeed, M., Elethawi, A. M. D., Al-Ani, Z., & Abdullah, R. A. (2016). Application of fractional microneedling radiofrequency and autologous platelet-rich plasma in managing facial acne scars. *British Journal of Medicine and Medical Research, 14*, 1–18. https://www.semanticscholar.org/paper/107bf45141cfd164fa3955f7dc5c1c0bf515aed6 (accessed on 11th June 2025).

41. Unal, M. (2017). *Platelet-Rich Plasma in Burn Treatment*. https://core.ac.uk/download/322432917.pdf (accessed on 11th June 2025).

42. Valentina, S., & Laksemi, D. A. (2025). Platelet rich plasma as a potential treatment for melasma: A review. *Siriraj Medical Journal*. https://www.semanticscholar.org/paper/f2dce882931105c443ac76e0b0c073488e95646b (accessed on 11th June 2025).

43. Wang, Z. Q., Lai, Q. W. S., Gao, X., Wu, Q. Y., Dong, T. T. X., & Tsim, K. (2025). Platelet-rich plasma extract derived from animals shows potential in promoting wound healing and suppressing inflammatory response in skin cells. *Cells, 14*. https://www.semanticscholar.org/paper/741e61cc6da0f8e3a251f25957fd017a1f75ab94 (accessed on 11th June 2025).

HAIR LOSS: DIAGNOSIS AND TREATMENT OPTIONS

2

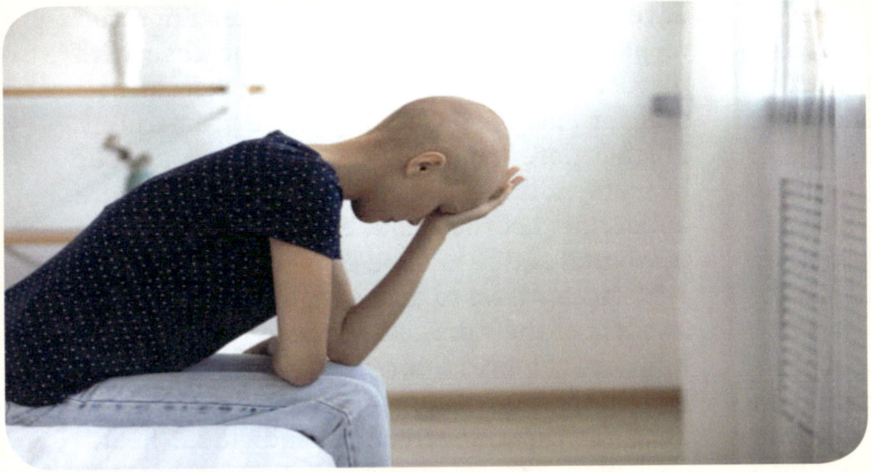

LEARNING OBJECTIVES

After studying this chapter, you will be able to:

1. Identify the types of hair loss
2. Explain the causes of hair loss
3. Explain how to diagnose hair loss
4. Summarize the treatments: medical treatment and surgical treatment
5. Emphasize alternative and complementary therapies

Introduction

Hair loss, also the medical condition referred to as alopecia, is a gigantic challenge to many millions of individuals worldwide. Alopecia can be categorized into various forms, such as androgenetic alopecia, alopecia areata (AA), and telogen effluvium, each having variations in etiology and patterns of hair loss. Hair loss is extremely prevalent, reaching both genders and varying with different age groups, making its etiology a crucial aspect to understand. Apart from genetic issues, additional driving causes like hormonal imbalance, stress, nutrition deficiencies, and associated medical conditions play a part in accelerated hair loss with accompanying physical and psychological impacts in affected persons. All these driving causes are important in the diagnosis of the underlying type of hair loss and, hence developing the right management. With numerous options of available managements of hair loss, they can be classified as medical, surgical, and alternative treatments. Medical therapies typically consist of topical creams, oral medications, and hormonal therapy aimed at encouraging hair regrowth and preventing future loss. The most familiar is minoxidil, which has shown efficacy in the stimulation of hair revival in both men and women. In contrast, surgery such as hair transplantation can provide permanent solutions for persons seeking enhancement of beauty. Other therapies, such as herbal treatment and lifestyle changes, have also become popular; however, their efficacy is often not strongly scientifically backed. Therefore, it is critical to ensure that the patient receives evidence-based therapy to maximize the outcome while avoiding undue side effects. In addition, the psychological influence of hair loss should not be ignored, as it will usually result in low self-esteem and higher anxiety. Hair loss patients feel a sense of loss of identity, which has a negative effect on social contact and quality of life. So, an immensely significant aspect of holistic care is addressing the psychological and emotional concerns about hair loss. Healthcare professionals are guided by this awareness in prescribing holistic treatment regimens that may include counseling or support groups along with other medical treatments. In the end, a combination of both clinical and psychosocial treatment is required to effectively treat hair loss so that patients can be empowered in their efforts to achieve renewed confidence and well-being.

Definition of Hair Loss

The alopecia clinical process of hair loss is a group of conditions that lead to partial or complete loss of body or scalp hair. Although traditionally considered to be a cosmetic issue, hair loss has important psychological ramifications for the individual, as it affects his or her self-esteem and quality of life. The condition can be categorized into various types, including androgenetic alopecia, telogen effluvium, and AA, each with its own etiology and pattern of development. Familiarity with these subtypes is of prime importance in the diagnosis and management, as they cover various mechanisms that demand specific therapeutic intervention. For instance, androgenetic alopecia, or male and female pattern hair loss, is primarily an outcome of genetic and hormonal factors and, therefore, emphasizes the intrinsic complexity involved in the diagnosis and treatment of hair loss conditions. In addition to the effect of genetic predispositions, environmental factors, stress, and some medical conditions can also contribute to the onset of hair loss. Studies have proven that psychological stress can result in hair loss or baldness, as is the case with diseases like telogen effluvium, wherein hair follicles enter the shedding phase prematurely. Furthermore, some illnesses, such as polycystic ovary syndrome (PCOS), are associated with endocrine disorders that cause hair loss issues in women and result in a growing social cost as women also have to deal with the psychological impacts of their disease (Annagur et al., 2018). Hair loss requires a comprehensive assessment that addresses not just the hair follicle's biology but the whole spectrum of individual health variables, taking particular care to identify where physical and mental health overlap. The proper definition of hair loss encompasses not just its medical characteristics but also its clinical applicability. An effective diagnosis typically includes a comprehensive patient history, physical examination, and potentially laboratory studies to rule out systemic causes. The psychological, as well as emotional, considerations of alopecia highlight a true public health concern, with patients with this condition frequently experiencing social stigmatization and mental illness. Novel therapies therefore, range from topical agents and oral agents to advanced procedures like hair transplantation. Finally, the end aim is to improve the quality of life of the affected individuals with full recognition that successful intervention would not only add value to the physical quality of hair restoration but also to the psychological coping of the people faced with hair loss problems (Anneliese et al., 2017).

Importance of Addressing Hair Loss

Treatment of baldness or hair loss is of paramount significance to psychological and social well-being. The patients experiencing baldness or hair loss exhibit low self-esteem and confidence, which has an impact on their mental status and social interactions. The direct consequence of hair loss is a cause of social stigma, and this encompasses depression as well as anxiety. Current evidence points towards the inadequacy of feelings resulting from physical appearance change being a cause of poor quality of life, and thus interventions are crucial. Being a multifaceted health condition, hair loss can be seen to imply its factors beyond cosmetic in nature. The importance of addressing these psychological and emotional factors is the possibility of improving the quality of life, leading individuals to take proactive measures, either through treatment programs, support groups, or counseling services. Second, addressing baldness is imperative on the clinical level because baldness can mean an underlying medical issue that should be addressed. Diseases such as alopecia areata (AA), thyroid function disorders, or malnutrition may present as hair loss, so proper treatment and diagnosis are crucial to overall health. Emphasizing hair loss allows healthcare providers an opportunity to perform a thorough evaluation that can actually reveal other underlying health conditions simultaneously. Further, the more that is known about hair loss, the more doors are opened to effective treatments for certain conditions. Pharmaceutical or surgical clinical treatments can significantly change the quality of life in a patient by restoring hair and thus enhancing self-esteem. Thus, recognizing the clinical relevance of baldness lends evidence to an integrated perspective for diagnosis and management. Finally, hair loss may be treated with significant benefits for society at large through greater inclusiveness and tolerance of diverse appearances. In an era where self-expression and mental health awareness are gaining immense popularity, the subject of hair loss is centered on embracing individuality. Portrayal in the media and exposure campaigns that bring attention to hair loss can assist in establishing an environment in which individuals become less stigmatized about their condition. Learning about the numerous causes and methods of treatment for hair loss can assist people in feeling more at ease seeking assistance without fearing judgment from others. Furthermore, the conversations emphasizing the emotional and psychological implications of hair loss can lead to an overall understanding of its effects and foster inclusive communities. Finally, the need to address hair loss extends beyond personal concerns, creating a societal transformation that focuses on health, acceptance, and well-being for all affected by this condition (Figure 2.1).

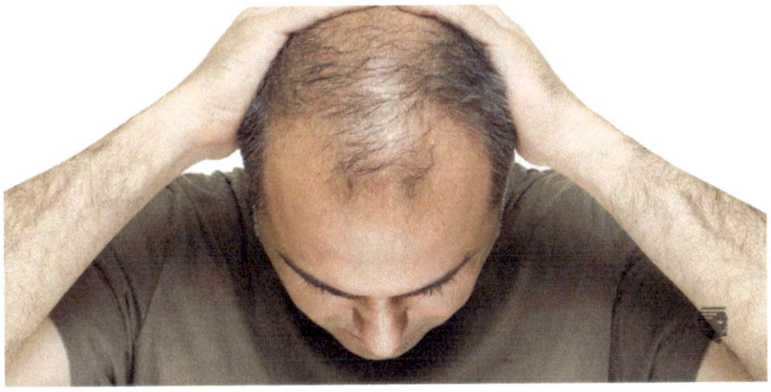

Figure 2.1. Male pattern baldness with visible thinning at the crown and frontal scalp.

Source: https://www.google.com/url?sa=i&url=https%3A%2F%2Fwww.advancedhairstudioindia.com%2Fblogs%2Ftips-for-hair-thinning-due-to-male-pattern-baldness&psig=AOvVaw2FE6EEc3LSgKzNPeQTZYHH&ust=1747839446698000&source=images&cd=vfe&opi=89978449&ved=0CBcQjhxqFwoTCKDv1MKnso0DFQAAAAAdAAAAABAE.

2.1. Types of Hair Loss

Learning Outcome

1. Define androgenetic alopecia
2. Explain telogen effluvium
3. Describe alopecia areata

The hair loss condition manifests in various presentations, with each having its own causative factors and characteristics. One of the most common is androgenetic alopecia (AGA), a hereditary condition that predominantly affects males but can also affect females. AGA presents as progressive thinning of the hair secondary to genetic and hormonal influences, that is, the effects of androgens, the male sex hormones that have a bearing on the hair cycle. With this condition remaining, chronic microscopic follicular inflammation also impacts hair follicle health, making the condition worse. Topical minoxidil and oral finasteride treatments have been developed to reverse these effects, emphasizing early intervention (Rossi et al., 2016). Telogen effluvium is another severe type of hair loss, characterized by temporary shedding of hair due to stress, disease, or hormonal changes. In this condition, a high number of hair follicles are driven into the resting phase early, leading to excessive hair loss within a short period of time. Telogen effluvium can be caused by many environmental or physiological stressors, and unlike AGA, it is generally reversible after the cause has been addressed. People may notice thinning of hair on the scalp, which is usually less centralized than in other forms of hair loss. Successful treatment generally entails the identification and removal of the causative factors, thus enabling hair to grow back naturally. Moreover, trichotillomania is a special type of hair loss due to psychological rather than genetic or medical causes. This is a compulsive disorder that induces individuals to pluck out their own hair, with visible bald spots being the resultant effect, as well as great emotional anguish. It has been discovered from research that trichotillomania often co-occurs with other psychiatric disorders and is influenced by social and behavioral determinants. In conventional therapy, the practices vary from cognitive-behavioral therapy to drug use. Understanding the complexities of trichotillomania and its ramifications can be of significant importance in effective treatment planning for not only the hair loss but also the causative psychological problems (Voth et al., 2009).

2.1.1. Androgenetic Alopecia

The AGA condition affects a large number of people from different demographics, making it the most common type of hair loss suffered by men. AGA is characterized by thinning hair with a progressive pattern, and in many cases, it is genetically inherited, with genetic factors playing an important role in its development and advancement. It is strongly associated with the action of androgens, the male sex hormones that affect the hair cycle of growth, along with an inflammatory response in the follicles of hair. Due to the multifactorial cause of its etiology with both hormonal and genetic influences, AGA demands a multidisciplinary treatment pattern that must be started early. Awareness of the progressive nature of AGA notifies both clinicians and patients of the importance of long-term treatment strategies to reverse the effect of hair loss and thinning (Rossi et al., 2016). In women, presentation of androgenetic alopecia can also differ significantly from men as female pattern hair loss. This state also has a high genetic foundation and is exacerbated by rising age, with estimates from studies that fewer than 45% of women ride out life with their full head of hair. Psychological implications are highly appropriate in the sense that women who experience hair loss are troubled and can appear to be seeking both medical and non-medical solutions for such conditions. Female pattern alopecia is typically diagnosed on clinical assessment and institution of treatment before advancement of loss to arrest it. As with men, hormonal imbalance plays a key role; therefore, oral antiandrogen treatment and topical minoxidil are the mainstays of treatment. Of significance, the effects of such treatments only become evident with time, requiring continuous maintenance to uphold any desirable effects (Dinh & Sinclair, 2007). Due to the intricacies and etiologies of androgenetic alopecia, therapy for the condition is diverse and ought to be customized for personal patient requirements. The main medications to date approved for the treatment of AGA are topical minoxidil and oral finasteride, both of which are aimed at slowing down hair loss and stimulating regrowth. Every treatment has its own set of potential benefits and risks, which clinicians and patients should study in turn. Besides, since AGA has a multifactorial etiology, adjunctive therapy such as counseling, cosmetic treatment, and hair transplanting may be added to maximize overall treatment. The emphasis on individual therapy is an expression of a growing recognition that patients can respond as individuals to the same treatment modalities and therefore encourage a more refined approach to the management of this chronic condition (Rossi et al., 2016) (Figure 2.2).

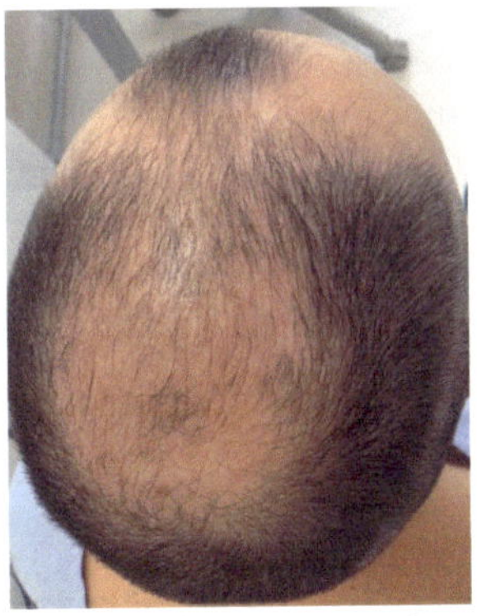

Figure 2.2. Male-pattern androgenetic alopecia. Hair loss from frontal, temporal, and central scalp areas.

Source: https://www.ncbi.nlm.nih.gov/books/NBK430924/figure/article-17526.image.f2/?report=objectonly.

2.1.2. Telogen Effluvium

Telogen effluvium (TE) is a very frequent reason for hair loss, and it is essentially produced by excessive shedding of the hair. It occurs when a substantial number of hair follicles enter telogen early, thus leading to a reduced density of the hair. The etiology of TE is multifactorial and can range from psychological stress and physiological trauma to side effects of drugs. It is important for clinicians to know the diverse etiologies of TE since the identification of the causes is most important in the establishment of effective therapeutic interventions. Acute forms of TE resolve spontaneously, while chronic TE may require more comprehensive diagnostic tests and therapies in a bid to prevent prolonged hair loss and psychological trauma from appearance changes (Aqeel et al., 2020). Telogen effluvium diagnosis involves an exhaustive evaluation consisting of a complete patient history and physical exam with special focus on causative type and duration. Patients are asked in general about potential precipitating causes such as recent life stresses, illnesses, or endocrine abnormalities that could be useful in appreciating the timeline and extent of hair loss. Diagnostic tools such as hair wash tests and trichograms may assist in measuring hair loss and ascertaining hair and scalp health. Awareness of the timing of telogen effluvium is crucial as it may direct diagnosis as well as treatment planning (Karadag et al., 2017). With prudent patient evaluation, healthcare providers can differentiate TE from other causes of hair loss, a crucial step towards effective management. In terms of treatment, the management plan for telogen effluvium is to address the underlying condition and provide symptomatic therapy. Lifestyle modification, stress mitigation techniques, and dietary support are typical interventions in the form of basics. Pharmacologic drugs such as corticosteroids and minoxidil may be added based on certain clinical situations. New evidence documents new therapies like caffeine, niacinamide, and dimethicone aimed at enhancing scalp health and promoting hair regrowth (Aqeel et al., 2020). A significant amount of the management process is patient education about the natural history of TE, which may decrease anxiety and engender proper recovery expectations. By integrating a multidimensional approach to treatment, healthcare professionals can enhance outcomes and quality of life for the person suffering from this debilitating condition (Figure 2.3).

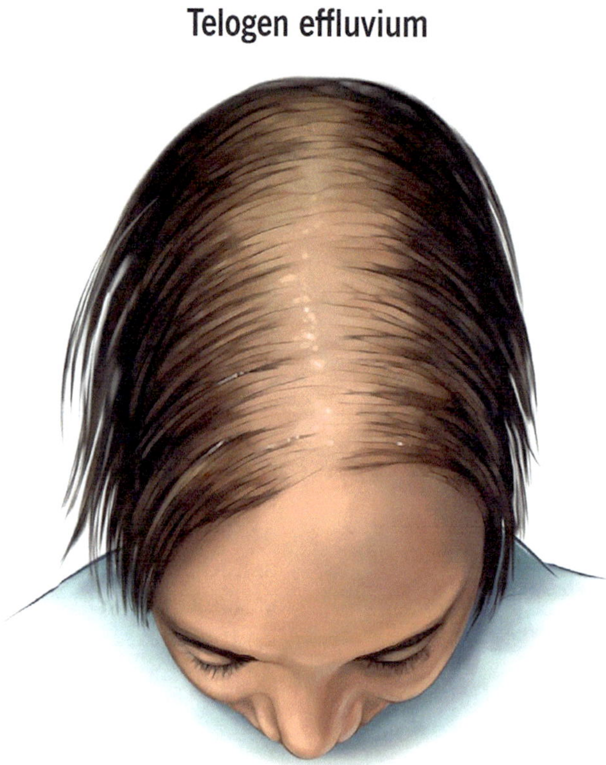

Figure 2.3. Telogen effluvium.

Source: https://my.clevelandclinic.org/-/scassets/images/org/health/articles/24486-telogen-effluvium.

2.1.3. Alopecia Areata

Alopecia areata (AA), an autoimmune condition, presents with acute loss of hair that can either be scattered in small patches or lead to complete baldness. Patients in question can suffer not only from bodily changes but also an enormous amount of psychological distress due to stigma and altered body image. The disease itself arises due to the immune system mistakenly attacking hair follicles, leading to secondary lymphocytic infiltrations around such structures. While its mechanism of action has become increasingly well understood, its etiology remains poorly characterized. Compounding this difficulty is the co-morbidity of AA with other autoimmune conditions, suggesting a complex relationship between genetics and the environment that culminates in predisposition to this hair loss condition (Butcher et al., 2019). The treatment of AA in the last decade has undergone a transition towards emphasizing the importance of being able to tailor it based on the extent of hair loss, as well as the unique needs of each patient. Topical corticosteroids are one of the first-line treatments, as they act to reduce inflammation within the hair follicles. However, these are unlikely to benefit all patients, particularly those with more diffuse patterns of hair loss. Recent research has generated new therapeutic strategies using Janus kinase inhibitors (JAKi) that have yielded promising results by selectively targeting certain inflammatory mechanisms shared among AA. The role of the JAK/STAT signaling pathways in hair follicle biology has it as a promising candidate for treatment, as its blockade can potentially reverse the autoimmune attack on hair follicles (Ghoreschi et al., 2019). Except for the medical procedures, counseling is an important function for individuals undergoing the emotional effects of AA. Sudden hair loss can be a cause of anxiety, depression, and social isolation in most cases. Multidisciplinary strategies, including counseling, support groups, and patient/family educational materials, treat these mental disorders. Tackling both the emotional and physical aspects of AA, doctors can now offer a better-rounded treatment regimen, and therefore improve the overall health. The continued research of the immunological etiology of AA will continue to allow for more focused interventions, thereby giving patients the best possible care options within the parameters of hair loss treatment (Butcher et al., 2019) (Figure 2.4).

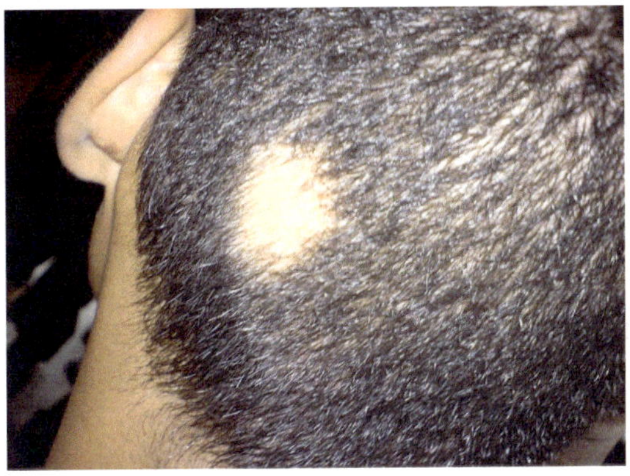

Figure 2.4. Alopecia areata seen on the back of the scalp.

Source: https://upload.wikimedia.org/wikipedia/commons/thumb/3/38/Allopecia_areata.JPG/1280px-Allopecia_areata.JPG.

Test Your Knowledge

1. What are the typical characteristics and symptoms of telogen effluvium, and what triggers this type of hair loss?
2. How does telogen effluvium differ from other types of hair loss in terms of the hair growth cycle, and what are some common triggers that lead to this condition?
3. What is the immune system's role in AA, and how does it lead to the sudden onset of hair loss, often in small, round patches?

2.2. Causes of Hair Loss

Learning Outcome

1. Describe the genetic factors causing hair loss
2. Explain how hormonal changes play a pivotal role in the manifestation of hair
3. Understand the contribution of environmental influences to hair loss

Hair loss is a complex disorder that could be caused by an assortment of biological and environmental factors. Its most prevalent etiology is androgenetic alopecia, also known as pattern baldness, in women and men. It is an inherited condition where there is a gradual hair thinning, most often linked with genetics and hormonal imbalances, particularly the effect of dihydrotestosterone (DHT). This hormone truncates the hair growth cycle and prevents the function of hair follicles to grow new hair. As the condition advances, individuals develop patches of thinning or even complete baldness, and hence the significance of early diagnosis coupled with appropriate treatments. Though genetics play a major role, other stimuli such as stress and endocrine disturbances may induce this type of hair loss, necessitating an adequate understanding of the causative factors for effective control. Nutritional deficiencies are another factor that could play a significant role in causing hair loss, apart from genetic susceptibility. Lack of essential nutrients such as iron, vitamin D, and proteins will stop the development of good hair and lead to hair shedding. For instance, iron deficiency, typically due to diet or health problems, can lead to telogen effluvium, which is reversible hair loss. This occurs when hair follicles skip the resting phase of the hair growth cycle prematurely. Also, protein deficiencies, such as keratin, which constitutes the structure of hair, may thin hair and accelerate loss. Correction of nutritional deficiencies through diet adjustment or supplements could be a basic process in not just preventing hair loss but also activating regrowth. Information regarding the nutritional aspect of hair health is crucial in patients with thinning hair since they may need to search and alter their diet to maximize outcomes. Additionally, various medical conditions and treatments induce hair loss, and it becomes difficult to diagnose. Autoimmune diseases such as AA result in acute hair loss due to the immune system attacking hair follicles mistakenly. In addition, systemic diseases like diabetes and endocrine disorders can disrupt the fine balance of hair growth. Treatment for the primary disease might involve modification of associated treatments to mitigate side effects in the form of alopecia. Diabetic patients, for example, have higher risks for idiopathic acute hearing loss that necessitates special care and customized treatment protocols that consider the patients' general health (Badiu et al., 2019). It is imperative for medical professionals to conduct thorough tests in a bid to find any such maternal health complications so that hair loss treatment can be thorough and effective. As with continuous research, awareness of such multifactorial etiology leads to more efficient diagnosis and treatment of hair loss, suggesting the use of a multidisciplinary approach in the treatment of such affected individuals.

2.2.1. Genetic Factors

The role of genetic factors in alopecia is pivotal, particularly in diseases such as male androgenetic alopecia (MAGA). This common condition of balding is characterized by an inherited element, manifest as a specific pattern of baldness and thinning. Investigations have established that MAGA is caused not only by genetic predisposition but also by hormonal effects, e.g., levels of DHT, on hair follicle susceptibility. The etiology of MAGA explains why some people lose hair at a younger age or with more severity than others. The genetic markers for MAGA have been researched intensively, resulting in findings that can help with early detection and individualized interventions, thus making it an essential and promising field of research in dermatology (Trilisnawati et al., 2021). Moreover, the impact of genetics is much more profound than balding alone, influencing the psychological and emotional condition of patients. Several studies have demonstrated that the experience of balding is most frequently linked with self-esteem as well as lifestyle impact in general, predominantly in younger populations. Patients increasingly experience significant shifts in their concept of themselves and dealing with society as balding progresses, creating a high demand for effective treatment options. Exhaustive understanding of the genetic aspect of baldness is necessary for strategizing interventions because it allows medical professionals to identify populations at risk and to promote preventive interventions. Besides enhancing the accuracy of diagnosis, knowledge of these genetic factors also allows for the development of successful treatment strategies intended to minimize the adverse effects of baldness on quality of life (Trilisnawati et al., 2021). Besides the traditional therapies such as topical minoxidil and oral finasteride, new therapeutic approaches are being designed every day with the help of breakthroughs in genetic research. For instance, agents that selectively inhibit mechanisms of hair follicle cycling and regeneration are being designed, which promise more personalized treatment approaches. Recent studies have indicated that awareness of a person's genetic background might lead to tailoring of treatment and hence, improved outcomes and patient satisfaction. Additionally, ongoing research on the genetics of alopecia may open doors to new modalities of intervention, including gene therapy and regenerative medicine modalities, a new frontier for the therapy of diseases like MAGA. Therefore, the discovery of the role of genetic factors not only shapes our understanding of hair loss but is also the introduction of a new era in the management of this disease (Figure 2.5).

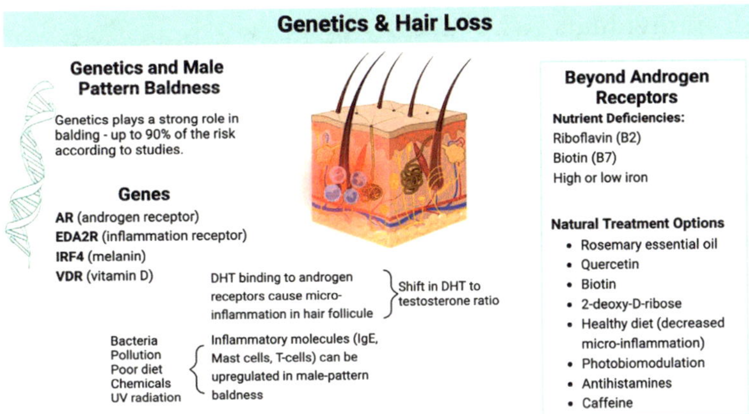

Figure 2.5. Genetics and hair loss.

Source: https://www.geneticlifehacks.com/wp-content/uploads/2023/06/Genetics-and-Hair-Loss.png.

2.2.2. Hormonal Changes

Hormonal changes are at the heart of the pathogenesis of alopecia, particularly in conditions such as androgenetic alopecia and endocrine dysfunction. Androgenetic alopecia, also referred to as male or female pattern baldness, is primarily stimulated by androgens, or the male hormones that can control hair follicle sensitivity. Along these lines, DHT, a potent derivative of testosterone, is the primary perpetrator that leads to miniaturization of hair follicles, which in turn leads to a progressive thinning of hair with time. The process demonstrates the entwined interplay between hormones and the regulation of hair growth, which is crucial for an understanding of different types of baldness. Furthermore, hormonal imbalances due to aging, pregnancy, menopause, and endocrine disorders can also become a cause of such conditions, leading to great psychological distress on the part of the afflicted people. Hormonal therapy for baldness cure, particularly for transgender individuals, has picked up significant pace in recent times. For instance, an individual on feminizing hormone treatment will be in a position to appreciate desired bodily changes like the development of breasts and a change in hair distribution by administering estrogens and antiandrogens that suppress the effect of androgens on the hair follicles (Arcelus et al., 2018). This approach addresses not only hair loss due to androgen dominance but also constitutes part of the general category of gender-affirming care. However, AFAB individuals who are considering masculinizing hormone therapy tend to experience increased facial and body hair growth according to the stimulating effects of the testosterones (Defreyne et al., 2019). Such knowledge about the effects of hormones is thus critical in managing patients to optimize both hair retention and overall well-being. Longitudinal studies also indicate that the psychological gains from appropriate hormonal treatments, such as improved mental health outcomes, are notable. Patients undergoing gender-affirming hormone therapy have been noted to suffer from high rates of depression and anxiety, which, coupled with physical alterations, enhance quality of life (Defreyne et al., 2019). It is also vital, however, to consider the dangers involved with these therapies, such as cardiovascular issues and changed fertility. Thus, doctors must approach from a multidisciplinary perspective to ensure full care that not only addresses the desired aesthetic outcomes but also the medical background of hormonal treatment. In this way, the hormonal variations can be adequately controlled within a broader plan for baldness treatment in diverse populations, necessitating ongoing discussion regarding health and wellness considerations (Figure 2.6).

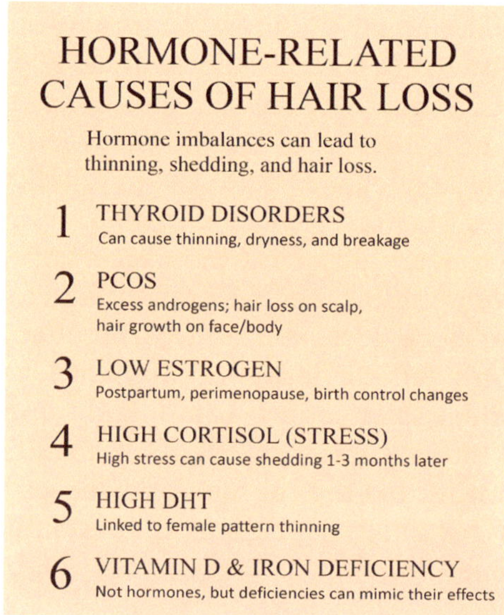

Figure 2.6. Hormone-related causes of hair loss.

Source: https://www.instagram.com/p/DInK0FSgBpU/.

2.2.3. Environmental Influences

Environmental factors contribute heavily to the multifactorial etiology of alopecia, intertwined with climate variables, environmental toxin exposure, and nutritional status. Chronic stressful environmental conditions, for instance, such as excessive heat or humidity, have been shown to disrupt the cycling of hair follicles. This can have the final consequence of hypertrichokinetic alopecia, or telogen effluvium. In addition, exposure to environmental pollutants, such as heavy metals or chemicals, may induce oxidative stress that is detrimental to the hair follicles. These types of pollutants can trigger inflammation and dysfunction in dermatological conditions and trigger or exacerbate hair loss conditions. Therefore, these factors must be taken into consideration when diagnosing as well as designing effective treatment strategies for patients who lose their hair, indicating the relevance of considering people's living conditions in therapeutic approaches. Moreover, some environmental aspects, such as diet, also play a significant role in hair well-being. Nutrient deficiency, especially vitamins and minerals that are required for hair development, can be attributed to dietary habits, which are also under the control of the environment. For instance, areas that don't have good access to healthy food can lead to a deficiency in proteins, iron, and essential fatty acids, leading to loss of hair. Moreover, the consumption of certain toxic plants or cereals, like toxic fescue in cattle that can affect physiological states, which can translate figuratively to human beings when talking about toxicity in diets. These factors in diets have been linked with alterations of hair thickness and texture, hence the importance of maintaining a balanced diet comprising vitamins and minerals to maintain healthy hair. Hence, rectification of nutritional deficiencies must form part of any therapy plan for the prevention of hair loss. Furthermore, psychosocial stressors, typically aggravated by environmental stressors, play an important part in hair loss. Stress may precipitate a hormonal imbalance that increases the predisposition to conditions such as AA or exacerbate chronic conditions of hair loss. Environmental circumstances, for example, living in highly stressful environments or experiencing sudden lifestyle changes, compel the victim to cope with baldness daily as a result of these stressors. For example, emotional distress brought about by socioeconomic uncertainty or relationship issues might lead to excessive levels of cortisol, which are detrimental to hair growth cycles. Moreover, chronic stress has been linked to systemic inflammation, which in turn drives hair follicle destruction. The link between hair loss and environmental stressors underlines the complexity of current treatments, the emphasis being on the priority of the numerous disciplinary treatment procedures encompassing psychological health alongside immediate medical interventions.

Test Your Knowledge

1. How do genetic factors contribute to hair loss, and what role do specific genes play in determining an individual's risk of baldness or thinning hair?
2. What hormonal changes, such as those related to pregnancy, menopause, or thyroid disorders, are commonly linked to hair loss?

2.3. Diagnosis of Hair Loss

Learning Outcome

1. Describe medical history assessment
2. Explain the importance of physical examination in the diagnosis of hair loss
3. Describe diagnostic tests and procedures

Diagnosis of hair loss involves a comprehensive examination that spans a patient's history, physical examination, and in certain instances, additional laboratory examination. A physician begins by questioning the pattern and mode of hair loss, symptoms accompanying hair loss, and possible underlying illnesses that could lead to the issue. This discussion is imperative since certain conditions like polycystic ovary syndrome (PCOS) can lead to loss of hair as part of other presentations like hirsutism and irregular periods, outlining a major aspect of diagnosis. Recognition of these associations illuminates the potential etiologies and guides more targeted treatment regimens.

Physical examination tends to include inspection of the scalp and hair density, which can show evidence for specific types of hair loss, e.g., androgenetic alopecia or telogen effluvium, to guide further investigation and treatment decisions. In a few cases, to clarify puzzling presentations of hair loss or rule out systemic illness, practitioners will prescribe laboratory studies, including blood tests to evaluate hormone levels, thyroid function tests, and iron studies. The role of endocrine disorders, especially in conditions like PCOS, is crucial because they can have a profound effect on hair growth and cycle patterns. Excessive androgen levels of PCOS, for instance, lead to hair loss and thinning in females, and treatment should be directed at correcting those imbalances (Bernier, 2012). The other etiologies, like nutrition deficiency, autoimmune diseases, and genetics, may also develop from these tests. In summary, thorough diagnostic workup is the foundation for revealing the pathogenic process of alopecia to enable treatment plans to be suited adequately based on the patient's specific requirement. Furthermore, scalp biopsy or trichoscopy can also be conducted for patients if the diagnosis remains unclear after initial evaluations. Scalp biopsy helps to distinguish between various forms of alopecia because it provides histological evidence of the integrity and position of the hair follicles. This method is particularly worthwhile when alopecia areata or other scarring alopecia is present, where the cosmetic significance is paramount. Trichoscopy is a harmless, non-invasive examination technique that yields graphical data regarding hair and scalp condition, allowing clinicians to identify follicular inflammation or hair shaft miniaturization typical of androgenetic alopecia or traction alopecia. Employing these diagnostic techniques, healthcare providers are able to specifically delineate causes of hair loss and create suitable intervention strategies. Diagnosis of hair loss, in general, requires a holistic approach integrating clinical presentation and patient history to optimize treatment outcomes and address underlying etiologies appropriately (Hussain, 2015) (Figure 2.7).

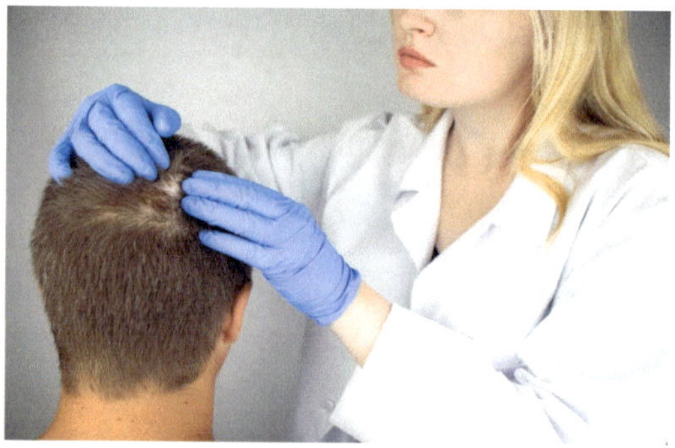

Figure 2.7. Hair loss diagnosis.

Source: https://upguys-images.s3.ca-central-1.amazonaws.com/prod/public/123326/conversions/hair-loss-diagnosis-thumb_retina.jpg.

2.3.1. Medical History Assessment

In the context of hair loss diagnosis and treatment planning, thorough medical history assessment remains a key foundation of efficacious intervention. Familiarity with a patient's complicated past, including previous medical illness, family history of hair loss, and medications they are currently taking, may provide insightful information regarding the etiology of their condition. For instance, hormonal imbalance due to endocrine diseases is typically responsible for causing alopecia and baldness. Information gathered from the medical history helps identify potential genetic and environmental factors contributing to baldness, and healthcare professionals can accordingly modify their diagnostic process and treatment plan. In addition, the psychological impact of alopecia is typically a function of extensive knowledge regarding a patient's psychiatric history as part of the history taking. Suffering on an emotional level about alopecia exacerbates the condition, thus rendering it a vicious cycle involving depression and anxiety symptoms. Studies indicate that alopecia patients have lowered self-esteem and social engagement. Therefore, the assessment of mental health not only aids in the formulation of a cohesive treatment plan, such as medical and psychiatric care but also highlights the importance of addressing the relationship between physical complaints and emotional state. As a result, the overall approach enables clinicians to facilitate a more effective recovery process in alopecia patients. Inclusion of gender identity and the corresponding medical considerations in the assessment is significant because newer evidence suggests differences in treatment requirements based on patients' gender identities. For instance, guidelines suggested by the Endocrine Society suggest that transgender individuals benefit from the offering of a multi-disciplinary course of treatment involving hormonal treatment to cause sought-after physical changes, which can be reflected in hair growth patterns as outcomes of such treatments. These subtleties underscore the need for personalized medical history assessment, taking into account gender identity and its impact on hormonal health. Ultimately, ensuring that all components of a patient's medical and psychological history are assessed enhances diagnosis accuracy and offers a pathway to effective, individualized treatment regimens for baldness, resulting in improved patient outcomes overall (Love et al., 2016; Arcelus et al., 2018) (Figure 2.8).

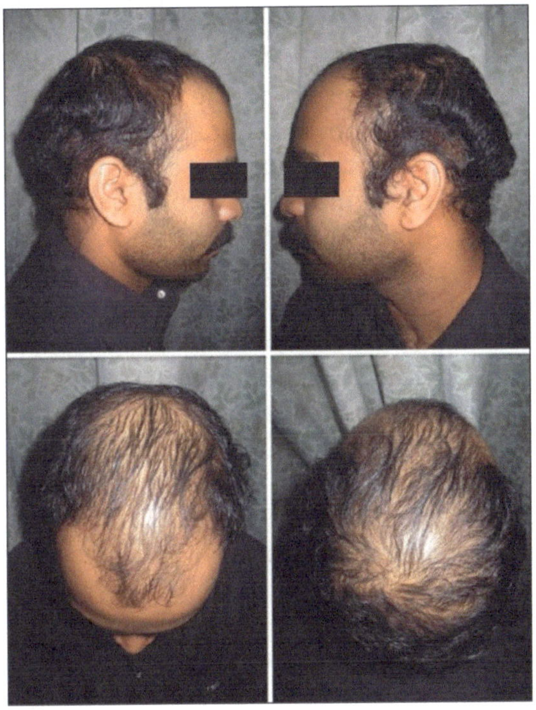

Figure 2.8. Androgenetic alopecia global assessment.

Source: https://www.researchgate.net/profile/Karalikkattil-Ashique/publication/51502289/figure/fig12/AS:203107855278130@1425436094834/Androgenetic-alopecia-global-assessment.png.

2.3.2. Physical Examination

The physical exam is a critical starting point for the diagnosis of alopecia since it provides valuable information regarding the details of the alopecia and the etiology. The clinician assesses the pattern, distribution, and severity of hair loss on the physical examination, and these can often provide clues to the underlying etiology. For instance, classic patterns such as androgenetic alopecia, the receding hairline and thinning crown may be suggestive of genetic predisposition. Patchy alopecia may suggest AA or tinea capitis, as opposed to the above illustration. Moreover, the presence of simultaneous clinical findings such as redness, scaling, or pustules on the scalp may aid in differentiating dermatologic conditions that cause alopecia. Hence, the full physical examination is a baseline that forms a bridge for the rest of the diagnostic tests and treatment interventions. Other than visual examination, certain diagnostic maneuvers can be incorporated into the physical examination to identify more accurately the etiology of hair loss. For example, the pull test is a rapid but diagnostic process where the clinician gently tugs on a small amount of hair is in a position to show over-shedding, indicative of telogen effluvium or traction alopecia. Further, even a physical exam of the nails and skin will be able to show signs of systemic disease or malnourishment, presenting as hair loss. As hair growth cycle and health are within the control of overall physiological states, any abnormality observed during this detailed examination can point to significant parameters that would need further investigation. This vigilance during the course of physical examination can lead to early intervention, which eventually leads to better patient outcomes. Patient history cannot be overruled in the context of physical examination for alopecia. Medical, family, and lifestyle history of a patient can reveal susceptibilities to diseases such as thyroid disease or autoimmune disease that may be a contributing factor to hair loss. In female patients, for instance, family history can be the deciding factor because predisposition for conditions such as androgenetic alopecia is a significant factor that depends on genetics. Lifestyle factors like stress, diet, and endocrine changes also must be addressed because they can play a role in exacerbating conditions leading to hair loss. Through integration of physical findings with detailed patient history, clinicians can formulate a complete representation of the patient's well-being. The holistically grounded process increases diagnostic precision and guides individualized treatment planning, ultimately improving hair loss management techniques (Dinh & Sinclair, 2007; Love et al., 2016) (Figure 2.9).

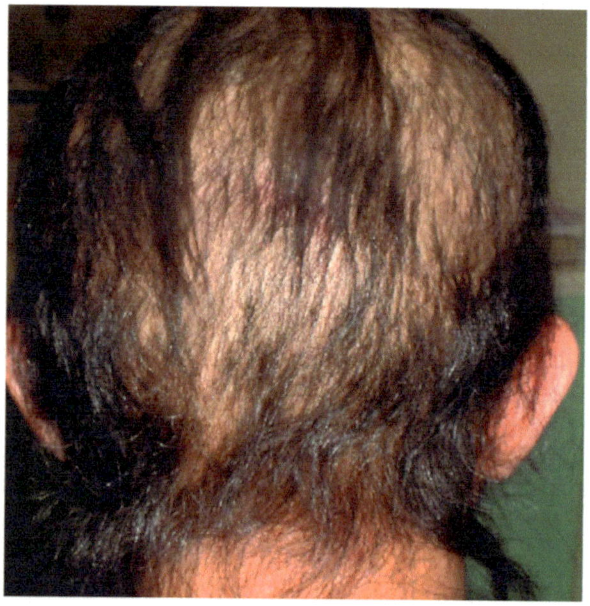

Figure 2.9. Physical examination showed a widespread and diffuse pattern of partial alopecia across all areas of the scalp.

Source: https://www.researchgate.net/profile/Khalid-Nagshabandi/publication/382031258/figure/fig1/AS:11431281270394703@1723043497229/Physical-examination-showed-a-widespread-and-diffuse-pattern-of-partial-alopecia-across.png.

2.3.3. Diagnostic Tests and Procedures

Diagnosis of hair loss entails a thorough assessment since the underlying causes may be diverse and multifactorial. Medical practitioners would normally start with a proper patient history and physical examination to determine whether there are any underlying medical conditions or lifestyle habits that may be causing thinning of the hair. Physical examination may also include a thorough evaluation of the pattern of hair growth and any accompanying symptoms, including itching or redness. Diagnostic tests tend to be utilized to determine the diagnosis; in the case of blood testing to determine hormone levels, iron deficiency, or thyroid condition. Scalp examination by dermoscopy can also determine some features of hair shafts and follicular conditions. Tests like the pull test can be utilized to measure how much hair loss has occurred and whether regrowth is possible, and these are of direct relevance to determining future treatment. In addition to further establishing a hair loss diagnosis, dermatologists can recommend a scalp biopsy. The test is particularly useful in differentiating among different types of alopecia, for example, androgenetic alopecia or autoimmune conditions such as AA. During a scalp biopsy, a sample of skin is removed and histologically examined. Results show hair follicle health status and whether or not there's inflammation or scarring, which can significantly influence treatment. In cases of suspected trichotillomania, psychiatric evaluation might be necessary since the condition is related to compulsive hair pulling and must be treated differently than other forms of balding. Through the integration of results from these inhomogeneous diagnostic tests, healthcare practitioners can create a tailored treatment plan that will consider both the somatic and psychological nature of hair loss (Arcelus et al., 2018). For some cases, patients with unexplained hair loss may be treated using advanced imaging technologies, such as high-resolution ultrasound or magnetic resonance imaging (MRI) of the scalp. These modalities enable noninvasive measurement of hair follicle density and scalp blood flow and provide information not evident on physical examination and laboratory testing. Further, procedures like measuring the tensile strength of hair or taking trichograms can better define the hair growth cycle and its aberrations. The findings of these tests are especially significant in determining the treatment regime, whether this is through pharmacological management, lifestyle modification, or surgery like hair transplantation. Overall, the blend of rigorous clinical assessment and cautious choice of investigational testing forms a solid foundation for management of alopecia for a variety of etiologies (Voth et al., 2009).

Test Your Knowledge

1. How does a thorough medical history assessment help identify potential underlying causes of hair loss, and what key factors are typically explored during this process?
2. What role does a physical examination play in diagnosing hair loss?

2.4. Treatment Options: Medical Interventions

Learning Outcome

1. Explain topical treatments
2. Describe oral medications
3. Focus on hormonal therapies for managing hair loss

Medical treatments for balding involve a variety of pharmacologic therapies aimed at treating a myriad of intrinsic etiologies. Most commonly prescribed perhaps, is minoxidil, an over-the-counter topical solution approved by the United States Food and Drug Administration (FDA). The medication is employed primarily for androgenetic alopecia, or baldness/male/female pattern baldness. Minoxidil enhances blood flow to the hair follicle, which stimulates hair growth and stops hair loss. Its efficacy is significantly enhanced when it is used continuously, with patients typically seeing observable effects within a few months. In addition, the oral prescription medication finasteride is also effective in inhibiting the conversion of testosterone to DHT, a hormone most commonly related to hair follicle loss. The combination of minoxidil and finasteride has been found to yield optimal effects, thus becoming an intriguing medical treatment for patients afflicted by baldness. In recent years, non-surgical forms of medical therapy such as low-level laser therapy (LLLT) have gained popularity in hair transplantation. LLLT is a procedure that employs some specific wavelengths of light to stimulate the follicles of hair to induce growth. LLLT is discovered to be effective and safe for the majority of forms of baldness, such as androgenetic alopecia and AA. Research has shown that LLLT can enhance thickness and hair density, hence a potential choice for those who require non-pharmacological therapies. In addition, numerous patients find the small side effects of this treatment preferable to conventional medications. Like all treatments, it is important for patients to undergo a detailed consultation with medical specialists to determine eligibility and possible results. The evolving landscape of medical therapies against baldness underscores the need for ongoing clinical research to strengthen guidelines and patient decisions. More recently, the advent of hormone therapy has also been recognized as a significant medical treatment for baldness, particularly in transgender individuals. Hormonal therapy, such as estrogen in trans women and testosterone in trans men, may cause physical changes that address issues of hair loss among them. Recent reviews indicate that feminizing hormone therapy can cause hair regrowth in some areas and alter facial and body hair distribution, which may enhance gender identity-related dysphoria. Besides, conversation regarding potential side effects, for instance, venous thromboembolism risk in women, is central in the decision-making process for initiating treatments. The multi-factorial etiology of hair loss coupled with the complexity of gender identity means that such interventions must be individualized, taking into account particular health needs and objectives, as the literature highlights (Love et al., 2016; Arcelus et al., 2018).

2.4.1. Topical Treatments (e.g., Minoxidil)

The science of hair loss therapy has developed a great deal, particularly with the introduction of topical medications such as minoxidil. First identified as an antihypertensive medication, minoxidil was discovered to stimulate hair growth, particularly in patients with androgenetic alopecia (AGA). Mechanism of action of minoxidil to cause hair re-growth is believed to be linked to vasodilation, which enhances blood supply to hair follicles and therefore causes an increase in the anagen phase of hair development. As AGA affects men and can induce serious psychological disturbance, the use of topical minoxidil is a highly attractive therapeutic option. However, such response can vary among subjects and necessitates an individual treatment regimen considering not only the degree of hair loss but also patient preference and medical history, as stipulated in treatment regimens for AGA (Rossi et al., 2016). The research highlights the necessity for initiating topical therapy early in the onset of baldness. Through studies, it is proven that minoxidil, which is approved by the FDA as well as the European Medicines Agency for AGA, must be used consistently for optimal results because cessation will lead to the loss of all hair growth achieved on treatment (Rossi et al., 2016). Clinical trials suggest that efficacy could be influenced by such variables as the concentration of minoxidil used, with more concentrated solutions being more effective. Notably, a systematic review of a range of non-surgical therapies made much of minoxidil's effectiveness, although it was noted that further studies are needed to inform its long-term safety and the side effects of long-term use. This lends support to the requirement of ongoing patient monitoring and an integrated approach to treating hair loss through topical treatments. Education and patient awareness are also key elements towards successful treatment with topical treatments like minoxidil. Patients will tend to observe initial shedding of hair, a condition likely to deter subsequent use; practitioners should therefore advise patients that this is a precursor to subsequent regrowth. Patient involvement in the discussion of realistic expectations and commitment for long-term use is fundamental to treatment compliance. Add-on topical minoxidil to a complete treatment plan, possibly including adjunct therapy such as oral finasteride or LLLT, may further enhance overall outcomes. Since hair loss is multifactorial, a multidisciplinary approach individualizing therapy to the patient's particular case will optimize the therapeutic potential of topical treatment like minoxidil (Figure 2.10).

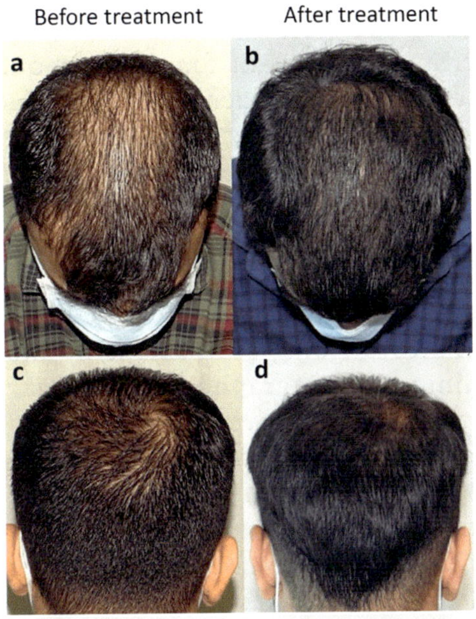

Figure 2.10. Clinical efficacy of 5% cetosomal minoxidil: a and c, before treatment; b and d, after treatment.

Source: https://www.researchgate.net/publication/374525966/figure/fig1/AS:11431281196420143@1696686833328/Clinical-efficacy-of-5-cetosomal-minoxidil-a-and-c-before-treatment-b-and-d-after.png.

2.4.2. Oral Medications (e.g., Finasteride)

Treatment of alopecia, androgenetic alopecia in particular, has extended to include many oral medications, one of the most common of which is finasteride. Finasteride is a 5-alpha-reductase inhibitor, which effectively slows down the conversion of testosterone to DHT, a hormone that causes miniaturization of hair follicles. By reducing DHT, finasteride can slow down alopecia and even cause hair growth in some cases. Its efficacy, although well documented to a large extent in men, has also provoked investigation into its potential therapeutic benefits in women, particularly those with female pattern hair loss. As a result of the progressive and chronic nature of hair loss, early intervention with oral drugs like finasteride is important for the best outcome (Dinh et al., 2007). Evidence suggests that oral antiandrogens like finasteride are a valuable therapeutic option in the treatment of alopecia in the medical setting. Therapeutic experience is that response varies significantly between patients, and 12 to 24 months is a typical time to measure efficacy. Such a delayed response necessitates ongoing assessment by methods like clinical photography and standardized severity scores. For women presenting with androgen-dependent hair loss, finasteride as a therapy is a consideration where there is close scrutiny of potential side effects and patient health profiles. While most of the patients have satisfactory results, it is important to consider that the therapeutic result is not uniform and thus some may seek other forms of treatment or complementary therapy to optimize their results (Dinh & Sinclair, 2007). Furthermore, the psychological impact of baldness necessitates an integrative approach to its management, over and above pharmacological intervention. Patients can be supplemented with services such as counseling and cosmetic treatment, which can adjust the emotional and social impact of hair loss. Therefore, the combination of oral drugs like finasteride with supportive therapy can potentially enhance overall treatment outcomes and patient satisfaction. The contribution of multidisciplinary treatment cannot be overstated, as it facilitates the customization of interventions according to clients' requirements, which not only improves the physiological effects of treatments but also the psychological elements of clients' health. Finally, oral drugs are a promising avenue of hair loss treatment, but an international strategy combining both pharmacologic and non-pharmacologic elements is the key for a holistic strategy towards management of this omnipresent disease (Dinh et al., 2007) (Figure 2.11).

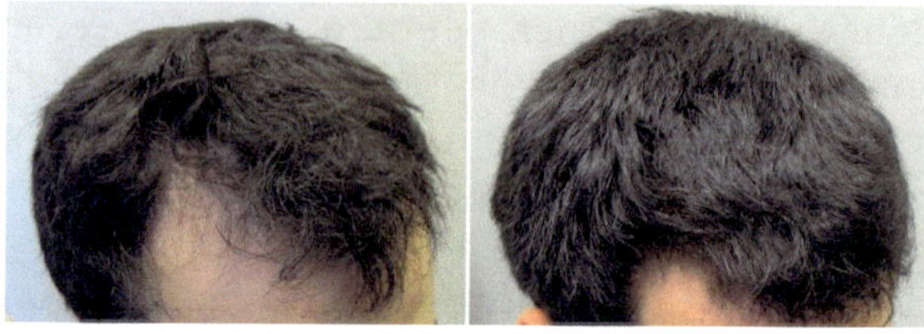

Figure 2.11. Finasteride: Before and after.

Source: https://innerbody.imgix.net/finasteride-and-minoxidil-before-and-after-photos-2-yr-2.jpeg?auto=format&ixlib=react-9.4.0&h=292&w=826.

2.4.3. Hormonal Therapies

Hormonal treatments are a significant advance in the management of alopecia, particularly androgenetic alopecia, which can be conveniently labeled as male pattern baldness. The causation of androgenetic alopecia is biological and involves genetic predisposition and hormonal dynamics, i.e., primarily androgens like DHT. The therapeutic window involves FDA-approved medications like finasteride, which intervenes through inhibition of the conversion of testosterone to DHT, thereby arresting hair loss. In addition, combination therapies like topical minoxidil have gained popularity due to their ability to induce hair regrowth. By the specific control of hormonal elements, they not only thwart further hair loss but also attempt to restore the thickness of the hair in the target population, thus improving their self-esteem and general well-being (Trilisnawati et al., 2021). Further research into hormone treatments also includes gender-affirming therapies in trans individuals who are going through hair loss due to hormonal fluctuations. For trans women, estrogen therapy with drugs that suppress androgens also contributes to the desired physical changes, e.g., lowering unwanted body and facial hairs, and this can also match the psychosocial presentation of gender. Transgender men, on the other hand, can be given testosterone treatment to induce virilization, and this also impacts hair patterning on the scalp. The problems arising from such therapy need multidisciplinary care, such as the coordination of endocrinologists and mental health professionals, to ensure complete treatment. The psychological benefits that patients derive from such therapy are significant, often bringing about decreased levels of depression and anxiety secondary to their gender dysphoria (Arcelus et al., 2018). While hormone therapies are encouraging, potential side effects have to be managed by patients and consented to. For instance, transgender patients undergoing hormone replacement therapy risk developing health complications like thromboembolism, cardiovascular disease, or sex steroid-related cancers, though these occurrences are rare. Such risks mean ongoing risk assessment and discussion of therapy and outcome. Moreover, human response diversity to hormonal therapy calls for individualized treatment modalities, particularly in special healthcare needs, such as nonbinary individuals. In the future, information regarding long-term effects and outcomes of these therapies will be crucial to ensure the optimization of hair loss treatment modalities so that it can improve patient satisfaction and enhance quality of life (Arcelus et al., 2018; Trilisnawati et al., 2021) (Figure 2.12).

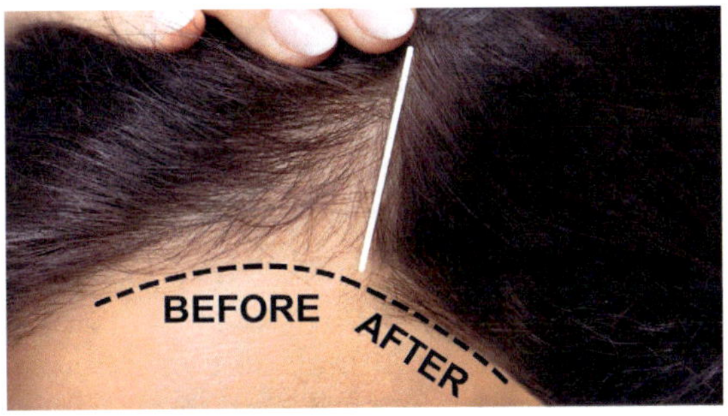

Figure 2.12. Result of hormone replacement therapy: before and after.

Source: https://hormonereplacementtherapyla.com/wp-content/uploads/2023/04/Natural-Alternatives-to-HRT-Can-They-Help-Prevent-Hair-Loss-Hormone-Replacement-Therapy.jpg.

Test Your Knowledge

1. How does minoxidil work as a topical treatment for hair loss, and what are the typical benefits and side effects associated with its use?
2. What is the mechanism of action of oral medications like finasteride in treating hair loss, and how effective is it in preventing further hair thinning or promoting regrowth?

2.5. Treatment Options: Surgical Procedures

Learning Outcome

1. Describe hair transplant techniques
2. Explain scalp reduction surgery
3. Understand the concept of follicular unit extraction (FUE)

Surgery has been an important remedy for patients with baldness, particularly where conservative treatment has been ineffective or inadequate. The most common surgical intervention is hair transplant surgical procedures, which harvest hair follicles from intensely growing regions and transplant them into balding or thinning scalps. Surgery has, over time, improved significantly due to advances in technology and surgical techniques, enabling more natural results. Follicular unit transplantation (FUT) and FUE are two procedures used most frequently. FUE, for instance, involves the removal of individual hair follicles, less scarring, and faster recovery, becoming a top favorite among several patients.

Surgical intervention can provide a one-and-done resolution to baldness problems, which not only enhances the physical but also the psychological and emotional well-being of patients. Another significant surgery in the treatment of hair loss is scalp reduction surgery. This consists of excising bald areas of the scalp, followed by closure and tightening of the surrounding hair-bearing skin. Scalp reduction is usually reserved for specific types of hair loss, such as androgenetic alopecia, in which patients have sufficient donor hair relative to the severity of baldness. While effective in covering obvious bald patches, the treatment is not for everyone and may be combined with hair transplantation for optimal results. Patient selection is also necessary, and psychological testing may be needed to determine realistic expectations. As demarcated in most studies, a combination of surgical treatments with psychiatric care can mirror change seen in other areas of medicine, such as growing recognition of transgender medical needs, including therapeutic techniques for improved quality of life among different groups (Defreyne et al., 2019). Lastly, advancements in procedures such as robotic-assisted hair restoration have provided an additional dimension to the surgical treatment of baldness. These newer systems enhance the precision of follicle extraction and implantation, producing more delicate and natural-looking results. Robotic systems can assess graft viability and density alone, further enhancing the transplants' outcome of surgery. Interestingly, even though intrusive procedures are constantly advancing, they still need to be done by experienced professionals to limit risks such as infection or poor aesthetic results. Furthermore, surgical alternatives must always be determined based on the individual's medical history and potential complications, as reported in trials of treatments like scalp cooling for associated scalp conditions. Ultimately, the integration of technology, patient-specific information, and skilled surgical technique emphasizes the evolving nature of hair loss therapy, as well as the significance of individualized, evidence-based practice.

2.5.1. Hair Transplant Techniques

The advancement of hair transplant techniques has significantly transformed the treatments for patients with baldness. FUE and FUT are the two prominent methods that dominate the market. FUE is the process of direct extraction of individual hair follicles from the donor area, which are then implanted into bald patches on the head. This method is favored for its minimally invasive character, which results in a shorter healing period and less visible scarring. FUT, on the other hand, involves the removal of a strip of donor's hair, which is dissected into follicular units and implanted. Each method has its own advantages and disadvantages, and patient selection and desired outcome are two important considerations in choosing the ideal method of proper hair restoration. The integration of new technologies in the conventional steps has increased efficiency and outcomes in hair transplantation. For instance, robotic technology can enhance the precision of follicle harvesting in FUE. Not only does this technology make the harvesting process more efficient, but it also reduces human error, resulting in improved graft survival. Also, these advancements have started the development of new methods for managing resultant complications, including scarring. In the treatment of conditions specific to different areas of the scalp, including the forehead, a step-by-step and algorithmic approach is most often practiced. Such a protocol typically includes intensive evaluation of single patient cases, thereby ensuring individualized plans for managing scarring, as documented in existing literature on scalp treatments (Bryant et al., 2017). Postoperative management contributes significantly to the success of hair transplant results, regardless of the technique employed. Patients must adhere to certain protocols to allow for optimal healing and hair growth, which generally involves staying out of physical activity and protecting the grafted area from direct sun exposure. Incorporation of follow-up observation allows health professionals to monitor progress and respond promptly if complications arise. Ensuring a good understanding of potential results and hair growth timelines is essential to offer realistic patient expectations. Lastly, the success of hair transplant surgeries is not just reliant on the practitioner's technical skill but also on the patient themselves in terms of following rigid postoperative directions, thus adopting a holistic attitude in solving baldness and being satisfied overall with the result of their treatment (Trilisnawati et al., 2021) (Figure 2.13).

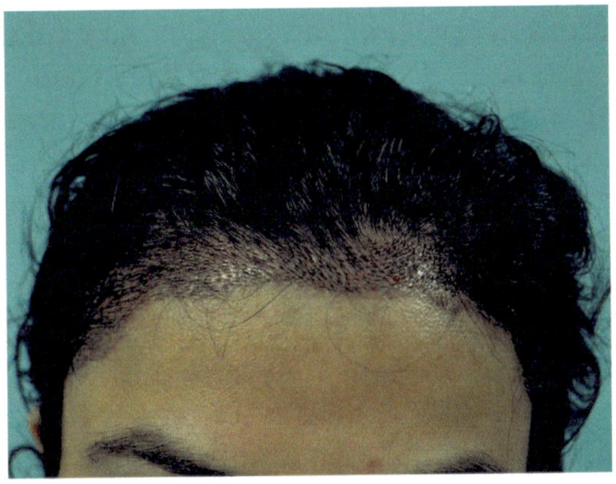

Figure 2.13. Hair transplant procedure of the frontal scalp.

Source: https://www.researchgate.net/publication/343167966/figure/fig4/AS:11431281173761360@1689045743369/Hair-transplant-procedure-of-the-frontal-scalp.png.

2.5.2. Scalp Reduction Surgery

Among all the various ways of treating baldness, scalp reduction surgery is one of the surgical processes that are specifically designed for individuals who have large bald areas. The surgical process involves the removal of the bald part of the scalp and expansion of the surrounding hair-bearing skin to cover the bald area and shrink the bald surface area. While scalp reduction does offer dramatic increases in hair density in the right patient, one must be aware that the procedure is not available to all individuals. Patient selection is crucial since only those patients with specific forms of balding, most notably those with androgenetic alopecia, will be disproportionately helped by such a procedure. Due to the danger of complications, including infection and scarring, thorough preoperative assessment must be done to determine the appropriateness of surgery for hair loss in a given case. Secondly, reduction surgery of the scalp is most successful as an adjunct to other hair replacement techniques. For instance, many practitioners favor simultaneous or follow-up hair transplantation to maximize the cosmetic outcome. This two-step approach allows the transplantation of follicular units within recipient sites of the residual hair-bearing scalp, thereby affecting the global fullness appearance as well as systematically targeting balding spots. Moreover, a mutualism of techniques requires a complete understanding of each patient's unique pathology, particularly in the case of androgenetic alopecia. Based on the statement, this disorder has its etiological foundation in genetics as well as hormones, which makes treatment on an individualized basis critical for success as well as longevity. If well integrated in an overall treatment plan, scalp reduction surgery plays a critical part in effectively treating baldness, especially when combined with medications such as minoxidil or finasteride that treat the underlying hormonal impacts on hair follicles (Rossi et al., 2016). Post-operative complications and scar maintenance also remain critical to the success of scalp reduction surgery. Because the forehead region presents unique challenges, effective scar management techniques are essential to minimize scarring as far as possible and facilitate ideal healing. Current best practices in treating surgical scars advocate a systematic, evidence-led approach tailored to each patient's specific needs (Bryant et al., 2017). Techniques can include the use of silicone sheets, laser treatment, and even steroid injections to minimize inflammation and maximize the cosmetic result of scars. For patients undergoing scalp reduction, attention to potential scarring serves not only their cosmetic interests but also helps their emotional and psychological well-being as they cope with baldness. Overall, a combined approach involving both surgical therapy and effective mechanisms of aftercare can raise patient satisfaction and the success of hair loss therapies considerably (Figure 2.14).

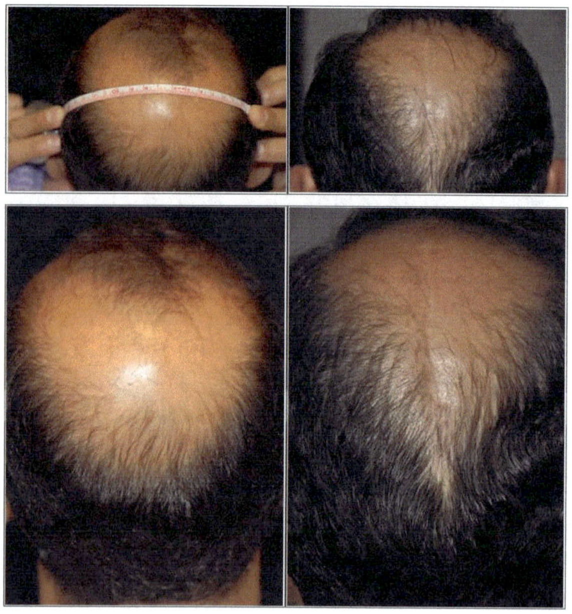

Figure 2.14. Scalp reduction hair transplant.

Source: https://www.plasticsurgery-sydney.com.au/wp-content/uploads/2013/12/scalp-reduction-hair-transplant-1.jpg.

2.5.3. Follicular Unit Extraction (FUE)

FUE is a breakthrough in hair restoration that offers a newer technique instead of the traditional hair transplantation procedure. FUE is a less-invasive procedure wherein hair follicles are removed individually from a donor site, usually located at the rear of the scalp, and implanted into areas that have been impacted by baldness or thinning. Unlike older strip harvesting methods, FUE does not leave a linear scar, which allows for less visible recovery and attracts patients who need a natural appearance following surgery. The procedural benefit and reduced downtime associated with FUE have made practitioners and patients more likely to select it as a viable option in the battle against baldness, making it possible to create novel diagnostic and treatment paradigms in alopecia treatment. The success of FUE in all forms of hair loss, such as androgenetic alopecia and cicatricial alopecia, accounts for its increasing popularity in clinical practice. It has been proven in studies that patients who undergo FUE have significant improvements in hair density and its restoration, which culminate in increased levels of satisfaction. As explained in available literature, the technicalities, such as the different extraction methods and the state of the received follicles, matter in order to generate successful outcomes. Moreover, the improvements in equipment and methods, such as the implementation of automated FUE machines, have been made to improve accuracy and efficiency in the extracting. With emphasis laid on the achievement of maximum hair growth, usually illustrated through comparison between before and after operation outcomes, FUE is a glowing embodiment of evolving treatment methods that are available for individuals who experience baldness. Although evolved, FUE is not immune to limitations. The success of the operation can be determined by numerous factors, including the patient's hair texture, the surgeon's competency, and post-operative care. Furthermore, while immediate results can be dramatic, long-term outcomes might be different, and there is a requirement for sound evaluation of patient expectations and potential for hair regrowth. Present evidence reflects that more research into the effectiveness of FUEs compared to other hair restoration technologies, such as platelet-rich plasma (PRP) treatments, would be beneficial. PRP has also shown potential in enhancing hair growth and density, and therefore, combined treatments could be even more valuable for patients. Since the understanding of hair loss continues to evolve, integrating diverse treatment modalities, e.g., FUE, into robust treatment plans could potentially maximize patient satisfaction and outcomes in the ever-growing field of hair restoration (Edaes & de Souza, 2023; Cyran et al., 2024) (Figure 2.15).

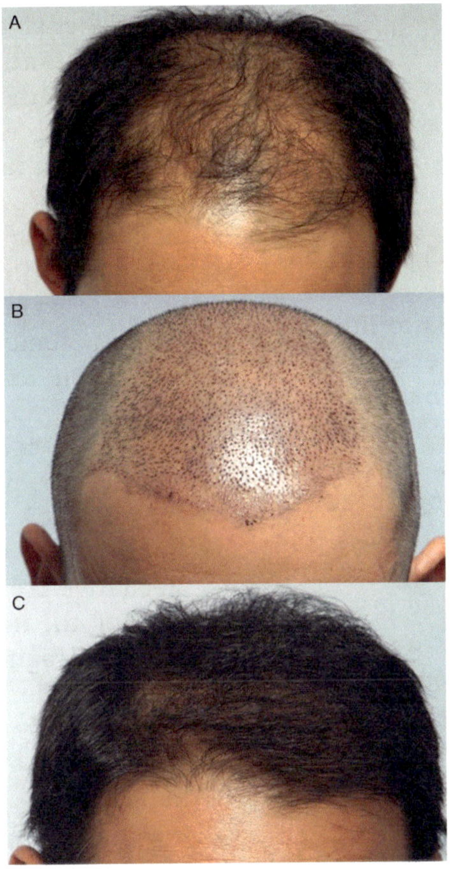

Figure 2.15. Good candidate patient for either follicular unit extraction (FUE) or the strip technique. A, Before transplant. B, Twenty-four hours after follicular unit extraction. C, Result a year after the intervention.

Source: https://www.researchgate.net/publication/317526710/figure/fig4/AS:974645427716097@1609384986766/Good-candidate-patient-for-either-follicular-unit-extraction-FUE-or-the-strip.jpg.

Test Your Knowledge

1. What are the different hair transplant techniques available, and how do they vary in terms of effectiveness, recovery time, and aesthetic results?
2. How does scalp reduction surgery work to treat hair loss?

2.6. Alternative and Complementary Therapies

Learning Outcome

1. Discuss the relationship between nutritional supplements and hair loss
2. Describe laser therapy for hair loss treatment
3. Explain herbal remedies

Alternative and complementary therapies have gained momentum in the last few years as individuals seek holistic remedies to illnesses, including baldness. These therapies encompass a host of practices such as herbal medicine, acupuncture, and nutrition supplements that aim to improve overall health rather than treating symptoms alone. Among these, the use of herbal supplements has a role to play in managing illnesses like AA, where immune dysregulation is the primary cause leading to baldness. Most of the patients have testified that adding these therapies to their regimen has led to an improvement in their general well-being, thus putting more importance on the holistic approach to the treatment of baldness. While scientific validation of these therapies is still in its infancy, users' reported perceptions require further investigation to define their mechanisms and efficacy more fully. More recent studies, including examination of the extracts of Agaricus blazei Murill (Sen-Sei-Ro), illustrate growing consumer interest among cancer patients for alternative therapies that would also likely be present among the alopecia afflicted. The patient questionnaires of cancer patients with this mushroom extract reported positive self-assessment of its impact on emotional as well as physical well-being (Clark et al., 2007). Although the perceived benefits were somewhat less specific than improvement for individual symptoms, they indicate a potential psychological effect that may be transferable to hair loss treatments. By enhancing overall quality of life and well-being, these therapies can eventually complement conventional treatments, giving patients a sense of control and satisfaction in the hair restoration process. This puts a value on practitioners honoring patients' wishes for more comprehensive care outside of conventional medical standards. The evidence supporting alternative therapies, though leaning toward anecdotal, shows extensive patient involvement and participation in non-pharmacological treatment. New treatment modalities, such as Janus kinase (JAK) inhibitors, are particularly highlighted in the treatment of AA because they represent a combination of conventional and complementary treatment methods to the assault on autoimmune processes to cause baldness (Brzozowska et al., 2025). The specialty, however, is complex, with treatments showing mixed outcomes in individual patients. This inconsistency emphasizes the need for rigorous clinical trials to validate the effectiveness of alternative treatments for managing hair loss. Through the implementation of a multi-faceted treatment regimen that includes both alternative and conventional methods, healthcare providers are potentially able to enhance results, revealing paths for personalized medicine directed toward the individual needs of every patient.

2.6.1. Nutritional Supplements

The relationship between hair loss and supplementation has gained substantial attention in the recent literature, reflecting heightened recognition of the implications of diet on hair health. Essential vitamins and minerals such as biotin, zinc, and iron are critical for the maintenance of hair follicle integrity. Deficiencies in these nutrients can lead to hair loss and thinning, necessitating the exploration of the utilization of supplements as a therapeutic intervention. For instance, biotin has been studied very intensely for its ability to fortify the keratin building, which is invaluable for promoting robust, healthy hair. Therefore, clients prefer using hair growth supplements containing these nutrients, anticipating they will reverse baldness. Insights into the biochemical processes by which these chemicals influence hair follicles may provide a scientific basis for their application in treatment protocols for patients experiencing baldness. Although there are possible advantages of nutritional supplements, they must be used cautiously and with good guidance. Not all supplements are identical; varying formulations, doses, and bioavailability can make a significant difference in their efficacy. The regulation of dietary supplements is also less rigorous than for drugs, and therefore, the quality can be greatly variable. Some supplements also contain increased concentrations of certain vitamins, which will lead to undesired side effects or toxicity. Therefore, it is necessary that individuals planning to utilize nutritional supplements for hair loss meet with health experts.

This will ensure that they are provided with specific guidance in accordance with their unique nutritional needs and medical circumstances. This method not only increases the chances of success in hair loss treatment but also lowers the risks associated with improper use of supplements. It can be further explored through inter-disciplinary research incorporating the fields of nutrition, dermatology, and pharmacology as a method of treatment for hair loss. Research studies may study diet habits that impact hair health, cross-pollinating ancient arts of healing and modern-day scientific knowledge. As an example, a study into the applications of omega-3 fatty acids and their anti-inflammatory properties presents a fascinating research field to explore, with a specific focus on diseases leading to hair loss. Addressing nutritional deficiencies holistically can contribute to increased success of hair loss treatments. Moreover, public education regarding the importance of balancing nutrition from sources such as (Masters & White, 1996; Banda-Nyirenda et al., 2025) can enable individuals to make educated food choices, potentially leading to enhanced hair loss control through nutritional therapy (Figure 2.16).

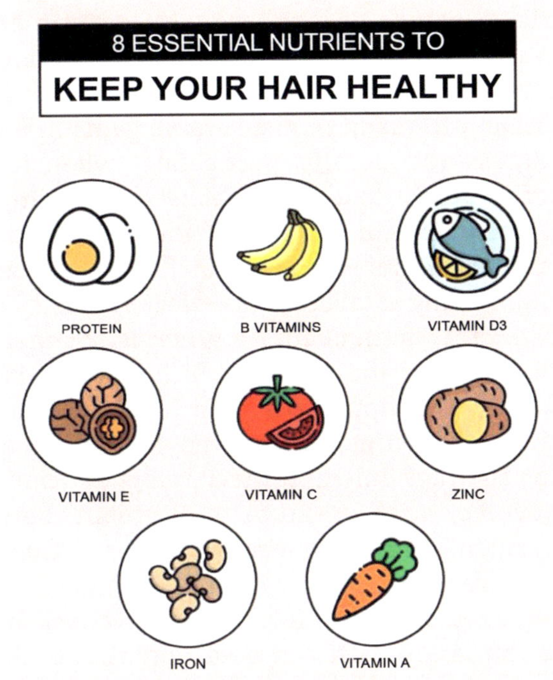
8 ESSENTIAL NUTRIENTS TO
KEEP YOUR HAIR HEALTHY
PROTEIN
B VITAMINS
VITAMIN D3
VITAMIN E
VITAMIN C
ZINC
IRON
VITAMIN A

Figure 2.16. Essential nutrients to keep your hair healthy.

Source: https://muskclinic.com/wp-content/uploads/2023/07/Must-have-nutrients.jpg.

2.6.2. Laser Therapy

The development of laser therapy has been a significant turn of affairs in the hair loss treatment scenario, particularly for androgenetic alopecia (AGA). AGA is the most frequent cause of hair loss and is characterized by continuous miniaturization of hair follicles with reduced hair density. Laser therapy attempts to stimulate hair follicles by way of specific wavelengths of light to enhance circulation and cellular metabolism in the scalp. The theory of this non-invasive treatment is based on the understanding that low-level laser light enhances the health of the follicles, potentially turning back the miniaturization process of the hair caused by AGA. Through encouraging blood flow to the follicles, laser therapy offers a promising addition to more traditional treatments, addressing the intricate nature of hair loss with genetic and hormonal factors (Rossi et al., 2016). Clinical studies have demonstrated the ability of laser treatment to result in measurable gains in hair thickness and density, particularly when it is incorporated into a comprehensive regimen of treatment. While traditional modalities such as topical minoxidil and oral finasteride are unequivocally established as effective, their use with laser treatment adds a synergistic benefit. Other studies indicate that individuals who utilize the equipment from a laser can have improved outcomes compared to individuals who use drugs only. Laser technology continues to evolve, with in-home equipment being convenient and easily accessible for patients. Therefore, laser treatment is increasingly being recognized not only for its effectiveness but also for safety, as it can be a potential option for patients seeking alternatives to conventional medications (Rossi et al., 2016). Furthermore, the use of laser therapy in combination with other treatments can maximize outcomes in patients suffering from hair loss. Other treatments like phototherapy have shown the potential to improve laser treatment effects by acting on inflammatory processes in the scalp. Research on the immunomodulatory effect of light treatment suggests that it may be beneficial in reversing causative conditions for hair loss, among which is chronic inflammation. For instance, localized diseases such as morphea, which have hair follicular implications, demonstrate how synergistic therapeutic approaches can lead to positive results. Through understanding and taking advantage of interfaces between adjunctive treatment methods, practitioners are better able to personalize interventions for patients, tailoring therapies to distinctive characteristics and needs in an attempt to maximize hair restoration (Figure 2.17).

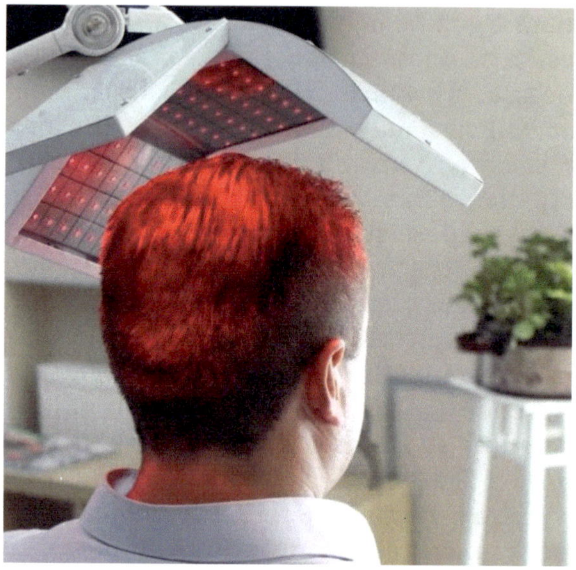

Figure 2.17. Laser therapy.

Source: https://vernonskinclinic.com/wp-content/uploads/2023/04/Untitled-design-25.png.

2.6.3. Herbal Remedies

Seeking effective treatment of baldness will more than likely drive the search to herbal treatments, which have gained much attention in the last decade. Historically, these natural treatments have been used in numerous cultures for their purported healing qualities, demonstrating a growing trend toward holistic application in modern medicine. Of the dozens of herbal remedies available, certain plants have been identified as potentially beneficial to the health of hair. For instance, Saw Palmetto and Ginseng products have been cited in studies for their inhibitory action on DHT formation, a key component in androgenetic alopecia. In addition, herbal therapies appeal to consumers because they have relatively lower side effect profiles compared to conventional medications, providing a viable alternative for individuals in need of milder, more natural remedies for hair thinning symptoms. Moreover, the integration of herbal treatments in the treatment regimen for hair loss can be made possible by understanding the conditions behind hair issues, for example, PCOS. PCOS has been noted to affect hair density and texture through hormonal imbalance, which will lead to excessive hair thinning and loss. Research on such products as OZiva® Plant Based HerBalance, which is a blend of herbal products, indicates potential benefits to both women with PCOS and those with accompanying hair loss. In research involving 153 patients with PCOS, there were significant improvements in the majority of the symptoms, including those related to hair care, after three months of supplementation with herbs. These findings infer that herbal therapies may not only serve as adjuncts to hair loss treatment but also as well-structured interventions that address the multi-dimensionality of diseases like PCOS, thus promoting overall well-being as well as hair growth. In light of evidence for herbal therapy, there is a need to investigate further to establish the efficacy and safety of herbal therapy for hair loss. While anecdotal evidence of success is abundant, it will be rigorous clinical trials that will validate therapeutic assertions regarding most herbal preparations. In addition, interactions with conventional therapies need to be carefully evaluated to prevent adverse effects. As popularity for natural products continues to grow, inclusion of herbal methodology in conventional treatment plans may offer patients a broader range of options. Lastly, embracing the benefits of herbal remedies, coupled with scientific discovery, can bring about better, patient-oriented solutions in addressing hair loss problems in the future.

Test Your Knowledge

1. How do nutritional supplements support hair health?
2. What is the role of laser therapy in treating hair loss, how does it work, and what are the potential benefits and limitations of using low-level laser devices for hair regrowth?

SUMMARY

Management of hair loss through correct diagnosis and autologous treatment is essential in improving the quality of life of patients with the condition. MAGA and AA are only two of the many etiologies of hair loss, each with its own therapeutic needs. MAGA, which is the most prevalent condition of hair loss among men, necessitates a full treatment course, comprising FDA-approved treatments such as minoxidil and finasteride, apart from newer treatments such as laser therapy and hair transplantation. The psychological effect of hair loss cannot be underestimated; patients experience lower self-esteem and social shame, requiring the application of total therapeutic regimens including physical rehabilitation and mental well-being, as evidenced by results outlined in Trilisnawati et al. (2021). Similarly, AA presents unique challenges, which are its autoimmune background and related psychosocial repercussions. Severe AA has severe impacts on patients as outlined in Bewley et al. (2024), whereby numerous patients suffer from anxiety, depression, and other comorbidities induced by the loss of hair. These should be addressed through a general treatment that takes into account the mental load of the condition, with information access and support systems being prioritized. Both medical and psychological treatments must work together in harmony for optimal success, underlining the importance of healthcare professionals addressing the complete scope of a patient's experience. Lastly, the context of hair loss treatment is changing, necessitating continued study and development in an effort to establish more efficient and personalized models of treatment. With an expanding understanding of hair loss disorders, fresh treatments are beginning to emerge, spurred on by advances in medical science and patient experience. It will be essential to integrate a holistic strategy that reunites proper hair restoration treatment with psychological counseling. Not only will this overall strategy seek to promote hair growth, but it will also attempt to promote greater overall patient satisfaction and well-being. As discussed, the impact of baldness extends beyond the physical, and as highlighted by the pressing need for quality and empathetic treatment modalities in clinical practice, supported by evidence from both (Trilisnawati et al., 2021; Bewley et al., 2024).

The investigation into hair loss includes a range of underlying causes and the related treatment plans, with the implication that this is a complex condition. Age, heredity, and the shift in hormonal balances are key factors that contribute to the development of hair loss, frequently leading to conditions in both men and women, such as androgenetic alopecia. It is an understanding of these determinants that is crucial to proper diagnosis, which will typically involve patient history, physical examination, and, where necessary, biopsy investigations to ascertain the exact nature of hair loss. This integrated approach enables clinicians to make educated suggestions for treatment, with interventions being especially individualized to the needs and situation of the person. Treatment approaches for baldness range from pharmacological treatments to surgical interventions, each for various alopecia types. Minoxidil and finasteride are, for instance, effective topical and oral medications, respectively, for the treatment of androgenetic alopecia. Furthermore, technological advancements in hair restoration surgeries, such as FUE and PRP therapy, offer patients other means of combating baldness. These therapies not only aim at restoring hair growth but also at improving patient satisfaction overall. Multidisciplinary management of baldness ensures that patients are given medical, psychological, and lifestyle management, highlighting the importance of dealing with both physical and psychological impacts of alopecia. Moreover, recent studies further clarify the intricacy of baldness and its treatment. Studies indicate that hormonal treatment can significantly benefit hair loss sufferers of conditions like PCOS, in which loss of hair is also a presenting symptom of underlying endocrine disease. As is discovered in studies investigating the endocrine basis of hair loss, an awareness of the hormonal context can lead to more effective treatment protocols when suffering from conditions like PCOS, in which insulin resistance is also a key component of symptomology. It is this integrated view that sheds light on the necessity of ongoing research and individualized treatment modalities that cater to the very specific hormonal and metabolic needs of the afflicted individuals, paving the way towards improved therapeutic outcomes in hair loss therapy (Bernier, 2012; Arcelus et al., 2018).

KEY TERMS FROM THIS CHAPTER

- Alopecia areata (AA)
- Androgen levels
- Baldness cure
- Co-morbidity
- Dermoscopy
- Dihydrotestosterone (DHT)
- Gender-affirming hormone therapy
- Hair follicles
- Hair transplantation
- Hormonal changes
- Alopecia clinical process
- Androgenetic alopecia
- Biotin
- Dermatological conditions
- Diagnosis accuracy
- Follicular unit transplantation (FUT)
- Hair follicle density
- Hair retention
- Holistic treatment regimens
- Hormonal imbalance

CRITICAL THINKING QUESTIONS

1. **What is the most common cause of hair loss in both men and women?**
   a. Alopecia areata
   b. Telogen effluvium
   c. Androgenetic alopecia
   d. Trichotillomania
2. **Which diagnostic test is most commonly used to evaluate hair loss and determine the stage of hair thinning?**
   a. Blood test for hormone levels
   b. Scalp biopsy
   c. Dermatoscopy
   d. Pull test
3. **Which of the following treatments is FDA-approved for promoting hair regrowth in androgenetic alopecia?**
   a. Minoxidil
   b. Vitamin D supplements
   c. Biotin
   d. Ketoconazole shampoo
4. **Which of the following conditions is characterized by patchy, sudden hair loss on the scalp or other areas of the body?**
   a. Telogen effluvium
   b. Alopecia areata
   c. Traction alopecia
   d. Male pattern baldness
5. **Which hair restoration procedure involves the removal of hair follicles from a part of the scalp and transplanting them to areas with thinning hair?**
   a. Platelet-rich plasma therapy (PRP)
   b. Follicular Unit Extraction (FUE)
   c. Laser hair therapy
   d. Hairpiece application

Short Answer Questions

1. What are the most common causes of hair loss in both men and women?
2. How is androgenetic alopecia diagnosed, and what are the hallmark features of this condition?
3. What are the main treatment options available for androgenetic alopecia, and how effective are they?
4. What is the mechanism of action of minoxidil in treating hair loss?
5. What are the potential side effects of finasteride, and which patient populations should avoid it?
6. How does a hair transplant procedure work, and what are the potential risks and benefits?
7. What are some lifestyle changes or home remedies that may help with hair loss prevention or treatment?

Answer to Critical Thinking Questions

1. (c); 2. (d); 3. (a); 4. (b); 5. (b)

REFERENCES

1. Abed, S. N., Al-Joufi, F. A., Asif, M., et al. (2022). Polycystic ovary syndrome: A disorder of reproductive age, its pathogenesis, and a discussion on the emerging role of herbal remedies. https://core.ac.uk/download/539616480.pdf (accessed on 11th June 2025).
2. Adelchi, C., D'Aguanno, V., De Vincentiis, M., et al. (2018). Audio-vestibular symptoms in systemic autoimmune diseases. https://core.ac.uk/download/188823057.pdf (accessed on 11th June 2025).
3. Annagur, A., Beck, B., Cronin, D., Dennett, D., et al. (2018). Polycystic ovary syndrome across the life span of women: A wellness-based integrative intervention. https://core.ac.uk/download/213088882.pdf (accessed on 11th June 2025).
4. Masters, David G. & White, C.L. (ed.), 1996. "**Detection and Treatment of Mineral Nutrition Problems in Grazing Sheep**," Monographs, Australian Centre for International Agricultural Research, number 118038.(accessed on 11th June 2025).
5. Rossi, A., Anzalone, A., Fortuna, M. C., Caro, G., Garelli, V., Pranteda, G., & Carlesimo, M. (2016). Multi-therapies in androgenetic alopecia: review and clinical experiences. *Dermatologic therapy*, *29*(6), 424–432. https://doi.org/10.1111/dth.12390(accessed on 11th June 2025).
6. Aqeel, R., Asghar, F., Farooque, U., et al. (2020). Telogen effluvium: A review of the literature. https://core.ac.uk/download/327082073.pdf (accessed on 11th June 2025).
7. Arcelus, J., Gooren, L., Klink, D., et al. (2018). Endocrinology of transgender medicine. https://core.ac.uk/download/162667742.pdf (accessed on 11th June 2025).
8. Ardeleanu, V., Constantin, V. D., Radaschin, D. S., et al. (2020). Laser therapy in superficial morphea lesions–Indications, limitations and therapeutic alternatives. https://core.ac.uk/download/304672910.pdf (accessed on 11th June 2025).
9. Badiu, D. C., Burcea-Dragomiroiu, G. T. A., Gherghiceanu, F., et al. (2019). Management options in the sudden hearing loss of a diabetic patient. https://core.ac.uk/download/216811037.pdf (accessed on 11th June 2025).
10. Banda-Nyirenda, D. & H^{n}sken, S.M.C. & Kaunda, W., 2009. "Impact of nutrition and fish supplementation on the response to anti retroviral therapy, Zambia: a literature review," Monographs, The WorldFish Center, number 38680, April.(accessed on 11th June 2025).
11. Barbara, M., Covelli, E., Filippi, C., et al. (2017). Intralabyrinthine vestibular schwannoma responsive to intratympanic gentamicin treatment. https://core.ac.uk/download/98349491.pdf (accessed on 11th June 2025).
12. Bernier, D. (2012). Polycystic ovary syndrome: Pathogenesis, health consequences, and treatment of PCOS in relation to insulin resistance. https://core.ac.uk/download/72048051.pdf (accessed on 11th June 2025).
13. Bewley, A., Blume-Peytavi, U., Chtourou, S., et al. (2024). Patient-reported burden of severe alopecia areata: First results from the multinational Alopecia Areata Unmet Need Survey. https://diposit.ub.edu/dspace/bitstream/2445/214052/1/CCID-445646-patient-reported-burden-of-severe-alopecia-areata--first-res.pdf (accessed on 11th June 2025).

14. Love, J. G., McKenzie, J. S., Nikokavoura, E. A., Broom, J., Rolland, C., & Johnston, K. L. (2016). The experiences of women with polycystic ovary syndrome on a very low-calorie diet. *International journal of women's health*, *8*, 299–310. https://doi.org/10.2147/IJWH.S100385 (accessed on 11th June 2025).
15. Bryant, L. M., Heffelfinger, R. N., & Sanan, A. (2017). Management of forehead scars. https://core.ac.uk/download/83049612.pdf (accessed on 11th June 2025).
16. Brzozowska, M., Furlepa, N., Jedlikowska, W., et al. (2025). Alopecia areata: Pathogenesis, current treatments, and future perspectives. https://core.ac.uk/download/646080111.pdf (accessed on 11th June 2025).
17. Butcher, J. P., Henriquez, F. L., Reid, S., et al. (2019). Alopecia areata: A multifactorial autoimmune condition. https://core.ac.uk/download/293865308.pdf (accessed on 11th June 2025).
18. Clark, J. A., Lee, I. P., & Talcott, J. A. (2007). Measuring perceived effects of drinking an extract of *Basidiomycetes Agaricus blazei Murill*: A survey of Japanese consumers with cancer. https://core.ac.uk/download/142041719.pdf (accessed on 11th June 2025).
19. Cyran, P., Jaroszyńska, A., Jaroszyński, F., et al. (2024). Platelet-rich plasma (PRP) in hair restoration treatments: A comprehensive review of existing literature. https://core.ac.uk/download/620863922.pdf (accessed on 11th June 2025).
20. de Souza, C. B., & Edaes, F. S. (2023). PRP in cicatricial alopecia: Unraveling mechanistic insights, assessing clinical efficacy, and paving future directions. https://core.ac.uk/download/652342091.pdf (accessed on 11th June 2025).
21. Defreyne, J., Iwamoto, S. J., Motmans, J., et al. (2019). Health considerations for transgender women and remaining unknowns: A narrative review. https://core.ac.uk/download/237010802.pdf (accessed on 11th June 2025).
22. Dinh, Q. Q., & Sinclair, R. (2007). Female pattern hair loss: current treatment concepts. *Clinical interventions in aging*, *2*(2), 189–199.(accessed on 11th June 2025).
23. Gadani, M. C., Tendulkar, N. S., & Upadhyay, R. (2024). Effectiveness of the OZiva® plant-based Her Balance supplement in the management of polycystic ovary syndrome: A real-world evidence study. https://core.ac.uk/download/620836195.pdf (accessed on 11th June 2025).
24. Ghoreschi, K., Meier, K., & Solimani, F. (2019). Emerging topical and systemic JAK inhibitors in dermatology. https://core.ac.uk/download/286097357.pdf (accessed on 11th June 2025).
25. Hussain, A. (2015). Polycystic ovary syndrome–Diagnosis and treatment. https://core.ac.uk/download/30820383.pdf (accessed on 11th June 2025).
26. Karadag, A. S., & Ozlu, E. (2017). Telogen effluvium. https://core.ac.uk/download/322430053.pdf (accessed on 11th June 2025).
27. Melin, S. A., Rugo, H. S., & Voigt, J. (2017). Scalp cooling with adjuvant/neoadjuvant chemotherapy for breast cancer and the risk of scalp metastases: Systematic review and meta-analysis. https://core.ac.uk/download/323062462.pdf (accessed on 11th June 2025).
28. Moreira, D. F. S. O. (2022). Non-surgical treatments for androgenetic alopecia in adult men: Indications, adverse effects and efficacy: Systematic review. https://core.ac.uk/download/554658806.pdf (accessed on 11th June 2025).

29. Ratton, A. (2018). Effects of toxic fescue exposure on vaginal microbial communities of crossbred beef cows. https://core.ac.uk/download/215461654.pdf (accessed on 11th June 2025).

30. Sharma, I. (2005). Psychosis in children: What is our present state of knowledge. https://core.ac.uk/download/pdf/86276.pdf (accessed on 11th June 2025).

31. Stell, A. J., Dorn, C. R., Hill, M., Bridges, J. P., Thornton, L. A., Michael, M., Cave, N., et al. (2017). Owner perceptions of their cat's quality of life when treated with a modified University of Wisconsin-Madison protocol for lymphoma. https://core.ac.uk/download/84659830.pdf (accessed on 11th June 2025).

32. Trilisnawati, D., Diba, S., Kurniawati, Y., Nugroho, S. A., Rusmawardiana, R., & Pamudji, R. (2021). Update Treatment of Male Androgenetic Alopecia. *Berkala Ilmu Kesehatan Kulit Dan Kelamin*, *33*(1), 63–71. https://doi.org/10.20473/bikk.V33.1.2021.63-71

33. (accessed on 11th June 2025).

34. Voth, D. (2009). *Trichotillomania: Educational Issues*. https://core.ac.uk/download/162575186.pdf (accessed on 11th June 2025).

HYPERPIGMENTATION AND MELASMA MANAGEMENT

3

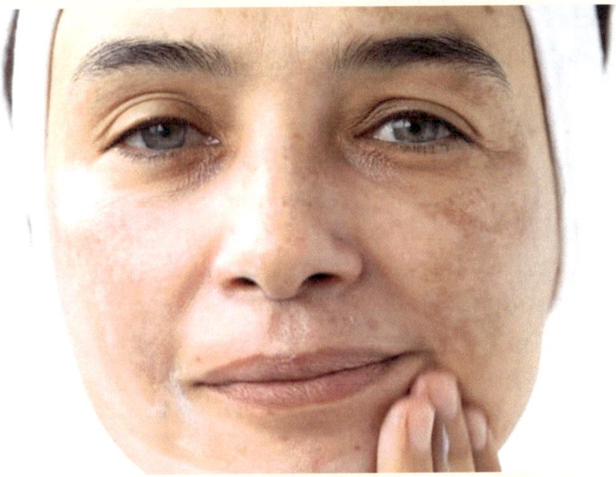

LEARNING OBJECTIVES

After studying this chapter, you will be able to:

1. Describe causes of hyperpigmentation
2. Discuss the forms of hyperpigmentation
3. Describe the process of diagnosing hyperpigmentation
4. Describe treatments used for hyperpigmentation
5. Emphasize lifestyle modifications to avoid it
6. Discuss the psychological impact of hyperpigmentation

Introduction

Melasma and hyperpigmentation are common skin diseases with overproduction of melanin, leading to skin coloration. The two diseases have a negative effect on the quality of life in the majority of individuals, particularly females. The prevalence of hyperpigmentation varies according to demographic characteristics of age, ethnic origin, and sun exposure and thus needs management in general. The severity of such disorders is not only due to their multi-factorial etiology but also to the varied response to treatment protocols. The effective treatment of hyperpigmentation involves a thorough understanding of the underlying mechanisms, including genetic predisposition, hormonal action, and environmental factors. With each discovery concerning these conditions, the importance of establishing targeted management strategies with a focus on efficacy and safety also increases. Recent advances in dermatologic research have introduced new therapeutic compounds with potential for the treatment of melasma and hyperpigmentation. Tranexamic acid (TXA), a plasmin inhibitor derived synthetically, originally as an anticoagulant for hemorrhage disorders, has been of specific interest because of its potential applications in dermatology. TXA has demonstrated anti-inflammatory properties and the ability to suppress tyrosinase activity, which is a critical enzyme in melanin synthesis. Research indicates that TXA is able to safely reduce hyperpigmentation and, for conditions like rosacea, inflammation too. Clinical research does, however, indicate limitations in the form of samples being too small, with uneven methodology, suggesting the need for more comprehensive research affirming its safety and efficacy in treating hyperpigmentation on a broader scale (Górska et al., 2025). In addition, sun exposure as a contributor to the aggravation of hyperpigmentation cannot be overestimated; it is linked with sunburn risk, photoaging, and skin cancer (Rodríguez-Luna et al., 2023). Recent studies highlight the role of UV light and visible light in the pathogenesis of the conditions. To counteract this, new photoprotection strategies are created to minimize these threats by employing natural extracts, for instance, Fernblock®, which is derived from the plant *Polypodium leucotomos*. This is proven to be effective and safe as a topical and oral treatment for a number of pigmentary disorders, including melasma. With advancing science, the combination of advanced treatments like TXA with intense photoprotection protocols offers an integrative approach to treating melasma and hyperpigmentation and reintegrating patients into a healthy regimen of skincare.

Definition of Hyperpigmentation

Hyperpigmentation is the name given to the darkening of specific skin areas due to overproduction of melanin, the pigment in the skin. It manifests as age spots, sunspots, and melasma, each with its own features and reasons. The condition may be caused by various reasons, like prolonged sun exposure, hormonal imbalances, and some medications. Ideally, hyperpigmentation could suggest a latent medical issue or response to environmental stressors, underscoring the significance of understanding its etiology. Identification of such different stimuli is crucial in formulating effective management since the cause goes a long way in determining treatment outcomes, calling for differentiation between types of hyperpigmentation to justify appropriate therapeutic interventions. Melasma, a specific form of hyperpigmentation, is most frequently observed in women and appears as symmetrical brown or gray-brown macules on the face. Melasma is frequently linked with hormonal factors, such as those of pregnancy or oral contraceptive use, and sun exposure. The physiology of melasma is complex and is founded upon the interaction between hormones and melanocytes – melanin-producing cells. Because melasma is so often refractory to therapy, treating the disorder poses numerous challenges to dermatologists. Various modalities, including topical therapy and laser therapy, are employed to treat the disorder, but relapse of melasma highlights the need for increased research on the pathogenesis of melasma and optimal treatment protocols. The recognition of melasma not only enhances the comprehension of hyperpigmentation as a whole but also directs clinical practice towards effective patient care and outcomes (Abadie et al., 2024). Hyperpigmentation and its variants, such as melasma, are not simply comprehended by being distinguished based on their visual characteristics; instead, comprehension of the biology of melanocyte function and the broader implications of pigmentary diseases is encompassed. There are recent findings that have given insights into critical aspects of melanocyte biology mechanisms, opening new possibilities for innovative treatment strategies. For instance, progress in the fields of immunotherapy and genomics indicates promising avenues for targeted therapies, which may offer better control of hyperpigmentation disorders. Furthermore, holistic care of the patient necessitates an accounting for the psychological impact of hyperpigmentation because skin appearance contributes significantly to one's self-esteem. Thus, not only does optimizing results in patients with hyperpigmentation rest on medical therapies, but also encourages extended understanding of the the quality of life consequences (Birlea et al., 2018) (Figure 3.1).

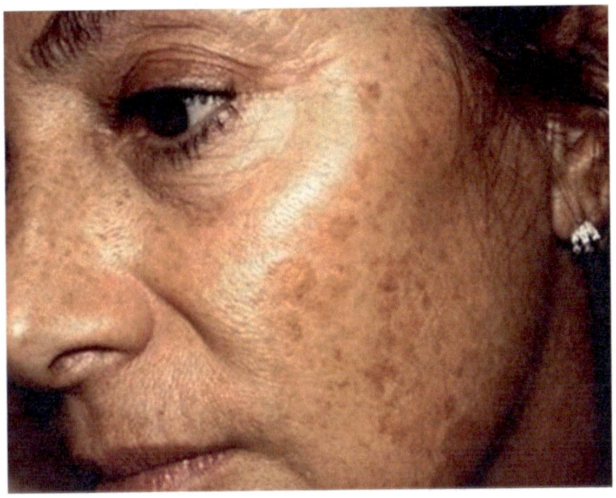

Figure 3.1. Facial hyperpigmentation with uneven skin tone and dark patches.

Source: https://www.drleah.co.uk/blog/image.axd?picture=/hyper-pigmentation.jpg.

Overview of Melasma

Melasma is a form of hyperpigmentation that appears as brown or gray-brown spots on the skin, usually on the face. Melasma is unequivocally more prevalent in women, particularly of childbearing age, suggesting a very strong role of hormonal factors and such hormones as estrogen and progesterone. The pathophysiology of melasma includes enhanced melanin production based on abnormal melanocyte proliferation, the cells that produce pigment. Environmental factors like exposure to UV radiation, which is known to worsen melasma, also make an essential contribution towards its onset. Not merely physically does melasma change the appearance of an individual, but it also can cause very strong psychological impacts, impacting self-esteem and quality of life, as evidenced by studies reporting the condition's association with heightened distress in individuals with melasma (Rodríguez-Luna et al., 2023). Treatment for melasma is often multifaceted in nature, involving both topical treatments and lifestyle modification. Topical treatments like hydroquinone, tretinoin, and corticosteroids attempt to reduce pigmentation by inhibiting melanin synthesis. Recent trends in dermatological research now point towards the inclusion of natural constituents that offer photoprotection along with helping to alleviate the ill effects of sun exposure, which is a requirement in melasma control. Fernblock®, for instance, a Polypodium leucotomos extract from a fern, has shown immense promise in offering both topical and oral photoprotection. This innovation opens up new avenues for treatment strategies that combine traditional treatments with natural agents, which can provide improved patient outcomes in melasma management while ensuring safety (Rodríguez-Luna et al., 2023). Preventive measures are also paramount when managing melasma, and the priority is sun protection. Because sun exposure can trigger the development and aggravation of melasma, adherence to regular broad-spectrum sunscreen application is vital. All patients should be encouraged to adopt a complete photoprotection regimen, such as the use of protective gear and sun avoidance during the peak sun hours. Patient education about the pathophysiology of melasma and sun avoidance can help empower patients to take control of their skin care regimens. Studies have revealed that patients who are actively involved in managing their skin condition, such as those with higher knowledge about hyperpigmentation, enjoy better health-related quality of life (Buainain et al., 2016). The integration of successful therapy and fastidious sun protection is the foundation for an overall approach to the therapy of melasma, which is promising for most victims (Figure 3.2).

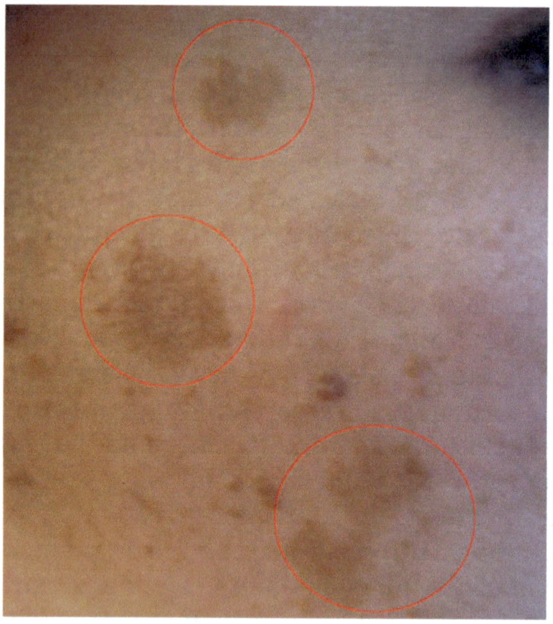

Figure 3.2. Melasma on the face.

Source: https://upload.wikimedia.org/wikipedia/commons/2/27/Melasmablemish.jpg.

Importance of Management Strategies

Successful management interventions are needed in the treatment of hyperpigmentation and melasma because they treat not just the physical presentation but also stem the psychosocial effects of such skin presentation. It has been proven that facial hyperpigmentation, which usually presents as dark patches, is not a cosmetic concern but can be a significant cause of emotional distress , such as depression and frustration, adversely affecting quality of life and self-esteem (Górska et al., 2025). By embracing an integrated management approach, dermatologists can offer individualized treatments that address the physical and psychological aspects of hyperpigmentation. Such an integrated management system not only enhances the patient outcome but also generates a supportive atmosphere that boosts individuals' confidence in actively engaging with their treatment process. The addition of innovative agents like tranexamic acid (TXA) to treatment protocols underscores the imperative of evidence-based management in dermatology (Górska et al., 2025). The effectiveness of TXA in the treatment of hyperpigmentation is a function of its ability to suppress the enzyme tyrosinase, which is involved in the production of melanin. Moreover, TXA's anti-inflammatory property positions it squarely as a choice for patients whose hyperpigmentation is a result of inflammatory-prone conditions. With the emphasis on evidence-based therapy, practitioners can make sure that their management strategies remain constantly effective, goal-focused, and aligned with the latest developments in dermatological science. This ongoing emphasis on exploring newer treatment options allows practitioners to adjust their strategy, leading to a better overall therapeutic field for those with melasma and hyperpigmentation. Inclusion of complementary modalities, such as lifestyle alterations and pharmacotherapies is another part of successful management strategies. Patients can benefit from lifestyle modifications that include sun protection measures and the use of topical agents with minimal side effects. As noted, certain treatments for facial hyperpigmentation can lead to adverse effects, prompting a shift toward plant-based alternatives that promise efficacy with fewer complications (Parveen et al., 2019). Empathy for the multifaceted nature of hyperpigmentation allows clinicians to develop care plans that not only result in maximal clinical outcomes but also match patients' desires for safe, effective, and less invasive procedures. Ultimately, these plans develop an integrative model of care centered on patient health and satisfaction.

3.1. Causes of Hyperpigmentation

Learning Outcome

1. Explain how sun exposure plays a crucial role in the development of hyperpigmentation and melasma
2. Understand the role of hormonal changes in the development and exacerbation of hyperpigmentation and melasma
3. Understand the pathophysiology of skin injuries and inflammation

Hyperpigmentation is a better-known condition, resulting from overproduction of melanin in the skin and appearing in various forms , such as freckles, age spots, and melasma. The primary cause of hyperpigmentation is increased activity of melanocytes, the cells responsible for the production of melanin. Causes of heightened activity are exposure to the UV radiation that triggers a protective reaction in the skin. In addition to environmental factors, hormonal imbalances , such as those that can occur during pregnancy or with the use of oral contraceptives, can exacerbate melasma, a type of hyperpigmentation. It is essential to know these triggers to develop effective treatment plans because addressing the causative factor itself can significantly improve the condition of those suffering from it. Genetic susceptibility can also play a significant role in determining the probability of individuals developing hyperpigmentation. Specific skin types, particularly Fitzpatrick skin types III to VI, are more susceptible to overproduction of melanin due to their inborn levels of pigmentation. The skin reacts to environmental stress factors due to genetic influences, which enhances the susceptibility to hyperpigmentation, as was concluded by research. Additionally, the role that is played by endocrine components cannot be overlooked; for instance, conditions , such as Addison's disease or hormone treatment can induce improved melanogenesis. Therefore, patients and healthcare workers alike need to realize the complex interplay between environmental and genetic components to create particular treatment plans for hyperpigmentation. More so, habits in lifestyle play a significant role in the development of hyperpigmentation, including dietary patterns and skin care. For example, excessive exposure to sunlight not only leads to initial pigment formation but also induces exacerbation of existing pigment disorders. Certain medications, e.g., anti-seizure or psychotropic drugs, are implicated in drug-induced hyperpigmentation and thus necessitate careful medication control.

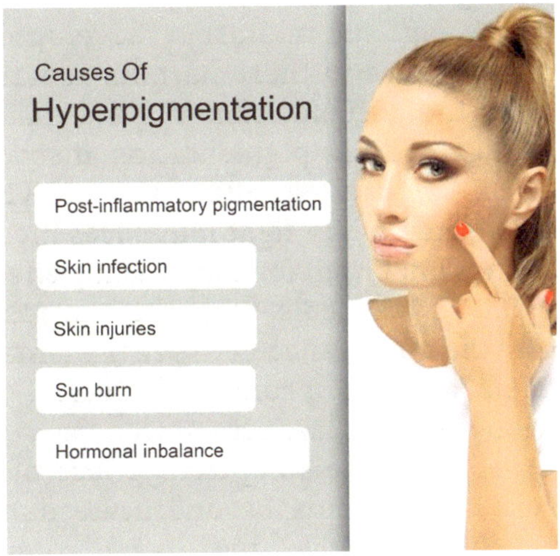

Figure 3.3. Causes of hyperpigmentation.

Source: https://blog.skinqure.in/wp-content/uploads/2023/04/Common-Triggers-for-Melasma-1.jpg.

Furthermore, exposure to inflammatory substances or excoriative skin conditions may induce post-inflammatory hyperpigmentation (PIH) and make treatment complex. Thus, an integrative treatment approach with consideration of personal lifestyle factors, besides therapeutic interventions like brightening creams and chemical peels, is justified in treating hyperpigmentation successfully, as suggested in respective literature (Khoo & Halim,2016; Camargo et al., 2021) (Figure 3.3).

3.1.1. Sun Exposure and UV Radiation

Sunlight is of primary concern to the formation of melasma and hyperpigmentation, two conditions that are characterized by hyperproduction of melanin. Sunlight ultraviolet rays are a known precipitant for these conditions that induce stimulation of melanocytes, leading to irregular pigmentation. There are studies that indicate both UVA and UVB radiations to be responsible for skin damage, with the UVA rays penetrating deeper into the skin and resulting in photoaging and melasma development. Chronic exposure to these harmful radiations results in the accumulation of gene damage, further aggravating pigmentation disorders. Consequently, understanding the individual pathways whereby UV light influences melanin formation is important for constructing effective management protocols with the purpose of reducing the appearance of hyperpigmentation and melasma and promoting overall skin condition and appearance. Moreover, recent studies identify the long-term effect of sun exposure that extends beyond acute damage to the skin. Even when the UV radiation has ceased, continuous DNA damage continues to affect skin cells, thereby complicating the treatment of melasma and hyperpigmentation. The interplay between solar radiation and skin response necessitates a thorough understanding of preventive measures against reversing pigmentation disorders. Practices , such as application of broad-spectrum sunscreens, application of protective clothing, and avoidance of sunlight are important in shielding the skin from UV-induced complications. Current advancements also allude to the possibility of natural photoprotective agents, such as Fernblock®, having demonstrated efficacy in clinical practice. These advancements are central to healthcare providers and patients who wish to more effectively manage conditions like hyperpigmentation, highlighting the importance of prudent photoprotection measures. Further, the impact of cosmetic treatments on hyperpigmentation conditions like Berloque dermatitis highlights the importance of informed sun exposure behavior. Cosmetics containing furocoumarins can interact negatively with exposure to UV light, causing further hyperpigmentation of photo-exposed skin. These interactions document the complexity of pigmentation disorders because they potentially worsen conditions associated with sun exposure. Although dermatologists endorse protection from the sun, they also need to educate patients regarding the special risks posed by photosensitizing cosmetic ingredients. Further research is needed to both establish interactions between products and UV exposure and to develop preventative and treatment regimens appropriate for these. By integrating these into a single management plan, patients suffering from hyperpigmentation and melasma can improve their epidermal health without having to relinquish possible psychological impacts associated with these quantifiable conditions (Figure 3.4).

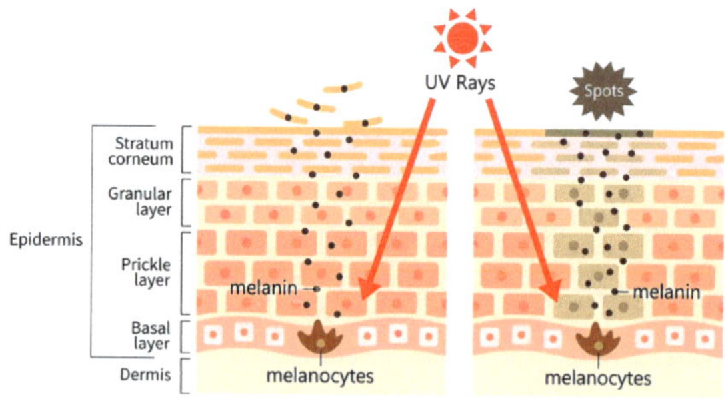

Figure 3.4. UV radiation for hyperpigmentation.

Source: https://thumbs.dreamstime.com/z/ultraviolet-light-can-cause-pigmentation-to-skin-diagram-human-skin-cell-isolated-white-background-sun-s-uv-radiation-270161207.jpg.

3.1.2. Hormonal Changes

Hormonal variations play a major role in the etiology and exacerbation of melasma and hyperpigmentation, particularly among women in their childbearing years. Upsurges and declines in estrogen and progesterone, commonly observed with pregnancy, hormonal contraceptives, or hormone replacement therapies, are known to stimulate the overproduction of melanin within the skin. This condition is caused by an upregulation of melanocyte activity as a result of multiple hormones binding to their respective receptors in the skin surface. Hence, patients with propensities towards melasma will experience dramatic pigment changes, particularly of sun-exposed areas of the skin. An understanding of the intricate interplay between hormones and skin pigmentation is crucial in the tailoring of effective treatment modalities that not only abate the hyperpigmentation process but also its hormonal triggers. In examining the impact of hormonal change on melasma, it is critical to examine the impact of inflammation. The relationship between inflammatory processes and hormonal change can enhance the impact of underlying skin conditions so that hyperpigmentation becomes a more common occurrence. For instance, hormonal fluctuation can cause an increased sensitivity to ultraviolet (UV) radiation, whose effect on melasma has been discovered to stimulate further melanocyte function. Additionally, pathologies , such as polycystic ovary syndrome (PCOS) can also elevate androgens, causing heightened skin pigmentation in vulnerable patients. The multifaceted role of hormonal influence provides a rationale for dermatological intervention that continues to be sensitive to these changes in endocrine dynamics, thereby enabling an integrated treatment of melasma and hyperpigmentation in patients. The therapeutic modalities for the treatment of hyperpigmentation caused by hormonal influences are gaining wider acceptance in dermatology. New treatments, , such as TXA, have proven effective in reducing the effects of melasma brought about by hormonal changes. TXA possesses the ability to inhibit melanin production and reduce inflammation, thereby effectively countering one of the key driving forces behind this skin condition. Also, topical photoprotective agent application and oral use, for example, Fernblock®, can deliver complementary benefits in terms of managing hyperpigmentation by limiting the exposure of the skin to UV and visible light, which have a propensity to exacerbate hormonal-induced pigmentation (Rodríguez-Luna et al., 2023). Complementary modalities highlight the importance of an integrative approach to the management of melasma, balancing hormonal treatment protocols with effective dermatological therapy (Górska et al., 2025).

3.1.3. Skin Injuries and Inflammation

It is crucial to know skin injury pathophysiology and inflammation in a bid to manage diseases like melasma and hyperpigmentation. Skin injury may be caused by various factors, , such as physical trauma, inflammatory response, or underlying illness. In case of skin injury, the body elicits an inflammatory cascade, leading to increased melanin production as a compensatory mechanism. This excess production commonly manifests as hyperpigmentation, particularly in darker skin types that are generally more susceptible to post-inflammatory pigmentation. Therefore, it is crucial to have an appreciation of the relationship between skin injury and inflammation when designing effective treatments for hyperpigmentation disorders. With the role of inflammation playing a part in pigmentary change, treatments that target both the injury to the skin and subsequent inflammatory responses are pivotal in the management of conditions like melasma and PIH. The use of TXA therapeutically is a testament to an innovative approach to healing skin wounds caused by hyperpigmentation. TXA is a synthetic plasmin inhibitor, originally used for its hemostatic property but also successfully applied for treating skin diseases as it possesses anti-inflammatory properties and can exert an inhibitory effect on tyrosinase, which is the primary enzyme responsible for melanin synthesis. Experiments demonstrate that TXA will assist in battling inflammation linked with skin injury and, simultaneously, suppress pigmentation, making it an all-in-one therapy for melasma and related hyperpigmentation. There is clinical evidence that TXA possesses the ability to enhance visibly inflammatory disorders of the skin by reducing hyperpigmented lesions induced by inflammation. Thus, TXA's twofold effect makes it an effective drug in the overall management of skin injuries and the resulting inflammatory sequelae they cause, particularly in the management of hyperpigmentation and melasma therapy (Górska et al., 2025). Apart from chemical modalities , such as TXA, laser modalities are an effective modality for the management of skin injuries and the subsequent inflammatory processes. The Q-Switched Nd: YAG laser, specifically, has proven effective in the removal of scars and PIH in different race groups, including Asians. Through its fractionated beam profile, this laser preferably treats the involved skin layers and minimizes hyperpigmented zones with minimal side effects. Not only does it help enhance the texture of the skin, but it also manages the inflammatory component by triggering the body's own healing pathways. The successful use of this treatment mode is a reflection of the necessity for an overall solution to skin damage, bringing together pharmacological and procedural interventions. With ongoing research and development, an overlap of these methods will continue to yield improved patient results in patients with melasma and hyperpigmentation (Bennardo et al., 2022) (Figure 3.5).

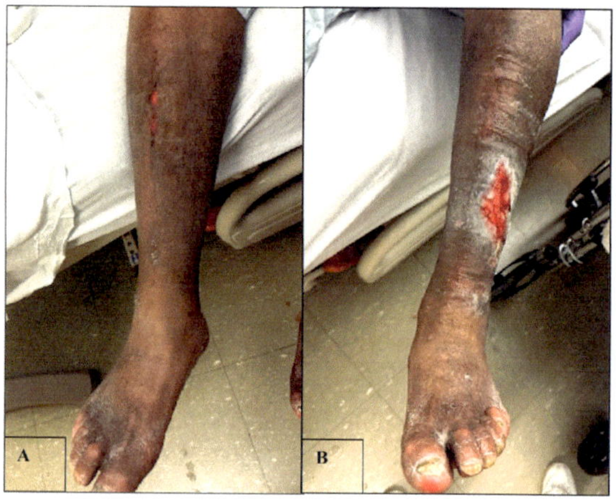

Figure 3.5. (A). Right leg showing skin hyperpigmentation and superficial, vertical open dry wound, around 3 centimeters on the anterior mid-leg; and (B). Left leg with skin hyperpigmentation and superficial, irregularly shaped dry wound, approximately 4 centimeters by 3 centimeters on the anterolateral mid-leg area.

Source: https://www.researchgate.net/publication/371407974/figure/fig1/AS:11431281203173991@1699202809319/A-Right-leg-showing-skin-hyperpigmentation-and-superficial-vertical-open-dry-wound.png.

Test Your Knowledge

1. How does UV radiation contribute to the development of hyperpigmentation?
2. What types of hyperpigmentation are most commonly associated with sun exposure?
3. Explain the role of hormonal changes in the development of melasma.

3.2. Types of Hyperpigmentation

Learning Outcome

1. Define melasma
2. Describe post-inflammatory hyperpigmentation
3. Focus on solar lentigines

Hyperpigmentation occurs in numerous varieties with individualized etiologies and clinical implications. Among the most prevalent is the solar lentigines, simply referred to as sun spots, which occur as a result of prolonged exposure to sunlight, particularly in fair individuals. These are lesions caused by melanin production confined to the site of UV stimulation that results in darkened patches of skin. Apart from sun exposure, solar lentigines can also be provoked by oxidative stress and inflammation. The cause of hyperpigmentation is important to recognize since this will determine the treatment modalities, which can vary from topical therapy, laser therapy, or chemical peeling. Understanding these subtypes enables dermatologists to tailor their approach to efficiently reduce the psychosocial impact with which such dermatoses are associated because hyperpigmentation will result in low-esteem and irritation among patients, and thus intervention at the right time becomes mandatory (Parveen et al., 2019). Melasma is another significant type of hyperpigmentation, where symmetrical facial brown patches in women, particularly those in their reproductive years, are commonly affected. Melasma is usually precipitated by hormonal fluctuations, specifically those associated with pregnancy or the use of oral contraceptives, in combination with environmental exposures like sunlight and heat. The pathophysiology of melasma is increased melanin production, which makes it a challenging condition usually not responsive to standard therapies. Treatment for melasma requires consideration of individual patient factors, with dermatologists using selective therapies that may involve topical agents , such as hydroquinone or the new therapeutic agent, TXA. TXA has been found recently to not only inhibit tyrosinase activity but also exhibit anti-inflammatory action, making it a good alternative for the management of melasma, which can greatly improve the outcome and quality of life (Górska et al., 2025). PIH is another common type of hyperpigmentation resulting from inflammation or injury to the skin. Common causes of PIH are acne, eczema, and psoriasis, where the reaction of the skin results in the deposition of excess melanin in the affected skin. In contrast to other types of hyperpigmentation, PIH is dark brown to purple and fades with the passage of time but, at times, persists. Management of PIH is usually aimed at prevention and adequate control of inflammation to minimize further damage. Besides, dermatologists are able to use therapies , such as topical corticosteroids, retinoids, and brighteners together to expedite the resolution of hyperpigmented lesions. Knowledge about the different types of hyperpigmentation, their causes, and treatment is necessary for healthcare providers to enhance patients' quality of life through effective treatment modalities (Parveen et al., 2019).

3.2.1. Melasma

Melasma, or the mask of pregnancy, is a common form of hyperpigmentation that most often affects women, particularly those of the reproductive age group. Melasma is an asymmetrical hyperpigmentation with dark patches typically found on the face, including the cheeks, forehead, and upper lip. Melasma is predominantly associated with hormonal imbalance, particularly pregnancy or through birth control, but the cause is multifactorial. Genetic predisposition, sun exposure, and oxidative stress are primarily accountable for the development and exacerbation of melasma. Furthermore, the psychosocial implications of melasma have a debilitating impact on self-confidence and overall quality of life for patients, with proper management techniques being needed to go far beyond simple cosmetic treatments, as they consistently fail to provide long-term outcomes. Over the past several years, the dermatology community has shown growing interest in the therapeutic application of TXA for the treatment of melasma. First designed as a hemostatic, TXA has found itself in the limelight due to its inhibitory effect on tyrosinase activity, an enzyme involved in melanin synthesis, and reduction of inflammation from hyperpigmentation. The research demonstrates that both topical and oral application of TXA can evoke significant amelioration in melasma symptoms, a great promise to traditional treatment. However, while clinical trials report its efficacy, they also identifies some limitations of sample size and study design, and therefore underscore the necessity for better-controlled studies to verify TXAs efficacy and refine treatment protocols for treating melasma (Górska et al., 2025).

Despite advances with pharmacologic options, effective management of melasma remains elusive in light of its multifactorial etiology. While TXA provides a valuable adjunct to treatment, an integrative approach of lifestyle modification, , such as sun protection and proper skincare routines, is also necessary. Not only does acceptance of these means cure the clinical presentation of hyperpigmentation, but it also works against risk factors driving the condition, , such as UV light exposure and hormonal shifts. Patients must be proactive in communication with dermatologists in order to construct individualized treatment plans that are tailored to specific needs and circumstances. Through this multi-dimensional strategy, it is possible to enhance the effectiveness of melasma treatments, leading to improved patient outcomes and quality of life (Fangmin et al., 2024) (Figure 3.6).

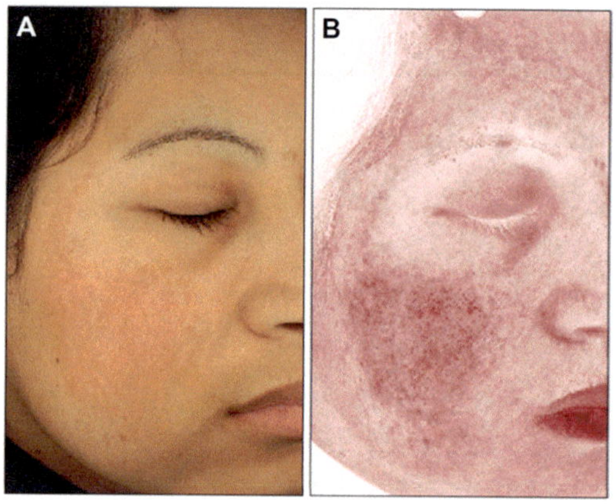

Figure 3.6. Vascular characteristics in melasma. Pronounced telangiectatic erythema noticed on melasma lesion. (A) Direct light; and (B) red zones from polarized photo.

Source: https://www.researchgate.net/publication/49690051/figure/fig1/AS:340831891410957@1458272063748/ascular-characteristics-in-melasma-Pronounced-telangiectatic-erythema-noticed-on-melasma.png.

3.2.2. Post-Inflammatory Hyperpigmentation

PIH is a common dermatological condition resulting from an inflammatory response to cutaneous damage, , such as acne, eczema, or other inflammatory skin diseases. PIH presents itself as pigmented spots following the resolution of the initial inflammation and typically incurs massive cosmetic and psychological morbidity. The pathophysiology of PIH is intrinsically linked with the enhancement of the production of excess melanin due to inflammatory cytokines, which causes the activation of the melanocytes and subsequent irregular pigmentation. Prevalence of PIH can vary significantly based on the skin type, and individuals with more melanin are likely to be affected. The condition not only impacts the outward appearance of the skin but also has the potential to lead to poorer self-esteem and social isolation, hence proper treatment modalities are vital in dermatologic practice (Górska et al., 2025). PIH treatment is a complex activity that involves preventive as well as therapeutic measures. An effective skincare regimen, with sun protection, is crucial as UV radiation worsens pigmentation. Topical treatment with products containing hydroquinone, retinoids, and azelaic acid has also been useful in lightening hyperpigmented marks, but no intervention is without potential side effects, making education of the patient a must. In recent years, TXA has gained limelight for its role in the enhancement of PIH, attributed to its anti-inflammatory potential and inhibiting property against tyrosinase, and thus reduced melanin production (Górska et al., 2025).

Merging of pharmacologic and processual interventions, such as laser therapy or peels, can also enhance the result, and thus reflects the need for a customized treatment based on the individual's skin type and response. While PIH management has been enhanced, there remain some issues, most notably in terms of recurrence and tolerability of therapy. Even though the majority of patients respond positively to established therapeutic interventions, a small number might manifest only partial improvement or recur upon termination of treatment. This warrants ongoing research to explain improved potential mechanisms of PIH and develop more effective and better-tolerated therapies. Further, the use of natural and herbal agents, which are reported to possess fewer side effects, could provide complementary treatment modalities in the management of facial hyperpigmentation in line with growing consumer interest in holistic treatment in dermatology (Parveen et al., 2019). To conclude, raising awareness and education of healthcare workers and patients is important to improve management and psychosocial impacts of PIH (Figure 3.7).

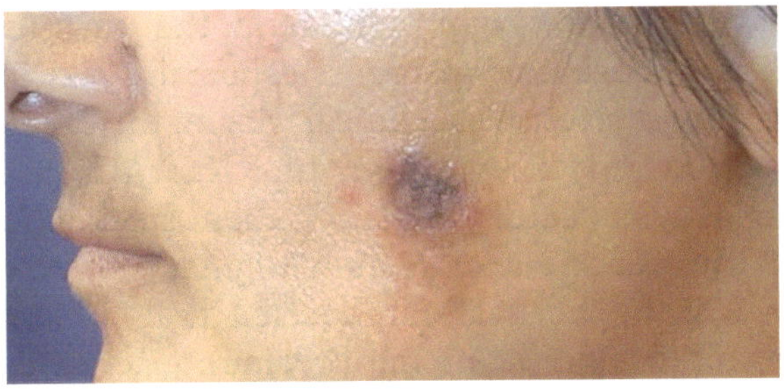

Figure 3.7. Post-inflammatory hyperpigmentation (PIH).

Source: https://dermnetnz.org/assets/Uploads/colour/hyperpig4.jpg.

3.2.3. Solar Lentigines

Solar lentigines, or age spots or liver spots, are an extremely common form of hyperpigmentation that typically results from cumulative exposure to the sun. Solar lentigines are level brown or black macules that most frequently present on sun-exposed areas of the face, hands, and forearms. The pathophysiology of solar lentigines involves excessive production of melanin, the pigment responsible for skin color, secondary to ultraviolet (UV) radiation. As the skin ages, it becomes less able to regenerate, so uneven pigmentation becomes more likely. Notably, while solar lentigines themselves are harmless and pose no health risk, they can produce a negative psychological impact on the affected individual, such that they feel less confident in themselves and unhappy with their appearance, so their removal is a significant issue in dermatology (Parveen et al., 2019). Effective treatment of solar lentigines involves a good understanding of the modalities of treatment available. A number of therapies have been formulated, ranging from topical treatments to procedural interventions. Topical agents are most typically hydroquinone, retinoids, and azelaic acid, which all have the effect of inhibiting melanin production and promoting skin turnover. Procedural treatments , such as chemical peels and laser treatments have also become increasingly popular in the past few years, with laser treatments especially proving to be most effective. A clinical trial on the carbon solution-amplified 1064 nm Nd:YAG laser showed satisfactory levels of patient satisfaction for the treatment of solar lentigines (Defne et al., 2023). The trial emphasized that patients exhibited significant improvement, i.e., these treatments are extremely effective in treating the observable manifestations of solar lentigines without inducing additional psychosocial distress associated with hyperpigmentation. Despite improvements in the treatments in place, prevention is still given priority. Daily use of broad-spectrum sunscreens is significant in the prevention of new solar lentigines, particularly among fair-skinned or those with a history of extensive sun exposure. Protective measures, , such as wearing hats or remaining under shades during the prime sun hours, are also viable preventive measures.

Psychosocial consequences should not be overlooked since instruction of the patients regarding the harmless nature of solar lentigines and counseling them towards proper management techniques can eliminate cosmetic-related concerns. By merging pre-emptive prevention with sound treatment habits, dermatologists can significantly improve the quality of life among the patients and regain confidence, thereby addressing the physical as well as the emotional dimension of this common skin condition (Parveen et al., 2019) (Figure 3.8).

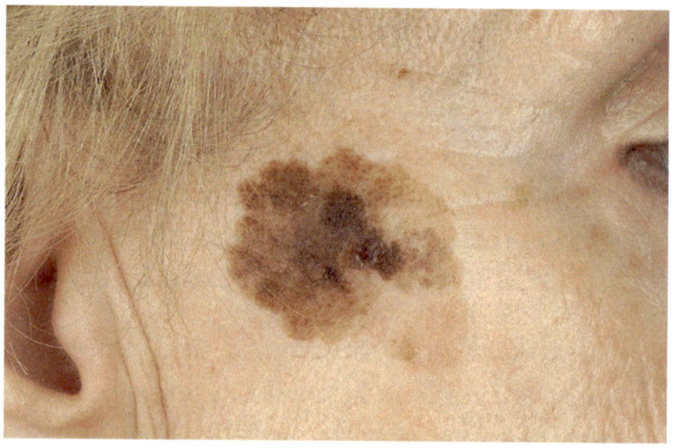

Figure 3.8. Solar lentigines.

Source: https://doctorsaestheticscentre.com/wp-content/uploads/2022/03/solar-lentigines-treatment-in-kochi.png.

Test Your Knowledge

1. What are the key clinical features and common triggers of melasma?
2. How does PIH differ in appearance and cause from melasma?
3. What are solar lentigines, and how are they typically caused and identified clinically?

3.3. Diagnosis of Hyperpigmentation

Learning Outcome

1. Explain the role of clinical evaluation in the management of hyperpigmentation and melasma
2. Define the term dermatoscopy
3. Understand the concept of biopsy and laboratory tests

Hyperpigmentation diagnosis is a latent process involving sensitive observation of the skin status and patient's medical history. Visual inspection is typically the first step followed by dermatologists in an attempt to identify the precise form of hyperpigmentation, i.e., idiopathic, post-inflammatory, or melasma-related hyperpigmentation. They differ in characteristics and etiology, and hence, accurate diagnosis is essential for successful treatment. Further, information on the patient's lifestyle, sunlight exposure, and potential genetic causes could prove helpful in terms of understanding the etiology of hyperpigmentation. Having such data allows health practitioners to tailor treatment plans accordingly, minimizing trial and error in disease management and maximizing patient satisfaction. Dermoscopy may become a diagnostic tool in everyday practice, as well, allowing thorough inspection of skin lesions, revealing underlying structural alterations that are invisible to the human eye. This technology assists in distinguishing among different forms of pigmentation, , such as lentigines or solar keratosis, thereby ensuring a better diagnosis. Furthermore, occasional skin biopsies are also justified, particularly in strange circumstances when malignancy is a consideration in the differential diagnosis. With new methods of diagnosis, dermatologists can identify hyperpigmentation as a separate entity from other dermatologic disorders so that appropriate treatment and management plans can be administered to the patient based on individual requirements. The psychosocial implications of hyperpigmentation, highlighted in recent studies, cannot be overlooked at the time of diagnosis. Conditions like melasma and facial hyperpigmentation often coexist with emotional distress, affecting the patient's self-perception and overall well-being. As has been explained, these signs can lead to significant psychosocial challenges, i.e., depression and anxiety, especially in patients with obvious skin alterations (Parveen et al., 2019). It is therefore important that dermatologists not only diagnose the skin condition but also consider its impact on the patient's psychological well-being. Treatment of these psychological factors can also bring us a more integrated treatment approach, enabling medical professionals to prescribe medicines like TXA, which have been promising in averting both hyperpigmentation and its consequent inflammatory reaction (Górska et al., 2025).

3.3.1. Clinical Evaluation

Clinical evaluation is paramount in the treatment of melasma and hyperpigmentation, and it provides a methodical approach to diagnosing these complex skin conditions. A thorough clinical evaluation begins with a comprehensive patient history with regards to skin type, family pigmentation disease history, and previous treatments. The nuances in a patient's unique clinical presentation are paramount in formulating an effective treatment regimen. Certain clinical features, including the pattern of pigmentation and the site involved on the face, set melasma apart from other pigmentary disorders. Provocative factors, such as hormonal fluctuations, sun exposure, and the administration of specific drugs are also assessed. These detailed evaluations form the basis for individualized therapeutic plans, which eventually enhance therapeutic outcomes in individuals with hyperpigmentation disorders. The process of clinical evaluation plays a critical role in the effectiveness of treatments for melasma and hyperpigmentation. New evidence has revealed positive results with treatments , such as TXA for the reduction of pigmentation due to its ability to block tyrosinase activity and its anti-inflammatory properties (Górska et al., 2025). However, the broad variation in individuals' responses demands ongoing monitoring at the clinical level to assess treatment efficacy and adjust accordingly. Periodic follow-up sessions enable the health care professionals to observe the patient's response, modify the dosages, or switch to other treatments based on the patient's response. The clinical evaluation process enables identification of potential side effects or complications so that the treatment regimen remains safe and effective. The continuous evaluation justifies the need for an individualized and responsive management approach to such challenging skin conditions. In addition to establishing the efficacy of drug therapy, clinical evaluation involves the evaluation of measures of photoprotection that are essential for the treatment of melasma. Sunlight's role in exacerbating pigment-related conditions has long been proven and highlights the need for proper photoprotective measures (Rodríguez-Luna et al., 2023). Avoidance of tanning and sun-induced damage calls for patient education on daily application of a broad-spectrum sunscreen and protective clothing. Furthermore, natural photoprotectant compounds like Fernblock® may be incorporated to provide additional protection against UV-induced injury and reduce the risk of hyperpigmentation worsening. Clinical evaluations should include consultations with respect to lifestyle changes that complement treatment modalities to ensure an overall approach to treating hyperpigmentation and melasma. Lastly, a thorough clinical evaluation not only supplements treatment but also empowers patients with the data necessary to maintain long-term cutaneous health (Figure 3.9).

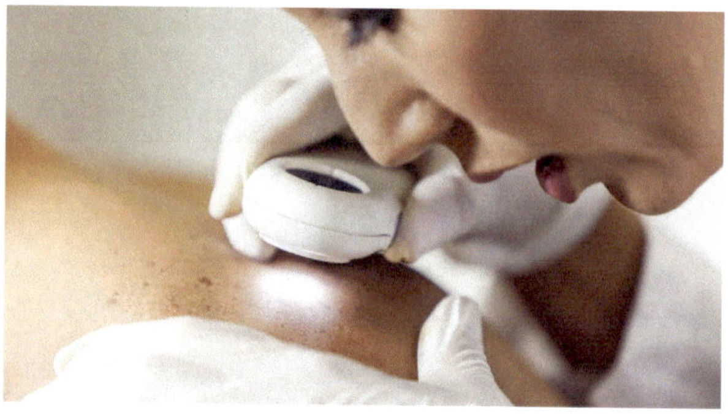

Figure 3.9. dermatologist examining hyperpigmentation.

Source: https://media.allure.com/photos/5e43262b4c93240009a30323/16:9/w_2560%2Cc_limit/hyperpigmentation-lede-1.jpg.

3.3.2. Dermatoscopy

Dermatoscopy is now an important tool for the management of hyperpigmentation and melasma, enabling dermatologists to assess skin lesions with greater precision. The non-invasive imaging technique makes it possible for practitioners to visualize subsurface skin structures, facilitating discrimination between benign and malignant lesions. Healthcare professionals can analyze pigmented lesions more thoroughly and select out characteristics , such as the presence of vessels, pigment distribution, and morphology using dermatoscopy. In cases of hyperpigmentation, the function of dermatoscopy is to assist in determining the depth and nature of pigmentation, significant in guiding appropriate treatment modalities. For instance, differential diagnosis between epidermal and dermal melasma can come a long way in determining the selection of therapeutic modalities, either laser therapy or topical drugs, whose aim is to reduce pigmentation. Utilization of advanced technologies like dermatoscopy can improve patient outcomes by enhancing diagnostic sensitivity. With the increasing prevalence of hyperpigmentation disorders, accurate diagnostic techniques have grown increasingly important. Dermatoscopic examination is capable of diagnosing most types of hyperpigmentation, including solar lentigo and other types of melanoses, which are usually challenging to diagnose visually. Research evidence indicates that dermatological clinics using dermatoscopy report higher levels of patient satisfaction due to improved diagnosis and associated treatment strategies. Furthermore, with a better understanding of physiologic changes in hyperpigmented lesions evolving continuously, dermatoscopy can give hints regarding the mechanisms of conditions like melasma and, hence, allow for better management.

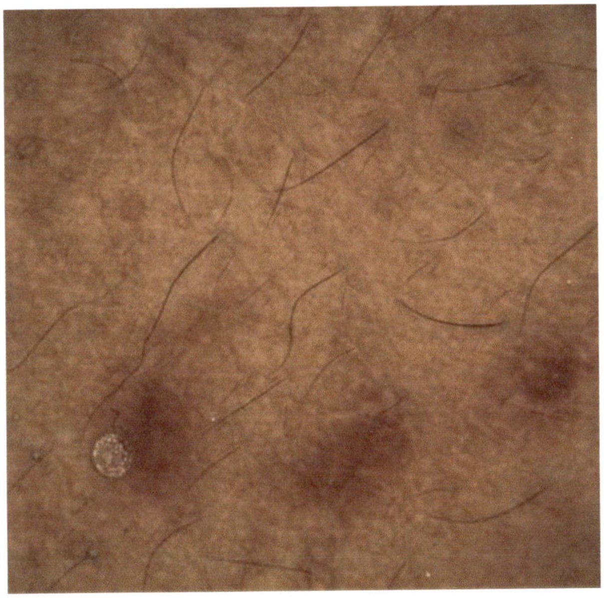

Figure 3.10. Dermatoscopy of a skin region affected by post-inflammatory hyperpigmentation.

Source: https://www.researchgate.net/profile/Ana-Martini/publication/334498049/figure/fig1/AS:781453264695297@1563324385824/Figura-1-Dermatoscopy-of-a-skin-region-affected-by-post-inflammatory-hyperpigmentation.jpg.

The conjunction of treatment modalities with dermatoscopic examination holds the potential to refine treatment protocols for hyperpigmentation. New treatments , such as Q-switched laser therapy, have been shown to yield positive results in the management of benign hypermelanosis, as mentioned in current studies using advanced laser technology for site-specific treatment. Additionally, the application of TXA has been promising in managing melasma with its anti-inflammatory and inhibitory properties on tyrosinase activity. Although promising, these therapies must be combined with precise diagnostic techniques like dermatoscopy in order to successfully customize treatment regimens. As dermatology continues to advance, the use of dermatoscopy as part of daily practice can maximize the treatment of hyperpigmentation and melasma and enhance therapeutic responses in patients (Figure 3.10).

3.3.3. Biopsy and Laboratory Tests

Diagnosis of hyperpigmentation, particularly melasma, typically requires an in-depth assessment with biopsy and lab tests. These diagnostic instruments are pivotal to differentiate among various forms of hyperpigmentation, , such as melasma, PIH, and other dermatoses. Biopsy can provide essential histopathological findings, which help confirm the diagnosis with the identification of changes in the epidermal and dermal layers that lead to increased melanin production. Laboratory testing, including serum hormone levels and fungal infection skin scrapings, may also be used to rule out secondary causes of hyperpigmentation. As knowledge of these diagnostic tests expands, so too does the ability of health care professionals to tailor treatment options and ultimately, improve patient outcomes by addressing the true type of hyperpigmentation. It is in the treatment of melasma that an understanding of the biochemical pathways involved in pigmentation is of utmost value. Hyperpigmentation disorders are characterized by their heightened production of melanin, whose manufacture can be regulated by various factors like hormonal changes, sun exposure, and inflammatory dermatosis. Laboratory tests measuring hormone levels, particularly during pregnancy, can help reveal the complex aspects of melasma. For example, excessive estrogen and progesterone levels are commonly cited to be associated with gestational melasma, as corroborated by studies reporting changes in the skin during pregnancy, whereby the majority of women exhibit extreme physiological hyperpigmentation (Gehlot et al., 2018). This information highlights the importance of integrating laboratory results into the clinical management plan for melasma, thereby making the treatment personalized and successful. Moreover, patient education on the significance of biopsy and laboratory tests is a must in the management of hyperpigmentation and melasma. Most patients have no idea how these diagnostic tests will impact their management and quality of life. For instance, patients with melasma have a serious psychosocial impact, as shown by studies that quantify the health-related quality of life (Buainain de Maymone et al., 2016). Through the involvement of patients in diagnostic tests, the compliance and satisfaction of patients with treatment can be enhanced by clinicians. Moreover, making patients aware of the potential outcome of their lab work provides them with a sense of control and understanding regarding their condition. Such care for biopsy and lab testing, along with a plan of communication, assumes an integral role under the holistic management of hyperpigmentation disorders (Figure 3.11).

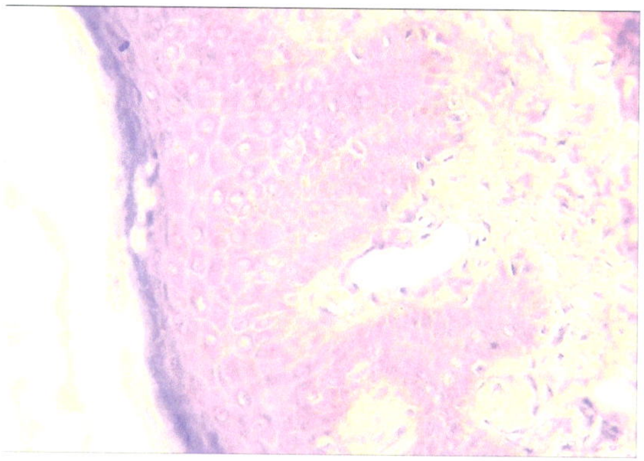

Figure 3.11. Skin biopsy (increased pigmentation in stratum spinosum and basal layer).

Source: https://www.researchgate.net/publication/258704332/figure/fig2/AS:411395154825216@1475095656111/Skin-Biopsy-Increased-pigmentation-in-stratum-spinosum-and-basal-layer.png.

Test Your Knowledge

1. What are the key elements of a clinical evaluation when diagnosing hyperpigmentation?
2. How can dermatoscopy aid in differentiating between melasma, PIH, and solar lentigines?
3. When is a skin biopsy indicated in the evaluation of hyperpigmentation, and what conditions might it help diagnose?

3.4. Treatment Options for Hyperpigmentation

Learning Outcome

1. Explain the role of topical agents in the management of hyperpigmentation disorders
2. Understand the use of chemical peels in the management of hyperpigmentation
3. Describe laser therapy in the management of hyperpigmentation and melasma

Treatment of hyperpigmentation is multifactorial, and each group of underlying pathophysiology and presenting patient has its own individual treatment. The most widely employed topical agents are hydroquinone, kojic acid, and azelaic acid. Hydroquinone, a well-established skin-lightener, is an inhibitor of melanin synthesis. One of its major disadvantages, however, of prolonged therapy is the risk of side effects , such as ochronosis, particularly in dark skin phototypes. Kojic acid has been a popular option, especially in formulations that have been formulated to enhance penetration in the skin by incorporating glycolic acid, since this is described to be effective and safe compared to traditional therapies. Dermatologists' preference follows a broad trend towards kojic acid blends, showing that they are becoming progressively more popular in practice as a safer way of treating hyperpigmentation, particularly prevalent in some populations, , such as in India (Gautam et al., 2023). Apart from topical treatments, procedural therapies provide useful tools for the treatment of hyperpigmentation. Chemical peeling, laser therapy, and microdermabrasion are finding growing use in dermatology. Chemical peels, which use agents , such as glycolic or salicylic acid, exfoliate the skin to better absorb topical medications and stimulate cellular turnover, thereby improving the look of hyperpigmented lesions. Lasers, specifically those that target melanin, provide a more invasive method. They are effective in lightening melasma and PIH but must be applied cautiously so as not to cause complications , such as paradoxical hyperpigmentation. While marked improvement can be achieved through procedural treatments, patient education on expectations and possible side effects is still important to maximize satisfaction as well as compliance with treatment regimens (Buainain et al., 2016). Patient education is fundamental in the management of hyperpigmentation, specifically in understanding the implications of the skincare regimen and lifestyle. Sunscreen use is essential, as exposure to the sun's UV rays can heighten pigmentation disorders, such as melasma and PIH. The presence of an important finding indicates a relationship between patient awareness and the regular use of protective measures; those with better educational levels tend to show greater awareness about their skin issues and preventive measures. Moreover, comprehensive treatment regimens consisting of a combination of topical and procedural treatments, along with robust patient education, have been shown to maximize therapeutic effectiveness and quality of life. Individualization of treatment as per the needs of the individual and patient education significantly improves management of hyperpigmentation and melasma (Buainain et al., 2016).

3.4.1. Topical Agents (e.g., Hydroquinone, Retinoids)

Topical agents are of critical importance in the management of hyperpigmentation conditions, particularly melasma. Hydroquinone is one such agent and has for years been referred to as the gold standard due to its ability to suppress melanin synthesis effectively. Hydroquinone acts by inhibiting the function of the enzyme tyrosinase, which is important in the synthesis of melanin. Though effective, concerns over potential side effects, , such as ochronosis, particularly in those with darker skin tones, led to the quest for other agents. With a changing world of dermatotheraphy, newer agents like kojic acid and licorice extract are surfacing as safer and superior options. Surveys of dermatologists highlight the utilization of such products, particularly those that involve a combination of hydroquinone with other synergistic ingredients to achieve enhanced efficacy and lower side effects, indicating the need for an optimized approach to melasma treatment (Gautam et al., 2023). Topical retinoids are another significant group of drugs for treating hyperpigmentation and melasma. From vitamin A, these medications cause turnover of cells and accelerate the sloughing of melanized epidermal cells, allowing for incremental depigmentation of the hyperpigmented lesion. Their anti-inflammatory effect makes them appealing, particularly for those patients with melasma associated with acne. There are preparations from retinol to more potent prescription retinoids like tretinoin available to dermatologists, allowing them to select an option from a range of treatments to suit each patient's needs. Additionally, newer studies emphasize the combination of retinoids with other medications—, such as hydroquinone or glycolic acid—to increase their effectiveness. Therefore, these combined therapeutic approaches have gained extensive popularity, particularly in groups with a tendency to develop darker skin tones, where careful attention to treatment protocols is necessary to avoid worsening pigmentation abnormalities (Callender et al., 2025). The use of several topical agents indicates the necessity for treatment modalities specific to the patient in managing hyperpigmentation and melasma. While hydroquinone and retinoids remain predominant, newer preparations employing a mixture of ingredients have been well received by dermatologists. Adding glycolic acid, for instance, was noted to enhance the penetration and activity of hydroquinone and kojic acid formulations, with the ability to bring about improvement in pigmentation more quickly. These survey results indicate a paradigm shift toward combination treatments, particularly within the clinic, as physicians increasingly embrace less likely-to-be side-effect-inducing regimens and more likely-to-be effective. With increasing realization of heterogeneous response to therapy in different skin types, the necessity to enhance the therapeutic modalities that appeal to both patients and physicians alike continues to rise. Individualized use of local agents is one of the cornerstones in the treatment of melasma and hyperpigmentation (Gautam et al., 2023) (Figure 3.12).

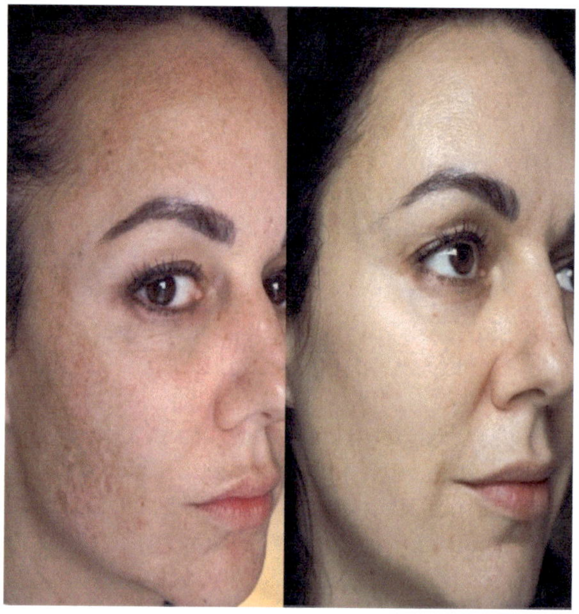

Figure 3.12. Hydroquinone 3 months before and after.

Source: https://i0.wp.com/skincarewithfriends.com/wp-content/uploads/2021/04/IMG_4049.jpg?w=640&ssl=1.

3.4.2. Chemical Peels

Chemical peels have been the center of significant attention in the treatment of both melasma and hyperpigmentation, and have been a very valuable modality for the treatment of both of these conditions. Chemical peels involve the application of chemical solutions that cause exfoliation of the skin layers, followed by removal of dead cells and thus the growth of newer, healthier skin. This process can depigment hyperpigmented lesions by targeting both epidermal and dermal pigmented lesions, thereby making chemical peels a multi-directed treatment for such conditions. Various chemicals , such as alpha-hydroxy acids (AHAs), beta-hydroxy acids (BHAs), and trichloroacetic acid (TCA) are employed based on the specific skin type and pigmentation depth. Response heterogeneity necessitates having individualized protocols to ensure optimization of efficacy and minimization of side effects, which is crucial for patient satisfaction and long-term outcome in the management of hyperpigmentation (Khoo & Halim,2016). Choice of chemical peel also needs to be made according to skin type, extent of hyperpigmentation, and the history of the patient. Light peels can be applied to individuals with superficial pigmentation, but a more serious case might need deeper peels. For instance, AHAs are commonly employed in bleaching superficial pigmentation, while TCA penetrates more invasively and can be employed as a concentrated solution for more severe melasma. It is important to mention that after treatment, follow-up with strict photoprotection is required to get the best results and prevent recurrence because unprotected sun exposure may aggravate hyperpigmented conditions. Also, chemical peeling can be followed by other treatments, for instance, topical retinoids or laser therapy, that target general skin texturing and coloring (Bińczyk et al., 2024). This integrated approach is increasingly important as practitioners strive to deliver comprehensive care in aesthetic dermatology. Despite their documented success, however, chemical peels are not without risk of ensuing dangers and complications. Some patients can develop brief erythema, peeling, or even hyperpigmentation following treatment, particularly if proper aftercare procedures are not taken or peels are done too frequently. Identification of these risks is crucial for medical practitioners in the planning of therapies for hyperpigmentation and melasma patients. The pre-treatment consultations that provide an assessment of skin sensitivity, history of pigmentation disorders, and overall dermatological health can prevent undesirable outcomes. Patient education regarding realistic expectations, aftercare, and potential side effects also facilitates an effective therapeutic partnership. Through the use of a balanced approach with chemical peels being used responsibly, practitioners are actually able to make a positive difference in the treatment of hyperpigmentation, thus improving patients' confidence and lifestyle (Khoo & Halim,2016) (Figure 3.13).

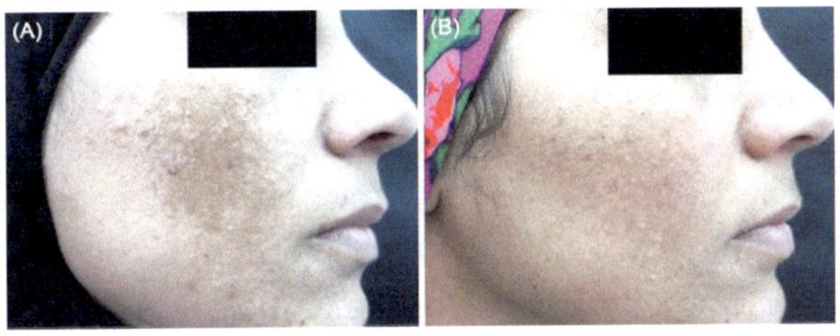

Figure 3.13. (A) Right side, before TCA 25% peeling; and (B) Right side, shows excellent improvement after 8 sessions with TCA 25% peeling.

Source: https://www.researchgate.net/profile/Doaa-Aboutaleb/publication/264396319/figure/fig1/AS:749023094910978@1555592430676/A-Right-side-before-TCA-25-peeling-B-Right-side-shows-excellent-improvement-after.jpg.

3.4.3. Laser Therapy

Laser therapy represents a breakthrough in the treatment of melasma and hyperpigmentation because it is a more concentrated modulation of skin pigmentation. It achieves this by using concentrated light beams to target melanin deposits on the skin and breaks them down before they are reabsorbed into the body. Clinical tests have already proved that laser therapy, whether fractional laser or pulsed dye laser (PDL), not only reduces the visibility of hyperpigmented lesions effectively but also stimulates collagen growth and therefore has a beneficial overall effect on the texture of skin. With the rising incidence of facial hyperpigmentation globally, particularly among women, laser therapy has become increasingly popular since it is highly effective in treating condition like melasma, which can be very hard to treat with usual topical medication.

The precision of laser technology allows for tailored treatment regimens, addressing the unique skin type and pigmentation concerns of each patient. Although favorable results associated with laser treatment are promising, practitioners must treat such procedures with a comprehensive understanding of the potential side effects and shortcomings involved. PIH or erythema can occur following treatment, particularly in darker skin types, which tends to further exacerbate present problems.

In addition, the need for return visits for repeated treatments can pose logistical barriers and may increase treatment costs, discouraging some patients' utilization. It is vital to balance the benefits of laser treatment against the risks, openly informing patients about post-operative care to minimize side effects. Application of laser treatment in a multimodal therapy can optimize outcomes, though continuous research into individualized protocols and selection guidelines will be required to enhance both safety and efficacy. Combining laser treatment with synergistic therapies can also provide an integrative treatment for hyperpigmentation. For instance, combining laser treatments with other therapies , such as TXA, has proven to be potentially useful for optimizing outcomes.

With emerging evidence regarding the anti-inflammatory properties of TXA and its ability to lower tyrosinase activity, dermatologists are increasingly examining its use in association with laser modalities as a method of treating melasma and hyperpigmentation more effectively (Górska et al., 2025). Also, while laser therapy is a valuable component of facial hyperpigmentation treatment protocols, therapists should also consider the psychosocial dimensions of such disorders since they were documented in research findings demonstrating the emotional burdens hyperpigmentation imposes on patients (Parveen et al., 2019). Having a multidimensional approach enables the effective management of the physical and psychological aspects of hyperpigmentation and melasma (Figure 3.14).

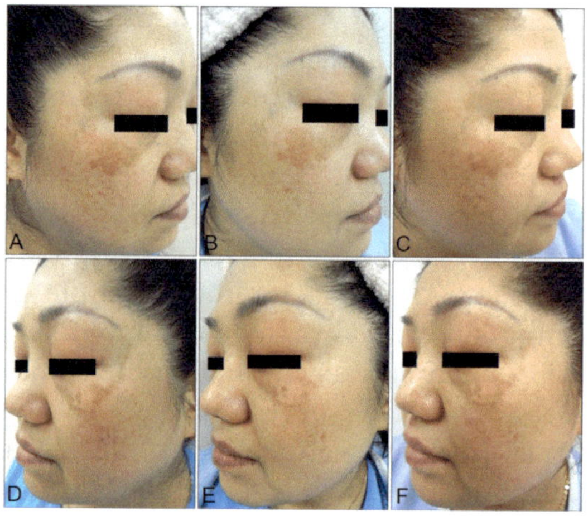

Figure 3.14. The patient who exhibited a rebound hyperpigmentation without purpura on pulsed-dye laser (PDL)+Q-switched Nd:YAG laser (QSNY) side at week 16. PDL+QSNY side (A, B, and C) revealed a great reduction of the melasma area and severity index score at week 9 (B) from the baseline (A), but rebound hyperpigmentation occurred at week 16 (C). QSNY side (D, E, and F) showed no rebound hyperpigmentation.

Source: https://www.researchgate.net/publication/322268979/figure/fig2/AS:669211873521666@1536563952246/The-patient-who-exhibited-a-rebound-hyperpigmentation-without-purpura-on-pulsed-dye-laser.png.

Test Your Knowledge

1. How do retinoids help in the treatment of hyperpigmentation, and what are the common side effects?
2. What types of chemical peels are commonly used for hyperpigmentation?
3. What are the advantages and risks of laser therapy for treating hyperpigmentation, especially in darker skin types?

3.5. Lifestyle Modifications for Prevention

Learning Outcome

1. Describe sun protection strategies
2. Focus on skincare routines in managing hyperpigmentation and melasma
3. Deal with dietary considerations

Treatment of hyperpigmentation and melasma calls for an aggressive multidisciplinary treatment consisting of successful lifestyle modifications. Prevention is a very important aspect, where one should maximize sun protection behavior since ultraviolet light is the prime culprit in causing color change in the skin. Patients should put significant importance on daily broad-spectrum sun use with a minimum SPF of 30, independent of skin type. Incidentally, while people with fair skin are more prone to sun damage, those with medium and darker skin are not exempt and can benefit as well from systematic sun protection. Current evidence suggests that visible light exposure can lead to pigmentary changes, particularly in dark skin. Therefore, wearing protective clothing and remaining in the shade during midday sun are also important components of a complete sun protection program that can stop the development of melasma and other pigmentary disorders (Bartonova et al., 2012; Dlova et al., 2024). Lifestyle diet is one of the key elements in managing hyperpigmentation and melasma. Antioxidant foods high in vitamins C and E, for example, may provide protective benefits against oxidative stress and therefore to skin health. Omega-3 fatty acid-rich foods , such as fish and walnuts also come in handy because they possess the ability to strengthen the integrity of the skin barrier and suppress inflammation that may exacerbate pigmentation disorders. Proper hydration is also important for skin elasticity and general appearance. The inclusion of a well-balanced diet that consists of fruits, vegetables, and whole grains holds the potential to improve skin health greatly and can even limit the onset of melasma. Proper circulation and nutrient delivery to the skin are also maintained through regular exercise, validating the role of an overall lifestyle in the prevention of hyperpigmentation (Bartonova et al., 2012; Dlova et al., 2024). Behavioral adjustments, including stress control and avoidance of certain stimuli, are components of a lifestyle adjustment plan to reduce the incidence of hyperpigmentation. Stress may cause hormonal changes that exacerbate melasma, and thus mindfulness, yoga, and other stress-controlling activities become essential. Additionally, one has to avoid exposure to potential irritants and inflammatory agents in some skincare products, which tend to exacerbate existing pigment dispositions. Steering clear of harsh chemicals and extreme heat treatments can significantly improve skin elasticity, which promotes a healthier condition for healing and recovery. Through adoption of such behavioral interventions as part of their regimen, individuals can minimize the aggravation of hyperpigmentation while at the same time promoting improved skin overall (Bartonova et al., 2012; Dlova et al., 2024).

3.5.1. Sun Protection Strategies

Effective sun protection strategies are core components of the management of hyperpigmentation and melasma, both conditions exacerbated by UV radiation exposure. Research has shown that UV light and visible light are both key players in the pathogenesis of these skin ailments, so photoprotection is the centerpiece of the lives of individuals involved. The application of broad-spectrum sunscreens protecting UVA in addition to UVB radiation is a recommended practice to monitor additional pigmentation changes. Recent articles bring to the fore high SPF products since they guard the skin against sunburn, and more importantly, avoid cumulative skin injury through prolonged exposure to sunlight, which is an etiology of hyperpigmentation. These protective measures should be complemented by the employment of shading and protective apparel, as these help to reduce further direct exposure to harmful solar radiation (Rodríguez-Luna et al., 2023). Sunscreens that are meant for individuals with darker skin colors represent a newer approach that is tailored to function within the particular constraints of hyperpigmentation and melasma. Skin of color patients possesses a variant melanin structure, which, even though it confers some degree of intrinsic protection, does not rule out the potential for sun damage and consequent pigmentation disease. The current evidence shows that dermatology consultation emphasizes the nuances of sun protection in skin of color patients because such groups may be less likely to adopt photoprotective behaviors. Also, the non-availability of appropriately formulated sunscreen products that are not whitening can discourage regular use among this group. Hence, the development of targeted sunscreens with appropriate cosmetic appeal and formulations that include broad-spectrum protection in conjunction with depigmenting agents can significantly promote compliance and effectiveness in preventing pigmentary disorders (Granger et al., 2023). Oral photoprotectants are also an emerging new frontier of sun protection protocols employed in the treatment of melasma and hyperpigmentation. Fernblock®, a natural compound extracted from the fern Polypodium Leucotomos, has been explored for its safety profile in both local and systemic usages to provide a safer photoprotective profile. There is clinical evidence to suggest that this extract can complement standard photoprotection by reversing sun action, including DNA damage that lasts after sun exposure. Routine intake of such photoprotective substances could strengthen the resistance of the skin to pigmentation change induced by UV exposure. With the development of knowledge in the area, it is important for healthcare practitioners to educate patients on the multifaceted practice of sun protection, encompassing oral and topical treatments alike, thereby optimizing treatment for melasma and hyperpigmentation (Rodríguez-Luna et al., 2023) (Figure 3.15).

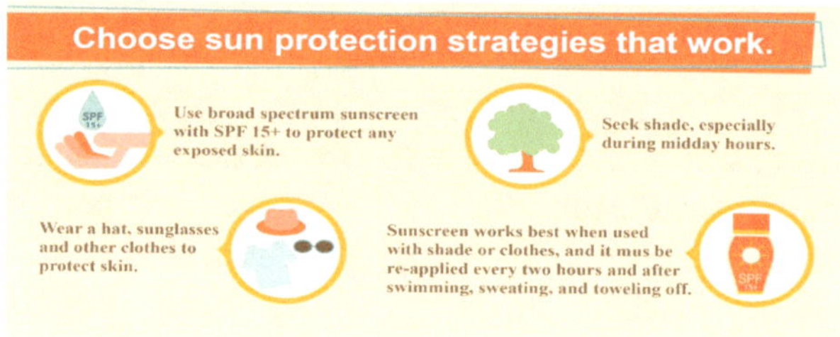
Choose sun protection strategies that work.
Use broad spectrum sunscreen with SPF 15+ to protect any exposed skin.
Seek shade, especially during midday hours.
Wear a hat, sunglasses and other clothes to protect skin.
Sunscreen works best when used with shade or clothes, and it mus be re-applied every two hours and after swimming, sweating, and toweling off.

Figure 3.15. Sun protection strategies.

Source: https://pbs.twimg.com/media/CFdahtqWoAAGq5Y.jpg.

3.5.2. Skincare Routines

Skincare routines are a critical part of managing hyperpigmentation and melasma because these conditions are usually exacerbated by improper skin care routines. Proper skincare routines can be utilized to reverse the effects of these forms of pigmentation, creating uniformity of skin tone. Effective routines usually consist of cleansing, exfoliating, treatment, and moisturizing. Gentle cleansing serves to remove impurities and prepare the skin for further treatment. Exfoliation helps remove dead skin cells that might harbor pigment. Regular exfoliant use can help enhance the efficacy of topically applied treatment to lighten skin dark spots, enabling active ingredients to better penetrate. Products possessing gentle exfoliating properties with moisturizing ingredients in this context can provide significant benefits, ultimately contributing to a brighter complexion. The selection of active ingredients plays a fundamental role in the efficacy of any hyperpigmentation skincare treatment. Progress in recent years has been enlightening on how ingredients , such as TXA, niacinamide, and vitamin C work together in synergy, with promising results in initiating skin lightening. Studies have indicated that when taken together, these compounds offer dramatic improvements to the appearance of dark spots, measured by high 13% reduction in color intensity after 8 weeks during clinical studies. The combination not only increases the overall efficacy of skincare but also gives a pleasing effect by increasing the luminosity of the skin. Besides, the addition of hyaluronic acid to formulas enhances product delivery, which means active ingredients permeate and penetrate skin layers efficiently, thus their full potential to act against melasma and hyperpigmentation is effectively (Abdel-Sayed et al., 2024). Furthermore, the role of dermocosmetics cannot be overlooked in the treatment of hyperpigmentation and melasma. They perfectly integrate into beauty routines and complement dermatological treatments with clinically recognized active ingredients. Dermocosmetics function by preserving the skin's lipid barrier, minimizing irritation, and promoting overall skin well-being, particularly applicable to patients undergoing a range of therapy for pigmentation conditions. Evidence suggests these products not only add to conventional treatments, but also improve cosmetic outcomes in addition to conventional drug treatment. Considering the difficulty of hyperpigmentation, an educated skincare regimen with the right dermocosmetics is a worthwhile approach for those wishing to improve the quality of their skin and control pigmentation problems effectively in the long run (Borkowska et al., 2024).

3.5.3. Dietary Considerations

The management of melasma and hyperpigmentation is significantly improved by proper knowledge of dietary elements that may exacerbate or ameliorate the conditions. A high-antioxidant diet is critical in the prevention of oxidative stress, which is also responsible for causing pigmentation diseases and skin damage. Dietary items that are high in vitamins E and C, i.e., citrus fruits, nuts, and greens, are responsible for keeping the skin healthy by inhibiting free radicals and inducing collagen production. Furthermore, incorporation of foods with high polyphenols , such as berries and tea, can render the skin resilient against environmental abuse. Hydration is also essential because it preserves the elasticity of the skin and facilitates the elimination of toxins, thereby indirectly influencing pigmentation patterns. In addition to antioxidant foods, some of the dietary fats and their sources also have a large influence on the health and color of the skin. Omega-3 fatty acids obtained from fish, flaxseeds, and walnuts are long recognized for their anti-inflammatory properties, which could reduce inflammation in melasma and other pigmentation types. Furthermore, an adequate balance of healthy fats in the diet can enhance cell membrane fluidity and aid nutrient absorption and intake to promote skin overall health. An overdose of processed sugar and unhealthy fats, however, can stress and inflame the body, most probably worsening the condition of hyperpigmentation. A balanced diet, therefore, primes the body for healthy internal function that aids the process of treating melasma and also makes the application of topical therapies effective. In addition, recent literature highlights the importance of some plant compounds that may either be used topically or ingested for the improvement of melasma outcomes. For instance, Polypodium leucotomos extract (Fernblock®) has been proven to be very useful in protecting the skin and is bound to provide an additive effect if combined with dietary interventions (Rodríguez-Luna et al., 2023). The potency of plant extracts, especially those that are flavonoid-dense, also confirms the regulation of pigmentation by dietary consumption. Research indicates that flavonoid-rich foods not only possess antioxidant potential but also play a part in preventing DNA damage, hence taking part in decreasing occurrences of hyperpigmentation (Almeida et al., 2021). These nutritional factors emphasize the conjunction of nutrition and cutaneous health, applying an integrative strategy for effectively treating hyperpigmentation and melasma (Figure 3.16).

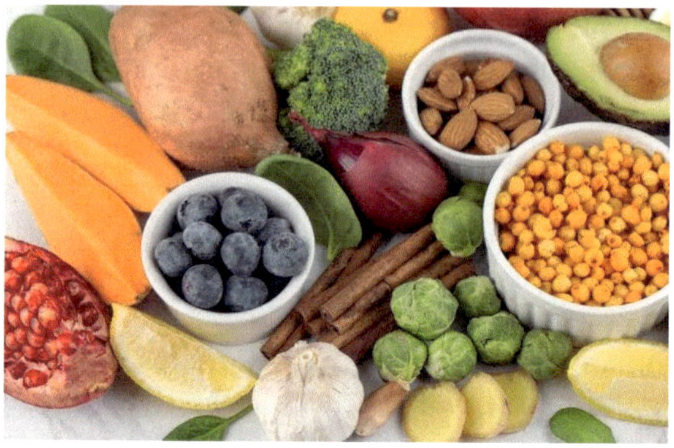

Figure 3.16. Best foods for pigmentation treatment.

Source: https://www.revitaliselondon.co.uk/wp-content/uploads/2024/10/image-18.jpeg.webp.

Test Your Knowledge

1. What are the key components of an effective sun protection strategy to prevent hyperpigmentation?
2. How can an appropriate skincare routine help prevent the worsening of hyperpigmentation?
3. What dietary habits may support healthy skin and potentially reduce hyperpigmentation risk?

3.6. Psychological Impact of Hyperpigmentation

Learning Outcome

1. Explain the impact of hyperpigmentation on self-esteem and body image issues
2. Describe social stigma and discrimination
3. Focus on coping strategies for hyperpigmentation and melasma

The emotional impact of hyperpigmentation, particularly such conditions as melasma, tends to be profound and multifaceted. Patients afflicted with the skin conditions tend to have to live through considerable emotional distress, which may manifest itself in several ways, such as anxiety, depression, and decreased self-esteem. The overt appearance of hyperpigmentation can lead to individuals afflicted with it modifying their social behavior and self-concept, ultimately resulting in social withdrawal and excessive preoccupation with perceived defects. This psychological weight is usually compounded by cultural standards of beauty emphasizing a pale, even complexion. As individuals adopt these standards, they can develop feelings of inadequacy and reduced self-esteem, making their emotional state even more challenging to navigate. It is vital to understand the psychological impact of hyperpigmentation since it points out the importance of an integrated approach to management that treats not only the physical manifestations but also addresses the emotional and psychological well-being of those suffering from it. Empirical studies have demonstrated that the lived experience of having hyperpigmentation can result in a diminished quality of life. Patients often react with heightened stress and body image dissatisfaction, which can have a negative effect on their daily interactions and mental well-being. Young adults and teenagers are particularly vulnerable to peer pressures and social comparison, with an intensified sense of body image concern as they navigate identity development. This frustration can lead to an unhealthy cycle of experimentation with various treatments, none of which typically produce expected results, thereby further perpetuating a negative self-image. In addition, the expense pertaining to treatment options, from dermatological treatments to cosmetics, may also contribute to stress, as individuals continually invest hope and money into coping with their situation. Such a confluence of economic and psychological distress underscores the importance of realistic communication and expectation during treatment planning. Furthermore, the social stigma attached to observable skin diseases can also serve to reinforce the psychological impact of hyperpigmentation. Patients become subject to discrimination or judgment on the basis of their appearance, with assumptions made about their lifestyle or character, leading to further intensification of feelings of isolation and vulnerability. Otherness of experience of skin conditions can hinder one's ability to engage in social and work environments, causing further consequent emotional suffering. In addition, as with Berloque dermatitis, which induces hyperpigmentation because of the use of cosmetics, the patient will also have feelings of betrayal or guilt toward his/her product usage, which also centers on blame. All such psychological effects call for an integrated management plan that goes beyond dermatological care to include mental health counseling and educational courses designed to reduce stigma and foster acceptance, thereby empowering individuals to better cope with their conditions.

3.6.1. Self-Esteem and Body Image Issues

The relationship between self-esteem and body image concerns is particularly important among individuals with hyperpigmentation and melasma. These skin conditions affect an individual's appearance severely, leading to a whole host of psychological effects. Individuals become more self-aware and lose some aspect of self-worth due to the perceived flaws. This is not merely a cosmetic problem; the harmful effect can insidiously penetrate all aspects of life, including social relationships, occupational opportunities, and sex relationships. Heightened practitioner sensitivity to the psychological effects of skin disease can lead to a more compassionate approach to patient care. Treating these issues holistically may involve combining dermatologic treatments with counseling or psychotherapy so that patients can restore their self-esteem and improve their overall well-being, demonstrating that effective treatment of melasma and hyperpigmentation is a matter of more than just skin. There is also evidence that visual cues, i.e., the color and contour of one's facial features, play an important role in influencing one's feelings of self and self-esteem in patients with skin disease. According to current research, facial shape can be linked to differences in skin colors, and these are what influence the degree to which individuals judge themselves positively (Matsumoto et al., 2025). Individuals with melasma or hyperpigmentation, for instance, may internalize cultural ideals of beauty that value even and clean skin. This internalization is what compounds the issue of body image to create a vicious cycle of negative self-esteem and ongoing psychological distress. By recognizing these correlations, clinicians are able to more fully understand the visual and emotional dynamic at play, allowing for treatments that not only act on the skin, but on empower individuals to have more confidence in their own skin. Body image issues related to conditions like hyperpigmentation and melasma are also compounded by both gender-based differences in societal expectations and individual experience. Research has indicated that women suffering from such skin conditions report a lower quality of life and greater psychological distress compared to their male counterparts (Abeni et al., 2023). The discovery reflects the unique needs of female patients, including societal pressure to maintain beauty standards that require blemish-free skin. The psychosocial burdens borne by these women necessitate certain interventions that address aesthetic as well as emotional aspects of control. Through developing a caring environment that acknowledges the gender-specific burdens, healthcare professionals can empower women to build resistance against societal pressures, ultimately ending up with a healthy sense of self and improved mental health (Figure 3.17).

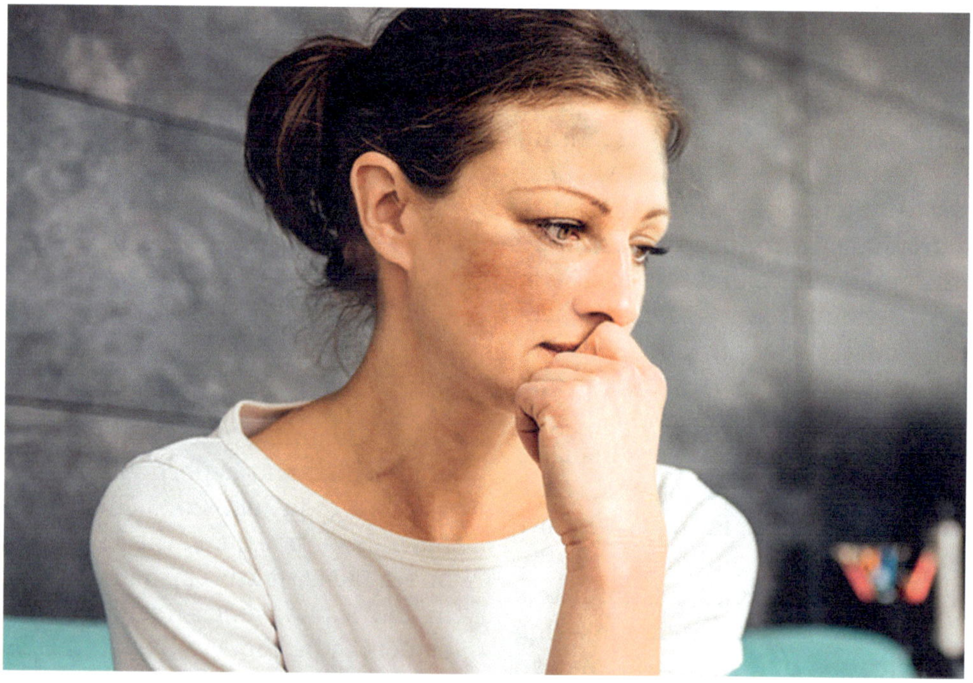

Figure 3.17. Emotional impact of facial hyperpigmentation on quality of life.

Source: https://www.reequil.com/cdn/shop/articles/The_Real_Impact_Of_Hyperpigmentation_On_People_s_Quality_Of_Life_desktop_reequil.jpg?v=1636445328.

3.6.2. Social Stigma and Discrimination

Social stigma and discrimination have a profound effect on patients with melasma and hyperpigmentation, generating negative social attitudes that tend to enhance psychological distress. Melasma and hyperpigmentation tend to produce perceptible discolorations, altering the affected person's appearance, inducing social prejudice and low self-esteem. Studies indicate that females, in particular, experience high levels of mental illness and a lower quality of life due to skin disease stigmatization. The psychological cost, added to social pressure to fit in with conventional beauty standards, usually amounts to isolation and social withdrawal. The social discredit can take various forms, from blatant discrimination to subtle prejudices, leading finally to interference in relationships and employment opportunities. In most societies, the process of dealing with hyperpigmentation is also made more difficult by the widespread practice of skin bleaching, driven by underlying beliefs in beauty and social status associated with lighter skin. In Nigeria, for example, the country has seen extensive use of skin bleaching products due to a cultural predisposition that associates lighter skin coloration with beauty and greater social standing. Despite the medical risks intrinsic in these products, women and even men, in some instances, will keep on using this practice so that they won't incur stigma by the color of their skin, showing the complex dynamics between social norms and personal health choices. This shows the need for public health initiatives that address not only the medical cases of hyperpigmentation treatment but also the cultural discussion leading to such behavior and eventually driving discrimination. Furthermore, increased education and awareness about hyperpigmentation can aid in overcoming social stigma. Affirmative skin representation campaigns that are initiated with a motive to overcome such unrealistic and damaging stereotypes are crucial in terms of redefining public opinion. As the psychological impact of discrimination upon patients suffering from diseases like melasma is profound, physicians must adopt a more comprehensive strategy that includes not just the physical condition but also the emotional and psychological sentiments revolving around such dermal ailments. In establishing an environment in which comprehension and acceptance are paramount, stigmatization of hyperpigmentation may be minimized, enhancing the quality of life for such patients as a whole. Hence, both public health interventions at the community level and broader public health strategies are important in avoiding discrimination and ensuring the successful treatment of melasma and hyperpigmentation among different populations.

3.6.3. Coping Strategies and Support

Management of melasma and hyperpigmentation is a multi-disciplinary approach as most of the patients seek both psychological and practical help to manage their conditions effectively. Patients can also experience emotional distress due to visible skin changes, which can affect self-esteem and lead to anxiety or depression. In preventing these psychological consequences, support groups and counseling services are relevant. Involvement in community resources allows patients the chance to offer support, validate feelings, and cope together. Positive reinforcement obtained through this interaction provides the individual with the resilience to view their skin condition in a positive manner and be strong and resilient as a whole. Additionally, healthy coping must include creating self-compassion, which can encourage an individual to seek proper medical consultation and treatment avenues appropriate for their needs. For treatment of melasma and hyperpigmentation, access to knowledgeable healthcare providers is essential for emotional and educational assistance. Not only do they treat, but also assist by providing useful information on dealing with daily activities. Open communication of potential side effects of treatment and realistic therapy expectations are essential components of patient assistance. This interaction assists in strengthening patient compliance with prescribed regimens and develops a sense of mutual partnership in the therapeutic endeavor. Second, educational material , such as pamphlets and online forums, can be employed to increase understanding, thereby dispelling myths about hyperpigmentation and melasma. This enlightened knowledge allows patients to make informed decisions concerning coping mechanisms, developing more control over their conditions. Maintenance care of melasma and hyperpigmentation often entails ongoing support and adaptation to shifting treatment settings. Frequent follow-up with dermatologists in an individualized approach can build confidence and promote ongoing discussion regarding the effectiveness of coping strategies employed. Additionally, formalized discharge processes , such as those outlined in recent studies, may facilitate a smoother transition from outpatient to self-care settings. For instance, utilizing standardized discharge information checklists would ensure patients are discharged with a clear awareness of their condition and care resources. These practices maximize healthcare outcomes while also enhancing the overall patient experience, thus allowing patients to manage their hyperpigmentation and melasma process better (Dlova et al., 2014; Harun et al., 2025) (Figure 3.18).

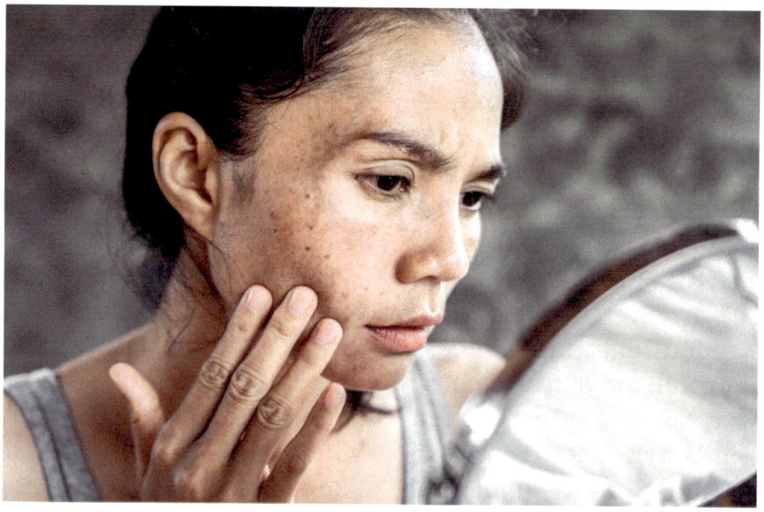

Figure 3.18. Self-examination of facial hyperpigmentation.

Source: https://healthaid.lemonaidhealth.com/wp-content/uploads/2024/08/Understanding-Hyperpigmentation_iStock-1171889653-1024x683.jpg.

Test Your Knowledge

1. How can visible hyperpigmentation affect an individual's self-esteem and body image?
2. What types of social stigma or discrimination might individuals with hyperpigmentation face?
3. What coping strategies can individuals use to manage the emotional impact of hyperpigmentation?

SUMMARY

The management of melasma and hyperpigmentation is a multidisciplinary one that is rooted in current dermatological literature and evidence-based interventions. The rising prevalence of these pigmentary conditions necessitates the application of effective therapies tailored to each patient's unique needs. Among all the therapeutic drugs, TXA has been a significant one due to its superior efficacy in reducing pigmentation and anti-inflammatory activities. Clinical trials have also shown that TXA not only decreases the apparent manifestation of melasma but also addresses the underlying inflammatory pathways responsible for hyperpigmentation, and therefore it is a promising candidate for overall management strategies (Górska et al., 2025). The role of photoprotection in the management of hyperpigmentation must not be underestimated either. UV radiation significantly contributes to the condition by causing melanogenesis and DNA damage, both of which play central roles in aggravating melasma. Emerging evidence verifies that photoprotection treatments, including the application of natural products like Fernblock®, provide additional protection from UV and visible light exposure. This not only avoids further pigmentation but also enhances ongoing therapies, enhancing patient outcomes for hyperpigmentation control (Rodríguez-Luna et al., 2023). Overall, on the basis of the literature and clinical experience, optimal results in hyperpigmentation and melasma will be achieved by an integrated treatment program that combines pharmacologic treatments with aggressive photoprotection. It is essential that further studies continue to evaluate and standardize these modes of treatment as more becomes known about their efficacy, safety, and mechanism of action. By coupling innovative treatments like TXA with preventive methods, healthcare providers can offer more effective, sustained relief for those with hyperpigmentation who are looking for an escape from the challenges it imposes (Rodríguez-Luna et al., 2023; Górska et al., 2025).

Treatment of melasma and hyperpigmentation demands a proper understanding of the underlying mechanisms of these diseases. Hyperpigmentation is increased melanin production determined by sun exposure, hormonal changes, and genetic predisposition. Melasma is a type of hyperpigmentation that predominantly affects women and is worsened by UV light exposure and endocrine imbalance, particularly during pregnancy or contraceptive use. Treatment of such conditions works best with a multi-modal approach that includes both pharmacologic treatments like TXA, as well as non-pharmacologic ones like sun prevention. Merging the etiology and pathophysiology, the clinician can better build individualized treatment plans targeting the specific etiology of pigmentation disorders. One important aspect of the management of melasma and hyperpigmentation is an exploration into a broad variety of different treatment modalities beyond conventional topical therapy. TXA has been the subject of research interest over the past several years as a drug with dual action as an anti-inflammatory and tyrosinase inhibitor, potentially providing considerable benefit to patients with such skin conditions. Clinical trials have proven the ability of TXA to successfully reduce hyperpigmentation and inflammatory responses, but published literature indicates that there is still a need for study into its longer-term safety and optimal dosing regimes. Other therapies like hydroquinone, laser treatments, and peels are each compounded by their respective limitations regarding efficacy, risk for side effects, and risk for recurrence, which illustrate the complexity of treating melasma (Górska et al., 2025). Technology also plays an important part in defining treatment strategies for melasma and hyperpigmentation. The application of nanotechnology in drug delivery systems presents a promising strategy for enhancing the effectiveness of topical treatment. Drugs can achieve better penetration within the skin and targeted delivery to areas of action through the application of nanoparticles, thus ensuring optimal therapeutic effects while limiting systemic absorption as well as side effects (Mokhtarzadegan et al., 2024). Further, as research continues to evolve, the integration of new formulations and innovative delivery methods could redefine current therapeutic regimens, improving patient compliance and satisfaction with the treatment of hyperpigmentation. The ongoing exploration of both pharmacologic and technological developments is a key shift towards more effective and personalized therapy in dermatology.

KEY TERMS FROM THIS CHAPTER

- Benign hypermelanosis
- Brightening creams
- Chemical peel
- Conventional drug treatment
- Dermatology community
- Facial hyperpigmentation
- Hormonal fluctuations
- Hyperpigmentation
- Hyperpigmented lesion
- Kojic acid
- Berloque dermatitis
- Broad-spectrum sunscreen application
- Chemical peeling
- Cosmetic-related concerns
- Dermocosmetics function
- Glycolic acid
- Hydroquinone
- Hyperpigmentation disorders
- Immunotherapy
- Kojic acid formulations

CRITICAL THINKING QUESTIONS

1. **Which of the following topical agents is considered the gold standard for treating melasma?**
   a. Azelaic acid
   b. Hydroquinone
   c. Kojic acid
   d. Tretinoin
2. **Triple combination therapy for melasma typically includes which three agents?**
   a. Hydroquinone, tretinoin, fluocinolone
   b. Azelaic acid, retinol, niacinamide
   c. Kojic acid, adapalene, clindamycin
   d. Tranexamic acid, retinoic acid, licorice extract
3. **What is the role of oral tranexamic acid in melasma management?**
   a. Tyrosinase inhibition
   b. Reduces UV-induced pigmentation directly
   c. Inhibits plasminogen activation and reduces vascular component
   d. Promotes desquamation of pigmented cells
4. **Oral tranexamic acid is thought to help in melasma by which mechanism?**
   a. Inhibiting tyrosinase activity
   b. Reducing mast cell degranulation
   c. Blocking plasminogen activation
   d. Enhancing dermal vasculature
5. **Which of the following lifestyle or environmental factors is most strongly associated with melasma exacerbation?**
   a. High-fat diet
   b. Smoking
   c. High humidity
   d. Ultraviolet and visible light exposure

Short Answer Questions

1. What are the primary differences between epidermal and dermal melasma in terms of clinical presentation and treatment response?
2. Which topical agents are commonly used in the treatment of melasma, and what are their mechanisms of action?
3. Discuss the role of sun protection in the management of hyperpigmentation and melasma. Why is it considered a cornerstone of treatment?
4. What are the indications and limitations of using chemical peels (e.g., glycolic acid, salicylic acid) in treating hyperpigmentation and melasma?
5. How do laser and light-based therapies work in the treatment of melasma, and what are the associated risks?
6. Explain the concept of PIH. What are the common causes and best practices for prevention and management?

Answer to Critical Thinking Questions

1. (b); 2. (a); 3. (c); 4. (c); 5. (d)

REFERENCES

1. Abdel-Sayed, P., Applegate, L. A., Hadjab, B., et al. (2024). Pilot clinical safety and efficacy evaluation of a topical 3% tranexamic acid cream and serum protocol for managing facial hyperpigmentation in Caucasian patients. https://core.ac.uk/download/631534027.pdf (accessed on 11th June 2025).
2. Abeni, D., Mattia, G., Matarrese, P., Alfani, S., Samela, T., & Malorni, W. (2023). Gender differences in vitiligo: Psychological symptoms and quality of life assessment description. https://core.ac.uk/download/596290287.pdf (accessed on 11th June 2025).
3. Adewoyin, A. A. (2020). Skin bleaching among female university students. https://core.ac.uk/download/346461990.pdf (accessed on 11th June 2025).
4. Al Abadie, M., Kubba, F., Patel, K. X., et al. (2024). Pathogenesis and update on the management of melasma. https://core.ac.uk/download/630039055.pdf (accessed on 11th June 2025).
5. Parveen, N., S. Ali, A., & A. Ali, S. (2019). On the Intricacies of Facial Hyperpigmentation and the Use of Herbal Ingredients as a Boon for Its Treatment: Cosmeceutical Significance, Current Challenges and Future Perspectives. IntechOpen. doi: 10.5772/intechopen.84257 (accessed on 11th June 2025).
6. Almeida, I., Ferreira, M., Magalhães, M. C., et al. (2021). Trends in the use of botanicals in anti-aging cosmetics. https://core.ac.uk/download/491506156.pdf (accessed on 11th June 2025).
7. Amoruso, G. F., Bennardo, L., Bennardo, S., Cannarozzo, G., Del Re, C., Negosanti, F., & Nistico, S. P. (2023). Q-switched Nd:YAG laser to manage hyperpigmentation in Asians: A multicenter study. https://core.ac.uk/download/590401236.pdf (accessed on 11th June 2025).
8. Bartonova, A., Bilanicova, D., Dusinska, M., et al. (2012). Associations between environmental factors and incidence of cutaneous melanoma: Review. https://core.ac.uk/download/622364720.pdf (accessed on 11th June 2025).
9. Bennardo, L., Cannarozzo, G., Fasano, G., Marigliano, M., Negosanti, F., Nistico, S. P., & Sannino, M. (2022). Fractional Q-switched 1064 nm laser for treatment of atrophic scars in Asian skin. https://core.ac.uk/download/592023342.pdf (accessed on 11th June 2025).
10. Bińczyk, W., Dróżdż, O., Lissak, K., et al. (2024). Topical treatment and aesthetic procedures in management of acne vulgaris. https://core.ac.uk/download/613694708.pdf (accessed on 11th June 2025).
11. Birlea, S., Bosenberg, M. W., Box, N. F., et al. (2018). Frontiers in pigment cell and melanoma research. http://arxiv.org/abs/1808.01869 (accessed on 11th June 2025).
12. Borkowska, A., Ciesielski, R., Izdebska, W., et al. (2024). Dermo cosmetics in the management of acne vulgaris. https://core.ac.uk/download/620863349.pdf (accessed on 11th June 2025).
13. Buainain de Castro Maymone, M. (2016). Skin hyperpigmentation disorders: Associations and impact on health-related quality of life. https://open.bu.edu/bitstream/2144/19513/1/BuainaindeCastroMaymone_bu_0017E_12224.pdf (accessed on 11th June 2025).
14. Callender, V. D., Dlova, N., Hollinger, J., et al. (2025). Updates in the understanding and treatments of skin & hair disorders in women of color. https://core.ac.uk/download/pdf/82678256.pdf (accessed on 11th June 2025).

15. Camargo, J., Mitjans Arnal, M., Maddaleno, S., et al. (2021). Melanogenesis and melasma treatment. https://core.ac.uk/download/479275602.pdf (accessed on 11th June 2025).

16. Dlova, N. C. N. (2014). *Ethnic Skin and Hair Disorders in Kwazulu-Natal: A Study of The Spectrum of Ethnic Skin and Hair Disorders, And the Composition and Use of Skin-Lightening Preparations, Traditional Cosmetics and Sunscreen.* https://core.ac.uk/download/196549925.pdf (accessed on 11th June 2025).

17. Dlova, N. C., Isaacs, T., Jacobs, T., et al. (2024). Integrated sun protection advice for the South African population. https://core.ac.uk/download/613869393.pdf (accessed on 11th June 2025).

18. Górska, A., Gniaź, N., Grela, W., Niewiadomska, J., Furtak, D., Tulej, D., ... Głogowska, P. (2025). Exploring the Role of Tranexamic Acid in Dermatology: A literature Review. *Journal of Education, Health and Sport, 77*, 56921. https://doi.org/10.12775/JEHS.2025.77.56921(accessed on 11th June 2025).

19. Fangmin, S., & Liu, L. (2024). Observation of the efficacy of different administration routes of tranexamic acid in the treatment of melasma. https://core.ac.uk/download/640063585.pdf (accessed on 11th June 2025).

20. Gautam, M. (2023). Management of epidermal hyperpigmentation with a novel depigmenting formulation: A research survey. https://core.ac.uk/download/588568112.pdf (accessed on 11th June 2025).

21. Gehlot, H., & Meena, M. (2018). A clinical study of skin disorders in pregnancy. https://core.ac.uk/download/543137095.pdf (accessed on 11th June 2025).

22. Rodríguez-Luna, A., Zamarrón, A., Juarranz, Á., & González, S. (2023). Clinical Applications of *Polypodium leucotomos* (Fernblock®): An Update. *Life (Basel, Switzerland), 13*(7), 1513. https://doi.org/10.3390/life13071513(accessed on 11th June 2025).

23. Granger, C., Krutmann, J., Lim, H. W., et al. (2023). Photoprotection for people with skin of color: Needs and strategies. https://core.ac.uk/download/555344410.pdf (accessed on 11th June 2025).

24. Khoo, Y. T., & Halim, A. S. (2021). Treatment modalities for hyperpigmented skin lesions: A brief overview. *Journal of Surgical Dermatology*, *7*(1), 29-37. https://doi.org/10.18282/jsd.v7.i1.35 (accessed on 11th June 2025).

25. Harun, N. A. (2025). Factors influencing discharge decisions in dermatology outpatients: Checklist and educational methods to support appropriate discharge. https://core.ac.uk/download/444030925.pdf (accessed on 11th June 2025).

26. Kim, T. H. (2021). *Depigmentation*. https://core.ac.uk/download/478113284.pdf (accessed on 11th June 2025).

27. Matsumoto, S., Nagashima, M., Tanikawa, C., et al. (2025). Association between the three-dimensional facial shape and its color in a boundary group of young to middle-aged Asian women. https://core.ac.uk/download/621342804.pdf (accessed on 11th June 2025).

28. Mokhtarzadegan, M., Kiafar, M. R., Ghasemiyeh, P., Fazlinejad, R., Rasekh, S., & Mohammadi-Samani, S. (2024). Different therapeutic approaches in melasma: Advances and limitations. https://core.ac.uk/download/614681802.pdf (accessed on 11th June 2025).

29. Özkoca, D., Hügül, H., Kirişçi, M., & Kutlubay, Z. (2023). Treatment indications of carbon solution-assisted Nd:YAG laser according to patient satisfaction: A retrospective study. https://core.ac.uk/download/591490855.pdf (accessed on 11th June 2025).

30. Tagua Moyolema, A. E., Toasa Zumbana, V. E., Velastegui Hernández, R. E., Velastegui Hernández, et al. (2024). Dermatitis de Berloque: Un problema estético en la dermatología moderna. https://core.ac.uk/download/620857060.pdf (accessed on 11th June 2025).

VITILIGO: COSMETIC CAMOUFLAGE AND SURGICAL OPTIONS

4

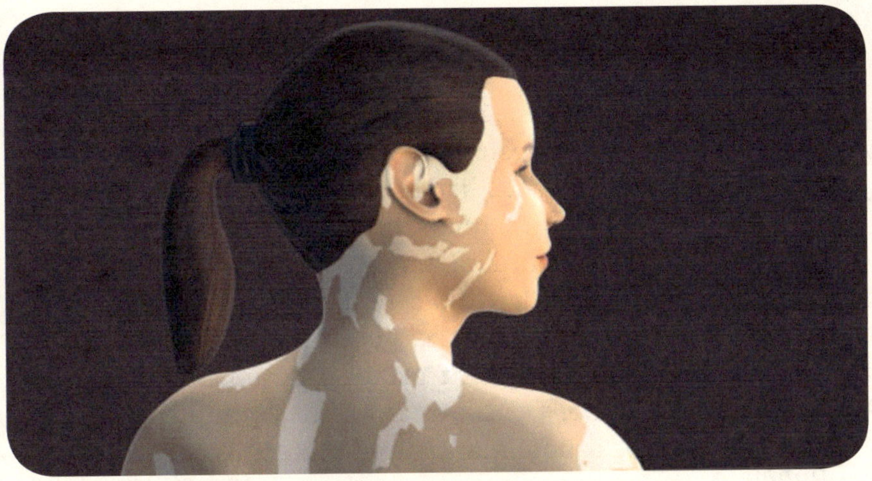

LEARNING OBJECTIVES

After studying this chapter, you will be able to:

1. Understand vitiligo
2. Describe cosmetic camouflage techniques
3. Explain surgical options for vitiligo
4. Focus on the effectiveness of cosmetic camouflage
5. Discuss the effectiveness of surgical options
6. Deal with societal perspectives on vitiligo

Introduction

Vitiligo is an illness that involves the progressive loss of melanocytes, the cells that produce skin pigment, with the formation of depigmented lesions of very variable size and distribution, often having severe psychological and social implications for the patient. The exact etiopathogenesis of vitiligo is not yet known, but it is commonly believed that both environmental as well as genetic factors, , such as physical trauma and stress, play an important role in its induction as well as progression. Understanding these background processes is essential not only to maximize diagnostic efficacy but also to maximize therapeutic approaches designed to manage the condition optimally, making research into vitiligo an important area of contemporary dermatological inquiry (Witek et al., 2025). Therapeutic management of vitiligo is multimodal and involves cosmetic as well as medical treatment. Available treatments range from topical, , such as corticosteroids, to systemic, , such as JAKis, each with variable success depending on the case in question. While some patients achieve adequate repigmentation with therapy, others remain resistant, a reflection of the disease's heterogeneity. Surgical options, like melanocyte transplantation, also form part of the options, even for segmental vitiligo. These developments underscore the ongoing need for evidence-based information to underpin understanding of the treatment modalities, considering that patient reactions may be implicit and difficult to predict (Witek et al., 2025). Apart from the existing surgical and medical interventions, the psychosocial impact of vitiligo cannot be overstated. The majority of patients with vitiligo experience concerns with identity, self-esteem, and social acceptance, which have a significant impact on the quality of life. Therefore, camouflage treatment of cosmetic concerns—like with the use of specialist makeup—is increasingly in the spotlight as a subsidiary treatment to medical intervention. This conflation of cosmetic camouflage and surgical treatment highlights the need for an integrated treatment plan for vitiligo sufferers that addresses both the physical and emotional concerns of those with vitiligo. Proceed with current research investigating these dimensions in order to enhance the quality of life and treatment response for individuals affected by this complex disorder.

Definition of Vitiligo

Vitiligo is a chronic skin condition that occurs with progressive loss of melanocytes, cells responsible for synthesizing melanin and is characterized by discrete lesions of depigmented skin. Loss of melanocytes occurs due to autoimmune destruction, genetic influences, or environmental influences, thus leading to diverse presentations in different individuals. It can affect any age group, but it often occurs in the initial three decades of life. Vitiligo significantly affects the general quality of life, transcending social relationships, psychological status, and patient self-esteem. Interestingly, understanding vitiligo is more than its clinical image because it typically signifies more inherent social problems involving beauty standards and stigmatization of skin imperfections. The classification of vitiligo is broken down into two main categories: generalized and localized. Generalized vitiligo is seen with large patches that are symmetrically distributed all over the body, while localized vitiligo is seen in the form of small areas of depigmentation but also showing a tendency to occur at specific sites, such as hands, face, or genital areas. Clinicians should be aware of the subtypes as they direct the treatment plan.

Treatment can vary quite significantly, from topical corticosteroids and phototherapy to more advanced types like surgical treatments aimed at repigmentation of the skin. According to the most current data, improving quality of life in patients with vitiligo remains a challenge for treatment, and it takes good communication and adapted treatment protocols from healthcare personnel (Atkar et al., 2022). Although this is not a potentially life-threatening condition, there are objections to the psycho-emotional load of vitiligo. The visible features of this skin pathology have a tendency to expand social exclusion, shame, and anxiety in patients. Consequently, the pursuit of cosmetic therapies, such as camouflage products, has been widely desired as a means to enhance self-perception and alter the aesthetic look of affected sites. Cosmetic camouflage conceals patches so that people can engage more freely in social activity; however, it is important to understand that this approach must not be regarded as a permanent solution. Instead, it is an addition to existing treatment, which may include surgical procedures like skin grafts for the management of severe vitiligo, creating an umbrella treatment for maximizing patient outcomes (Lai et al., 2018) (Figure 4.1).

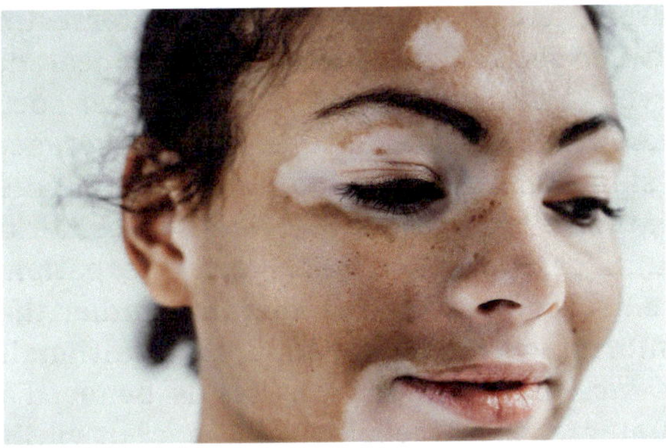

Figure 4.1. Facial depigmentation in a patient with vitiligo.

Source: https://www.verywellhealth.com/thmb/7Z6GNskwIsIqcGf8EG-ZDRN8pb4=/1500x0/filters:no_upscale():max_bytes(150000):strip_icc()/GettyImages-1310862767-eabc3042c93e44939122c50a7b89a0f7.jpeg.

Prevalence and Demographics

Its incidence varies worldwide, and prevalence is estimated to affect one to two percent of the global population. Vitiligo is beyond color, age, and sex, and it presents a unique dermatological challenge. Interestingly, though vitiligo equally affects populations in demographically diverse groups, its psychosocial impact can differ vastly according to culture. Regions with higher stigmatization of more apparent skin ailments tend to suffer more from the mental well-being and health of individuals. For instance, vitiligo has been known to lead to embarrassment, stress, and anxiety and thus becomes hard to handle and calls for a combined measure in its treatment that involves both medicine and psychological treatment (Witek et al., 2025). Understanding demographic aspects surrounding such experiences is critical to delivering care that is shaped to meet the needs of vitiligo patients from various backgrounds. Demographically, vitiligo has been observed to occur in quite even gender distribution, with occasional male predominance reported in some populations in studies. Age at onset is also relevant, with vitiligo most often developing in individuals during childhood or adolescence and having continuing impacts on self-esteem and social adjustment throughout their lifetime. The psychological impact is particularly important; those with early diagnosis might struggle with body image issues, extending into adulthood. In addition, in light of certain ethnic groups, the prevalence may appear higher based on environmental factors or genetic susceptibility, further complicating the epidemiological landscape of vitiligo. This population's awareness allows the medical professional to set individualized support systems and regimens (Witek et al., 2025), hence striving for better outcomes for each patient afflicted by the condition. A thorough examination of population parameters is needed for a thorough understanding of the magnitude of the effect of vitiligo on quality of life (QoL). It has been reported by research that patients with vitiligo experience moderate impairment of QoL, which can be attributed to both cosmetic concerns and social stigmatization (Agaba et al., 2017). The lack of existing research studies that focused on residents of specific regions, , such as Sub-Saharan Africa, indicates a significant gap in the literature. Understanding differences in prevalence and societal attitudes towards vitiligo across regions can inform interventions addressing both the medical and psychosocial determinants of the condition. Through heightened awareness and effective communication in clinical practice, health practitioners can strengthen support networks for patients and help them receive holistic care in which the psychological dimensions of their vitiligo experience are addressed.

Importance of Addressing Cosmetic Concerns

The requirement to correct cosmetic defects in patients with vitiligo extends beyond mere looks; it encompasses the severe psychological effects of the disease. Vitiligo affects not just the skin but also the self-worth and social lives of individuals. Patients report embarrassment and isolation due to their disfigurement, generating increased anxiety and depression. As highlighted by research, the psychosocial impact of such a visible illness has a drastic impact on quality of life that necessitates interventions aimed at emotional well-being as well as physical health care. Incorporating cosmetic interventions like camouflage therapies, the patients will be in charge of their looks once again and therefore sustain a better self-perception and lessen the psychological pressure put upon them by vitiligo (Eleftheriadou, 2013). Thus, cosmetic management of these problems becomes not only preferable but also important in overall management. In recognition of the importance of the treatment of cosmetic problems, the use of effective treatment for vitiligo becomes indispensable. While treatment procedures , such as topical corticosteroids and phototherapy have already been recognized, there is an imperative need to combine these treatments with cosmetic camouflage techniques, which have already proved useful in supporting patients' emotional resilience. The investigations of treatment uncertainties among patients clearly indicate that many of these patients desire beautiful results, indicating a shared need for treatments that balance functionality and appearance (Eleftheriadou, 2013). Second, it is critical to improve the quality of evidence that precedes those treatments to make effective clinical recommendations. Thus, there needs to be further study in developing strict evaluation systems that will be able to assess the effectiveness of cosmetic treatments in addition to standard therapies, so that patients will be given the tools to deal with the physical and psychological aspects of vitiligo. In addition to this, knowledge of the sociocultural associations of vitiligo can also enlighten one on the importance of treating cosmetic concerns in a larger sense. Individuals suffering from vitiligo are prone to face the social views that weigh heavily on conforming to mainstream traditional definitions of beauty, thereby feeling inadequate. This intersection between social identity and physical appearance serves to underscore the need to foster social awareness and tolerance towards differences in skin complexion. By promoting combined treatment approaches, including cosmetics, health care providers can facilitate patients to embrace their unique identities rather than conforming to societal models. Additionally, the fact that cosmetic therapy is believed to counteract the psychological impact of vitiligo highlights the need to treat not only the visible aspects of the disease but also the social and emotional ramifications of the condition, paving the way for future research and intervention strategies centered on holistic patient care (Khalid et al., 2025).

4.1. Understanding Vitiligo

Learning Outcome

1. Explain the causes and triggers of vitiligo
2. Understand the types of vitiligo
3. Describe the psychological impact on individuals

Vitiligo is a multifactorial disorder of the skin caused by depigmentation of the cells of the skin known as melanocytes. It results in abnormal pigmentation of the skin, with various sizes and positions of patches on the body. The etiology of vitiligo remains multifactorial, encompassing genetic predispositions, autoimmune reactions, and environmental triggers. It is noteworthy that the psychological impact of vitiligo can be widespread, often causing self-consciousness, distress, or social stigma in the case of those with darker skin, where the color contrast of depigmented sites is maximized. Cosmetic concerns in such cases create inquiry into several cosmetic and therapeutic modalities, reflecting a desire to normalize skin tone and minimize the emotional cost of this disease. In the pursuit of treatment for therapy, cosmetic camouflage techniques and surgical interventions have been well developed. Using cosmetic camouflage technique , such as specially designed cosmetics and pigmenting products, people can conceal depigmented skin and feel more normal and self-assured when socializing. Therapeutic depigmentation can also be seen as a type of therapy for individuals seeking a more even appearance. Additionally, surgical procedures like melanocyte–keratinocyte transplantation have emerged as potential repigmentation strategies, varying by patient success rate. Knowledge about these differing approaches is important not just for excellent patient management but also for the establishment of correct expectations for outcome, particularly when navigating the complexities of this disorder (Eleftheriadou, 2013).

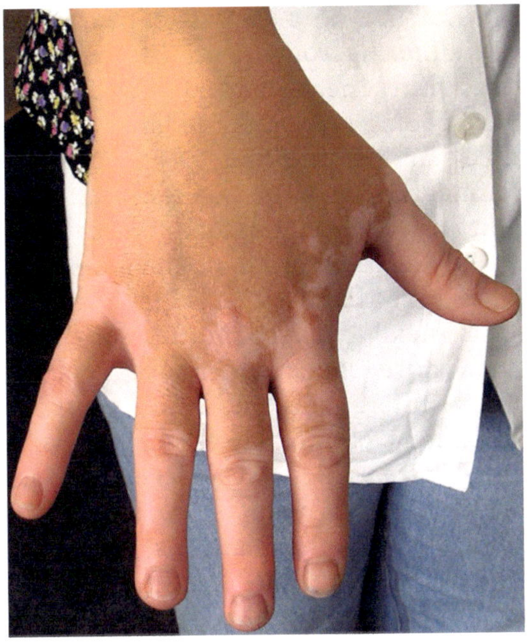

Figure 4.2. Vitiligo on lighter skin.

Source: https://upload.wikimedia.org/wikipedia/commons/thumb/6/64/Vitiligo03.jpg/800px-Vitiligo03.jpg.

New research offers further insight into vitiligo and its treatment techniques. More advanced methods, such as co-culturing melanocytes and keratinocytes, attempt to maximize cellular interaction and melanin production to improve surgery. For instance, investigating the broad spectrum of ratios and responses of these cells to biochemical stimuli , such as αMSH, emphasizes the intricate biological processes at stake with treatments for vitiligo. Apart from that, clinical trials are on-going assess the quality of life of patients who suffer from vitiligo, as well as the efficacy of treatments, acknowledging the strong emotional resonance this disease carries. By focusing on whole treatment modalities that consider both psychological and somatic influences of the disease, scientists and practitioners seek to develop integrated approaches that consider complex meanings (Shetty,2020) (Figure 4.2).

4.1.1. Causes and Triggers

The precise etiology of vitiligo is not known, though it is widely accepted to be an autoimmune condition with multifactorial causation of the progressive loss of melanocytes, the cells responsible for the production of pigment. Genetic factors play an important part, as there is evidence that people who have a history in their family of vitiligo or of other autoimmune diseases are at higher risk of developing this skin condition. Environmental factors make things all the more complicated; precipitants , such as skin trauma, ultraviolet rays, and certain psychosocial stresses have also been implicated in the onset or exacerbation of vitiligo. What this suggests is that there is a synergistic relationship between endogenously based genetic vulnerabilities and aberrant external environmental stressors that synergistically work together to play a part in the disease pathogenesis, suggesting the subtle interrelationship between heredity and environmental lifestyle in the development of vitiligo (Witek et al., 2025). Of all the environmental precipitants, stress is likely the best-documented precipitating or aggravating factor in vitiligo. Not only is psychological stress unhealthy in general, but it may also induce inflammatory reactions that have a tendency to destabilize the immune system and cause autoimmune disease to continue. The discoloration of the skin, which can be seen, may bring about great psychological distress in patients, leading to a cycle of stress and withdrawal, thereby aggravating their condition. In addition to stress, cuts and sunburn may be observed to cause depigmentation in susceptible patients. This suggests that while the genetic background provides a stage upon which vitiligo is played out, environmental precipitants with particular reference to stress and cutaneous trauma are major determinants of disease onset and course (Li et al., 2024).

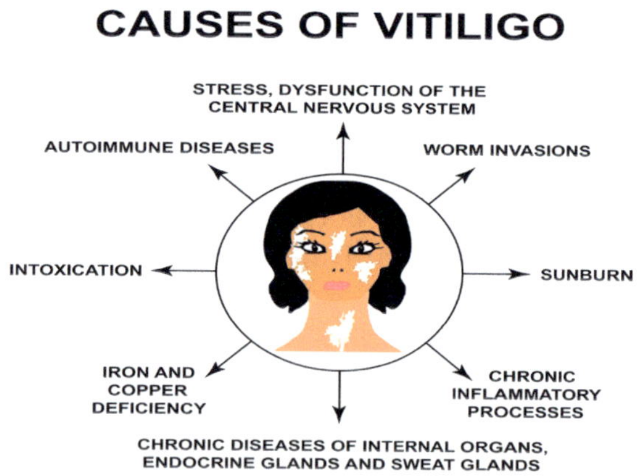

Figure 4.3. Causes of vitiligo.

Source: https://drdeepikashomeopathy.in/wp-content/uploads/elementor/thumbs/Causes-of-Vitiligo-r4q8wc5upv9b6jhjzp4p8rw0zgmnwrwa20oauyplly.jpg.

The identification of vitiligo as a condition influenced by both genetics and the environment requires an integrative management approach with goals not merely towards treatment but towards healthy coping behavior on the part of patients. Evidence indicates that interventions , such as JAKis have demonstrated efficacy in curing refractory vitiligo, most so on very conspicuous locations like the face and hands. Coupled with pharmacological therapy, managing psychological impacts with counseling or support groups can go a long way in enhancing the quality of life of those who are suffering from the emotional implications of having vitiligo. Furthermore, the inclusion of cosmetic camouflage techniques provides an instant repair for patients who must conceal depigmented spots until the outcome of long-term therapy is achieved. Both these multi-faceted solutions aim to improve not only physical looks but overall quality of life in patients with vitiligo (Witek et al., 2025) (Figure 4.3).

4.1.2. Types of Vitiligo

Vitiligo, characterized by well-defined skin depigmentation, can be broadly classified into two main types: non-segmental vitiligo and segmental vitiligo. Non-segmental vitiligo is the most prevalent type, occurring in nearly 90% of patients suffering from the disorder. It is further classified into generalized and localized vitiligo, the latter being presented as large patches in multiple parts of the body, while the former is confined to specific smaller regions. The volatility of non-segmental vitiligo typically brings significant psychological challenges, to the extent that it affects patients of any age and racial background, thereby making patients more concerned about appearance and social interaction. The emotional effect is higher among children, who may experience lower self-esteem and social acceptance under perceptible skin change, correlated with findings showing the disease's psychological stigma in child patients (Lai et al., 2018). Segmental vitiligo, on the other hand, has a patchier distribution and tends to precede the occurrence of white patches which are uniformly distributed in certain segments bordered by normally pigmented zones. Segmental vitiligo progresses more rapidly than non-segmental vitiligo and stabilizes in a few months to a few years. Segmental vitiligo typically occurs in young people, thereby particularly significant in the context of therapeutic considerations, as the physical symptoms play a major role in socialization. The relative stability of this pattern over time can offer some reassurance to patients and caregivers; however, the cosmetic implications are increasingly a worry that is too commonly followed by consideration of both cosmetic camouflage techniques and surgery to re-establish skin coloration (Lai et al., 2018).

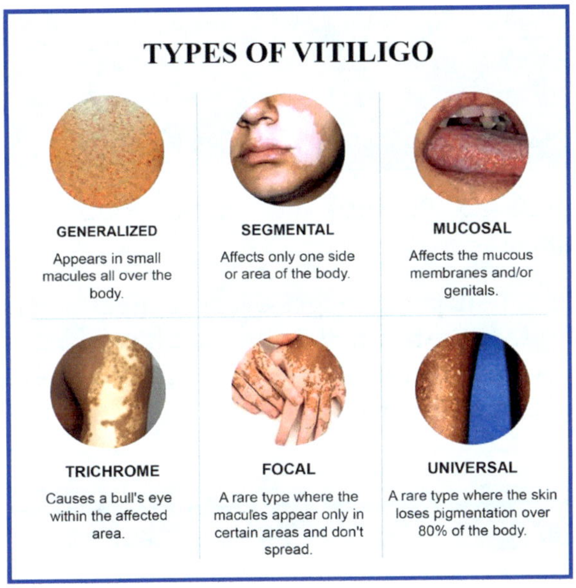

Figure 4.4. Types of vitiligo.

Source: https://www.mehektaguldermaclinic.com/template/mehektaguldermaclinic_com/images/Infographics/Types-of-Vitiligo.webp.

An understanding of the different types of vitiligo is paramount in planning treatment that addresses both the physical and psychological requirements of the disease. While cosmetic camouflage offers instant visual assistance in the management of vitiligo appearance, operation through skin grafting or micropigmentation can be performed in people who seek more permanent interventions. The selection of these treatments typically considers the type of vitiligo, the patient's age, and the degree of skin involvement, which underscores the significance of individualized treatment protocols. As emphasized in recent publications, the integration of therapeutic interventions that incorporate surgical and non-surgical methodologies can significantly contribute to the improvement of the quality of life of vitiligo victims, given the potential for psychological trauma associated with the disease (FranÃ§a et al., 2018) (Figure 4.4).

4.1.3. Psychological Impact on Individuals

The psychological impact on the individual of vitiligo can be profound, extending to self-esteem, body image, and general mental health. Most of the patients are extremely upset by perceptible changes in the skin, which embarrass them and lead to social apprehension. Studies have shown that individuals with vitiligo keep themselves away from social dealings to avoid stigmatization or judgment from others. The unpredictable and autoimmune nature of vitiligo can then act to exacerbate these emotions, as the afflicted must cope with an illness that is both perceptible and not well understood. Witek et al. (2025) point out that the psychological effect extends beyond concerns of appearance, becoming strongly entangled in the self-concept of the afflicted. This can thus precipitate depression and anxiety disorders, and so a clear need exists for appropriate psychological intervention in combination with the medical treatment of vitiligo. In contemplating interventions for vitiligo, one should note the efficacy of cosmetic camouflage and surgery as interventions, both of which can significantly influence an individual's mental status. Products for cosmetic camouflage serve as a non-surgical option through which patients can disguise differences in their skin, thus potentially enhancing self-esteem and social ease. But while such products can cover up the condition, they do nothing to alleviate the underlying emotional trauma that many individuals endure. On the other hand, surgical intervention , such as melanocyte transplant, are more permanent but then maybe have their own psychological strings attached, such as concern about efficacy and recovery. Lai et al. (2018) mentions that the importance of weighing these alternatives has not only to do with physical outcomes but also with the manner in which these affect the quality of life as well as the mental well-being of patients. Psychological care as part of the treatment protocol for vitiligo is essential. Health care providers must realize that effective treatment for vitiligo is not just based on clinical management; it also encompasses counseling and psychiatric care. Support groups, where shared wisdom will contribute to the construction of coping skills, can benefit from the participation of patients. Health care providers ought also to be educated in the psychology of chronic cutaneous illnesses in order to be able to provide holistic care. As emphasized in Witek et al. (2025), the evolving definition of vitiligo must include the psychosocial nature of the condition to help broaden therapeutic care addressing both physical and emotional needs. Integrated approaches of this type can alleviate the psychological strain and allow individuals to embrace their identity in spite of skin differences (Figure 4.5).

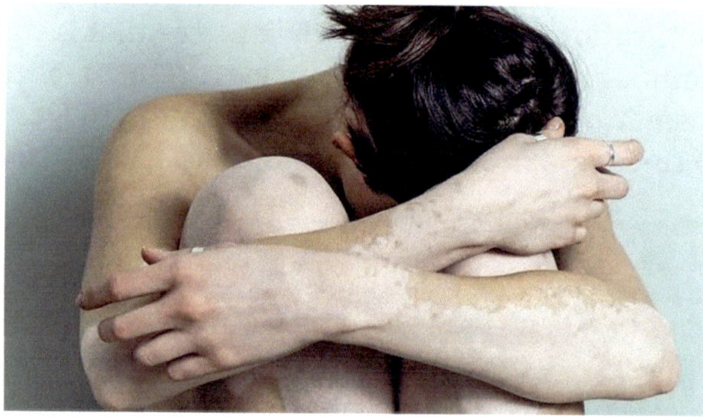

Figure 4.5. Physical and emotional burden of vitiligo.

Source: https://images.everydayhealth.com/images/skin-beauty/vitiligo/vitiligo-physical-and-emotional-complications-722x406.jpg?sfvrsn=5886b434_1.

Test Your Knowledge

1. What are the primary causes of vitiligo, and how does the immune system contribute to its development?
2. What are the main types of vitiligo, and how do they differ in terms of appearance and distribution on the body?
3. How does vitiligo affect self-esteem and social interactions, especially in adolescents and young adults?

4.2. Cosmetic Camouflage Techniques

Learning Outcome

1. Describe makeup products for vitiligo
2. Understand tanning lotions and sprays
3. Discuss skin dyes and pigments

Cosmetic camouflage techniques have emerged as crucial tools for those afflicted with vitiligo, a disease that entails depigmentation of the skin and may cause great psychological discomfort. Such techniques involve the application of expertly designed makeup that is employed to conceal effectively depigmentation patches, thereby enhancing the aesthetic look of the subject as well as general self-confidence. Some products, , such as dermablend foundations and water-resistant creams, have also been specially made to match the natural shade of the user's skin. This personalized application allows users to continue with their day without the hassle of evident patches on the skin, particularly critical among children and youths because the social pressures of these years of development tend to further activate feelings of inadequacy regarding one's skin. Moreover, not only does cosmetic camouflage have practical applications, but it also provides emotional rewards to vitiligo patients. With these methods, patients can perhaps experience some relief from the psychological burden of their illness, typically including low self-esteem and social withdrawal. Actually, the method of blending skin colors and lowering visibility enhances the confidence level of the wearer during social encounters such that they can participate more fully in daily interactions without the ever-present fear of color-based discrimination. The psychological advantages gained from camouflage procedures are also instrumental in enhancing quality of life because they enable individuals to show themselves in a way that makes them feel like themselves, promoting a more favorable self-perception (Lai et al., 2018). Aside from the psychological effects, consideration should also be given to the fact that cosmetic camouflage is sometimes combined with other treatments for vitiligo. While there are medical therapies and surgical treatments, the success of the treatments is variable and not every patient wants to seek out invasive treatment. For some, use of non-invasive therapy and cosmetic camouflage may be a comprehensive plan for treating the condition. This combined treatment plan speaks to the need for ongoing education and resources available that allow one to make informed choices about his or her appearance and health. With increased awareness being generated about cosmetics, it can help raise overall health awareness about how vitiligo impacts patients and guide healthcare professionals in delivering complete care that addresses physical and psychological needs (Lai et al., 2018).

4.2.1. Makeup Products for Vitiligo

The use of makeup materials as a cosmetic camouflage for vitiligo is a pressing field that promises more self-esteem and confidence to the individuals who undertake it. Vitiligo or depigmentation patches on the body tend to affect the psychological state of mind in addition to its visible impact. Thus, cosmetic interventions in terms of makeup that camouflage the patches can be an important aspect in a human's life. Many beauty firms have taken heed of this need and produced specially formulated products like concealers, foundation, and dermatologically approved cosmetics that are both effective in coverage and non-irritating on sensitive skin. The treatments tend to aim to match perfectly with surrounding skin color to reduce the visual contrast of depigmented areas. This practice is also evident in the growing realization of the need for beauty products that provide inclusivity towards diverse skin conditions, hence empowering individuals with vitiligo and making them more accepted in society. Choice of makeup products among people with vitiligo must also take priority in maintaining skin health as well as cosmetic functionality. Most of the product line today uses innovations in formulation technology, so they are not only effective for camouflage on depigmented skin but also as low-irritancy and reaction-reducing as one can get. Data on safety and tolerability are useful because vitiligo patients may sometimes be overly sensitive. It should be noted that such cosmetics may contain ingredients that are not only moisturizing and nutritious, providing overall skin care, but also functioning in their planned cosmetic function. Also, encouraging dermatological testing of cosmetics helps users to safely rely on these products without worrying that their condition might worsen or their skin deteriorate. These are important in fostering an integrative way of living with and depicting vitiligo. The profound role that cosmetics play in regulating the appearance of vitiligo also necessitates ongoing discussion on how society perceives and embraces vitiligo. Most individuals affected by this skin condition are plagued by feelings of self-consciousness, particularly when dwelling in societies where depigmented skin is not welcomed. As cosmetic camouflage gains popularity, it is no longer a means of covering up skin blemishes but also a statement of empowerment and self-acceptance. The increasing visibility of makeup products specifically formulated for vitiligo challenges conventional beauty standards, making society adapt to a changed perception of diverse presentations of the skin. Furthermore, this innovation is evidence of increasing recognition of the psychological effects of skin diseases and the call for diversity in the beauty industry. By proper application of makeup commodities, vitiligo patients are more able to socialize, thus creating a sense of tolerance and understanding towards skin diversity within public discourse (Eleftheriadou, 2013; Witek et al., 2025) (Figure 4.6).

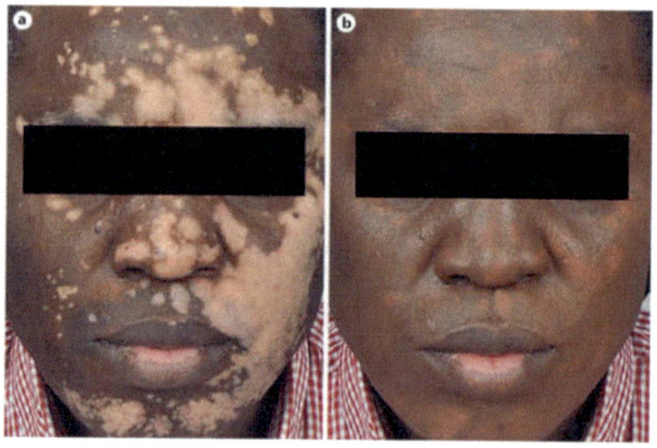

Figure 4.6. Patient with vitiligo before (a) and at the end (b) of the medical corrective make-up lesson.

Source: https://www.researchgate.net/profile/Lucie-Peuvrel/publication/228114439/figure/fig3/AS:280409016422407@1443866127132/Patient-with-vitiligo-before-a-and-at-the-end-b-of-the-medical-corrective-make-up.png.

4.2.2. Tanning Lotions and Sprays

The use of tanning sprays and lotions is fast becoming popular as a cosmetic procedure among people suffering from vitiligo who seek to have an equalized skin tone. The said products, which are often made up of active ingredients , such as dihydroxyacetone (DHA), act on the amino acids present in the skin to give the skin a bronzed appearance without exposing it to harmful ultraviolet (UV) radiations. This non-invasive approach is of most interest to those with vitiligo since it allows temporary camouflage of mottled pigmentation. Second, products targeted at inducing evenness and camouflage of skin color can increase the self-esteem of shoppers, providing a psychological boost in social situations where one's skin appearance is subject to scrutiny. However, the efficacy of the tanning lotions and sprays can be quite variable among buyers. Skin type, existing pigmentation levels, and manner of application could all influence the end result. Additionally, results aesthetically could differ vastly from one person to the next and could lead to potential dissatisfaction. As noted in Brazil, where cultural beliefs concerning sun exposure and skin color are diverse, the popularity of tan products shows an interest in embracing the sun-kissed look while coping with diversity in the skin color. Consensus of the Brazilian Society of Dermatology promotes the need for educated use of the products, particularly in sun-exposure zones with high levels of exposure, where skin cancer incidence is rising amazingly (Abarca et al., 2014). Safety is also an important aspect of the tanning lotion and sprays debate. Even though such products are a replacement for sunbathing, the user must be mindful of the necessity for nonsensitizing and hypoallergenic preparations, especially in sensitive skin or pre-existing conditions like vitiligo. Not being tested as extensively as drugs, most over-the-counter tanning products are of low risk if applied properly. Nevertheless, sensitivity to potential allergic reactions or abnormal application must be appreciated. The dermatology world is increasingly acknowledging the importance of educating users with proper application skills and how to take care of their skin so that aesthetic desires do not compromise dermatological safety (Adaskevich et al., 2016) (Figure 4.7).

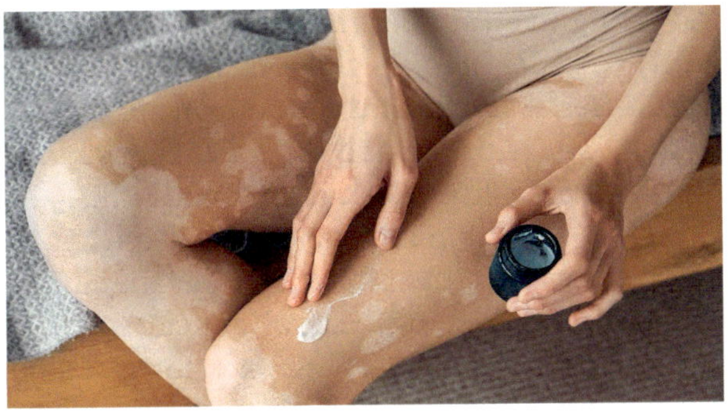

Figure 4.7. A woman applying cream for skin with vitiligo.

Source: https://media.post.rvohealth.io/wp-content/uploads/2024/02/woman-applying-cream-skin-vitiligo-1296x728-header.jpg.

4.2.3. Skin Dyes and Pigments

Local application of skin pigments and dyes is now a major focus in cosmetic management of vitiligo, a procedure that involves destruction of melanocytes and consequently skin pigment. Because individuals with vitiligo form visible patches of depigmentation, the only way to enhance their quality of life is through cosmetic camouflage. The traditional methods of pigment repigmentation, like topical repigmentation, have certain drawbacks, particularly in darker-skinned patients who have more contrasted patches. Thus, skin dyes resembling natural skin pigmentation have been a topic of interest in the field of dermatology. They are not only designed to deliver an aesthetically attractive look but also prioritize durability as well as skin compatibility, providing patients with a stable choice to use daily to manage the condition (Witek et al., 2025). In addition, the performance of skin pigments and dyes can be strongly connected to cultural definitions of beauty and skin color. Depigmentation is, in the majority of communities, particularly darker skin complexions, not just a medical condition but also a psychological and social concern. The association between identity and skin color has led to a market that is full of products that are cosmetic in nature and designed to provide solutions to the different skin types (Eleftheriadou, 2013). Patients tend to seek products that are not only effective in a practical sense but also provide emotional solace and social acceptance. Hence, understanding the cultural meaning of cosmetic solutions to vitiligo treatment enhances the process of product development such that the solutions offered are not only effective but also desirable to the diverse experiences and needs of the afflicted individuals. While cosmetic therapy, including skin dyes, represents a less invasive means of managing vitiligo, it is not complication-free. The addition of surgical procedures, , such as melanocyte transplantation, adds an important complement to cosmetic camouflage, particularly in patients in need of more definitive therapy. The suitability of surgical procedures will frequently be related to issues of depigmentation size, the patient's skin and general health. New treatments are also being created, merging cosmetic and surgical methods to yield comprehensive treatment plans focusing on patient-specific needs. With each advancement in knowledge in comprehending vitiligo, studies still examine where cosmetic treatments and surgery intersect, eventually converging into holistic care that will treat aesthetic and emotional themes of managing vitiligo (Witek et al., 2025).

Test Your Knowledge

1. What types of makeup products are most effective for concealing vitiligo patches, and how should they be applied for long-lasting coverage?
2. Are tanning lotions and sprays safe and effective for people with vitiligo, and what precautions should be taken when using them?
3. What are the differences between temporary and semi-permanent skin dyes or pigments used to camouflage vitiligo?

4.3. Surgical Options for Vitiligo

Learning Outcome

1. Describe skin grafting procedures
2. Understand depigmentation therapy
3. Discuss laser treatments in the management of vitiligo

The surgical procedures for vitiligo are mostly utilized for improving cosmetic outcomes of patients, particularly if other conventional therapies are ineffective. Among the therapies, skin transplantation, in the form of split-thickness or full-thickness grafting, is quite commonly applied. It entails taking healthy skin from a healthy donor site and transplanting it to the depigmented zone. Success rates do vary, and the size of lesions, their location, and the age of the patient all affect outcomes. While skin grafting can restore color in localized vitiligo, it also can result in mismatched colors and textures, which complicates the overall appearance. Considering these potential drawbacks, it is of utmost importance that patients receive thorough consultation from dermatological specialists so they can effectively comprehend the advantages and disadvantages of undergoing surgical treatment. Another novel method of surgery is melanocyte transplantation, a more advanced process wherein melanocytes are extracted from patients' healthy skin and cultured in a lab setting before applying them to areas with vitiligo. The technique has been popular because it can restore the pigmentation more consistently than grafts. Melanocyte transplantation is extremely suitable for stable vitiligo patients because it decreases the chances of repigmentation failure. Its technicality and the requirement of special skills can however, be obstacles to its mass application. Given the psychological impact of vitiligo on individuals, especially children, this method may be an interesting avenue to enhance self-esteem and quality of life in patients. As noted, vitiligo impacts self-esteem and quality of life greatly, which means learning about surgical procedures in individuals who have it is critical (FranÃ§a et al., 2018). In balancing the surgical option for vitiligo treatment, the efficacy and availability of such surgeries remain central concerns. While laser treatment, , such as the excimer laser, has emerged as a non-surgical alternative, surgery has special advantages in terms of how long the treatment lasts and how certain the outcome can be. Adding surgery to the regimen as part of a combination treatment may be the best option, particularly when coupled with counseling to provide psychotherapeutic support. Finally, as the practice develops further, it's critical that further research attends to how these surgical procedures are improved, whether they work effectively in the long term, and how patients' inevitable emotional reactions to alterations in their skin appearance are better understood. In addition, research , such as the suggested non-randomized trial of surgical excision versus laser therapies is evidence of the necessity for evidence-based guidance to direct clinical practice more effectively (Lai et al., 2018).

4.3.1. Skin Grafting Procedures

Skin grafting procedures are now well known to be an effective surgery in patients suffering from vitiligo, particularly when other treatment methods do not yield much progress. Skin grafting is performed by transferring the skin from a donor area, usually a healthy pigmented area, to the depigmented areas on the skin due to vitiligo. This technique is not only aimed at reversing typical pigmentation but also at the significant psychosocial morbidity associated with the disease. As mentioned, Vitiligo is a substantial childhood skin condition that could lead to psychological trauma and decreased quality of life (FranÃ§a et al., 2018). Skin grafting is therefore cosmetic and psychological as well, improving the health and wellbeing of those afflicted by it. Of various skin grafting techniques used in treating vitiligo, punch grafting and split-thickness grafting are the most effective. Relative to others, punch grafting was found to achieve repigmentation of over 75% in certain cases, which was in agreement to restore aesthetic symmetry to the skin (Sureka et al., 2017). This technique involves the excision of small, rounded sections of normal skin and translocation to the sites of depigmentation. While punch grafting has been documented with promising outcomes, one should be aware of the side effect of cobblestone skin or hyperpigmentation developing, which can mar the good-looking outcomes achieved (Sureka et al., 2017). Hence, while being effective, care providers must weigh the benefits and potential drawbacks of this procedure. This combination of skin grafting with a complete therapy regimen for vitiligo can maximize the potential for successful therapy. The optimal cosmetic results are obtained by most practitioners using surgical interventions plus adjunct therapy , such as phototherapy or topical agents, as noted in comparisons to punch grafting in studies.

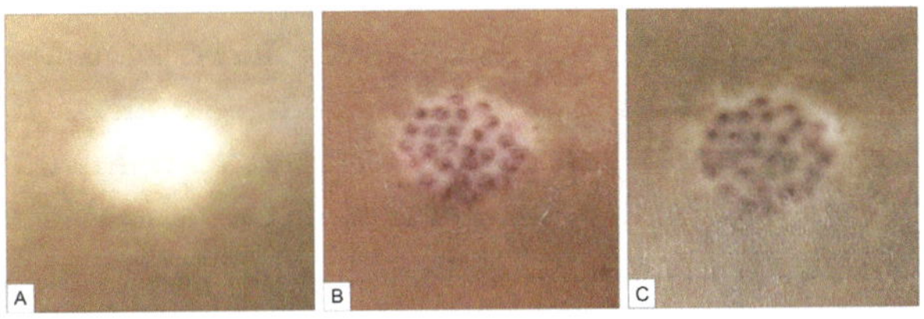

Figure 4.8. Punch grafting (a) patch of vitiligo; (b) punch grafting after 1 week; and (c) after 6 months showing almost complete repigmentation.

Source: https://www.researchgate.net/profile/Vishal-Thakur-8/publication/352319651/figure/fig2/AS:1056551825575937@1628912993962/Punch-grafting-a-patch-of-vitiligo-b-punch-grafting-after-1-week-and-c-after-6.jpg.

These adjuncts can improve repigmentation and patient satisfaction with cosmetic results. Interestingly, a survey of patients' responses revealed that the patients who received combination treatments were more satisfied with their cosmetic outcome (Sureka et al., 2017). Thus, a multidisciplinary treatment involving skin grafting procedures in association with other therapies provides an integrated solution to treat vitiligo effectively, addressing both physiological and psychological effects of the disorder (Figure 4.8).

4.3.2. Depigmentation Therapy

Depigmentation therapy becomes a necessary component of therapy in vitiligo, especially if the patient has widespread skin involvement. Depigmentation therapy is employed to depigment the pigmented residual skin evenly in such a manner that it can match the color of the depigmented skin, thereby achieving an even appearance. Although repigmentation therapy can help most patients, patients with widespread vitiligo may seek depigmentation in an attempt to achieve cosmetic satisfaction . The treatment itself also typically utilizes topical medications, , such as hydroquinone or corticosteroids, and may further utilize laser therapy or chemical peels to bring more effectiveness. The psychological impacts of the treatments may also be complex since patients may have difficulty with external perceptions of beauty as well as their sense of self in terms of changing skin color. Although having some utility, depigmentation therapy does present controversies and hazards. There have been accounts of many patients reacting intensely emotionally to being treated with this, with mixed feelings of jealousy towards their otherwise depigmented skin against the ongoing social stigma that still clings to vitiligo. Furthermore, the treatment is a long-term process, with patients needing to maintain the coloration of the skin that has been achieved with constant application and checkup. Depigmentation is also known to lead to increased susceptibility to exposure to the sun, necessitating intense photoprotection to shield against the harmful effects of ultraviolet light. Taking these considerations into account, physicians and patients need to have intensive discussions to understand the complexities of depigmentation and its role in a multi-faceted treatment regimen for vitiligo (Witek et al., 2025). Therefore, opting to receive depigmentation therapy warrants serious consideration, emphasizing the need for individually designed treatment plans that address the physical and psychological features of vitiligo. Practitioners are challenged to balance demands for cosmetic improvement with a recognition of potential emotional implications and bodily damages associated with skin lightening. With so much more research being discovered, it is possible to have dermatologists, psychologists, and support groups included within a multidisciplinary treatment, informing patients in their entirety about their options and providing an affirmative environment. In the end, the goal is to empower patients with vitiligo to make informed choices about their skin, balancing clinical efficacy with personal values and social context (Witek et al., 2025) (Figure 4.9).

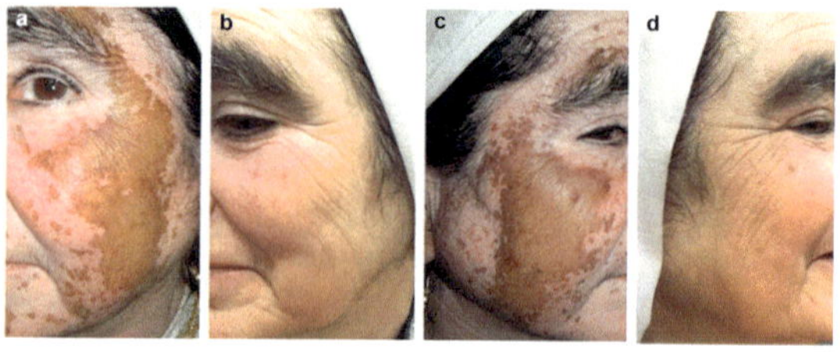

Figure 4.9. (a, b) Residual pigmentation on the face in universal vitiligo. (c, d) Persistence of therapeutic results after 4 years of follow-up.

Source: https://www.researchgate.net/publication/314279473/figure/fig2/AS:960344830783510@1605975458840/a-b-Residual-pigmentation-on-face-in-universal-vitiligo-c-d-Persistence-of-therapeutic.gif.

4.3.3. Laser Treatments

Laser therapies have become a viable option in treating vitiligo, especially among those patients who want cosmetic camouflage and surgery. Laser therapies, employing intense beams of light to cure pigmented or depigmented skin, can stimulate repigmentation by encouraging melanocyte proliferation and migration. Research has identified that certain lasers, , such as the 308 nm excimer laser, are found to be beneficial in treating vitiligo patches. This form of treatment is particularly helpful for patients who have been refractory to standard therapy , such as phototherapy or topical corticosteroids, thereby increasing the repertoire of possible treatments for patients with this debilitating illness. The addition of laser treatment to an adequate management plan can thus significantly enhance the total aesthetic outcome for vitiligo patients, effectively enhancing their quality of life. In a practical sense, the laser therapies are an elegant way of treating vitiligo that is both aesthetically and psychologically gratifying. Evidences show that laser treatments can create visible improvements in complexion and are often followed by minimal downtime. Compared with more invasive surgical alternatives, laser treatment is conducive to being performed as an outpatient, which appeals to the majority of patients. Furthermore, ongoing clinical studies aim to define the most effective laser protocols to gain superior repigmentation results. By analyzing these lasers' precise mechanisms and optimal applications, dermatologists are able to enhance their treatment strategies for vitiligo, offering a customized therapy that responds to the distinct requirements of their patients. This adaptability provides laser therapy with an essential role in the changing landscape of vitiligo therapy. While the potential benefits of laser treatments are significant, there are also limitations and various patient responses that need to be considered. Not all vitiligo patients will experience equally good outcomes with laser therapy, since duration of disease, skin type, and extent of depigmentation are significant predictors of treatment outcome. Furthermore, as reflected in the current literature, laser treatment comparisons with other modalities, e.g., surgical removal, emphasize an ongoing need for further information on each treatment's impact on the patient's quality of life. Clinical studies, e.g., measurements of the total well-being before and after treatment, will help determine evidence-based protocols for the application of laser therapy in dermatological practice. As research continues to advance, future breakthroughs are likely to bridge knowledge gaps that exist as of the writing and, ultimately, clinicians will have guidance to develop comprehensive treatment modalities for vitiligo patients (Witek et al., 2025; Lai et al., 2018) (Figure 4.10).

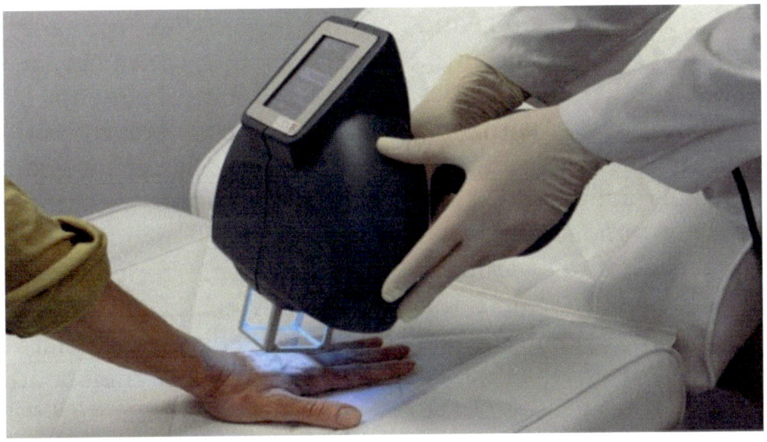

Figure 4.10. Excimer laser for vitiligo treatment.

Source: https://drgeetanjalishetty.in/wp-content/uploads/2023/10/1520164073021.jpg.

Test Your Knowledge

1. What are the different types of skin grafting procedures used in vitiligo treatment, and which patients are considered suitable candidates?
2. How does depigmentation therapy work, and when is it recommended as a treatment option for vitiligo?

4.4. Effectiveness of Cosmetic Camouflage

Learning Outcome

1. Describe short-term and long-term results
2. Focus on user experiences and testimonials
3. Deal with the limitations of cosmetic solutions

Cosmetic camouflage is a valuable tool in managing the visible effects of vitiligo and proves to be an essential factor in the emotional and psychological well-being of patients. As vitiligo is an occurrence of disappearance of skin color due to melanocyte destruction, the patients not only experience physical change but also social stigma and self-image issues. Cosmetic commodities that replicate the inherent color of skin are useful at this juncture. The success of such products is that they have the potential to carry instant visual improvement with them, and the patient can return to being confident in the manner in which they appear. Additionally, effective cosmetic camouflage has the potential to enable patients to engage in more active social contact without fear based on their skin disorder (Witek et al., 2025). Consequently, not only is cosmetic camouflage practical, but it also offers positive body image and social integration for those who have vitiligo. While cosmetic camouflage offers advantages, its use can be significantly varied between individuals, based on skin type, extent of depigmentation, and personal application ability. The formation of these products is crucial; good-quality cosmetics that are water-resistant and possess sufficient opacity will cover better and be more durable throughout the span of daily activities (Lai et al., 2018). More importantly, patient education on the proper use of the technique and product selection is necessary in order to realize the maximum benefit of cosmetic camouflage. Dermatologists and skin therapists can enhance patient results by being able to prescribe individualized products and provide application methods that suit individual needs. It must be said, however, that cosmetic camouflage, as beneficial as it is, does not resolve the condition of vitiligo, a fact that reinforces the necessity for the full treatment strategies alongside cosmetic therapy. In reality, while cosmetic camouflage is a basic part of the therapy for vitiligo, it is secondary to, but not a replacement for, medical treatment. Patients can find that a dual strategy provides the ideal result as today's research continues to explore more fully the numerous forms of treatments, including surgery and topical therapy. Methods like laser therapy and melanocyte transplantation, although being surgical methods, have the function of replenishing the pigmentation and can potentially enhance the utility of cosmetic camouflage in long-term management of vitiligo (Lai et al., 2018). Thus, a team of medical professionals, dermatologists, and cosmetics experts can provide all-around care to the patients. By integrating cosmetic camouflage into care together with surgical therapies and other therapies, healthcare workers are more likely to manage the cosmetic as well as the psychological components of having vitiligo, and this ultimately equates to an improvement in the quality of life for the sufferers.

4.4.1. Short-Term vs. Long-Term Results

Treatment of vitiligo by cosmetic camouflage and surgery has a duality of short- and long-term results, which have a dramatic effect on the quality of life of patients. Short-term treatments, , such as cosmetic camouflage, produce instant cosmetic satisfaction and enhance self-esteem. The preparations allow individuals to temporarily camouflage depigmented lesions, so they appear more evenly toned. This short-term remedy typically achieves psychological benefits, giving victims relief from social stigma and emotional pain attached to their condition. However, these are naturally transitory; camouflage's efficacy relies on consistent usage and can be erased, necessitating constant effort and upkeep from the victim. On the other hand, long-term measures like surgical intervention, , such as melanocyte transplant and depigmentation therapy, provide an opportunity for further long-term change of skin pigmentation. Prolonged, taxing, and expensive though these may be, they also hold the potential to remain effective longer in changing the look of the skin and have been hailed for their capability to redefine a more natural skin color. But the road to achieving successful long-term results could be fraught with risk, including complications and the possibility of subtotal repigmentation. The psychological scenario of such decisions also complicates decision-making, as patients must weigh the prospect of permanent change against the risks and challenges of taking such decisions. Thoughtfully assessing short-term and long-term results shows a complex interplay between immediate gratification and long-term outcomes of vitiligo treatment. The psychological impact of vitiligo is high, and this has resulted in many people looking for treatments that provide quick aesthetic satisfaction. As seen, there is evidence of the emotional burden of living with vitiligo, especially among children, where low self-esteem is a product of their condition (FranÃ§a et al., 2018). Meanwhile, long-term therapy techniques can sometimes elicit a paradoxical response, such that cosmetic success can spark jealousy from those who want the same outcome, highlighting the dynamic tension between cosmetic treatments and self-concept (Eleftheriadou, 2013). Ultimately, intervention choice must be weighed in an integrated approach, with consideration of personal preference, psychological impact, and varied levels of efficacy for both time-limited alternatives (Figure 4.11).

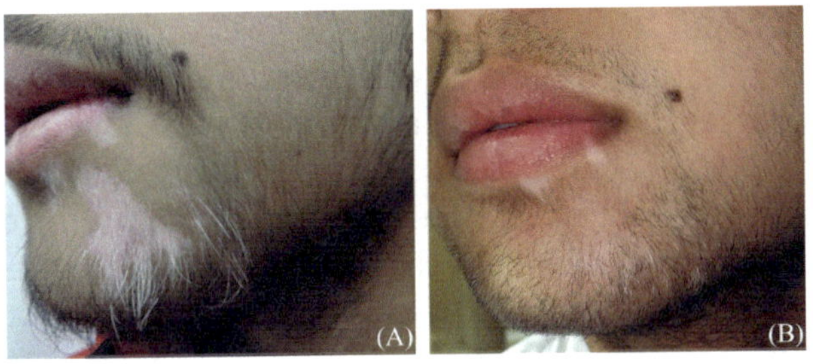

Figure 4.11. (A) Segmental vitiligo with leukotrichiasis; and (B) Excellent response after 28 doses of excimer light therapy.

Source: https://www.researchgate.net/publication/340736693/figure/fig1/AS:1143128117381472 6@1689056470921/A-Segmental-vitiligo-with-leukotrichiasis-B-Excellent-response-after-28-doses-of.png.

4.4.2. User Experiences and Testimonials

Perceptions and feedback from the users are critical to understanding the impact of vitiligo on an individual's life, particularly in terms of cosmetic camouflage and surgery. The majority of vitiligo patients describe their feelings of discomfort and isolation due to the visibility of their skin condition. For instance, anecdotal evidence suggests that clients who have used cosmetic camouflage measures find that they experience a boost in confidence, which enables them to engage more confidently in social interactions. Testimony highlights how products utilized for concealing skin not only provide beauty enhancement but are also a psychological defense against the stigma attached to skin color discoloration. Such criticism facilitates user involvement in product design and highlights the wider social importance of cosmetic interventions, which can radically alter the self-perception of individuals with vitiligo. In addition to cosmetic camouflaging, surgical interventions , such as skin grafting or depigmentation therapy are now available as options for vitiligo treatment. User responses are likely to range from satisfaction to disenchantment based on the procedure's success and the patient psychological set. As noted in wide-ranging reports on scar management, patients undergoing therapy for vitiligo are likely to undergo increased anxiety and expectation, developing a complex psychological picture in their process of healing. While there are individuals empowered by surgical interventions, others face challenges in the recovery process and still need to be supported by medical providers. Understanding such varied experiences is important for researchers and clinicians who seek to maximize treatment processes and inform patients on realistic outcomes of surgical interventions. Notably, the contribution of support from the community to user experiences of vitiligo should not be downplayed. The majority of individuals find comfort and camaraderie in sharing their experiences via forums, support groups, or social websites. The sites provide a platform where the participants can exchange reviews regarding cosmetic and surgical options that play a major role in decision-making. Furthermore, anecdotes that prove the treatment of vitiligo through camouflage or surgery have a strong motivating effect on individuals who have recently been diagnosed with the condition. The experience of the patients collectively provides meaningful lessons that are used to improve the treatment policies and education of the patients. Such community narrations are not anecdotal; they belong to common sense used in advancing knowledge and care of vitiligo, focusing on cosmetic and surgical treatments, compared with procedures described in books like Textbook on Scar Management (Gauglitz et al., 2021).

4.4.3. Limitations of Cosmetic Solutions

Cosmetic products, , such as camouflage cosmetics, are frequently employed by individuals with vitiligo to achieve a more uniform coloration of the skin. While these products can provide short-term appearances that can serve to increase one's confidence, several significant disadvantages are involved in their use. Some of the notable limitations include high maintenance on such solutions, wherein they need to be reapplied several times during the course of a day, particularly for active individuals or in hot climatic conditions, which could lead to smudging or wear and tear. Moreover, these cosmetic treatments are not generally found to blend the shifting hues of the skin naturally, particularly for individuals with progressive vitiligo, thus leading to an unnatural appearance. These issues highlight the functionality and impermanence of cosmetic concealment as a definitive solution for vitiligo, highlighting the urgent need for more stable strategies for dealing with the cosmetic concerns of individuals affected by this condition. No less concerning is the psychological burden typically associated with the reliance on cosmetic treatment in vitiligo patients. Even though these products aim to empower the users, they will perpetuate feelings of inadequacy or self-consciousness if the intended cosmetic appearance is not achieved. From studies, individuals with vitiligo will tend to experience higher anxiety and social retreat, where they are relying solely on camouflage products to conceal their condition. This psychological load comes on top of the societal beauty and appearance standards of the skin, leaving the affected individual trapped in a never-ending cycle of dissatisfaction. The constraints of cosmetic therapy, therefore, extend beyond matter-of-fact issues, , such as profound mental health impacts that disrupt the overall well-being of individuals afflicted by vitiligo, in which there is a requirement for a prolonged intervention incorporating psychological care in addition to cosmetic therapy. Cosmetic therapies are also less effective in altering the underlying pathology of vitiligo. Pharmacological or surgical procedures are treatments that hold the promise of repigmentation, whereas cosmetic treatments merely camouflage the condition and never address its causes or effects. While evaluating outcomes of treatment, studies now emphasize more patient-report measures, which assess patients' satisfaction with appearance alongside the effectiveness of treatments (Batchelor et al., 2014). For instance, clinicians' varying perceptions of what constitutes treatment success are likely to highlight the limitations of isolated use of cosmetic camouflage. How noticeable the vitiligo is and how well the skin tone matches become crucial issues, and these are areas where cosmetic interventions may fall short. Thus, it is crucial to combine cosmetic treatments with comprehensive treatment plans that prioritize holistic health and address both cosmetic and psychological dimensions of existence with vitiligo.

Test Your Knowledge

1. How do the short-term results of cosmetic camouflage compare to long-term outcomes in managing the appearance of vitiligo?
2. What do user testimonials and personal experiences reveal about the day-to-day effectiveness and confidence boost provided by camouflage products?

4.5. Effectiveness of Surgical Options

Learning Outcome

1. Understand the success rates of surgical interventions for vitiligo
2. Describe risks and complications using surgical options for vitiligo
3. Deal with patient satisfaction and follow-up care

The success of surgical treatments in vitiligo has gained popularity due to the failures of the conventional treatment methods. Among various methods, melanocyte transplantation has become the leading operation among the best surgical treatments for those with localized vitiligo who have failed to receive proper treatment through medicine. It involves the transfer of healthy melanocytes from pigmented skin to depigmented skin. The success of this process is subject to factors , such as the nature of the recipient site, the process used, and the surgeon's experience. Studies confirm that patients with non-progressive, stable vitiligo have better results from the process, which highlights the importance of selecting appropriate candidates for the process to achieve optimal therapeutic gains (Witek et al., 2025). Apart from melanocyte transplantation, other surgical techniques like skin grafting have been researched as possible treatments for vitiligo. Skin grafting is accomplished by the excision of depigmented skin and covering the site with grafts of the patient's normal skin. While cosmetically acceptable outcomes may be achieved through skin grafting, the invasive nature of the procedure might dissuade certain patients. Furthermore, it entails careful consideration of the risk of donor site complications and the need for scrupulous postoperative care. The success of grafting can vary with recipient site parameters, including skin texture and color compatibility, and this can complicate long-term results. These are considerations that both patient and clinician must keep in mind when surgical therapies are being considered for managing vitiligo (Witek et al., 2025). Even current studies continue to broaden the range of surgical treatments, offering promises to the victims of vitiligo. Current research continues to aim for more specific guidelines and more precise patient selection criteria for surgical interventions. For instance, newer studies have proposed comparing the success rates of different approaches, , such as surgery versus laser treatments, not only in terms of achieving desired cosmetic outcomes but also in terms of the well-being of patients. As the medical profession continues to develop its knowledge base regarding the pathophysiology and reaction to different treatment regimes, surgical interventions will continue to adapt in their design and efficacy, offering more tailored and effective solutions for sufferers of this troublesome condition (Witek et al., 2025).

4.5.1. Success Rates of Surgical Interventions

The outcomes of surgical treatments for vitiligo, in that they are melanocyte–keratinocyte transplantation procedures (MKTP), lend credence to the essence of the challenge of treating this skin condition effectively. Research indicates that while current methods are capable of yielding positive results, there is variability in results that offers justification for better techniques. Factors , such as the patient's skin type, the extent of depigmentation, and prior emotional impact on the individual are all significant in determining the overall success of such treatments. A recent systematic review highlighted the scarcity of good-quality literature, citing that the majority of studies reporting discrepant success rates are confounded by low sample size and heterogeneity, making it challenging to have uniform clinical guidelines (Eleftheriadou, 2013). These limitations call for more tightly controlled trials to provide an effective basis for the effectiveness of surgery in vitiligo treatment. Increased research into combining new technology with surgical methods will undoubtedly improve success rates significantly. Recent attempts at simplifying the MKTP procedure bring cell-based technology to the point of identifying melanocytes and keratinocytes, which are thereafter co-cultured with one another in various combinations (Shetty,2020). This novel approach not only aims to enhance repigmentation outcomes but also tries to address the psychological effect of vitiligo in patients. The enhancement observed in early pilot trials implies that optimizing cellular preparation can potentially succeed in restoring pigmentation better. However, larger trials are necessary to validate these initial observations. With the progressing discipline, it becomes necessary that researchers place patient-based outcomes at the forefront in rewriting the success tale of surgical procedures for robust decision-making in clinics.

The evolving situation of vitiligo surgery also brings forward the component of long-term follow-up and judicious measurement of outcomes. Traditional approaches, e.g., percentage repigmentation, are not often capable of measuring patient satisfaction and cosmetic acceptability variability, of most significance for establishing the surgical success of such treatment (Eleftheriadou, 2013). Outcome measures based on cosmetically acceptable repigmentation are suggested in the present research to be used as a primary objective, more in line with patient and physician needs. While these new standards become a reality, it becomes evident that surgical procedures must not only aim towards visible alteration in skin pigmentation but also enhance the quality of life among vitiligo patients. This broad perspective establishes success in surgical procedures more universally, implying that effective treatments go beyond cosmetic alteration to encourage emotional health (Figure 4.12).

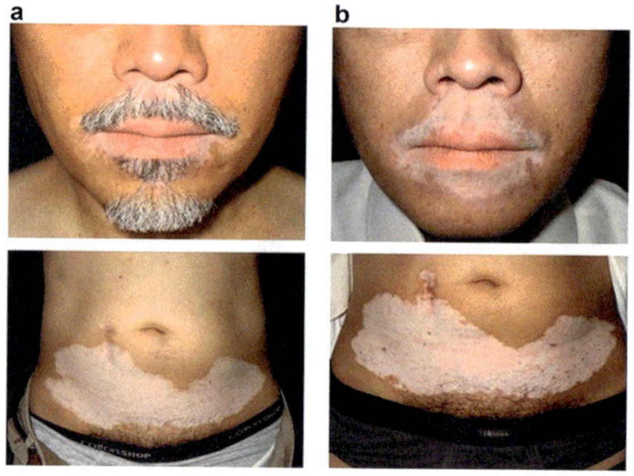

Figure 4.12. Treatment of generalized vitiligo in case 24. (a) Before surgery. (b) One year after treatment of the upper and lower lips, abdomen, and both hands (not shown). The outcome was assessed as no change.

Source: https://www.researchgate.net/publication/256613839/figure/fig5/AS:195810353520644@1423696234548/Treatment-of-generalized-vitiligo-in-case-24-a-Before-surgery-b-One-year-after.png.

4.5.2. Risks and Complications

In evaluating cosmetic camouflage and surgery for vitiligo, one must be aware of the several risks and complications that could result. Cosmetic camouflage preparations, while generally safe, have the potential to cause skin irritation or an allergic response in a few patients. Repeated use can also induce changes in skin texture or may worsen underlying disease, such as eczema, and thus good selection and a physician's advice are imperative. Additionally, camouflage efficacy is not always identical, and at times it can lead to dissatisfaction when the appearance is not as anticipated by the patients. Individuals must be educated regarding the extent of the products, supporting the need for an open discussion with doctors so that they choose the options based on their preference and skin type, avoiding unwanted reactions and enhancing general satisfaction with treatment outcomes. Surgical therapies of vitiligo, , such as melanocyte transplantation, also carry their share of potential risks and complications. Though the procedures have been successful in inducing significant cosmetic alteration in segmental vitiligo, they are invasive and carry a risk of scarring or infection at the donor site. Moreover, the success of transplantation is unreliable, with a lot of factors influencing the degree of repigmentation, , such as the skin type, and the length of time that they have had vitiligo. Postoperative morbidity can also include alterations in skin texture or mismatches of pigmentation, leading to cosmetic discontent. The patients must have an adequate pre-surgical interview to be informed of these risks and weigh these against advantages, which would help them in informed decision-making for their treatment plan. Furthermore, the psycho-emotional consequences of undergoing cosmetic camouflage and surgery cannot be overlooked. Treatment for vitiligo often becomes conflated with cosmetic concerns and psychological state, as societal pressures can foster feelings of inadequacy or concern about appearance. Social reintegration after treatment is often an emotional process, potentially solidifying beliefs of isolation or frustration if expectations are not met. Mental health intervention, alongside dermal care, is essential to address these complications in an integrated manner. Multidisciplinary approach, as highlighted in contemporary research to improve outcomes in treatment, emphasizes incorporating psychological well-being into the discussions of vitiligo management and treatment (Lai et al., 2018; Witek et al., 2025). This method ensures that patients are given integrative care directed at their physical as well as emotional needs in the context of this often stigmatized disease.

4.5.3. Patient Satisfaction and Follow-Up Care

Patient satisfaction is paramount in the treatment of vitiligo, particularly regarding interventions available to them, ranging from cosmetic camouflage to surgery. Patients' personal experience often hinges on their perception of the effectiveness of treatment and aesthetic outcomes achieved. Research indicates that patients tend to focus more on the psychological impact of vitiligo, prioritizing an acceptable cosmetic outcome of repigmentation over basic dermatologic parameters, i.e., percentage repigmentation. This is also in line with findings that emphasize the need for treatments that not only address the visible features of vitiligo but also improve the overall quality of life and self-esteem of individuals with the condition. Patient satisfaction measurement should, therefore, extend beyond clinical parameters to include holistic outcome parameters that are a true reflection of patients' perceptions and expectations. Follow-up is crucial in the maintenance of patient satisfaction and control of patient expectations in vitiligo patients. Follow-up attendances offer patients an opportunity for clinicians to assess the effectiveness of treatment modalities chosen, different protocols to achieve optimal patient outcomes. Research shows that open communication during these follow-up consultations is imperative in bringing treatment goals in line with patient expectations. Additionally, the use of institutionalized feedback mechanisms, in the guise of questionnaires measuring treatment satisfaction, will be able to guide clinicians towards better practices. These measures not only help monitor the efficacy of cosmetic camouflage and surgical interventions but also promote patient involvement, enabling them to voice their concerns and preferences. Accordingly, a robust follow-up care program is critical in creating a therapeutic alliance between healthcare workers and patients. Moreover, the lack of standardized treatment protocols for managing vitiligo highlights the need to develop evidence-based guidelines that meaningfully include patient experience. Research studies funded by the National Institute for Health Research highlight the need to prioritize the development of patient-reported outcomes as an immediate priority in clinical trials. By actively engaging patients in the creation of the research agenda, the medical community can identify and address important uncertainties around treatment choice. Such engagement not only promotes patient involvement but also guarantees that future studies consider the actual needs and concerns of individuals with vitiligo. Incorporating evidence from pilot trials and systematic reviews can enhance informed treatment choices and patient satisfaction. Lastly, reinforcing the correlation of adequate follow-up care, patient participation, and clinical research has the potential to introduce more effective management systems in vitiligo treatment (Eleftheriadou, 2013) (Figure 4.13).

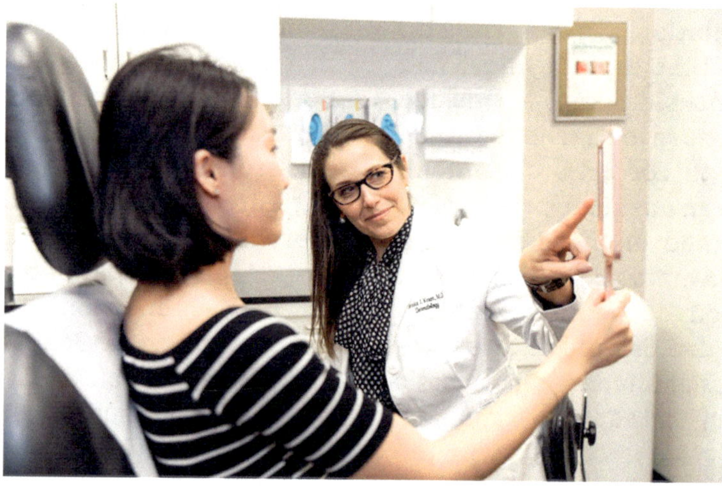

Figure 4.13. Dermatological consultation for facial aesthetic evaluation.

Source: https://www.laserskinsurgery.com/wp-content/uploads/2020/03/Dr_Krant_Filler_Female_Cheeks_New_York_NYC_55468-scaled.jpg.

Test Your Knowledge

1. What are the reported success rates of various surgical interventions for vitiligo, , such as skin grafting and melanocyte transplants?
2. What are the most common risks and complications associated with surgical treatments for vitiligo, and how can they be minimized?
3. Are surgical treatments more effective for certain types or stages of vitiligo, and how does patient selection influence the results?

4.6. Societal Perspectives on Vitiligo

Learning Outcome

1. Describe the stigma and discrimination associated with vitiligo
2. Focus on representation in media and culture
3. Understand support networks and advocacy

Vitiligo is not only a medical disorder; it is a social issue that affects and is affected by beauty and normalcy constructs. Vitiligo patients often face stigma, discrimination, and ignorance from society, which further increases the mental load of the disease. The visibility of the skin condition presents a unique challenge, where individuals may receive negative reactions or unwanted comments regarding their appearance. This social perspective is one element within a story that attaches physical appearance to self-esteem. The psychological effects of such stigma are extensive, encouraging individuals towards various coping mechanisms, some of which include cosmetic camouflage and surgery. Awareness of the social environment is necessary to grasp the lived realities of individuals with vitiligo, particularly when it comes to their mental well-being and self-perception, as acceptance and self-esteem are most likely associated with social perceptions of normalcy and beauty (Khalid et al., 2025). Social perceptions of vitiligo have profound implications extending beyond personal experience; they impact cultural beauty values. Conformity to some aspects of beauty is deeply ingrained in most cultures, and physical skin differences in the guise of vitiligo can go against these. Therefore, people with vitiligo might feel pressured to change their appearance to conform to society's standards more desirably through cosmetic methods or operations. These kinds of decisions are often laden with various emotions, indicative of a tug between embracing one's uniqueness and the desire to be accepted in society. Furthermore, the process of self-acceptance is potentially enormously hampered by such societal pressures, thereby necessitating greater awareness and education about vitiligo. The analysis of these social narratives not only makes clear the challenges of those with the condition but also provides a way of understanding how we can create a more tolerant and accepting environment (Smith et al., 2025). Support systems, including counseling and community groups, assist in shaping social opinion about vitiligo. By creating awareness and knowledge, these support groups can diminish the stigma of the condition and promote acceptance. The lives of individuals with vitiligo can be significantly influenced by how they engage with such support networks, as these provide space for discussion and mutual experience. For instance, qualitative studies have illustrated how discussing the diagnosis and its impact can help individuals accept their feelings and adopt resilience coping strategies. The practice of Counselling Psychology aimed at the emotional impact of visible differences can be part of the process of self-acceptance, turning around negative societal attitudes into empowering opportunities. Thus, working on societal attitudes towards vitiligo not only assists individual processes but also recycles society's concept of beauty and acceptance, moving towards an embracing history (Khalid et al., 2025).

4.6.1. Stigma and Discrimination

The visibility of vitiligo has the tendency to subject people to discrimination and stigma, with serious psychological effects. The beauty standards that exist in society tend to equate homogenous skin color with beauty, where those suffering from visible skin disease are starkly contrasted. It is not just skin-deep discrimination but also carries effects that are deep-seated in individuals and society. Virtually all those with vitiligo report experiences of social rejection, which further enhances the sense of loneliness and lack of self-esteem. The quality of such experiences calls for a heightened sense of awareness and sensitivity towards skin illnesses since societal attitudes determine not only self-concept but also mental well-being. Coupled with superficial judgments, the effects of such stigma necessitate adaptive coping strategies and interventions to foster acceptance within wider social spaces, so much so that one cannot over-emphasize the necessity for empathetic health care and support community systems (Atkar et al., 2022). Moreover, the treatment guidelines for vitiligo also point to the necessity of dealing with psychological well-being as part of treatment. Though cosmetic camouflage and surgery provide physical solutions for hiding or minimizing the appearance of vitiligo, they do not address the social stigmas behind the psychological impact of the illness. It has been established that control should aim not only at the visible manifestations of the disorder but also at resulting relief from associated stigma. Thus, health professionals are urged to adopt the holistic approach, integrating cosmetic therapy with psychological guidance. As a multi-faceted approach, this is necessary since it gets the patient to react positively towards the condition as well as reduces the impact of outside judgment towards self-perception (Atkar et al., 2022). Lastly, respect for the man's perspective of vitiligo is particularly significant in developing bespoke supportive interventions. While large bodies of research have explored stigma for women with skin disease, research on men's experiences is limited. The absence of such reporting not only limits our knowledge base but also signifies a critical deficiency of support resources specifically tailored for men. Through the application of qualitative approaches, understanding of how men cope with their diagnosis and navigate relationships can inform clinical practice. Treating the unique stigma that men who suffer from vitiligo have would improve outcomes by using specially tailored counseling methods, confirming the notion that psychological impact transcends gender. Therefore, a multimodal approach to vitiligo must take into account the varying experiences of all victims, emphasizing the intersection of stigma, discrimination, and personal identity (Khalid et al., 2025) (Figure 4.14).

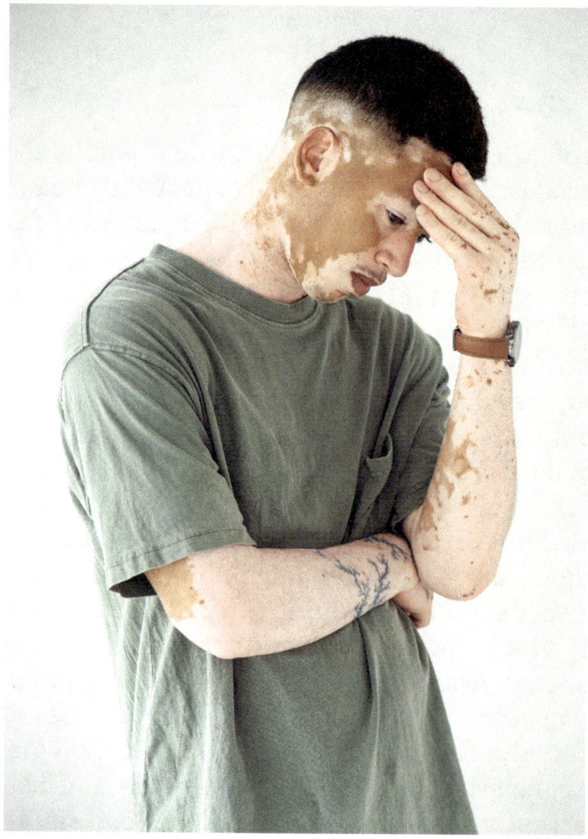

Figure 4.14. Psychosocial impact of vitiligo in a young adult.

Source: https://www.vipoc.org/wp-content/uploads/2023/06/studio-shot-of-a-young-man-with-vitiligo-looking-u-2023-01-10-22-52-57-utc-scaled.jpg.

4.6.2. Representation in Media and Culture

Media and cultural depictions significantly affect society's view of skin diseases like vitiligo. The media tend to support certain notions of beauty, and people who do not meet them tend to be excluded. For patients with vitiligo, this depiction may manifest in a variety of ways, from invisibility to stereotyping. Conversely, instances of positive depiction can empower people to foster acceptance and normalcy for the condition. The portrayal of individuals with vitiligo in ads, social media campaigns, and films can shatter traditional notions of beauty, thereby influencing the public's perception and acceptance of varied skin tones. Through various media platforms, society has a chance to redefine the concept of beauty by opening doors for diversity and inclusion in the representation of people with skin differences. The psychological impact of vitiligo has been highlighted in studies that investigate the various ways in which this skin ailment affects an individual's self-concept and social interaction. Investigations have shown that individuals suffering from vitiligo are likely to develop severe emotional disturbance, augmented by a scarcity of representation in dominant culture. Men are particularly disprivileged in the sense that lackluster narratives tend to deny their experience of vitiligo. Male sufferers' experiences give immense insight into the relationship between masculinity, self-concept, and social expectation around appearance. Integrating these voices into the mainstream conversation allows culture to develop a richer understanding of vitiligo. In media portrayal, it is essential to magnify these voices in an attempt to establish broader discourses about mental health and individual identity through vitiligo and other skin disorders, as authenticated by studies of individual narrative and psychological health (Khalid et al., 2025). With evolving cosmetic technology and surgeries for vitiligo, portrayal in the media also influences public acceptance of such treatments. Cosmetic camouflage is a popular choice; however, the manner in which it is showcased in media will affect perceptions of its effectiveness and popularity. On one hand, the depiction of individuals with vitiligo embracing the application of camouflage products can empower them to use such products without shame or remorse. Also critical is the fact that the media counteract this by hosting true stories about the necessity of self-acceptance and also the psychosocial implications entailed in the use of cosmetic intervention. With academic exploration of the emotional aspects of managing vitiligo emerging, discussion around media representation can deconstruct such experiences and support a better understanding of the options available for individuals living with the condition (Shetty,2020). This all-inclusive representation eventually results in a culture embracing diversity and supporting the emotional thriving of all its members.

4.6.3. Support Networks and Advocacy

Support systems are crucial in alleviating the psychological distress faced by vitiligo patients. Because this is a chronic condition of the skin that leads to noticeable differences, individuals end up experiencing body dissatisfaction and social anxiety, which lead to severe impacts on their mental health. If well utilized, such systems can provide emotional support, belonging, and shared experiences with others who have similar problems. Organizations like the Vitiligo Society offer spaces through which individuals can interact and share personal experiences, thus establishing a community that reduces loneliness. Support groups can also initiate coping mechanisms, enhance awareness of the disease, and enhance the advocacy required in the quest for greater public understanding of the impact of vitiligo on quality of life (Khalid et al., 2025). This kind of public backing galvanizes a strong force that can influence individual attitudes as well as broader societal opinion regarding skin disease. The advocacy forms the core of raising awareness and knowledge about vitiligo, particularly in the eradication of myths and misconceptions regarding the condition. Health workers are in a prime position not only to provide medical care but also to advocate for the psychosocial needs of the affected individuals. As highlighted in the literature, most children and young people with noticeable differences suffer extreme psychosocial challenges as a result of stigma and body image concerns (Bellew et al., 2019). By raising awareness about cosmetic camouflage and surgery as forms of treatment, medical practitioners can empower individuals to make educational choices about their treatment while supporting efforts to mainstream mental health services into dermatology. This advocacy not only highlights the necessity to care for the emotional health of patients but also calls for the creation of integrated models of care that promote coping behavior and resilience for vitiligo sufferers. Furthermore, internet websites and social media platforms have become significant sources of advocacy and support for vitiligo sufferers. Such mediums extend support networks geographically to allow multicultural groups to meet up, share resources, and demand visibility in the virtual community. Emerging virtual communities are opportunities for awareness campaigns and education campaigns that create de-stigmatization of the condition. The interactivity of web-based campaigning enables sufferers to articulate their experiences, and this has the power to fuel public interest and drive systemic change in perceptions of, and responses to, vitiligo. Through the optimization of these sites, affected individuals, as well as their support networks, can create a strong story that inspires awareness and acceptance and, in turn, emphasizes the importance of solidarity in more thoroughly understanding the complexity of living with vitiligo (Witek et al., 2025) (Figure 4.15).

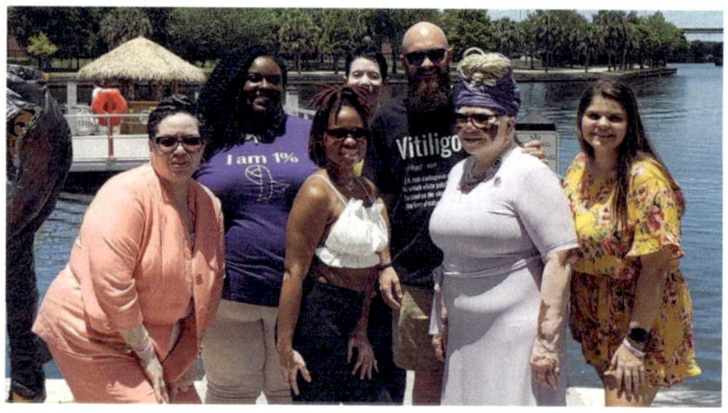

Figure 4.15. A support group helps people with vitiligo come together.

Source: https://ewscripps.brightspotcdn.com/dims4/default/3c74e37/2147483647/strip/true/crop/1280x720+0+0/resize/1280x720!/quality/90/?url=http%3A%2F%2Fewscripps-brightspot.s3.amazonaws.com%2Fd0%2F39%2Fc656858843ad861a32ea4d178f89%2Fbeautifully-unblemished-wfts-boyd.jpg.

Test Your Knowledge

1. How do stigma and societal misunderstanding affect the daily lives and mental health of individuals with vitiligo?
2. In what ways has the representation of vitiligo in media, fashion, and popular culture evolved over the past decade?
3. How effective are support networks, both online and offline, in providing emotional and practical help to individuals living with vitiligo?

SUMMARY

Finally, the intricacies involved in vitiligo require awareness as well as creative strategies when it comes to treatment and care. Since vitiligo is an autoimmune disease resulting from melanocyte loss, how the condition manifests can be so varied among patients that it presents distinctive challenges in diagnosis as well as management. The importance of knowing its etiopathogenesis has become greater for those who practice medicine and want to offer effective interventions based on specific patient requirements. Today's practices , such as topical treatment and phototherapy, are just a small fraction of the possibilities; ongoing research holds more effective therapeutic methods. In addition, applying evidence-based practice not only teaches higher patient outcomes but also provides a platform for future therapeutic discovery (Witek et al., 2025). Moreover, cosmetic camouflage products have also become integral to the majority of individuals with vitiligo, particularly those wishing to deal with societal attitudes and gain confidence. Patients usually resort to cosmetic treatments , such as skin lightening and camouflage creams that can easily conceal depigmented spots. These treatments address both short-term and psychological requirements by allowing patients to deal with society more comfortably. However, illogical reactions that are seen in some patients indicate the psychological implications that are attached to the desire for even skin color. The feeling of jealousy experienced by others who have undergone depigmentation treatments adds to the varied individual impacts of having to endure and cope with the disease (Witek et al., 2025). Surgical intervention is also worth a seat of acceptance as a valid action, particularly in situations where traditional treatments are found to be insufficient. Methods like melanocyte transplantation present hopeful avenues for the restoration of skin pigmentation and significantly enhance the quality of life for individuals involved. Our understanding of not only treatments but also the emotional and social impact of vitiligo increases over time. With the ongoing investigation, it is important that practitioners remain vigilant in offering holistic care that not only covers physical and psychological dimensions of vitiligo living but also explores more. The integration of surgical interventions with cosmetic camouflage opens a broader scope of choice for patients, and therefore, there is a call for multiple planes of approach in the management of vitiligo (Witek et al., 2025).

Cosmetic treatment of the patient with vitiligo plays a significant role in increasing self-esteem and quality of life. They range from basic topical medication to more sophisticated preparations. The most common among them are cosmetic camouflage products that effectively cover depigmentation patches, allowing patients to have an improved, more uniform skin tone. These products are typically specifically designed for sensitive skin and are water-resistant, providing a long-lasting solution. Many patients also find that these products not only camouflage the patches but also boost their self-esteem levels in public or social interactions. This is particularly so for those patients with Fitzpatrick skin types that are most visibly affected by vitiligo, as these topical cosmetic products are specifically formulated to meet various skin tones and textures, thereby promoting their reliability in everyday use. Surgical intervention is another alternative for individuals who seek to address the physical appearance of vitiligo. Methods , such as grafting techniques, where autologous skin grafting takes place, are gaining ground as a choice for patients with stable vitiligo. Such procedures involve transferring the skin from pigmented regions to depigmented ones to induce a more homogenous appearance. Laser therapy is also in the meanwhile researched for its potential to induce repigmentation in the affected parts of the body. Despite the advances in these surgical procedures, caution is needed when providing such procedures since outcomes are extremely variable among patients. A recent recommendation noted comparison of laser therapy with surgical excision for lesions imitating vitiligo, which necessitates broad measurement tools, including the Children's Dermatology Life Quality Index, to measure the global quality of life of patients in such treatment (Lai et al., 2018). In contrast, therapeutic depigmentation offers a second intervention, specifically for severely affected patients with vitiligo. Chemical depigmentation agents, for the explicit purpose of bleaching residual pigmented skin to create an homogeneous skin color, can be employed. Despite many individuals being relieved and satisfied by the achievement of an even color via this treatment, it can actually lead to psychological complexities, , such as feelings of jealousy regarding their fully depigmented skin (Witek et al., 2025). It is essential that healthcare professionals understand the psychological influences and driving forces for such treatments. The union of cosmetic procedures and surgery is to be able to provide an overall treatment plan that not only targets the physical aspect of vitiligo but also addresses the psychological and quality-of-life concerns that accompany many skin conditions.

KEY TERMS FROM THIS CHAPTER

- Autoimmune destruction
- Camouflage technique
- Cosmetic camouflage
- Cosmetic commodities
- Cosmetic management
- Depigmented lesions
- Dihydroxyacetone (DHA
- Etiopathogenesis
- Holistic care
- Keratinocytes
- Beauty industry
- Co-culturing melanocytes
- Cosmetic camouflage techniques
- Cosmetic improvement
- Cosmetic treatments
- Dermatological testing
- Effective management systems
- Genetic susceptibility
- Individualized support systems
- Laser therapy

CRITICAL THINKING QUESTIONS

1. **Which of the following is a commonly used method for cosmetic camouflage in vitiligo patients?**
   a. Skin grafting
   b. Microdermabrasion
   c. Cosmetic camouflage using makeup
   d. Chemical peeling
2. **What is the primary surgical option used for vitiligo patients with stable depigmentation?**
   a. Laser treatment
   b. Skin grafting
   c. Phototherapy
   d. Cryotherapy
3. **Which type of skin grafting technique is commonly used for vitiligo treatment?**
   a. Full-thickness skin graft
   b. Split-thickness skin graft
   c. Punch grafting
   d. Composite grafting
4. **Which cosmetic camouflage product is often recommended for patients with vitiligo for covering depigmented areas?**
   a. Foundation
   b. Tinted sunscreens
   c. Self-tanners
   d. Pigmented creams or lotions
5. **What is the main advantage of using surgical options for vitiligo, , such as skin grafting or melanocyte transplant?**
   a. They are non-invasive and pain-free
   b. They provide permanent color restoration
   c. They work only on small vitiligo patches
   d. They do not require post-surgical care

Short Answer Questions

1. What are the main components of cosmetic camouflage used in vitiligo management?
2. What are the benefits and limitations of using cosmetic camouflage in vitiligo treatment?
3. Which types of camouflage products are recommended for use on large or exposed vitiliginous areas?
4. Which surgical techniques are commonly used in the treatment of stable vitiligo?
5. What are the main criteria for selecting a vitiligo patient for surgical treatment?
6. What is the primary advantage of using camouflage makeup for vitiligo over other treatment options?
7. What criteria must be met for vitiligo to be considered stable enough for surgical treatment options?

Answer to Critical Thinking Questions

1. (c); 2. (b); 3. (c); 4. (d); 5. (b)

REFERENCES

1. Abarca, J., Abdel-Malek, Z., Abel, E., Acosta, L. R., Adam, J., Ahmed, A. M., Alaluf, S., et al. (2014). *Brazilian Consensus on Photoprotection.* https://core.ac.uk/download/293550918.pdf (accessed on 11th June 2025).
2. Adaskevich, V. P. (2016). *Skin Diseases and Sexually Transmitted Infections.* https://core.ac.uk/download/80150454.pdf (accessed on 11th June 2025).
3. Agaba, E. (2017). *Quality of Life Among Vitiligo Patients Attending Dermatology Out-Patient Clinics in Johannesburg.* https://core.ac.uk/download/188770332.pdf (accessed on 11th June 2025).
4. Atkar, R., Batchelor, J., Eleftheriadou, V., Exton, A., et al. (2022). *British Association of Dermatologists Guidelines for the Management of People with Vitiligo 2021.* https://core.ac.uk/download/467106966.pdf (accessed on 11th June 2025).
5. Batchelor, J. M., Leighton, P., Thomas, K. S., Tour, S., et al. (2014). *Survey and Online Discussion Groups to Develop a Patient-Rated Outcome Measure on Acceptability of Treatment Response in Vitiligo.* https://core.ac.uk/download/pdf/81628894.pdf (accessed on 11th June 2025).
6. Bellew, B., Bessell, T., Bessell, N., Braun, V., et al. (2019). *Opening a Pandora's Box That Can't be Salvaged: Health Professionals' Perceptions of Appearance-Related Care in An Australian Pediatric Specialist Hospital.* https://core.ac.uk/download/323907070.pdf (accessed on 11th June 2025).
7. Witek, A., Parys, J., Mikosińska, A., Kaźmierczak, M., Mossakowski, M., Kałuziak, P., ... Bieś, R. (2025). Vitiligo Review: etiopathogenesis, diagnosis and treatment. *Quality in Sport, 37,* 57367. https://doi.org/10.12775/QS.2025.37.57367(accessed on 11th June 2025).
8. Chunying, L., Jianru, C., Shuli, L., Wei, W., & Xinju, W. (2024). *Management of the Refractory Vitiligo Patient: Current Therapeutic Strategies and Future Options.* https://core.ac.uk/download/597897754.pdf (accessed on 11th June 2025).
9. Eleftheriadou, Viktoria (2013) *Setting priorities and reducing uncertainties for the treatment of vitiligo.* PhD thesis, University of Nottingham. (accessed on 11th June 2025).
10. França, K., Gianfaldoni, S., Lotti, J., Lotti, T., et al. (2018). *Vitiligo in Children: A Review of Conventional Treatments.* https://core.ac.uk/download/162147389.pdf (accessed on 11th June 2025).
11. Gauglitz, G. G., Middelkoop, E., Mustoe, T. A., Téot, L., et al. (2021). *Textbook on Scar Management.* https://core.ac.uk/download/478135440.pdf (accessed on 11th June 2025).
12. Gauglitz, G. G., Middelkoop, E., Mustoe, T. A., Téot, L., et al. (2025). *Textbook on scar management.* https://core.ac.uk/download/362226683.pdf (accessed on 11th June 2025).
13. Khalid, S. J. (2025). *An Exploration of Men's Subjective Experience of Vitiligo: A Qualitative Study.* https://core.ac.uk/download/76979685.pdf (accessed on 11th June 2025).
14. Kim, T. H. (2021). *Depigmentation.* https://core.ac.uk/download/478113284.pdf (accessed on 11th June 2025).
15. Lai, Y. (2018). *Comparing Congenital Melanocytic Nevus Treatment Effect on Children's Health-Related Quality of Life.* https://core.ac.uk/download/475688229.pdf (accessed on 11th June 2025).

16. Shetty, N. 2020. *Developing methods of measuring and manipulating melanocyte/keratinocyte ratios to inform potential treatment of vitiligo vulgaris.* PhD Thesis Canterbury Christ Church University School of Allied and Public Health Professions(accessed on 11th June 2025).

17. Smith, F. (2025). *Shame and the Body*. https://core.ac.uk/download/5230562.pdf (accessed on 11th June 2025).

18. Sureka, D. (2017). *A Comparative Study on The Degree of Regimentation of Punch Grafting and Topical 5-Fluorouracil on Dermabrader Skin in The Treatment of Vitiligo*. https://core.ac.uk/download/327695973.pdf (accessed on 11th June 2025).

NAIL AESTHETIC CONDITIONS AND TREATMENTS

5

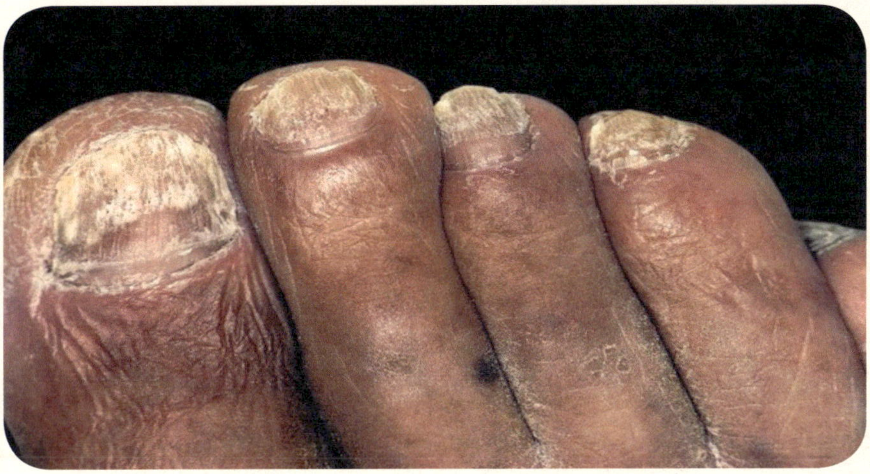

LEARNING OBJECTIVES

After studying this chapter, you will be able to:

1. Describe common nail aesthetic conditions
2. Identify symptoms that are associated with nail aesthetic conditions
3. Describe treatment for nail conditions
4. Highlight home remedies and prevention
5. Describe the role of nutrition in nail condition
6. Discuss professional treatments and procedures

Introduction

Nail aesthetics has increasingly been identified as an integral component of dermatological practice, particularly in terms of beauty and health enhancement of the nails. Aesthetic nail disorders typically arise from an amalgamation of local pathologies, systemic diseases, and lifestyle factors, inducing physical discomfort as well as psychological injury. Deformities, discoloration, and brittleness are distressing for patients and prompt them to seek effective treatments. As the literature has evoked, growing awareness about nail enhancement means more engagement of dermatologists in this field, raising aesthetic treatments from the traditional salon experience to more clinically-based settings (Bansal et al., 2024). This model is a shifting view of how aesthetic treatment modalities can both address functional impairment and improve quality of life for the patient at the same time. In addition, despite major advances in nail aesthetic treatments, one needs to appreciate the spectrum of causative conditions that can lead to nail disease. These disorders are likely to be a result of local conditions, e.g., fungal infections, and systemic disease-related abnormalities, which make clinical assessment and the following therapeutic approaches challenging (Dalave et al., 2024). The problem of accurate diagnosis of such disorders is further compounded by the lack of investigative modalities that lead to misdiagnosis or under-treatment of nail disorders. This background points to an exploration of successful treatments aimed at restoring not only the cosmetic looks of nails but also underlying health issues. Interestingly, the application of aesthetic treatments , such as nail peels and laser therapy can have a two-way function—providing cosmetic relief while also feeding into therapeutic value in patients with nail ailments. Aesthetic therapy, when practiced under the guidance of experienced dermatologists, can yield much benefit, particularly in instances of chronic nail disease. A combination of various methods, from nail peels that seek to remedy surface abnormalities to gel nails that enhance the cosmetic appearance of deformed nail plates, has been promising in the literature (Bansal et al., 2024). In addition to this, lasers are emerging as innovative treatments for certain aesthetic disorders, whereas their use is just in its primary stages. Through increasing research, full assessments, including histological examination, are needed for the appropriate management of nail disorders and to ensure the safety of aesthetic treatments (Dalave et al., 2024). Finally, by integrating cosmetic and therapeutic modalities, the profession of nail aesthetics can contribute importantly to elevating patient care, enhancing the health and beauty of nails in a clinically sound way.

Definition of Nail Aesthetic Conditions

The phrase nail aesthetic conditions is used to describe a wide range of physical disorders of the nails, primarily in terms of appearance and integrity. They can appear in many different forms, , such as color changes, nail deformities, and texture irregularities. Some of the examples are ridges, brittleness, and lifting of the nail plate off the nail bed, not only altering the cosmetic outlook but also potentially being indicative of an underlying condition. Aesthetic disorders are also often worsened by environmental factors like repeated water or harsh chemical exposure, which can irritate brittle nails more and become cosmetically bothersome. Proper understanding of these definitions matters since it aids in deciding likely treatments and informs individuals about the necessity for preventive care to maintain healthy, aesthetically pleasing nails. Ascertaining the beauty status of nails is a keen sense of its formation and function. The nail apparatus consists of various structures, that is, the nail plate, nail bed, and surrounding tissues, each of which can be affected by internal and external factors. Diseases , such as onychomycosis, a fungal infection that displaces nail color and texture, are a prime example of how beauty and health issues are interdependent. The appearance of nails is visually reflective of systemic health because alterations would then reflect diseases like conditions of psoriasis, or even respiratory disease. It thus becomes important to adhere to an approach that not only examines the beauty of nails but also their connectivity with health as a whole, in order to examine further treatments that take care of both beauty and health problems on a holistic level. Increased nail aesthetics visibility has also introduced the use of sophisticated treatments designed to improve the appearance of nails as well as internal conditions. Nutritional supplements and medicated nail lacquers are some of the treatments that have been praised for improving nail aesthetic appearance as well as nail health. For instance, nanoparticles incorporated into cosmetic formulations have been discovered to enhance penetration and bioavailability of active ingredients, thus enhancing the moisturizing capacity of nail care products and enhancing the general nail look (Salvioni et al., 2021).

Furthermore, having standardized measures of nail assessment helps healthcare professionals implement personalized interventions appropriate for every patient's needs, improving the patients' experience and satisfaction with the healthcare services. The interplay between beauty and health highlights the importance of comprehending the state of the nails holistically when developing effective treatment protocols (Robbert et al., 2021) (Figure 5.1).

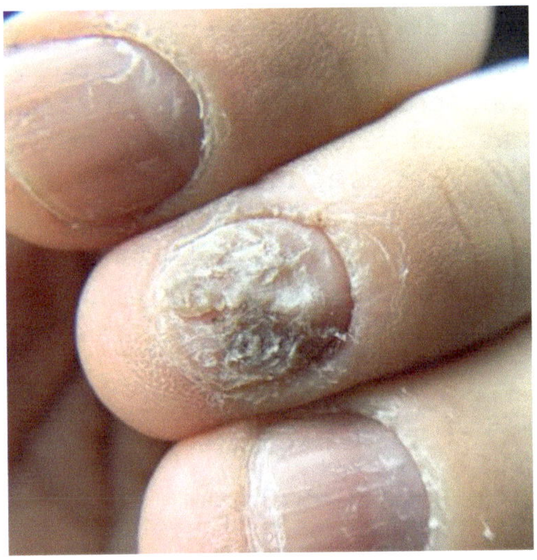

Figure 5.1. Nail dystrophy associated with dermatological conditions.

Source: https://illinoisderm.com/wp-content/uploads/2021/11/Nail-Problems-Square-1-450x475.jpg.

Importance of Nail Health in Overall Well-Being

The significance of nail health extends beyond mere its cosmetic significance; it is a vital indicator of one's overall well-being. Nails reflect the health status of the body from within and can indicate signs of nutritional deficiency, systemic disease, and even some dermatological conditions. For instance, color, texture, and growth rate changes in the nails could indicate conditions, such as anemia, diabetes, or thyroid disease. Therefore, regular monitoring of the nail status can assist in identifying possible health problems at an early stage, and individuals are given appropriate medical advice. While traditional thinking would view nail maintenance as shallow, it is actually true that healthy nails can assist in deriving improved overall health advantages, like better self-esteem and mental health. For that reason, gaining knowledge about and giving attention to nail health is necessary for a holistic approach to individual health following the interdependent nature of physiological processes. In the process of achieving nail health, nutrition comes into play as a very important aspect. Micronutrients like vitamins and minerals can greatly affect nail strength and beauty. For instance, vitamin C has also been observed to promote skin and nail health in general, and the contribution of nutritional absorption to the integrity of the nail was emphasized. Supplements like multivitamins and vitamin C have also been discovered to be beneficial to skin and potentially nail health, as evidenced in some of the studies on micronutrients and skin conditions (Akram et al., 2025). Therefore, the incorporation of a well-balanced diet containing such essential nutrients may not only promote skin health but also strengthen to make nails stronger and more resilient. Health care professionals ought to encourage patients to appreciate the correlated relationship between diet and the cosmetic condition of skin as well as nails, so that they value the wholesome character of health care. Psychological elements for nail care cannot be overstressed either. The health of one's nails generally follows in tandem with self-esteem and confidence levels. Individuals who have well-maintained nails often perceive their body image positively, promoting socialization and life satisfaction. Conversely, diseases , such as fungal infections or nail brittleness may prompt individuals to feel embarrassed or shy, resulting in withdrawal from social interaction (Shelke et al., 2024). Recognition of this dynamic can impact treatment in nail disorders and aesthetics, as clinicians consider both physical and psychological concerns in treatment. By promoting nail health as integral to integrated aesthetic care, health professionals are able not only to improve the aesthetic appearance of nails but also the well-being of patients, and hence have a more holistic approach to health care.

Overview of Common Nail Conditions and Treatments

Nail disorders frequently indicate more widespread health concerns and may have a profound effect on an individual's looks and self-image. Onychomycosis, psoriasis, and nail trauma are frequent disorders, each with its own unique difficulties. Onychomycosis, or fungal infection of the nail, causes discoloration, thickening, and potential nail loss, thus necessitating both systemic and topical antifungal medications. Alternatively, psoriasis appears as pitting, ridging, and inflammation of the nails and is treated with specific therapies like corticosteroids or phototherapy. Nail trauma, from superficial trauma to infection, usually needs protective therapy and, in severe cases, surgery. A good treatment of such disorders hinges on an acute understanding of their pathogenesis, clinical manifestation, and the provision of the best therapy to reinstate nail function and integrity. Treatment of nail disorders varies from conservative to more ablative modalities. Topical treatment is usually the first line, particularly for superficial fungal infections and cosmetic problems like pigmentation of the nails. Antifungal lacquers have also been found useful in the management of mild onychomycosis with consistent application over a duration of time. In more severe infection or in the event of refractory disease to topical therapy, oral antifungals can be considered, but with knowledge of their side effects. Other than pharmacologic treatment, prevention and control are also dependent on lifestyle modification in the form of greater nail care and the use of protective coverings. Proper identification and early treatment play crucial roles in halting complications of advanced nail health diseases. Cosmetic considerations do play a role over medical ones in some instances. Patients are often prompted to receive treatments not only to alleviate pain but also to beautify their nails. This looks-oriented treatment has spawned other cosmetic procedures, including gel polish and nail artwork, which are often applied as a way of covering up conditions rather than curing their causes. However, this raises an important question about the connection between medical treatment and cosmetic treatment. It is essential that health practitioners teach patients safe nail care and ensure effective treatment without sacrificing aesthetic ideals that the majority of individuals pursue. By encouraging holistic approaches to nail care, we can satisfy medical and aesthetic needs successfully in the realm of nail aesthetic conditions and treatments.

5.1. Common Nail Aesthetic Conditions

Learning Outcome

1. Understand fungal nail infections
2. Define nail psoriasis
3. Describe ingrown nails

Nail aesthetic disorders consist of a variety of diseases that compromise both the appearance and the health of the nails. Onychomycosis, paronychia, and brittle nail syndrome are the most prevalent of these disorders. Brittle nail syndrome is typified by brittle or splitting nails, which are typically caused by systemic disease or environmental exposures. Onychomycosis, or fungal infection of the nails, leads to coloration and thickening of the nails, thus detracting from their appearance. Paronychia, swelling and discoloration caused by inflammation of the skin of the nail, may lead to painful swelling. All these ailments not only hamper the aesthetic appeal of the nails but also mirror and could represent underlying pathological states, requiring proper diagnosis and treatment strategies for improving both aesthetic as well as functional outcomes. Apart from the cosmetic concerns, the frequency of common nail diseases may also be an indicator of systemic conditions, which explains the need for meticulousness in taking histories and performing physical examinations. Certain presentations, such as longitudinal melanonychia or Beaus lines, may signal conditions as dangerous as subungual melanoma or other systemic disease. The diagnostic approach for these nail disorders calls for diligent history and clinical evaluation of every nail unit to rule out malignancies and establish appropriate therapy. New research indicates an early diagnosis can significantly improve diagnosis as well as patient outcomes, alerting healthcare professionals to potentially dangerous conditions requiring prompt intervention. Thus, the understanding of the clinical importance of these nail disorders is more than mere cosmetic presentations and is a critical component of comprehensive patient care (Lee et al., 2022). Treatment of nail aesthetic disorders is very variable based on the specific disorder, etiologic factors, and severity. Onychomycosis may be treated with topical antifungals, nail psoriasis with intralesional steroid therapy, or paronychia by surgical intervention in advanced cases. Management typically necessitates the application of pharmacological therapy in addition to modifications in lifestyle, , such as improved nail hygiene and protective devices to prevent future damage. Patient education is also very crucial to facilitate compliance with therapy and good nail hygiene. By addressing the different aspects of nail aesthetic conditions, medical professionals can not only make the nails look beautiful but also enhance the well-being of individuals with such conditions by enhancing the quality and color of the nails, thereby providing greater patient satisfaction and better health (Lee et al., 2022).

5.1.1. Fungal Infections

Fungal infections take a great toll on nail appearance, with one of the most prevalent types being onychomycosis. This infection is mainly caused by dermatophyte fungi, in this case, species of the Trichophyton genus, which prefer warm, damp conditions. As the infection advances, discoloration, thickening, and ultimately separation of the nail from the nail bed occur, not only affecting the appearance of the nails but also their integrity. Their global dissemination poses an enormous challenge to public health, and recent epidemiological trends reveal an increase in resistant strains. This tendency has increased the threat of treating these infections as the inappropriate use of antifungal agents increases the resistance of such pathogens. Management of nail cosmetic disorders due to fungal infection necessitates a keen understanding of their causative agents and the evolving trends in response to treatment protocols, which also continue in flux in the face of rising resistance (Chanyachailert et al., 2023). Treatment and diagnosis of fungal infections require specific diagnostic techniques to separate dermatophyte from non-dermatophyte pathogens. The management varies significantly based on the causal organism. For instance, although infections due to dermatophytes can typically be managed with systemic or topical antifungals, non-dermatophyte infections are more challenging due to their higher rates of treatment failure. This is even more intensified in those who also have other skin diseases , such as psoriasis, in which the compromised barrier of the nail plate also going to improves fungal penetration. The relationship between onychomycosis and psoriasis describes this dynamic most accurately since onycholysis and nail structural alteration afford a fertile environment for fungal colonization and development. Thus, intensity-orientated interventions must contend with the multi-factorial nature of these infections, incorporating patient-specific assessment of the fungal pathogen as well as the epidermal status of the host (Kyriakou et al., 2022). Evolution of prevention and therapeutic interventions is crucial in the management of the aesthetic effects of fungal infections of the nails. Apart from pharmacologic intervention, lifestyle modification , such as good foot hygiene and ventilation of footwear, is crucial in averting infection. Generation of awareness on early signs and symptoms of onychomycosis also leads to timely intervention and averts the advancement of the disease. With advances in the treatment of antifungals and growing understanding of the mechanisms for resistance in fungi, more effective treatments that meet the unique circumstances of each patient are now available. Lastly, at the point where aesthetic beauty and effective treatment meet, there is a need for an integrated treatment of nail health, addressing both the physical appearance of the nails as well as the pathological conditions that aggravate fungal infections (Kyriakou et al., 2022; Chanyachailert et al., 2023) (Figure 5.2).

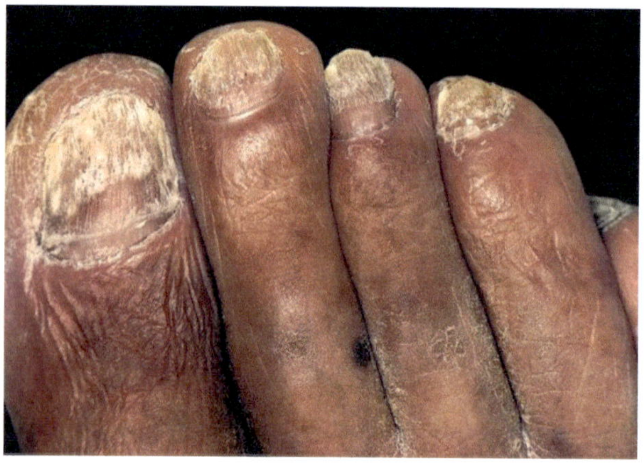

Figure 5.2. Fungal nail infection.

Source: https://assets.nhs.uk/nhsuk-cms/images/C0509911-Fungal_nail_infection_copy.max-600x600.jpg.

5.1.2. Nail Psoriasis

Nail psoriasis, a symptom of the chronic skin disorder known as psoriasis, significantly impacts the physical appearance of nails and the quality of life for its sufferers. The condition is characterized by pitting, ridges, and discoloration, which result in pain and discomfort caused by nail loss or injury. The relationship between nail condition and psoriasis has been the target of recent research, which proved a complex relationship, indicating the need for personalized therapeutic approaches. Therefore, knowledge of the pathophysiology of nail psoriasis is paramount since it directs aesthetic and therapeutic management that could be provided to patients. By managing not only the physical symptoms but also the psychological effects, professionals can provide holistic care that includes counseling, skincare routines, and lifestyle changes to optimize both nail health and self-esteem. New advances in the treatment of psoriasis of the nails have led to the exploration of various therapeutic modalities, from topical treatments to systemic approaches. Topical corticosteroids and vitamin D analogs are standard therapies to reduce inflammation and maximize nail health. Because the disease is often resistant to standard therapies, phototherapy and biologic agents are very popular among physicians because of their efficacy and ability to modulate the key inflammatory pathways of psoriasis. Notably, contemporary studies indicate that micronutrient supplementation, as described in the literature, can complement the effectiveness of such treatments through stimulation of skin barrier function and inflammation reduction. Integration of these nutritional interventions into treatment protocols shows evolving knowledge in treating nail psoriasis and indicates better hope for patients with nail psoriasis seeking cosmetic and functional improvement (Januszewski et al., 2023). Recent research has also brought forward the possibility of fungi playing a role in controlling inflammatory skin conditions, including nail psoriasis. Fungal compounds have shown promise as therapeutic agents owing to their unique biological activities, including anti-inflammatory and antimicrobial activity.

This is a significant trend, particularly because development efforts are repeatedly moving away from conventional therapies. For instance, certain fungal derivatives may be utilized synergistically with existing treatments in an attempt to enhance outcomes. As the science matures, these new modalities of therapy need to be evaluated critically on the basis of efficacy versus safety and patient acceptability. In doing so, exploring the benefits of fungi in the treatment of psoriasis of the nails not only sheds new light on the field of treatment but also adheres to the growing movement toward holistic and integrative dermatology (Corbu et al., 2023) (Figure 5.3).

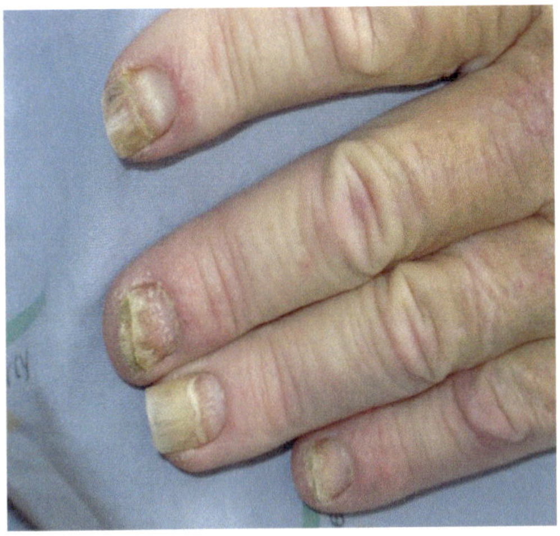

Figure 5.3. Nail psoriasis.

Source: https://www.ncbi.nlm.nih.gov/books/NBK559260/figure/article-27962.image.f1/?report=objectonly.

5.1.3. Ingrown Nails

Ingrown nails, or onychocryptosis, are a common but often painful nail condition. This is the growth of a nail into the surrounding skin, leading to pain, swelling, and redness. Even though the condition can affect any nail, it most often affects the large toe. There are various reasons for the occurrence of ingrown nails, including cutting the nails inappropriately, injury to the nail, and shoes that compress the toe region. Individuals who engage in activities that subject their feet to constant stress, , such as athletes and individuals who wear rigid footwear, are particularly vulnerable. Apart from the subjective pain, there is also a cosmetic complication in relation to ingrown nails as they are bound to result in a distorted appearance of the nail and ultimately lead to infections that further compromise the aesthetic value and health of the nail, thus necessitating early intervention and treatment. Treatment of ingrown nails also ranges from conservative to aggressive, based on the severity of the condition. For less severe conditions, self-care like soaking the foot affected with warm water and washing the area around the nail can treat the symptoms. Over-the-counter medication may be applied to manage pain, providing a sense of relief without visiting a physician. However, in more severe instances, surgical options may be necessary. One commonly employed technique involves chemical matricectomy using phenol, which has proven effective in reducing recurrence rates and accelerating healing. The application of 30 seconds of phenol has been shown to provide a significantly shorter healing time compared to the 60-second application, without an increase in complications (Coheña et al., 2021). This underlines the significance of employing appropriate treatments based on individual patient history and condition. Preventive therapy has come a long way in curing ingrown nails and preventing recurrence. Informing individuals about proper nail care procedures, like straight cutting and not curving the corners too much, can simply avert the development of this disease. Also, wearing appropriately fitting shoes with sufficient toe room can reduce tension that may result in nail encroachment upon the skin. Regular inspection of the feet and prompt action are called for, particularly in patients with predisposing factors like diabetes or circulatory disease that can complicate nail pathologies. On the whole, while ingrown nails pose both health and beauty issues, a combination of preventive care actions and targeted treatments will be able to successfully manage this condition. Treatment of ingrown nails not only cures the nail look but also benefits the overall health of the foot, showing the complementarity of beauty and health in the context of nail care (Eekhof et al., 2012) (Figure 5.4).

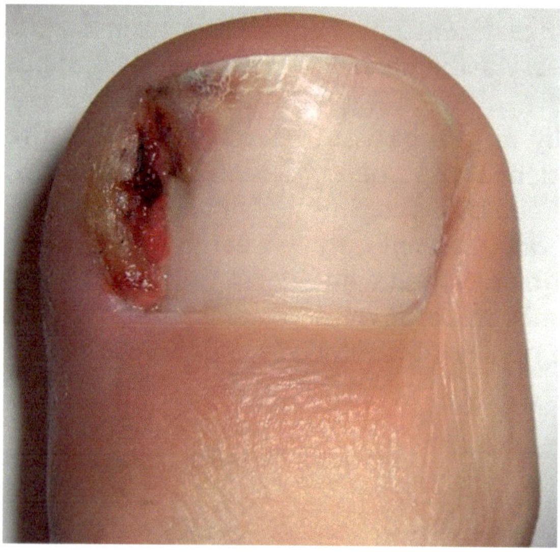

Figure 5.4. A clear picture showing the ingrown nail and the wounded infected nail bed.

Source: https://upload.wikimedia.org/wikipedia/commons/a/a5/Ingrown_nail_002_cropped.jpg.

Test Your Knowledge

1. What are the key visual differences between fungal nail infections and nail psoriasis?
2. How can poor nail hygiene contribute to the development of fungal infections and ingrown nails?
3. Are nail fungal infections contagious, and what precautions should be taken to prevent their spread?

5.2. Symptoms and Diagnosis

Learning Outcome

1. Describe visual signs of nail conditions
2. Understand diagnostic procedures for nail issues
3. Explain the importance of early detection

Symptom assessment compared to nail aesthetic disorders is of fundamental importance in accurate diagnosis and subsequent treatment. Classical symptoms that are significant are those related to the color, texture, and shape of the nail. For instance, disorders like fungal infection will present with nail color alteration and thickening, while psoriasis will cause pitting and separation from the nail bed. The psychological and emotional impact of these symptoms and signs on the individual, particularly one who is in the aesthetic profession, creates a necessity for an early assessment. Practitioners also should be vigilant for underlying systemic illness that may manifest via alteration of the nail, such as anemia or thyroid disease, with nonspecific manifestations. A comprehensive understanding and detection of these symptoms provides a very essential foundation for an appropriate diagnosis and a treatment plan in the domain of nail aesthetic disorders. Diagnosis of nail aesthetic disorders greatly relies on careful clinical examination as well as the patients' medical history. Dermatologists and physicians utilize various diagnostics to determine appropriate reasons for nail symptoms. This may include naked eye inspection, in which the form, color, and surface irregularities of the nail are assessed. Laboratory tests can also be done to rule out infections or systemic conditions; for instance, fungal culture can confirm the presence of an infection, while hematologic studies can demonstrate nutritional deficiencies that cause nails to be deformed. Diagnostics within this area are sometimes complicated by the fact that different conditions present similar symptoms, underlining the importance of specialized training and education within dermatology. Added awareness of the correlation between internal health and nail health can also go a long way in terms of accurate diagnosis and result in more effective treatments that are tailored to each person's individual case. Care also has to be taken to the limitations and barriers associated with diagnosing nail aesthetic conditions. Fragility of symptoms is most often the reason for misdiagnosis, with unnecessary interventions undertaken by patients or long periods of misery lived through. Underreporting of symptoms, particularly in stigma-induced cases—, such as in the case of nail disorders caused by hygiene or personal care practice, comprises some of the chief barriers to accurate diagnosis. Also, the unawareness of primary practitioners about the complexities of nail health can make referrals too late. It is emphasized in the present literature that the early detection of symptoms is of utmost importance in the management of conditions like nail psoriasis or onychomycosis because delayed referral will result in chronic disease or irreversible damage (Mikulska et al., 2025). Thus, a holistic and empathic diagnostic method is required whereby the patients receive appropriate management methods with respect for both the psychological and physical aspects of their nail beauty disorders (Gilbert et al., 2025).

5.2.1. Visual Signs of Nail Conditions

One should understand the visual signs of nail diseases when diagnosing associated underlying diseases and enhancing nail beauty treatments. Fingernails can show a range of alterations that are indicative of general health or many conditions. For instance, pitting, ridging, or coloration changes can be caused by a range of dermatologic or systemic conditions. These visual cues are capable of sparking sensitivity towards potential health problems, since the nails tend to reflect the body's internal condition. Specifically, changes , such as yellowish coloration that can signify fungal infection or blue coloration that is representative of lack of oxygen are evidence of the interplay between beauty and health. Detection of such signs enables individuals to seek early medical visits and appropriate treatments, thereby maximizing the aesthetic appearance of the nails and general health. The texture and form of nails can also provide crucial evidence regarding nail health. A healthy nail is normally even and smooth, while conditions, such as onycholysis or clubbing show up in the form of discernible abnormalities. Onycholysis involves the loss of adhesion of the nail from its nail bed to reveal a smelly appearance, which can also be a sign of trauma, infection, or thyroid diseases. Similarly, clubbing, or a more marked curvature of the nails and fingertips, has been associated with pulmonary and cardiovascular ailments. Such changes not only affect the look of the nails but also raise concerns for the overall health checkups. The ability to detect them early can make interventions and preventive measures easier and therefore enhance the effectiveness of treatments for restoring nail aesthetics and health. Apart from form and texture, the overall well-being of the nails is also influenced by various environmental factors and individual habits. Prolonged exposure to chemicals, water, and harsh detergents makes them brittle and assume the shape of cracks or splits. Such changes will lose their beauty and therefore raise concerns regarding appropriate protective care and treatments. Also, inappropriate nail care measures—, such as over-filing or misuse of nail products, may further aggravate such issues. By embracing the full understanding of these visual signals and the influencing factors upon them, individuals can best coordinate treatments. A combination of awareness of visual signs, precautionary care measures, and treatment to rectify underlying health conditions impacting overall nail appearance is finally needed to promote healthier nail appearances.

5.2.2. Diagnostic Procedures for Nail Issues

Diagnostic examinations for nail conditions are essential in making the correct diagnosis and developing a proper treatment plan. Routine procedures include visual examination, microscopy, and imaging studies. A thorough visual examination allows health workers to identify such visible findings as discoloration, brittleness, or change of the nail's surface that may indicate underlying conditions. Further, dermoscopy with a specially designed hand-held instrument provides even better visualization of the nail and nail bed structures so that the clinician can detect subtle differences not apparent with the naked eye.

Microscopy may be employed to inspect nail clippings or scrapings and help diagnose fungal infections or other pathologies. Finally, accurate diagnosis relies on a combination of these approaches, each yielding valuable information to assist in the decision regarding appropriate treatment of patients who present with complaints regarding their nails. In addition to basic examinations, specific diagnostic procedures are essential to the assessment of nail disorders. For instance, cultures and biopsies are often necessary in the diagnosis of certain dermatologic diseases, e.g., onychomycosis or psoriasis of the nail. Cultures may be utilized to identify fungal organisms causing infection of the nail, thereby informing the targeted antifungal therapy. Biopsy entails amputation of a tiny piece of the nail bed or surrounding tissue to permit histopathological evaluation. It is a highly valuable tool in differentiating benign and malignant lesions and in identifying the exact etiology of unexplained nail changes. Application of these diagnostic techniques should ensure that practitioners are positioned to effectively handle the intricate nature of nail aesthetic conditions, which essentially means a tailored therapy following specific patient requirements.

Finally, clinical correlation and patient history form important aspects of the diagnostic process for nail conditions. A proper assessment requires consideration of the patient's medical history, lifestyle, and previous aesthetic treatments received. For instance, individuals who have a background of trauma or who are chronic nail-pickers may have some deformities or changes that come into play during the diagnosis. Furthermore, the psychosocial impact of nail disease is what determines the treatment regimen since such cosmetic impairments have significant effects on the individual's self-esteem. As the literature has emphasized, the evolution of nail aesthetic treatments, such as gel and laser treatments, involves an intense understanding of both the underlying pathologies and the patient's aesthetic goals (Bansal et al., 2024). Introducing these seemingly disparate elements into medical practice enables clinicians to have a better appreciation of the nuances of nail diagnosis, and thus the success of treatment for patients who have aesthetic-related issues of the nails (Figure 5.5).

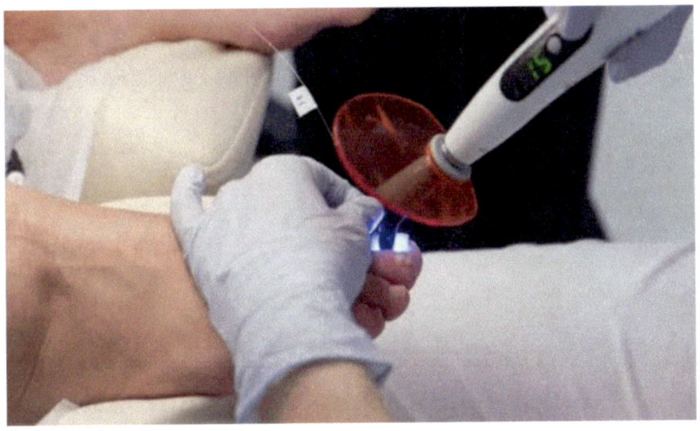

Figure 5.5. Diagnostic for nail issues.

Source: https://www.shutterstock.com/shutterstock/videos/3727055235/thumb/1.jpg?ip=x480.

5.2.3. Importance of Early Detection

The significance of early diagnosis in nail cosmetic disease cannot be overstated, as this directly impacts on treatment and patient satisfaction. The majority of nail ailments, , such as fungal infections and skin diseases, can lead to more serious systemic complications if not detected. Early detection is thus crucial to ensure the employment of therapeutic measures to prevent progression. For instance, nail fungal infection may not only affect appearance but also be painful and lead to secondary infection if not attended to. Further, early diagnosis of the conditions means that early information on available care options is relayed to the patients, enabling them to make informed decisions regarding their treatment, as well as overall improved health and well-being. The visual appearance of the nail is usually a sign of one's overall health, and hence brings into focus the significance of early detection. Certain abnormalities, such as color changes, texture modification, or lifting and separation from the nail bed, could signal underlying systemic health problems, including autoimmune diseases or vitamin deficiency. By identifying these changes in their initial stages, doctors can start testing that might in fact, detect important conditions, thereby allowing for preventive action. Raising public consciousness of the connection between health and the appearance of nails will enhance the feeling of the importance of early diagnosis. General benefits of early diagnosis extend beyond the cosmetic aspect to encompass preventive medical care and improved quality of life for the patients. Incorporation of regular nail checks into the individual's care routine not only assists in early detection but also encourages a preventive approach towards the preservation of health. By making individuals more conscious of their nail health, practitioners can provide early intervention and, as a result, have a considerable impact on the overall healthcare system. For example, early management of nail conditions could possibly reduce the incidence of advanced infection that requires more intensive intervention or admission to the hospital. In addition, education about nail appearance and the consequences can lead to increased involvement in self-care activities among individuals. Thus, the emphasis laid on early diagnosis of nail aesthetic disorders finds coherence with the latest models of health that focus on preventive practices, ultimately aiming to enhance patients' overall health outcomes and beauty satisfaction in the field of nail care (Figure 5.6).

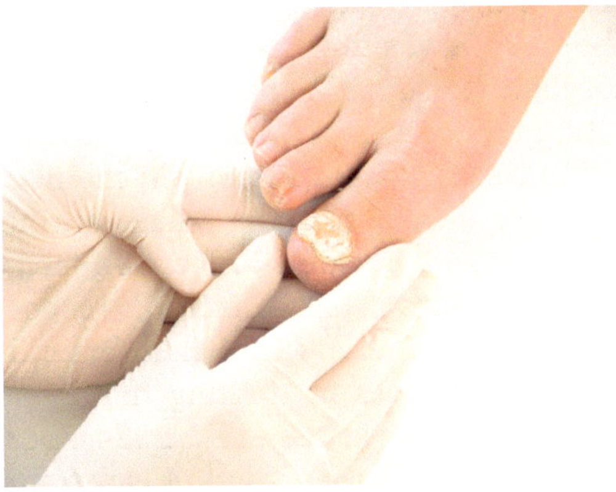

Figure 5.6. Clinical examination of toenail onychomycosis.

Source: https://familydoctor.org/wp-content/uploads/2001/02/nail.jpg.

Test Your Knowledge

1. What are the key visual signs that may indicate underlying nail aesthetic conditions?
2. What diagnostic procedures are used to identify the causes of abnormal nail appearance?

5.3. Treatment Options for Nail Conditions

Learning Outcome

1. Discuss topical treatments for nail aesthetic conditions
2. Define oral medications for nail aesthetic conditions
3. Focus on surgical interventions

The multifaceted nature of nail disease necessitates a multidimensional treatment approach with both topical and systemic therapy. Perhaps the most prevalent of these diseases is onychomycosis, a fungal infection of the nail that poses especially recalcitrant therapeutic challenges due to its propensity for recurrence and growing resistance to standard antifungal medications. Emerging therapies , such as nonthermal atmospheric plasma (NTAP) may be the answer to these difficulties. Recent studies indicate that NTAP has been successful in inhibiting the growth of Trichophyton rubrum, a common causative agent of onychomycosis. With more studies exploring NTAPs antifungal properties, it will provide an effective alternative for those patients still unsatisfactorily responsive to conventional therapy and thus extend the scope of alternatives in treating this common nail disease, as seen in Lee et al. (2024). Besides fungal disorders, nail aesthetic disorders also encompass an array of congenital disorders, , such as the ectodermal dysplasias (ED), which impart profound effects on the function and appearance of the nails. ED are expressed in multiple ways, including nails, hair, and teeth, leading to remarkable clinical presentations, such as abnormal morphology of the nails and tooth agenesis. Although complete management of EDs is still largely symptomatic, inclusion of aesthetic and functional considerations in the management plan is of prime importance. For instance, the application of cosmetic nail treatments has the added effect of beautifying while at the same time repairing structural flaws within. This can further be complemented by prosthetic options that consequently improve the quality of life in patients with EDs. The treatment implications of the treatment of nail disorders that come with ED illustrate the importance of an individualized approach, as stressed by Boutrid et al. (2022). Lastly, advances in laser treatment and photodynamic therapy (PDT) are expanding the scope of treatments for nail disorders. These non-invasive technologies are beneficial in the management of a variety of nail disorders, including nail psoriasis and fungal infection. Laser treatment works by concentrating on the compromised tissues and causing them to heal while minimizing damage to normal skin in the surrounding area. Patients also notice significant improvements in nail appearance and comfort, thus testifying to the importance of such a modality in aesthetic nail treatment. As more research continues to evaluate the long-term outcome and potential side effects of such treatments, providers need to remain informed on these emerging treatment modalities. Evolution of the treatment modalities reflects a broader movement towards integrative treatment of nail disorders to make patient care sensitive and dynamic to emerging evidence.

5.3.1. Topical Treatments

Among cosmetic nail disorders, topical treatment has been a crucial component in the management of many disorders, most notably fungal infections and dermatological responses. Topical treatments are formulated to directly reach affected areas, providing a focused approach with fewer side effects systemically. As an example, antifungal lacquers formulated for onychomycosis, or infection by fungi like Trichophyton rubrum, have been widely in demand due to their ease of application and efficacy. Moreover, these agents are also often used in conjunction with other therapies to achieve maximum total effectiveness. As the prevalence of nail disease grows, especially in patients undergoing systemic therapy with agents , such as chemotherapy, the role of local agents in the prevention or minimization of incidental nail disease is increasingly significant, ensuring improved quality of life and adherence to primary treatments (Bukvić et al., 2022). Moreover, the mixture of various active ingredients in topical preparations enhances their therapeutic value. For instance, the incorporation of moisturizing components can successfully alleviate manifestations of xerosis and pruritus that frequently accompany oncologic treatment. Certain emulsions containing urea or lactic acid even facilitate nail hydration and soften hardened nails for better cosmetic appearance. These adjuvant therapies are crucial to patients who are experiencing dermatologic side effects since they can prevent further complications and provide comfort during their broader course of treatment. Aggressive skin and nail integrity management through these topical medications enables patients to maintain their self-esteem and psychological well-being in challenging circumstances (Bukvić et al., 2022). Furthermore, new technologies , such as PDT are transforming the practice of topical treatment of nail diseases. PDT uses a photosensitizer, visible light, and oxygen to produce reactive oxygen species that kill infection-causing pathogens , such as Trichophyton rubrum. New research has emphasized the potential of treatments involving the combination of Protoporphyrin IX with light treatment as powerful agents against infection without helping in the development of microbial resistance, a key problem with systemic drugs. The shift to these newer techniques is particularly promising, with patients being treated effectively but with fewer side effects. Owing to more research, PDT can potentially give a valuable adjuvant to the traditional topical preparations, widening the therapeutic possibilities to effectively treat nail aesthetic disorders (Figure 5.7).

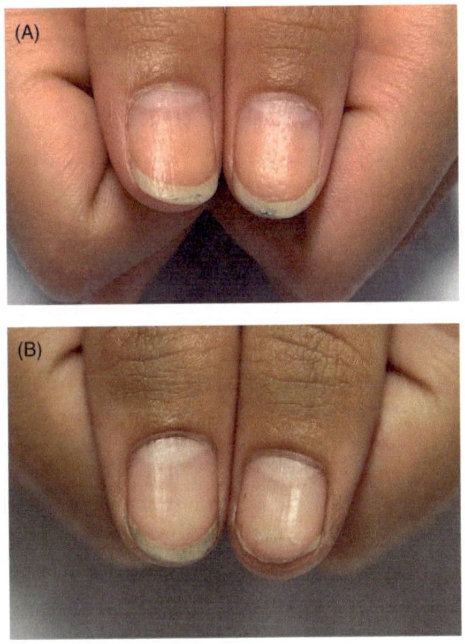

Figure 5.7. (A) Bilateral thumbnails after treatment with topical corticosteroids demonstrate recalcitrant nail matrix disease, with irregular pitting and nail plate fragility; and (B) Four months after a single dose of intralesional triamcinolone, bilateral thumbnails show significant improvement in nail matrix features, with only a few remaining solitary pits on the right thumbnail.

Source: https://www.researchgate.net/publication/361228996/figure/fig1/AS:11431281173864384@1689056768626/A-Bilateral-thumbnails-after-treatment-with-topical-corticosteroids-demonstrate.png.

5.3.2. Oral Medications

Within the specialty of nail cosmetic disease, oral medications are the foundation for the treatment of most disorders, particularly fungal infections. Fungal infection of the nails, known as onychomycosis, is one of the more prevalent nail disorders and occurs in a high percentage of the population. Though there are topical drugs in the form of antifungal lacquers, these struggle with drug permeation through the nail plate, and their efficacy is therefore compromised (Bhowmik et al., 2025). Oral antifungal medicines have therefore taken over as the treatment of choice for more severe or recalcitrant cases that cannot be controlled using topical therapies. Yet, systemic application of such drugs is not without risk, as they have the potential to elicit side effects ranging from gastrointestinal discomfort to more severe complications like liver damage. This highlights the need for careful patient selection and follow-up on therapy. Oral drug pharmacokinetics are frequently confounded by concurrent administration of other therapies, , such as glucagon-like peptide 1 receptor agonists (GLP1RAs). These medications are commonly utilized in the management of diabetes and obesity and may impact the absorption of certain oral medications, like those utilized in the management of nail disease (Calvarysky et al., 2024). Data indicate that the use of GLP1RAs has been implicated in delayed gastric emptying, hence modifying the peak plasma concentration and time to peak concentration of co-administered oral drugs. Despite that such interactions are not likely to dramatically alter the overall exposure to drugs, they ought to be reported, particularly for those with a narrow therapeutic index, and may have significant clinical implications. The complex interactions among these drugs necessitate continued research and patient-specific treatment approaches to maximize efficacy and safety. Novel drug delivery methods also address traditional oral therapy for the treatment of nail aesthetic disorders. For instance, new technologies , such as iontophoresis and ultrasound-assisted drug delivery systems are studied to enhance the delivery of antifungal drugs through the nail plate (Bhowmik et al., 2025). These technologies can potentially reduce the consumption of systemic drugs, thereby diminishing associated risks. Electrical or ultrasonic wave technology is employed by these technologies to deliver drugs into the affected tissue more efficiently, which may translate to a more localized treatment modality. With the development of the field of nail aesthetics, the use of such sophisticated delivery systems could potentially usher in a new era in the treatment of nail disorders that is both effective and safe.

5.3.3. Surgical Interventions

Surgery plays a significant role in the treatment of several nail cosmetic disorders, particularly after failure of nonsurgical interventions. The most common surgery is matrixectomy, which entails excision of the nail matrix to avoid regrowth of the ingrowing nail. This treatment is usually performed under local anesthetic and involves the meticulous excision of the nail plate and matrix tissue, thereby alleviating pain and reducing the risk of subsequent infections. Reconstruction of the nail bed may also be needed for traumatic nail loss due to injury. Surgical treatment offers good remedies to such disorders as onychomycosis, in which severe fungal infection compromises the nail. The decision of the appropriate surgery should consider the individual patient parameters and aesthetic aims for optimal results in nail reconstruction. In certain instances, surgical treatment is not only required for aesthetic reasons but also to enhance the function and health of the hand. Digital mucous cysts or subungual exostoses could be further challenged by being tender and altering the mechanical digit function. Surgical removal of such lesions can potentially dramatically improve not only the cosmetic aspect of the nail, but also alleviate pain, which would enhance patients' quality of life. In addition, in extreme circumstances where surgery is indicated, multi-disciplinary approaches can be utilized. Cooperative practice with dermatologists, orthopedic surgeons, or plastic surgeons can lead to comprehensive treatment plans considering the aesthetic as well as the functional aspects of nail disorders, thereby offering a holistic solution to patient care. The advancement in techniques and equipment employed in surgery has greatly enhanced the efficiency of intervention in nail aesthetic disorders. Minimally invasive procedures, for instance, have become equally effective as traditional open surgeries, resulting in shorter recovery times and reduced scarring. Innovations , such as laser therapy and endoscopic surgery are standard examples of how the industry continues to advance, pushing the boundaries of traditional surgical procedures. Also, integration of predictive modeling, as has been outlined in studies of other types of surgical procedures, might similarly be useful for nail surgery in a bid to further optimize patient outcomes. Through an understanding of the complex interplay between beauty desires and necessary medical procedures, surgical processes can make a lot of difference in the management of nail diseases, ultimately contributing to improved patient satisfaction and psychosocial well-being (Christopher et al., 2024; Netala et al., 2024) (Figure 5.8).

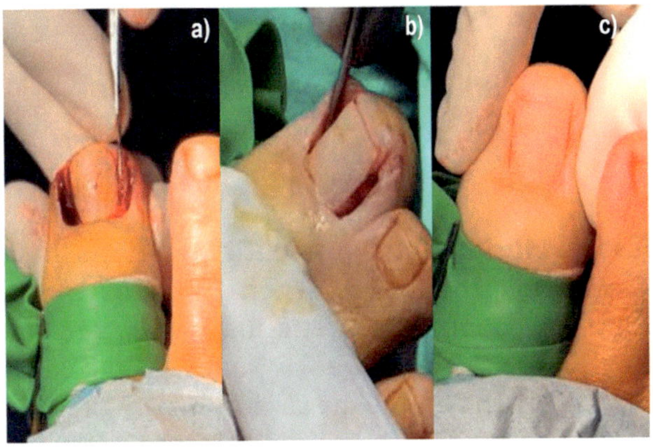

Figure 5.8. Aesthetic reconstruction: (a) Subeponychial wedge excision; (b) curettage of the matrix zone and the nail bed; and (c) coapting the folds.

Source: https://www.researchgate.net/publication/340069619/figure/fig1/AS:11431281213117451@1702971056372/Aesthetic-reconstruction-a-Subeponychial-wedge-excision-b-curettage-of-the-matrix.tif.

Test Your Knowledge

1. What are the most common topical treatments for nail conditions, and when are they most effective?
2. When are oral medications preferred over topical treatments for nail disorders?
3. What surgical interventions are available for nail conditions?

5.4. Home Remedies and Preventive Measures

Learning Outcome

1. Deal with natural treatments for nail health
2. Explain the role of daily care routines for nails
3. Focus on lifestyle changes to prevent nail conditions

Home solutions and prevention options have come into prominence when it comes to the treatment of nail aesthetic disorders, because they usually provide a readily available remedy without the need for much medical intervention. Many individuals seek natural options in the belief of strengthening nail health, an activity that aligns with a long-standing tradition that involves shared information and personal experience. Research has shown that these remedies can be derived from an extensive variety of cultural traditions, some of which existed before the modern medical understanding. Through the use of materials like coconut oil, tea tree oil, and vitamin E, it is possible to enhance the hardness and softening of the nails. However, it is important to handle these remedies with caution, as they may have vastly different degrees of potency and not cure diseases. Therefore, the balance between home remedies and expert health guidance is necessary for optimal nail care, particularly in cases where appearance conditions are indicators of overall health issues. The interaction between indigenous and contemporary practices in health care emphasizes the imperative role of preventive measures in deriving healthy nails. Scholars have contended that the synthesis of different health belief systems increases the understanding of nail care and beauty. For instance, preventive measures , such as moisturizing, avoiding harsh chemicals, and keeping the nails clean in a proper manner have their root in folklore as well as modern health education. It may avoid common issues, such as brittleness and discoloration. Furthermore, by establishing a sense of awareness regarding the determinants of nail health, such as nutrition and environmental factors, people are capable of making better-informed choices. This integrative approach not only takes advantage of rising patterns of individual wellness but also respects cultural histories that long ago ordained preventive care as a first priority in sustaining overall well-being, as emphasized in the work of scholars reviewing synergies across alternative health paradigms (Brady et al., 2001). To enhance the effectiveness of home treatments and preventive measures, nail care education needs to be incorporated into settings in the community. Educational outreach can help demystify the secrets of the aesthetics of the nails so that individuals are empowered with the tools to achieve and take care of their nails. Initiatives that combine ancient knowledge and modern practices, , such as workshops or webinars, can empower individuals to gain healthier habits on a constant basis. Moreover, as highlighted in Tanya Langtree's study of previous nursing methods, a science-based methodology can create healthier outcomes. It throws into relief the necessity for the integration of proven historical practices with new nail care breakthroughs. Through encouraging a people-oriented way that accepts diverse sources of knowledge, we can encourage sustained nail health practices that are effective and respond to the varied experiences of individuals seeking to improve nail beauty (Langtree et al., 2020).

5.4.1. Natural Treatments for Nail Health

The quest for natural treatments for nail care has gained much momentum as consumers grow more sensitive to the potential negative impacts of synthetic chemicals that are commonly employed in commercial nail treatments. Of the most valuable natural treatments is the application of essential oils, which have antifungal and antibacterial properties that make nails harder and battle diseases, such as fungal infection. For instance, tea tree oil kills off pathogens and also promotes general nail health. Moreover, the combination of essential oils with a carrier oil like coconut or almond oil can introduce moisture so that nails do not crack and become brittle. The integrated use of such natural resources does not merely restore present nail imperfections but also promotes the preventative approach, creating long-term care and cosmetic enhancement for the nails, a movement toward healthy beauty in general. Aside from essential oils, dietary changes also contribute significantly to the nail condition. Nutrients , such as biotin, zinc, and protein are necessary in nail strengthening and promoting their growth. Inserting foods rich in these nutrients, , such as eggs, leafy greens, nuts, and fish, will also fortify the nail matrix and enhance the look of nails. Science shows that adding biotin supplements to one's diet has a notable improvement in the thickness as well as overall strength of nails. Furthermore, staying properly hydrated is essential, as nails usually reflect the level of hydration in the body. Through a balanced diet and proper fluid intake, individuals are not only able to feed their nails but also their bodies, demonstrating the interconnectedness between diet and the look of nails. This integrated approach is part of growing trends centered on holistic health, manifesting an aesthetic worldview that appreciates that beauty is a quality within. Though the majority of natural treatments owe their origins to the centuries of common practice, contributions made by the topical application cannot be overlooked. Various natural remedies, such as garlic and lemon juice, have also received much acclaim for their beneficial effects on nails. Garlic, selenium-enriched, will work towards growth and firmness, while lemon juice, replete with vitamin C, imparts a shiny natural sheen to the nails. Application of these substances on a consistent basis can help keep nails healthy and discoloration-free. Moreover, the use of a combination of olive oil and vinegar as a soak can potentially create a healing environment that restores moisture and elasticity. These treatments not only correct acute cosmetic illnesses, but they also create a preventative protocol for nail health. By incorporating such natural remedies into everyday life, individuals can not only enhance their nails but also gain a better sense of appreciation for natural ingredients, aligned with contemporary orientations toward sustainability and health in personal care routines (Figure 5.9).

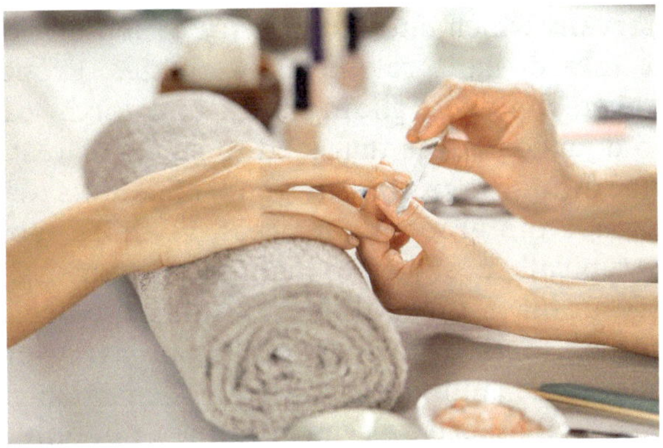

Figure 5.9. Natural nail care.

Source: https://images.squarespace-cdn.com/content/v1/66620d8447d7562ea9de8bcc/b2b1521b-f84f-432d-b02e-ecc7de9b8680/natural-nail-spa-treatments-asheville.jpg.

5.4.2. Daily Care Routines for Nails

Developing an effective day-to-day care routine for nails is central to ensuring their well-being and cosmetic attractiveness, especially in the prevention of different nail disorders. It is vital to practice frequent cleansing since it clears waste and possible irritants that may cause infections or disorders. People should use a mild soap and warm water to wash their hands and nails before they dry well. In addition, the use of moisturizers for nails and cuticles plays a significant role in preventing nails and cuticles from drying up or becoming brittle. This moisturizing method is particularly effective because nails are usually exposed to unfavorable environmental factors, something that tends to worsen nail health. Additionally, the incorporation of nail strengtheners in regular grooming can act as protection, hardening the nails against daily stresses (Dalave et al., 2024). Such advanced maintenance is vital for maintaining the aesthetic appeal and functionality of the nails. Apart from overall hygiene, an entire care program for nails should include regular, systematic trimming and filing of nails to maintain nail shape and prevent breakage. Regular trimming is advisable at fixed intervals, which one should vary depending on the rate of nail growth and activities. Proper filing techniques, gliding back and forth, can avoid jagged edges that lead to snags or tears. In addition, investing in good nail tools will enhance the grooming process, as those tools are typically designed to maintain healthy nails and not harm them. Lastly, avoiding the use of nails as tools to open packages or carry out other tasks minimizes the risk of mechanical damage. By these everyday routines, not only is the physical appearance of the nails preserved, but also the potential for future nail aesthetic disorders (Coli C-Iță et al., 2024). Even applying and removing nail polish should be done carefully in everyday care tasks. Although nail polish may make a person appear more presentable, constant application can lead to staining of the nails and weakening if precautions are not taken into consideration. Therefore, the application of a base coat is recommended to act as a covering to protect the nail from the polish. Use of no acetone-containing nail polish removers is also recommended to prevent nails from drying out. Breaks from polish usage from time to time to allow the nails to "breathe" can also help to maintain healthy nails overall. Also, regular inspections of nails for signs of infection or color alteration are important, which will enable early action if there is any cosmetic disorder. In summary, the incorporation of these extensive daily routines can contribute significantly to improving nail health and cosmesis, thereby reducing the occurrence of nail disorders (Dalave et al., 2024). Through constant practice, an individual is able to learn not only good nails but also a profound understanding of personal grooming and care (Figure 5.10).

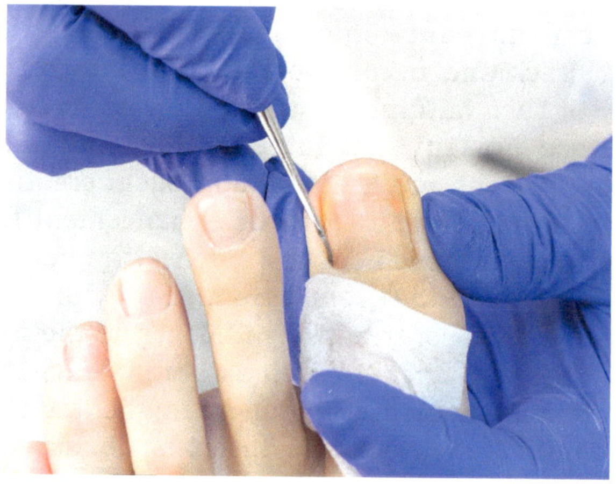

Figure 5.10. Treatment of an ingrown toenail by a podiatrist.

Source: https://sanderspodiatry.com.au/wp-content/uploads/2022/08/toenails-health.jpg.

5.4.3. Lifestyle Changes to Prevent Nail Conditions

The inclusion of lifestyle changes is central to the prevention of many nail diseases since these changes have a direct impact on the improvement of nail appearance and health. A simple step involves proper hygiene practices. Proper washing of hands with soap and keeping the nails short and clean can decrease the risk of fungal infections and other nail disorders. In addition to that, hydration plays an important role; proper intake of fluid not only enhances general health but also prevents nails from becoming brittle and on the brink of breakage. In general, the adoption of sustainable hygiene practices is a beginning towards safeguarding against conditions of nail appearance. Dietary modifications are another significant lifestyle change that enhances nail wellness. Consumption of a balanced diet rich with sufficient vitamins and minerals contributes to strengthening and nourishing the nails. Biotin, zinc, and omega-3 fatty acids have been proven to be contributory to nail health. Further, use of dietary supplements has gone up steadily during periods of health crises, most of which was during the COVID-19 pandemic, and also reflects rising public interest in preventive health aspects (Djaoudene et al., 2023). There needs to be a focus on nutrient-dense foods , such as leafy greens, seeds, and nuts to achieve the best outcomes, which might decrease the incidence of nail disorders due to deficiencies. Lastly, preventive action can also stop the incidence of nail disorders. Frequent use of moisturizers, particularly on the cuticles and surrounding skin, can avoid dryness and cracking, both precursors to nail disorders. Also, the use of gloves when cleaning the house or when handling harsh chemicals is essential in preventing nails from being disfigured. These preventive measures, together with healthy living and proper nutrition, constitute a full-scale prevention program against nail aesthetic disorders. Implementing these lifestyle changes first results in both the health and beauty of the nails, which is part of the bigger goal of effectively treating nail disorders (Antoine, 2023).

Test Your Knowledge

1. What natural treatments can support nail health and help manage common aesthetic nail conditions?
2. What daily nail care routines can help maintain healthy and aesthetically pleasing nails?

5.5. The Role of Nutrition in Nail Health

Learning Outcome

1. Describe essential vitamins and minerals for nails
2. Understand dietary recommendations for strong nails
3. Explain the impact of hydration on nail aesthetics

Nail care falls under a broad category where nutrition plays a significant role, impacting the structure and appearance of nails. Nutritional factors , such as proteins, vitamins, and minerals play a vital role in the survival and appearance of nails. The most vital among them are biotin, zinc, and B vitamins, which contribute to nail strength and growth. For instance, biotin, which is mostly associated with hair, also plays a role in the thickening of nails and in preventing brittleness as well as breaking. Vitamin E, which belongs to the antioxidant class, contributes to the maintenance of moisture, a key contribution to preventing nail fragility. Thus, a diet lacking these necessary nutrients could lead to some nail diseases , such as discoloration and ridging, highlighting the importance of dietary awareness in the pursuit of healthy, good-looking nails. Further, recent studies highlight the link between nutritional deficiencies and a number of nail diseases. Diseases , such as koilonychia, which involve spooned nails, can be caused by iron deficiency, whereas white nail spots may indicate zinc or other essential mineral deficiencies. These conditions are external manifestations of the body's internal nutritional imbalance that, in this case, signifies that diet has an important influence on nail health. In this case, the use of a balanced diet that includes vitamins and antioxidants becomes important not only for appearing good but also for good health. This holistic strategy on nutrition brings out the fineries of nail care and emphasizes the point that cosmetic treatments cannot replace the role played by a vitamin-supplemented diet. In addition, the consumption of some nutritional supplements has proven to be a probable method for maximizing the health of nails. According to studies, such supplements, , such as vitamin C and biotin, have been effective in therapeutic uses, influencing nail growth and appearance. Of particular significance is vitamin C, with a key role in collagen synthesis, a critical component in strengthening nails. In addition, variable results from research demonstrate the necessity for adapting supplement use based on specific health profiles and specific deficiencies (Bayar et al., 2025). Local treatments may produce short-term improvement or cosmetic enhancement of nail appearance, but cannot correct underlying nutritional imbalances. In general, a profound understanding of the role of nutrition enables individuals not only to enhance their nails but to invest in their general health in the long term, showing the intricate interaction between inner nutrition and external appearance (Akram et al., 2025).

5.5.1. Essential Vitamins and Minerals for Nails

The health and cosmetic condition of nails is directly attributed to dietary intake, i.e., essential minerals and vitamins. For example, biotin, a B-vitamin, has been recognized for centuries as having the role of strengthening and promoting growth of nails. Scientific evidence indicates that biotin supplementation increases nail thickness and reduces brittleness and is therefore a fundamental nutrient for anyone experiencing nail cosmetic issues. Additionally, vitamins A, C, and E play a role in maintaining healthy nails overall by facilitating keratin development and combating oxidative stress to the nails. This vitamin combination not only enhances nail outlook but also contributes towards the preventative care of many nail afflictions, further endorsing the concept that nutrition is the foundation for achieving and maintaining nail aesthetics as exposed in ongoing research that identifies the significance of diverse nutrient intake in maintaining skin and nail health (Januszewski et al., 2023). In addition to vitamins, minerals , such as zinc and iron play equally crucial roles in nail health. Zinc, being a "beauty mineral," is essential in the metabolism of cells and tissue growth, and this converts directly into the health of the nails. A zinc deficiency may cause alterations in the nails' texture and a higher susceptibility to contracting conditions , such as white spots on the nails. Iron is another necessary mineral since it allows oxygen to be transported to cells, like those in the nail matrix. Iron deficits lead to anemia, which leads to brittle or spoon-like nails, also affecting nail appearance.

Therefore, having adequate amounts of these minerals is not only important to systemic health but also healthy, cosmetically beautiful nails as part of an overall approach to nail health and treatment interventions (Castro et al., 2023). For optimal bioavailability of these vitamins and minerals, the addition of a balanced diet with sufficient whole foods is essential. Protein foods , such as fish, meat, and legumes provide the building blocks for keratin, while nuts and leafy greens may provide both minerals and vitamins required for nail care. Inclusion of antioxidant vegetables and fruits can also serve to buffer oxidative damage implicated in nail care. Recent studies suggest beneficial roles of antioxidants for skin integrity, which would suggest an equivalent protective role for nail care. Further, supplementing the diet with omega-3 fatty acid-containing foods can help to keep the body hydrated and thus enhance nail flexibility and minimize brittleness. Through customization of food intake to include these essential nutrients, patients can improve their nail appearance and condition considerably, in line with the latest tendencies in holistic well-being and cosmetics (Januszewski et al., 2023) (Figure 5.11).

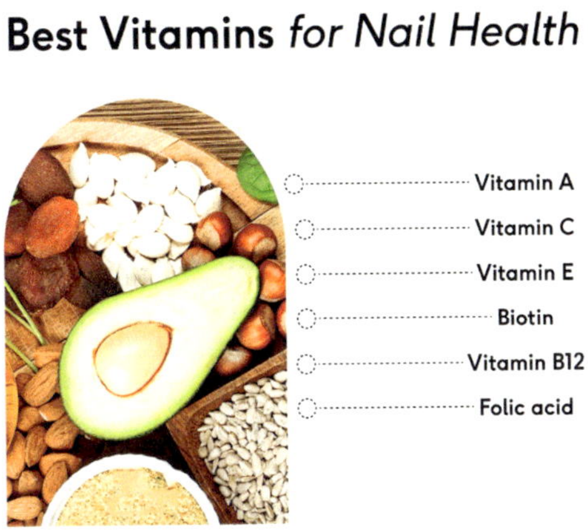

Figure 5.11. Best vitamins for nail health.

Source: https://cdn.shopify.com/s/files/1/0024/7123/1534/files/Vitamins_for_nail_health_2x_ef462e77-e119-44be-89ac-dafbd87fd547.jpg?v=1680786485.

5.5.2. Dietary Recommendations for Strong Nails

Healthy, well-fed nails are normally taken to be a significant indicator of overall health, and diet is crucial in their achievement. Vitamins, proteins, and minerals are all important nutrients that constitute part of nail health and development. A biotin-supplemented diet, for instance, is beneficial in strengthening keratins and nails. Eggs, nuts, and whole grains are rich dietary sources of biotin. Furthermore, the presence of proteins from fish, poultry, and legumes brings amino acids that support the development of the structure of nails. This nutritional basis not only makes the nails stronger but also inhibits common conditions like brittleness and splitting, thus enhancing the link between food choices and the appearance of the nails. Apart from biotin and protein, hydration cannot be excluded from food recommendations for healthy nails. The state of body hydration has a direct impact on the color and well-being of the nails. Dehydration results from water deficiency, which compromises the structural supporting system of the nails and makes them susceptible to breakage. Consuming adequate amounts of water, together with hydrating foods like cucumbers and oranges, can assist in keeping the body sufficiently hydrated. Electrolytes contained in foods like bananas and avocados also play an important role in ensuring fluid balance. A well-hydrated body promotes the health of the nails as well as general physiological function, thus highlighting the importance of an appropriate diet with sufficient hydrating factors to promote improved nail appearance.

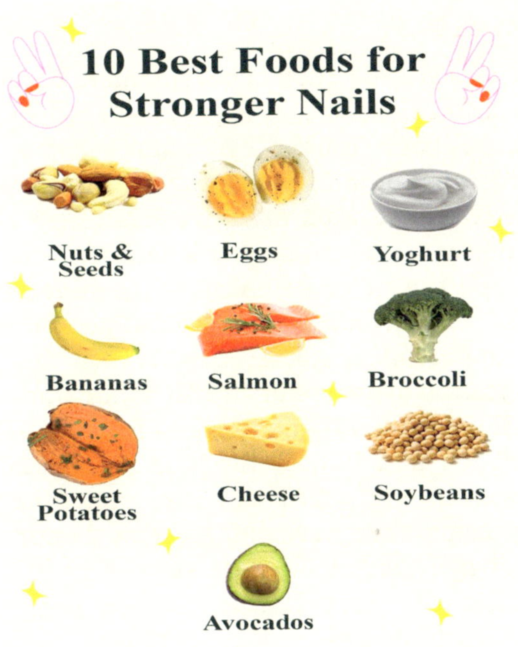
10 Best Foods for Stronger Nails
Nuts & Seeds
Eggs
Yoghurt
Bananas
Salmon
Broccoli
Sweet Potatoes
Cheese
Soybeans
Avocados

Figure 5.12. 10 best foods for stronger nails.

Source: https://i.pinimg.com/736x/66/7c/1b/667c1b93f6db49a6783030ffda015c12.jpg.

Moreover, some micronutrients like zinc and iron have significant functions in the prevention of nail aesthetic issues, particularly involving weakness or color. Zinc, which is present in shellfish, beans, and seeds, plays a crucial role in cell production, as it influences the growth and repair of nails. Iron, rich in red meat, lentils, and green leafy vegetables, is necessary for carrying oxygen in the blood, which consequently impacts the nails. Deficiency in any one of them may manifest as white spots, ridges, or even nail plate cracking. Therefore, emphasis on the ingestion of foods comprising these micronutrients is paramount for individuals seeking to enhance the texture of their nails, as part of broader therapies of nail treatment amidst overall aesthetic states and treatments (Al-Zyoud et al., 2023; Gopalakrishnan et al., 2023) (Figure 5.12).

5.5.3. Impact of Hydration on Nail Aesthetics

The look of nails extends beyond mere cosmetic appearance; nails can express overall health and wellness. Proper hydration plays a key role in maintaining the integrity and look of nails. Well-hydrated nails are less likely to be brittle, which eventually will lead to cracking and splitting. This emphasizes the function of moisture in avoiding ailments that detract from nail appearance. Studies have shown that the application of some nutritional compounds can enhance the quality of skin and nails by better hydration and barrier function. For instance, micronutrients , such as biotin and Omega-3 fatty acids have been linked with firmer and better-hydrated nails, thus suggesting proper nutrition is essential to having gorgeous nails without any beauty concerns, such as coloration or texture defects (Januszewski et al., 2023). In addition to nutritional aspects influencing hydration, exogenous factors play a role in determining the optimal appearance of the nails. Exposure to environmental harsh chemicals and frequent hand washing leads to the nails losing natural oils, leading to dryness and a weakened appearance. Vegetable-based moisturizers, e.g., Aloe vera or Jojoba oil, are effective in rebalancing moisture content and gaining additional advantages through their antioxidant effect (Michalak, 2023). These biological compounds not only moisturize but also impart protective benefits against stress from the environment. Adequate moisturizing of nails is thus a multi-faceted approach—one that unites hydration inward with nutrition and outward through skin care practices that prefer agreeable aesthetic states conducive to healthy-looking nails. Where hydration overlaps with aesthetic appeal to the nail, the necessity for an integrated or holistic approach to caring for nails necessitates attention. Adequate hydration levels also foster not only cosmetic beauty but functional healthiness, affecting the general nail bed and the surrounding tissue health. Neglecting proper hydration will cause unsightly nail health, so it is crucial to attend to both internal and external hydration sources consistently. In addition, understanding what dehydration symptoms look like can make individuals proactive with their nail care regimen. Through a focus on hydration by way of dietary habits and conscious application of moisturizing products, individuals can improve the aesthetics of their nails while avoiding possible conditions that would interfere with their overall look (Januszewki et al., 2023; Michalak, 2023).

Test Your Knowledge

1. Which essential vitamins and minerals are most important for maintaining healthy nails?
2. What dietary recommendations can help promote stronger, healthier nails?

5.6. Professional Treatments and Procedures

Learning Outcome

1. Explain the terms manicures and pedicures
2. Understand the concept of nail enhancements and artificial nails
3. Describe laser treatments for nail conditions

Nail beauty exists beyond the realm of mere cosmetic appearance to encompass a diverse array of professional procedures for an equally wide array of nail ailments. Nail technicians more and more incorporating newer methods into their practice, treating issues with fungal infection, brittle nails, and nail pigmentation. Treatments commonly involve both systemic and topical methods, from antifungal medication to nail-care specialty products, which not only restore the nail's health but also beautify its appearance. Of special significance, aesthetic therapies are increasingly being added to patient care, , such as the outcomes of an experimental trial highlighting how aesthetic treatments alleviated distress and improved skin-related quality of life in patients with cancer undergoing treatment. This evidence suggests that those techniques could also benefit individuals suffering from cosmetic nail disorders, towards the convergence of medical processes and cosmetic beautification procedures to ensure overall wellness (Faccio et al., 2019). Besides the treatment of some nail diseases, professional treatments usually involve the application of advanced technologies to enhance the aesthetic appeal of nails. Techniques , such as PDT and laser therapy are utilized more in the nail care industry, solutions to difficult problems that conventional techniques cannot address. Furthermore, the training in the somatology and beauty markets has to be standardized for the use of these sophisticated techniques. As highlighted in somatology profession studies, there has been a need for more training in aesthetic treatments that can encourage practitioners to administer such high-end treatments confidently. The emphasis on education and skill acquisition is particularly significant in understanding the science behind nail aesthetics and applying new techniques effectively and safely (Ambrosio et al., 2018). Lastly, the integration of multidisciplinary methods in nail aesthetics increases not just the standards of care rendered but also answers rising client demands for comprehensive aesthetic treatments. What is needed to create and provide an appropriate course of treatment for both the functional and aesthetic requirements of nail care are professionals from multiple disciplines—either licensed nail technicians or dermatologists. By providing better treatment outcomes and higher client satisfaction, this team effort is achieved. Besides, acknowledgment of the need for aesthetic training, as sworn by somatology students and professionals, justifies the view that further training will equip practitioners with the needed skills to deal with different client requirements. As nail aesthetic continues to develop and expand, fostering an attitude of innovation and continuous learning will enhance the efficacy of treatment and client achievement (Ambrosio et al., 2018).

5.6.1. Manicures and Pedicures

Manicures and pedicures form the fundamentals of nail beauty treatments and do not merely address the beauty of nails but also hand and foot health. Manicures and pedicures feature many techniques like shaping, buffing, and polishing nails, which contribute to a gorgeous appearance while supporting hygienic practices. The art of a manicure or pedicure can also be seen as a form of self-care, a way for individuals to sit back and indulge themselves. Further, as used within the beauty community, these treatments can enhance one's confidence by improving the outwardly visible state of one's nails, which are in direct correlation with femininity and business image. Thus, the meaning of manicures and pedicures goes beyond superficial beauty treatment, as they are central to personal grooming narratives. The cultural meaning of manicures and pedicures further emphasizes their role in nail beauty treatments. These treatments tend to blend with cultural demands on beauty, particularly for women, who are subjected to repeated treatments to accord with traditional expectations. A fresh ethnographic examination has appeared of the way that vocational training in beauticians, particularly in urban India, reflects broader social processes whereby the business of beauty is understood as one of empowerment and self-actualization for women. This empowerment is, however, made complex by the socio-economic and familial duties many of the actors have to contend with. The study brings forth the fact that while beauty routines promote a higher level of agency, they are typically placed within traditional roles and shared responsibilities, making independent beauty challenging in neoliberal settings (Donner, 2023). In addition to aesthetic benefits, manicures and pedicures can be a part of physical well-being and self-esteem (Figure 5.13).

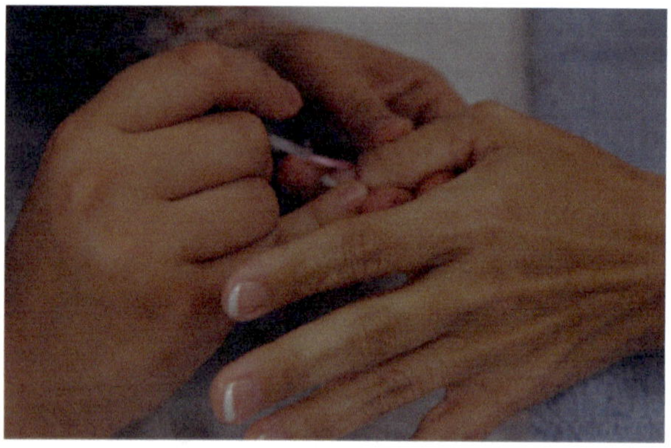

Figure 5.13. Manicure closeup – clear nail polish being applied.

Source: https://upload.wikimedia.org/wikipedia/commons/8/80/Manicure_closeup.jpg.

Recent evidence indicates that self-practices , such as yoga for inner beauty place great importance on women having greater awareness for complete well-being and self-care (Karuniati et al., 2022). Caring for inner beauty is appealing to the belief that manicure and pedicure are self-care activities for well-being. By practicing these beautification methods, women become more confident and well-accepted in society, a factor that contributes significantly to their psychological well-being and self-esteem. Hence, manicures and pedicures are far from being mere superficial beauty procedures; they contribute significantly to psychological health by seeking to correct aesthetic ailments with improved nail care and pristine cleanliness (Figure 5.14).

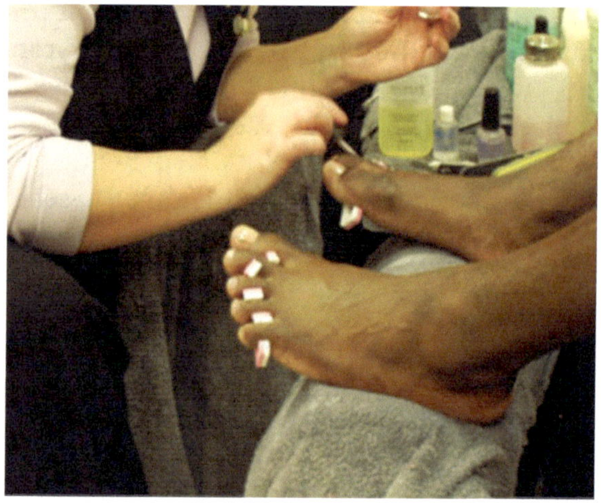

Figure 5.14. A pedicure in progress.

Source: https://upload.wikimedia.org/wikipedia/commons/9/98/Pedicure_1.jpg.

5.6.2. Nail Enhancements and Artificial Nails

The popularity of artificial nails and nail enhancements has taken center stage in contemporary beauty culture. With continued advances in cosmetic technology, artificial alternatives are in greater demand to improve the appearance of the nail. High-gloss effects and fancy designs are not only means of communication but also remedies to various aesthetic conditions affecting the nail. For others, being ideally shaped nails is not about vanity; it is representative of wider societal patterns towards self-betterment and empowerment. To this extent, the psychological impact of well-groomed nails cannot be overstated since they serve to boost individuals' confidence and self-esteem regarding their appearance. Moreover, the application of artificial nails entails a range of methods that vary from gel nails, acrylics, and nail wraps. These advances are able to effectively hide innate imperfections, thereby seeking cures in instances like brittle nails and nail deformities. Methods of nail enhancement are primarily embraced by individuals who suffer from afflictions like onychotillomania, where nail biting causes excessive breakdown. New techniques, , such as the use of nail peels and lasers, have emerged to offer cosmetic benefits while at the same time working to deliver treatment for the resultant nail disorders. These procedures adhere to modern dermatologic practice that emphasizes both cosmetic satisfaction and clinical efficacy, highlighting the importance of professional advice in aesthetic nail procedures (Bansal et al., 2024). While widespread, the application of artificial nails needs to be supplemented with a sophisticated understanding of adverse effects and complications. A defective application or inadequate after-care can result in adverse effects ranging from nail infection or allergic responses. Furthermore, the majority of individuals opt for these procedures in salons in which professional medical expertise is lacking, compromising the issue of long-term nail health. The integration of dermatological procedures into nail beauty would close this gap by requiring skilled professionals to carry out procedures in a bid to enhance overall safety and efficiency. As research and technology keep advancing, the profession can explore artificial nail enhancements that are not only pleasing aesthetically but also support and protect natural nail health (Bansal et al., 2024) (Figure 5.15).

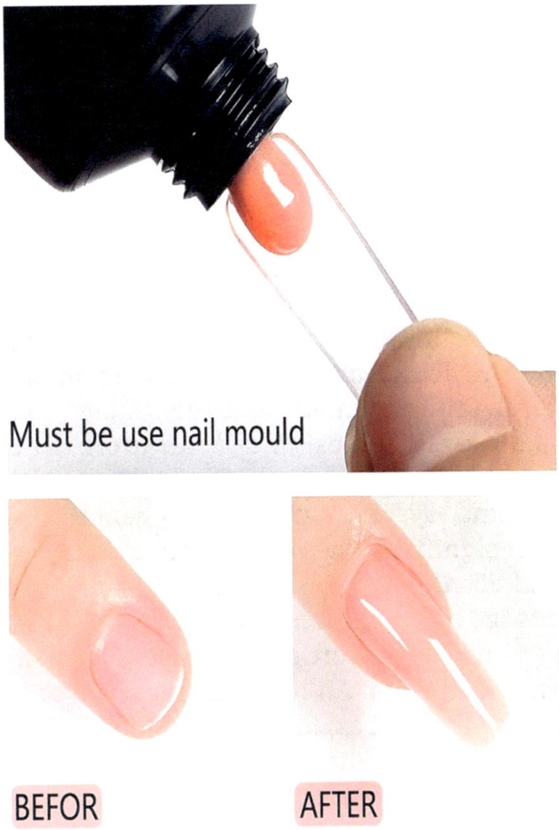

Figure 5.15. Nail enhancement.

Source: https://www.gosupps.com/media/catalog/product/cache/25/image/1500x/040ec09b1e35df139433887a97daa66f/6/1/61yIEZd8hTL._AC_SL1500__1.jpg.

5.6.3. Laser Treatments for Nail Conditions

Application of laser treatments for nail conditions has emerged as a major advancement in the area of dermatology, particularly for the condition of onychomycosis and other nail disorders. Traditional treatment of fungal infections is generally reliant on systemic antifungal agents or topical medication, which can have lower efficacy and side effects. Conversely, laser treatment utilizes concentrated light energy to specifically target and damage the cellular structure of infections that develop on the nail bed. Clinical trials have demonstrated the effectiveness of lasers like Nd:YAG and CO_2 lasers in successfully eliminating the fungus that causes nail fungus, as well as the encouragement of regrowth of healthy nails. Moreover, the non-surgical nature of laser treatments is a significant advantage, reducing the occurrence of side effects typically associated with the application of pharmacology, thereby enhancing patient compliance and effectiveness. Besides their use in fungal infections, lasers have also been found useful in the management of several other cosmetic nail disorders , such as nail dystrophies and coloration. These disorders are most frequently the consequence of trauma, systemic disease, or genetics and cause significant psychological distress for the affected patient. Laser therapy effectively treats the pigmentation and vascular alterations caused by such disorders to enable a return to normal nail color. An important feature of this modality is that it exploits the specificity of laser energy, which allows the treating clinician to selectively target diseased tissue without injury to surrounding tissue. Clinical reports show an excellent safety profile, further solidifying its place as a suitable therapy for those who wish to improve the beauty of their nails and self-esteem. The incorporation of laser treatment into regular practice in nail care is a testament not only to the progress of technology in medical aesthetics but also a move towards improved, patient-centered treatment. With the ongoing development of lasers, their applications in nail diseases will find further impetus through research and clinical studies. It is notable that although laser therapy does have a very strong potential to achieve nail health and appearance, clinicians must also comment on overall patient evaluations to tailor individualized treatment programs. Addressing the underlying systemic causes, such as diabetes or other long-term diseases, alongside laser treatment will make the treatment more effective and give long-term outcomes, paving the way to life-altering results in nail aesthetic conditions and treatments (Figure 5.16).

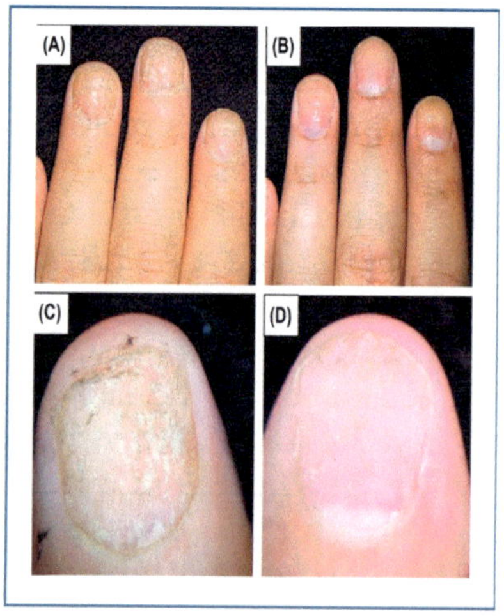

Figure 5.16. Psoriatic nails treated with fractional CO_2 laser-assisted delivery of methotrexate. (A) At baseline, the nails showed marked pitting; (B) At Week 12, the nails showed marked improvement; (C) Evident pitting by dermoscopic examination before treatment; and (D) At Week 12, dermoscopic examination showed marked improvement.

Source: https://www.researchgate.net/profile/Rania-Alakad-2/publication/359475721/figure/fig4/AS:11431281163072651@1685486964319/Psoriatic-nails-treated-with-fractional-CO-2-laser-assisted-delivery-of-methotrexate-A.png.

Test Your Knowledge

1. How can professional manicures and pedicures contribute to both nail health and aesthetics?
2. What are the potential risks and benefits of using nail enhancements and artificial nails?
3. How are laser treatments used in managing nail conditions, and what are their advantages?

SUMMARY

In summarizing the above discussion regarding nail aesthetic conditions and therapies, it is evident that the conditions impact far beyond the physical appearance of the nails themselves to the overall well-being and health of the individual. Nail disease can range from superficial esthetic issues to more profound health-related ones, hence the need for both patients and clinicians to address them in an integrative fashion. Recognition of the multifaceted nature of such disorders allows for more comprehensive treatment, which is optimized for patient satisfaction and promotes enhanced health results. To this measure, understanding the subtleties of numerous nail conditions facilitates successful treatment programs and patient education. Success of treatments for cosmetic conditions of the nails is to a great extent dependent on accurate diagnosis and individualized methods of management. As discussed throughout the chapter, various treatment modalities, including topical therapies, systemic medications, and surgical interventions, must be chosen based on individual patient needs and the specific characteristics of their nail conditions. Moreover, regular monitoring and follow-up are essential to assess treatment success and make necessary adjustments. Of special interest is the application of innovative techniques , such as free vascularized fibular flaps for the treatment of more complex conditions, and it indicates the crucial role played by innovation in the treatment of aesthetic nail conditions. This means that there is research and development poised to improve patient care in this area. Due to the complexity that comes with aesthetic nail conditions, identification of the importance of preventive factors also becomes necessary. Prophylactic interventions, , such as education regarding proper nail care and prompt treatment of problems in the developmental stages, can decrease the risk of progressing to a severe stage. Application of tools , such as the individualized fingertip injury outcome score (FIOS) also directs toward better management and assessment of nail injuries by taking into account the functional as well as esthetic outcomes. This integration of such evaluation instruments and proactive measures can bridge the gap between surgery and esthetic recovery, resulting in overall improvement in the quality of treatment provided to patients with varying nail challenges (Cavola et al., 2024; M et al., 2024).

The study of nail cosmetic conditions and their associated treatments includes several conditions that affect the look and health of nails. Key issues in this field are the identification of common nail disorders, , such as fungal infection, psoriasis of the nail, and onychocryptosis, that can significantly influence appearance as well as functional capability. Through the grouping of these disorders based on their underlying pathophysiology and clinical picture, a cohesive system emerges that encourages accurate diagnosis and targeted treatment methods. This methodical understanding is useful to practitioners and patients both, as it facilitates the selection of effective interventions, which can range from topical remedies to surgical corrections. The precision in the definition of these conditions ensures optimal communication in clinical practice, such that patients and health professionals communicate effectively on a broad range of treatment objectives and management of nail disease. A key component of the treatment of nail aesthetic conditions is the growing awareness of advanced treatment modalities that have been fashioned in contemporary dermatology and cosmetic therapy. With the progress made in laser treatments, PDT, and application of bioengineered products, patients are now able to select a range of procedures for improving nail aesthetics. For instance, laser therapy has been demonstrated to reduce fungal infection and improve the health of the nail with minimal damage to surrounding tissues. Progress in cosmetic procedures not only focuses on treating the condition at hand but also on care prevention, which emphasizes frequent nail care and hygiene practices. Furthermore, the inclusion of regenerative strategies with stem cell technologies and biomaterials highlights the emerging arena of nail therapies, offering a new horizon for the restoration of nail appearance and function. This dualistic aspect of treatment modalities indicates the necessity for ongoing research and development in the arena. The fusion of nail aesthetic conditions and treatment expertise requires evidence-based clinical practice. The development and revision of appraisal criteria, , such as those issued by the FDI for dental restorations, furnish a helpful analogy with the standardization of nail treatment protocol (Hickel et al., 2022). Accurate guidelines ensure consistency of evaluations to the greatest extent possible and offer a common language among professionals. Besides, similar to what happens with advancements in 3D printing technology applied in biomedical areas (Palmquist et al., 2022), the continuously evolving methods for nail aesthetics provide a way for the personalization of treatments according to the individual patient's needs. The focus on evidence-based treatments not only improves the outcome for the patients but also encourages interdisciplinary relations among dermatologists, podiatrists, and cosmetic professionals, ultimately contributing to the advancement of aesthetic medicine.

KEY TERMS FROM THIS CHAPTER

- Aesthetic states
- Anemia
- Brittle nail syndrome
- Chronic nail-pickers
- Cosmetic disorders
- Diagnostic techniques
- Dietary supplements
- Ectodermal dysplasias (ED)
- Full-scale prevention program
- Fungal infection
- Aesthetic training
- Antimicrobial activity
- Chemical matricectomy
- Cosmetic appearance
- Cosmetic impairments
- Dietary sources
- Disease-related abnormalities
- Fingertip injury outcome score (FIOS)
- Fungal derivatives
- Gastrointestinal discomfort

CRITICAL THINKING QUESTIONS

1. **What is the primary cosmetic treatment for yellow nail syndrome when secondary infection is not present?**
   a. Oral antifungals
   b. Topical corticosteroids
   c. Vitamin E supplementation
   d. Laser therapy
2. **Which of the following lasers is commonly used for the treatment of onychomycosis in cosmetic dermatology?**
   a. CO_2 laser
   b. Nd:YAG 1064 nm laser
   c. Pulsed dye laser
   d. Alexandrite laser
3. **Which of the following treatments is most commonly used for managing fungal nail infections (onychomycosis)?**
   a. Topical corticosteroids
   b. Oral antifungal medications
   c. Retinoids
   d. Cryotherapy
4. **Which of the following is a characteristic feature of psoriasis affecting the nails?**
   a. Brittle nails
   b. Splinter hemorrhages
   c. Horizontal ridges
   d. Thickening of the nail plate with pitting
5. **Which cosmetic dermatology procedure is commonly used for treating nail discoloration caused by fungal infections or trauma?**
   a. Laser therapy
   b. Nail polish application
   c. Manicure
   d. Pedicure

Short Answer Questions

1. What are common aesthetic nail conditions treated in cosmetic dermatology?
2. What is onychomycosis and how is it treated in an aesthetic setting?
3. What is the recommended treatment approach for brittle nails?
4. How is nail psoriasis treated to improve cosmetic appearance?
5. What role does laser therapy play in aesthetic nail treatments?
6. Discuss the importance of proper nail care and hygiene in aesthetic dermatology.
7. What are the cosmetic concerns related to artificial nails and how are they managed?

Answer to Critical Thinking Questions

1. (c); 2. (b); 3. (b); 4. (d); 5. (a)

REFERENCES

1. Muneeb Akram, Dr Adnan Hafeez, SAbir, S., & Imad Ud Din Khan. (2025). The Role Of Nutritional Supplements in Enhancing Skin Health and Aesthetic. *Journal of Biological and Allied Health Sciences*, *5*(1), 88–96. https://doi.org/10.56536/jbahs.v5i1.95(accessed on 11th June 2025).
2. Eekhof, J. A., Van Wijk, B., Knuistingh Neven, A., & van der Wouden, J. C. (2012). Interventions for ingrowing toenails. *The Cochrane database of systematic reviews*, *2012*(4), CD001541. https://doi.org/10.1002/14651858.CD001541.pub3(accessed on 11th June 2025).
3. Al-Zyoud, W., Haddadin, D., Hasan, S. A., Jaradat, H., & Kanoun, O. (2023). Biocompatibility testing for implants: A novel tool for selection and characterization. *Materials*, *16*, 6881–6881. https://doi.org/10.3390/ma16216881 (accessed on 11th June 2025).
4. Ambrosio, D. V. (2018). *Incidence and Need of Advanced Aesthetic Somatology in South Africa*. https://core.ac.uk/download/222968033.pdf (accessed on 11th June 2025).
5. Andreol, A., Greco, A., & Todaro, M. (2021). *Dermo Cosmetology and Breast Cancer Patients: Effectiveness on Physical and Mental Wellbeing*. https://core.ac.uk/download/630989145.pdf (accessed on 11th June 2025).
6. Araujo, F. G., Boer, N. C. P., da Silva, W. R., de Aquino, S. A., et al. (2022). *Protoporphyrin IX Associated with Visible Light for The Treatment of Trichophyton Rubrum Causing Onychomycosis–An updated review*. https://core.ac.uk/download/591028582.pdf (accessed on 11th June 2025).
7. Bambara, L., Cardarelli, E., Kari, V., Valtinen, J., Pacheco, R., et al. (2013). *The Baptist Church in Warren: Rehabilitation and Preservation Report*. https://core.ac.uk/download/56706186.pdf (accessed on 11th June 2025).
8. Bansal, S., Nanda, S., Bansal, S., & Grover, C. (2024). Dermatologist driven aesthetic nail enhancement. *Indian Dermatology Online Journal*, *16*, 72–80. https://www.semanticscholar.org/paper/ca1261c74508df7a0fc055cf6b00ee0a19ff6826 (accessed on 11th June 2025).
9. Bayar, E., & Besler, H. (2025). The importance of nutrition before and following metabolic/bariatric surgery. *Trends in Surgical Sciences*. https://www.semanticscholar.org/paper/6cbdb5ac3c11e2d35c31547adaf82ea13bb31105 (accessed on 11th June 2025).
10. Bhowmik, D., Gopinath, H., Kumar, B., Duraivel, S., Aravind, G., & Kumar, K. S. (2025). Nail drug delivery system–A novel approaches for drug delivery system. *International Journal of Pharmamedix India*. https://www.semanticscholar.org/paper/cc773b32153aa2ba1c861fa4ba3cc6e1da7ea4f0 (accessed on 11th June 2025).
11. Boutrid, N., Rahmoune, H., Bioud, B., & Amrane, M. (2022). 64 Conical teeth? Think outside the box! *Rheumatology (Oxford, England)*, *61*. https://www.semanticscholar.org/paper/d362608238148bc1f53d6d8e2d4496b70f94c15f (accessed on 11th June 2025).
12. Brady, E. (2001). *Healing Logics*. https://core.ac.uk/download/32550161.pdf (accessed on 11th June 2025).
13. Bukvić Mokos, Z., Kovačec, L., Marinović, B., Čeović, R., et al. (2022). *Dermatologic Adverse Events in Oncologic Therapies*. https://core.ac.uk/download/565935341.pdf (accessed on 11th June 2025).
14. Calvarysky, B., Dotan, I., Shepshelovich, D., Leader, A., & Diker Cohen, T. (2024). Drug-drug interactions between glucagon-like peptide 1 receptor agonists and oral medications: A

systematic review. *Drug Safety*, *47*, 439–451. https://www.semanticscholar.org/paper/6e5ae3e69330f52feee900b3e7ffbf9c6f31ca04 (accessed on 11th June 2025).

15. Cavola, F., El Motassime, A., Maccauro, G., Ziranu, A., et al. (2024). *Recent Advances in The Surgical Management of Radiation-Induced Fractures Following Soft Tissue Sarcomas*. https://core.ac.uk/download/655041529.pdf (accessed on 11th June 2025).
16. Chanyachailert, P., Leeyaphan, C., & Bunyaratavej, S. (2023). Cutaneous fungal infections caused by dermatophytes and non-dermatophytes: An updated comprehensive review of epidemiology, clinical presentations, and diagnostic testing. *Journal of Fungi*, *9*. https://www.semanticscholar.org/paper/fb499ff982bd22e1264584f83ddf3530861f1c4e (accessed on 11th June 2025).
17. Christopher, M., Gonzalez, R., Huynh, J., Walker, E., Saseendrakumar, B. R., Bowd, C., Belghith, A., et al. (2024). Proactive decision support for glaucoma treatment: Predicting surgical interventions with clinically available data. *Bioengineering*, *11*. https://www.semanticscholar.org/paper/22b5621ecd9dd8a67f87f4cebdbbdcdcde73aafd (accessed on 11th June 2025).
18. Coheña Jiménez, M., Montaño Jiménez, P., & Muriel Sánchez, J. M. (2021). Effect of phenol application time in the treatment of onychogryphosis: A randomized double-blind clinical trial. https://core.ac.uk/download/560385938.pdf (accessed on 11th June 2025).
19. Coliţă, C. I., Hermann, D., Fîlfan, M., Colita, D., Doepnner, T. R., Tica, O., Glavan, D. G., et al. (2024). Optimizing chronotherapy in psychiatric care: The impact of circadian rhythms on medication timing and efficacy. *Clocks & Sleep*, *6*, 635–655. https://www.semanticscholar.org/paper/2aaee4cba5c98db75f7e7e29e1ec6c85400da3fd (accessed on 11th June 2025).
20. Corbu, V. M., Gheorghe-Barbu, I., Dumbravă, A. Ş., Vrâncianu, C. O., & Şesan, T. E. (2023). Current insights in fungal importance—A comprehensive review. *Microorganisms*, *11*, 1384–1384. https://doi.org/10.3390/microorganisms11061384 (accessed on 11th June 2025).
21. Dalave, K., Raman, T., Patil, P., & Buccha, Y. (2024). A clinico-histopathological study of nail dermatoses in a tertiary care hospital. *Cureus*, *16*. https://www.semanticscholar.org/paper/2731590b78a6dd4c6526fdef6190f2fa47dd5709 (accessed on 11th June 2025).
22. Djaoudene, O., Romano, A., Bradai, Y. D., Zebiri, F., Ouchene, A., Yousfi, Y., Amrane-Abider, M., et al. (2023). A global overview of dietary supplements: Regulation, market trends, usage during the COVID-19 pandemic, and health effects. *Nutrients*, *15*, 3320–3320. https://doi.org/10.3390/nu15153320 (accessed on 11th June 2025).
23. Donders, G. G. G., Akinosoglou, K., Massie, Z., & Özçelik, S. (2025). Review of current and emerging estrogen receptor agonists for vaginal atrophy. *Expert Opinion on Pharmacotherapy*, *26*, 249–255. https://www.semanticscholar.org/paper/49194ad2bc5c4b783ba1419a55e0e9fa95350846 (accessed on 11th June 2025).
24. Donner, H. (2023). 'The girls are alright': Beauty work and neoliberal regimes of responsibility among young women in urban India. *Critique of Anthropology*, *43*, 399–421. https://doi.org/10.1177/0308275x231216255 (accessed on 11th June 2025).
25. Faccio, F., Indino, M., Monzani, D., Oliveri, S., Pizzoli, S., Pravettoni, G., & Redaelli, C. (2019). A pilot study on aesthetic treatments performed by qualified aesthetic practitioners: Efficacy on health-related quality of life in breast cancer patients. https://core.ac.uk/download/512043573.pdf (accessed on 11th June 2025).

26. Gopalakrishnan, R., & Thamaraiselvi, B. (2023). Immunotherapy: Breakthrough in cancer treatment. https://doi.org/10.22192/ttdls.2023.010 (accessed on 11th June 2025).

27. Gulati, K., Chopra, D., Kocak-Oztug, N. A., & Verron, É. (2023). Fit and forget: The future of dental implant therapy via nanotechnology. *Advanced Drug Delivery Reviews*, *199*, 114900–114900. https://doi.org/10.1016/j.addr.2023.114900 (accessed on 11th June 2025).

28. Hennion, A. (2023). *Sensing Collectives. Transcript Verlag eBooks*. https://doi.org/10.1515/9783839457450 (accessed on 11th June 2025).

29. Hickel, R., Mesinger, S., Opdam, N., Loomans, B., Frankenberger, R., Cadenaro, M., Burgess, J., et al. (2022). Revised FDI criteria for evaluating direct and indirect dental restorations—Recommendations for its clinical use, interpretation, and reporting. *Clinical Oral Investigations*, *27*, 2573–2592. https://doi.org/10.1007/s00784-022-04814-1 (accessed on 11th June 2025).

30. Hong, Z., Zhu, S., Li, H., Luo, J. Z., Yu, Y., An, Y., Wang, X., et al. (2023). Bioengineered skin organoids: From development to applications. *Military Medical Research*, *10*. https://doi.org/10.1186/s40779-023-00475-7 (accessed on 11th June 2025).

31. Januszewski, J., Forma, A., Zembala, J., Flieger, M., Tyczyńska, M., Dring, J. C., Dudek, I., et al. (2023). Nutritional supplements for skin health—A review of what should be chosen and why. *Medicina*, *60*, 68–68. https://doi.org/10.3390/medicina60010068 (accessed on 11th June 2025).

32. Karuniati, N. N., Suda, I. K., & Utama, I. W. B. (2022). Yoga inner beauty as a lifestyle woman in Ghanta Yoga Asram Kertalangu Village, East Denpasar. *International Journal of Social Sciences*, *5*, 15–23. https://doi.org/10.21744/ijss.v5n1.1821 (accessed on 11th June 2025).

33. Kyriakou, A., Zagalioti, S. C., Trakatelli, M., Fotiadou, C., Apalla, Z., Lazaridou, E., & Patsatsi, A. (2022). Fungal infections and nail psoriasis: An update. *Journal of Fungi*, *8*. https://www.semanticscholar.org/paper/e2e1f7af33e1e605bd2d813dc869189fb4b7818f (accessed on 11th June 2025).

34. Langtree, T. G. (2020). Notes on pre-Nightingale nursing: What it was and what it was not. https://core.ac.uk/download/385849274.pdf (accessed on 11th June 2025).

35. Lee, A. K. W., Chan, L. K. W., Lee, C. H., Cerón Bohórquez, J. M., Haykal, D., Wan, J., & Yi, K. (2025). Artificial intelligence application in diagnosing, classifying, localizing, detecting and estimation the severity of skin condition in aesthetic medicine: A review. *Dermatological Reviews*, *6*. https://www.semanticscholar.org/paper/40baea047d537dbed284a2af94546c49c33ab015 (accessed on 11th June 2025).

36. Lee, D., & Lipner, S. R. (2022). Optimal diagnosis and management of common nail disorders. *Annals of Medicine*, *54*, 694–712. https://doi.org/10.1080/07853890.2022.2044511 (accessed on 11th June 2025).

37. Lee, Y. J., Kim, K. S., Ahn, H. J., & Shin, M. K. (2024). Non-thermal atmospheric plasma for the treatment of onychomycosis: *In vitro* and *ex vivo* ultrastructural study. *Journal of Mycology and Infection*. https://www.semanticscholar.org/paper/254916c6f761be077a5c0f656f43617e587df540 (accessed on 11th June 2025).

38. Leonor Castro, M., Ferreira, J. P., Pintado, M., Ramos, Ó. L., Borges, S., & Baptista-Silva, S. (2023). Grape by-products in sustainable cosmetics: Nanoencapsulation and market trends. *Applied Sciences*, *13*, 9168–9168. https://doi.org/10.3390/app13169168 (accessed on 11th June 2025).

39. Lynch, A. J., Cooke, S. J., Arthington, A. H., Baigún, C., Bossenbroek, L., Dickens, C., Harrison, I., et al. (2023). People need freshwater biodiversity. *Wiley Interdisciplinary Reviews Water, 10*. https://doi.org/10.1002/wat2.1633 (accessed on 11th June 2025).

40. Malik, S., Muhammad, K., & Waheed, Y. (2023). Nanotechnology: A revolution in modern industry. *Molecules, 28*, 661–661. https://doi.org/10.3390/molecules28020661 (accessed on 11th June 2025).

41. Michalak, M. (2023). Plant extracts as skin care and therapeutic agents. *International Journal of Molecular Sciences, 24*, 15444–15444. https://doi.org/10.3390/ijms242015444 (accessed on 11th June 2025).

42. Mikulska, J., Lewandowski, M., Kurkiewicz, W., Woźniak, O., Wąsik, J., Gryboś, K., Sepioło, W., et al. (2025). Eating disorders among athletes: Causes, symptoms, and health consequences. *Quality in Sport*. https://www.semanticscholar.org/paper/acc9968f0cbe7d32b830cf3082772697d471ff6e (accessed on 11th June 2025).

43. Morningstar, B. J., Xu, J., Gauthier, C., Scott, D., Gross, C., Jackson, M. M. J. B., & Gonzalez, T. (2025). Examination of preoperative conditions and treatment techniques on outcomes following tibiotalocalcaneal arthrodesis. *Foot & Ankle Orthopaedics, 10*. https://www.semanticscholar.org/paper/7afd23d127bce28c50c7213f8451cc0efd1d5385 (accessed on 11th June 2025).

44. Netala, V. R., Teertam, S., Li, H., & Zhang, Z. (2024). A comprehensive review of cardiovascular disease management: Cardiac biomarkers, imaging modalities, pharmacotherapy, surgical interventions, and herbal remedies. *Cells, 13*. https://www.semanticscholar.org/paper/308135f5cf36d96b4e2d99c8fad92729ba89260d (accessed on 11th June 2025).

45. Palmquist, A., Jolic, M., Hryha, E., & Shah, F. A. (2022). Complex geometry and integrated macro-porosity: Clinical applications of electron beam melting to fabricate bespoke bone-anchored implants. *Acta Biomaterialia, 156*, 125–145. https://doi.org/10.1016/j.actbio.2022.06.002 (accessed on 11th June 2025).

46. Pussetti, C. (2023). Life comes first, but lifestyle also matters: Aesthetic responses to pandemic angst. https://core.ac.uk/download/565358070.pdf (accessed on 11th June 2025).

47. Rani, M., Ducoli, S., Depero, L. E., Prica, M., Tubić, A., Ademović, Z., Morrison, L., et al. (2023). A complete guide to extraction methods of microplastics from complex environmental matrices. *Molecules, 28*, 5710–5710. https://doi.org/10.3390/molecules28155710 (accessed on 11th June 2025).

48. Salvioni, L., Morelli, L., Ochoa, E., Labra, M., Fiandra, L., Palugan, L., Prosperi, D., et al. (2021). The emerging role of nanotechnology in skincare. *Advances in Colloid and Interface Science, 293*, 102437–102437. https://doi.org/10.1016/j.cis.2021.102437 (accessed on 11th June 2025).

49. Shelke, S. S., Shinde, A. D., Shinde, V. L., Swami, A. L., Ashture, N. R., & Borkhede, P. K. (2024). Assessment of parental attitude, knowledge and awareness towards preventive dentistry in south zone of Chhatrapati Sambhajinagar: A questionnaire based cross sectional survey. *International Journal of Science and Research Archive*. https://www.semanticscholar.org/paper/d07cc063f7526a224da46b44e7f6d9332af63db9 (accessed on 11th June 2025).

50. Soujanya, M., & Rajput, D. (2024). A comprehensive study of fingertip injuries at a tertiary care center–Fingertip injury outcome score subset pilot. https://core.ac.uk/download/635339062.pdf (accessed on 11th June 2025).

51. Wouters, R. M., Jobi-Odeneye, A. O., de la Torre, A., Joseph, A., Hovius, S. E. R., Shin, A. Y., MacDermid, J. C., et al. (2021). A standard set for outcome measurement in patients with hand and wrist conditions: Consensus by the International Consortium for Health Outcomes Measurement Hand and Wrist Working Group. *The Journal of Hand Surgery*, *46*, 841–855.e7. https://doi.org/10.1016/j.jhsa.2021.06.004 (accessed on 11th June 2025).

THREAD LIFTING AND SKIN TIGHTENING TECHNIQUES

6

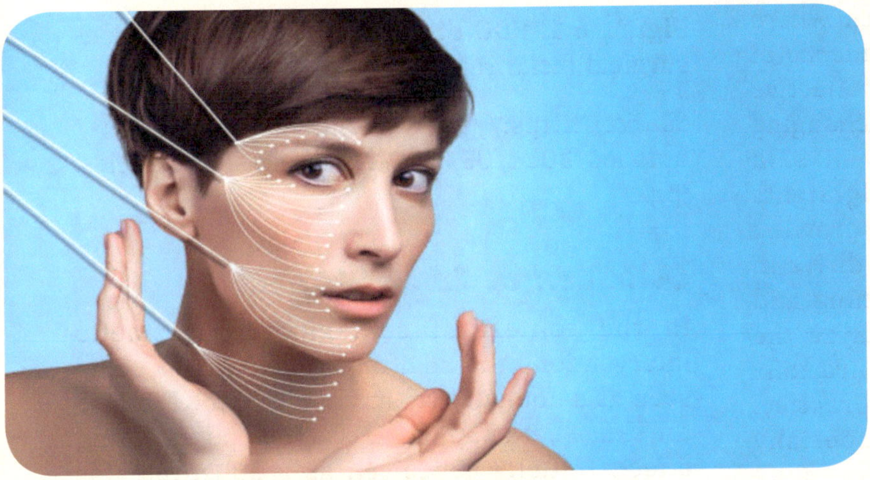

LEARNING OBJECTIVES

After studying this chapter, you will be able to:

1. Explain the different forms of thread lifting
2. Explain the mechanism of action for thread lifting and skin tightening treatments
3. Define skin tightening treatments
4. Describe about benefits of thread lifting
5. Discuss risks and considerations

Introduction

The search for youthful and elastic skin has driven significant development in aesthetic medicine, particularly in thread lifting and skin tightening. Our understanding of changes in the structure of aging skin has progressed through the years, leading to more effective and less aggressive interventions for the rejuvenation of the face. Thread lifting, in particular, is the added benefit of giving patients instant lifting with a long-term skin tightening that occurs with collagen stimulation. With the continuing progress of aesthetic improvement, it is increasingly necessary to research the multi-faceted approaches that not only aesthetically enhance their appeal but also improve the well-being of patients treated with these procedures. These advances have brought about new possibilities in the practice of cosmetic surgery and dermatology, bridging the generation between non-invasive treatments and invasive surgical procedures. The visually oriented society today has necessitated an enormous demand for treatments that produce natural outcomes without the recovery time required of traditional facelift surgeries. With universal beauty standards constantly evolving, particularly influenced by trends in the likes of South Korea, the global demand for such cutting-edge processes like thread lifting has gained international popularity. The combination of cultural sentiments with the procedures marks a further integration of Western populations towards minimally invasive treatments. South Koreas ascendant leadership in beauty enhances the stakes on these methods global reach, where advanced technology and quality standards of healthcare attract those in search of effective solutions to cosmetic treatments. This changing culture not only drives innovation in skin tightening technologies but also highlights the vast economic opportunity of the growing market for aesthetic care globally. To thrive in the ever-evolving field of skin tightening and thread lifting, one must critically analyze the various methodologies and the implications of their application in cosmetic practice. Significantly, thread lifting utilizes specially designed materials , such as polydioxanone (PDO) and polylactic acid (PLA) threads that have been proven to achieve great lifting while inducing long-term collagen synthesis. The growing popularity of the procedure is a function of a broader cultural shift toward less-invasive procedures as an alternative to routine surgical procedures, allowing shorter recovery times and fewer opportunities for complications. Through the knowledge of such advanced procedures' details, both patients and practitioners can better make educated decisions optimally suited to aesthetic success. As the research continues to improve and develop such methods, the specialty is poised to embrace new technology, setting standards of excellence for cosmetic revitalization, as witnessed in the ongoing innovation in the field (Marques, 2023; Portilla et al., 2024) (Figure 6.1).

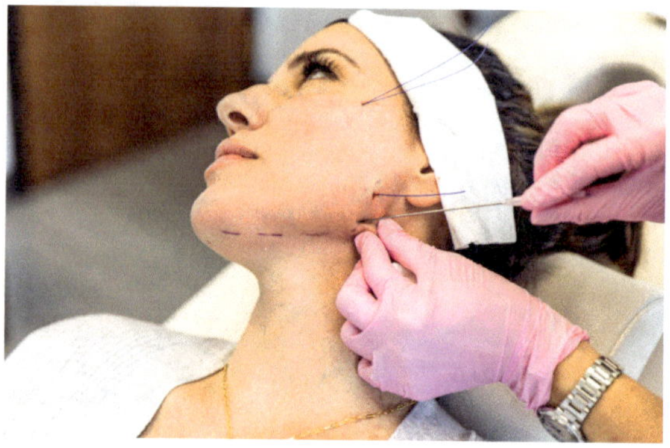

Figure 6.1. PDO thread lift procedure for non-surgical facial rejuvenation.

Source: https://www.hushla.net/wp-content/uploads/2024/05/PDO-Thread-lift-Los-Angeles.jpg.

Definition of Thread Lifting

In the context of contemporary cosmetic interventions, thread lifting is increasingly being seen as a non-surgical method intended to give the skin a better appearance and impose a lifting effect. Initially conceived as a substitute for a facelift, thread lifting utilizes biocompatible threads that are injected subdermally in a predetermined pattern in order to establish a mesh support. When these strands are inserted into the subcutaneous layer, they stimulate the production of collagen and induce tightening of the tissue, ultimately resulting in a younger appearance. The minimally invasive technique of thread lifting maintains recovery time very low as opposed to conventional facelifts and thus provides an appealing choice for most patients seeking desired outcomes without downtime from more invasive treatments. Modern developments show a complex array of thread materials and structures, which allow therapists to personalize treatments based on individual anatomical considerations and specific aesthetic goals (Kyu-Yi et al., 2024). The technical effectiveness of thread lifting requires experience and precision, as the placement of threads and choice of material can potentially affect the success of the treatment. Filaments are typically made of PDO or polytetrafluoroethylene (PTFE) that are well known for their biocompatibility and collagen-stimulating properties. The insertion method often utilizes specially designed needles or cannulas in order to minimize tissue trauma and patient pain. Aside from that, the treatment can be employed to correct a series of conditions, which include drooping in the facial region, marionette lines, and laxity of the jawline. With increased levels of expertise and technique among practitioners, thread lifting becomes further refined through the use of it, with ongoing research reaffirming its safety and efficacy in aesthetic medicine (Beiu et al., 2023).

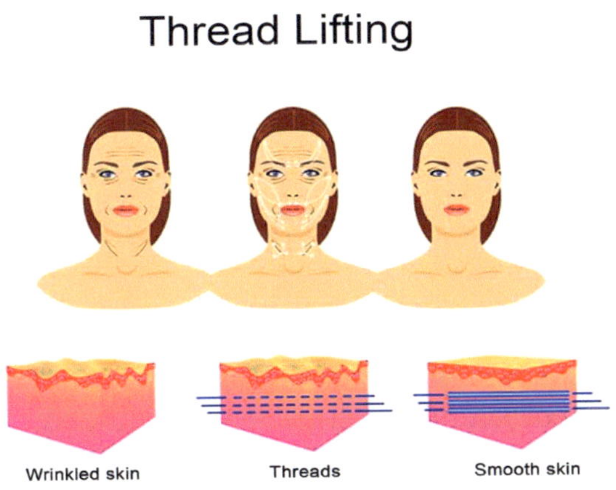

Figure 6.2. Thread lifting.

Source: https://polylactide.com/wp-content/uploads/2023/09/how-thread-lifts-work.jpg.

The growing popularity of thread lifting is part of a greater trend in cosmetic surgery, where patients are gravitating toward less invasive procedures that yield good results with fewer risks. As societal expectations of beauty continue to evolve, there remains demand for procedures that offer subtle improvement without extreme alteration. Thread lifting not only minimizes noticeable signs of aging but also works as an empowerment agent for people who want to regain the confidence in their appearance. The use of high-quality threads and the potential for combining the treatments with other aesthetic treatments, such as fillers, contributes to the patient's outcome. Herein, professionals in the subject point out the necessity of extensive consultation with patients and rich acquaintance with individual needs for obtaining the highest degree of satisfaction from thread lifting treatments (Kyu-Yi et al., 2024) (Figure 6.2).

Overview of Skin Tightening Techniques

The skin tightening treatments field has undergone a radical shift in recent years, a sign of technological advancements as well as evolving preferences. Non-invasive techniques , such as ultrasound and RF have gained immense popularity due to their safety profiles and short recovery times. They work by stimulating collagen synthesis within the dermis, giving a tightening effect that is achieved over a period of several months. Also, they cater to patients willing to observe subtle adjustments without the time factor of surgical commitments. With these new techniques being embraced by various cultures, particularly South Korea, the sale of minimally invasive beauty therapy has gained roots worldwide where patient demand for effective yet minimal procedures continues to grow (Marques, 2023). Consequently, the weather of skin tightening is increasingly characterized by innovation in both effectiveness and patient comfort. In addition to non-invasive intervention, surgery has always been part of the dialogue in skin tightening procedures. Surgical techniques like facelifts and thread lifts present immediate gratification, potentially not found in non-invasive treatments. Thread lifting, in particular, has carved out its own niche with its minimally invasive nature and success at lifting. The technique involves implanting specialized threads that lift the skin with a lift upwards in sagging areas, also stimulating collagen formation. While surgery is traditionally associated with more extended recovery times and visible scarring, it remains a favorite among patients looking for dramatic, instant results (Gulbitti et al., 2022). The relative efficacy of surgical against non-surgical methods drives a debate within the aesthetic medicine industry, with patients and practitioners weighing the advantages and disadvantages of each process. Patient satisfaction is still a crucial indicator of the efficacy of skin tightening treatments, regardless of the treatment employed. Contrasts between treatments highlight that although surgical techniques are known to create more extreme results, satisfaction with non-surgical techniques is also high. Patients have been found to report that, as non-invasive treatments do not produce significant downtime, they become more preferable even though they create smaller changes. Notably, the risk-benefit ratio between improving aesthetics and possible negative impacts should be addressed; patients tend to favor measures that reduce risks while enhancing outcomes. With growing consciousness and evolving tastes towards minimally invasive therapy, especially in those geographies under the domain of South Korean beauty, the future of skin tightening therapy shall move towards an intersection of innovation and cultural consciousness in aesthetic therapy (Gulbitti et al., 2022;Marques, 2023).

Importance of Non-Surgical Cosmetic Procedures

The explosion of non-surgical cosmetic procedures is one of the biggest paradigm shifts in the beauty market, fueled by technology advances and changing attitudes about beauty. Thread lifting and skin tightening are some of the procedures that enable individuals to enhance their beauty with minimal downtime and invasiveness, as opposed to traditional surgical procedures. With growing need for such treatments, the professionals are then faced with the dilemma of satisfying the patients' requirements while providing high standards of care. The significance of non-surgical treatments lies not only in their immediate cosmetic value but also in the provision of a less daunting option for the fearful candidates. As advances in technology continue to develop, the types of non-surgical means increase, ensuring greater patient satisfaction and acceptance in the pursuit of aesthetic outcomes. Thread lifting, for example, is a prime illustration of the advantages of non-surgical procedures through the use of innovative ways of intervening in order to create a lifted appearance without undergoing major surgery. The process involves the insertion of threads into the skin that are anchored to form a support structure for sagging tissues, basically lifting and tightening the skin. The process, highlighted in a recent article on the benefits of lateral face lifting with an anchoring technique, points to its efficiency in enhancing facial contours with safety and minimal recovery. Moreover, with more attention given to short-term results and less procedural risk, thread lifting is a popular choice among those patients in need of rejuvenation. The very high effectiveness of such procedures is in harmony with contemporary aesthetic goals, coinciding both patient satisfaction and availability within the broadening realm of cosmetic modification. With increasing pace in non-surgical interventions, the practitioners' learning curve gains momentum, particularly in the context of integrated plastic surgery training. Specifically, the deficit in actual life exposure that residents receive in non-surgical procedures is most strikingly observed from the low confidence in carrying out complex facial cosmetic operations reported by trainees. The incorporation of non-surgical procedures into educational processes is critical due to the documented 19% increase in overall cosmetic procedures since the pandemic. Junior cosmetic fellowships are just one example of how this potential for enhancing residents comfort and familiarity with such procedures can ultimately bridge the learning foundations and clinical application gap. This approach can not only improve the skill level of future plastic surgeons, but also meet the rising need for non-surgical procedures for the face, that it can develop a future when patient aesthetics care remains strong and effective, as seen in present statistics on procedural trends (Kelsey et al., 2024) (Figure 6.3).

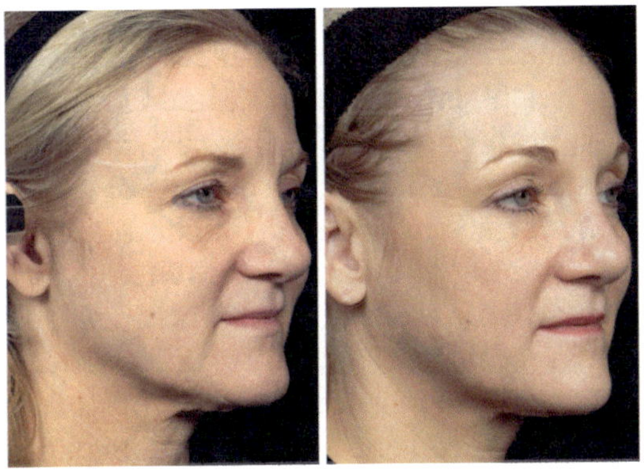

Figure 6.3. Before and after pictures of a patient treated with thermage to the full face.

Source: https://www.researchgate.net/publication/357176194_Non-surgical_skin_tightening.

6.1. Historical Background

Learning Outcome

1. Understand the evolution of thread lifting
2. Discuss the development of skin tightening technologies
3. Focus on cultural perceptions of aging and beauty

The history of tightening the skin is richly interwoven in historical methods of beauty treatments that have varied across cultures and centuries. Historically, the desire to remain young has been a common pursuit, with ancient civilizations employing different means , such as herbal preparations, cosmetic creams, and unsophisticated surgical techniques. The ancient Egyptians, for instance, employed natural oils and infusions to enhance the elasticity of the skin and lessen the appearance of aging. As beauty standards in society have evolved, so too did the means to achieve them. The invention of surgical facelifts marked a milestone, introducing more invasive procedures with superior outcomes for aging than less invasive ones. This era laid the groundwork for today's advanced skin rejuvenation systems that now go beyond the cutting-edge offerings of thread lifting that combine technology with patient safety and satisfaction factors. In the late 20th and early 21st centuries, the aesthetics market experienced a boom of minimally invasive cosmetic procedures as part of society's overall movement toward non-surgical interventions. Thread lifting as a specific type of skin tightening evolved from the demand for shorter recovery times, reduced costs, and more minimally invasive techniques than traditional surgical facelifts. This greater demand for subtle enhancements rather than radical makeovers is part of cultural transformations where there is a greater focus on natural beauty. The nation that has set the pace in this kind of transformation is South Korea, a country known for setting trends in beauty standards. As Marques (2023) notes, the rise of Korean beauty regimes, characterized by their focus on achieving a naturally flawless look, has gained an audience globally looking for non-surgical solutions. This cross-cultural exchange also expanded the trend of thread lifting techniques across borders, establishing new aesthetic standards worldwide. With the evolution of the technical foundation of thread lifting, mastering such methods through empirical results and patient experience became a necessity. Structural dynamics of facial aging are diverse and involve changes in skin elasticity, muscular tone, and the overall facial structure, as discussed in Pourdanesh et al. (2016). Characterization of such anatomical changes has witnessed increased practice in skin tightening, allowing clinicians to individualize procedures according to the patient's needs.

The individualized process not only optimizes healing and aesthetic results but also optimizes satisfaction levels among patients. Through the marriage of ancient ideals of beauty and modern advances in technology, thread lifting is a beacon in the history of aesthetic medicine that addresses a wide swath of the population and their shifting beauty ideals yet maintains a rich heritage in cosmetic treatments.

6.1.1. Evolution of Thread Lifting

Thread lifting is a significant advance in minimally invasive facial aesthetic procedures. Facelifts, which were once the norm, represented extensive surgical intervention, resulting in patients having a lot of downtime, as well as potential complications. With the disadvantages of the invasive methods, the introduction of thread lifting has ushered in a new alternative that tries to balance effectiveness with less downtime. This technique involves the application of meticulously crafted threads, for instance, polydioxanone (PDO) or polylactic acid (PLA), and they are placed inside the skin to trigger the formation of collagen while simultaneously offering the lifting of sagging tissues as well. Therefore, thread lifting is a breakthrough in dermatological and surgical practices, which is headed towards patients' increasing demands for natural results without the invasiveness offered by traditional methods (Portilla et al., 2024). Thread liftings gain in popularity can be also explained by broader cultural shifts surrounding beauty ideals and standards. South Korea has been among leaders in the world of beauty, focusing on an aesthetic of natural augmentation rather than dramatic transformation. Korean beauty ideals are not only gaining traction domestically but are also gaining acceptance among international consumers, like in Europe and North America. This social trend has paved the way to the mass popularity and acceptance of minimally invasive procedures like thread lifting (Marques, 2023). The quest for rejuvenated, youthful skin without the scarring that is typically associated with surgical facelifts has catapulted this trend into the limelight of contemporary cosmetic procedures. With the progression in thread lift technology, knowledge and practice of these treatments within the science of aesthetic medicine improve too. Progress in materials adopted for threads and techniques of insertion has resulted in improved results and patient satisfaction. Treaters have been able to personalize treatment based on individual needs, with more personalized treatment. Further, with ongoing studies regarding thread lifting's long-term effects, matters of durability and efficacy are now being touched upon. With proper training and enough knowledge of facial anatomy, professionals can optimize results, enhancing the overall safety and efficacy of the procedure. Therefore, the history of thread lifting not only reflects a large move towards less invasive options but also reflects a broader trend on the dermatology and anti-aging strategy landscape (Portilla et al., 2024).

6.1.2. Development of Skin Tightening Technologies

The evolution of skin tightening technologies has witnessed remarkable innovation, particularly in minimally invasive procedures that seek to address the signs of aging. Historically, skin laxity was primarily managed through surgical facelifts, a method that, while effective, often involved significant recovery times and risks. Over the past two decades, the development of thread lifting techniques has emerged as a viable alternative that combines aesthetic enhancement with reduced invasiveness. This new technique uses special materials, which differ from the conventional sutures, to allow tissue manipulation without having to undergo major surgery. Advances in thread material, , such as polydioxanone and poly-L-lactic acid, have popularized thread lifting, allowing doctors to give patients solid solutions for tighter and more youthful-looking skin without compromising safety or convenience (Gi-Hong et al., 2024). Apart from thread lifting, advancements in non-surgical skin tightening equipment have offered more treatment options for individuals seeking facial renewal. Radiofrequency (RF), ultrasound, and laser treatments have emerged as widely used methods, utilizing energy-based techniques to stimulate collagen regeneration and enhance skin elasticity. These treatments are used in conjunction with thread lifting to enhance overall facial shape while smoothing skin texture and tone. The integration of such technologies in aesthetic treatments reflects an overall aesthetic philosophy of skin rejuvenation that allows practitioners to tailor treatments based on the individual needs of each patient. Thus, the practice of non-invasive and minimally invasive aesthetic treatments is further evolving, with practitioners having more tools at hand to effectively treat skin laxity (Gi-Hong et al., 2024). Advancement and refinement of skin tightening technology promote the necessity of selecting appropriate treatment based on individual condition. Tissue laxity, desired outcomes, and patient anatomy dictate thread lift versus the adjunct procedure of energy-based treatments. Understanding the interaction between variations in thread properties, ranging from composition to cog design positions the provider optimally to achieve maximum results. Current trends reflect a trend towards multi-modality treatment approaches that utilize multiple thread types and other devices to maximize outcomes. Such a balanced perception not only maximizes esthetic outcomes but also minimizes complications and recovery time associated with skin tightening treatments. Ultimately, the ongoing development of these technologies has transformed the aspect of aesthetic medicine to offer innovative solutions to meet the evolving needs of patients seeking younger, fresher-looking skin (Gi-Hong et al., 2024) (Figure 6.4).

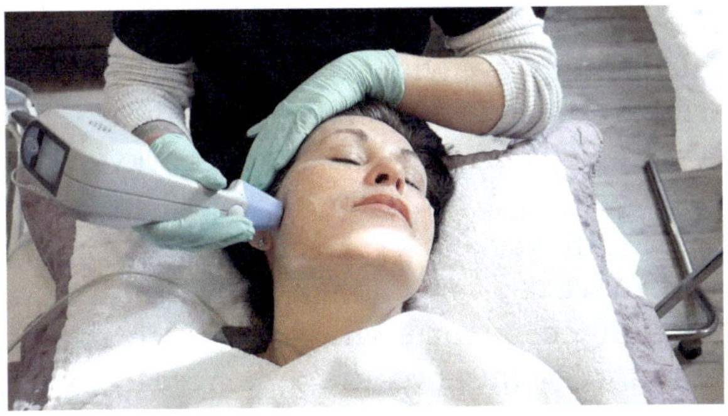

Figure 6.4. Non-invasive facial skin tightening using a radiofrequency (RF) device.

Source: https://purplepearlskin.com/wp-content/uploads/2019/05/Sequence-01.01_17_28_41.Still095.jpg.

6.1.3. Cultural Perceptions of Aging and Beauty

The intersection of cultural beauty and aging attitudes has been of substantial interest, particularly where aesthetic treatments are becoming a norm. Aging is often regarded negatively by most cultures, influencing beauty and aging views within society. For instance, in South Korea, emphasis on appearing young produces a substantial market for non-surgical procedures , such as thread lifting and skin tightening. These procedures are not merely choices of beauty; they are components of a cultural conversation that equates body appearance with social acceptance and individual success. Thus, the quest to maintain a youthful face reflects broader cultural pressures, in which one's value is frequently linked to conformity to ideals of beauty. The global spread of South Korean conceptions of beauty underscores the dynamic process of cultural sentiments towards aging. As such ideals increasingly gain traction in Western cultures, they reflect an attitude shift in relation to beauty and aging. Adding technology to such treatments for beauty has placed procedures like thread lifting within reach of the masses, attracting a populace that values efficiency and results. These advances have placed South Korea as the leader in the beauty industry, with a unique culture that perfects an already perfect look, one which not only sells well in one's own backyard but is also gaining popularity abroad. The growth potential in markets like Switzerland highlights the effective capitalization of this cultural trend, in that higher income and growing acceptance of minimally invasive therapies create a rich field for Korean cosmetic therapy (Marques, 2023). As these cultural values around aging and beauty evolve, so too do they have implications on the healthcare environment, inviting into the conversation an ethical discussion around issues in cosmetic therapy. While many seek these augmentations to become part of today's beauty standards, these urges can lead to talks about self-esteem and societal pressures. Stigmatizing the process of aging as a disease rather than an inevitable process can end up perpetuating unhealthy standards. It is thus crucial that practitioners and societies foster discussions about inborn beauty and self-acceptance. By addressing these issues, there is an opportunity to reframe the discussion of aging and engage in a more holistic approach that respects the both experiential and aesthetic aspects of beauty. This assists in the creation of a more balanced perception of aging, offsetting harmful stereotypes while respecting the value of life's changing phases (Silva et al., 2023).

Test Your Knowledge

1. What have been the major milestones in the development of skin tightening technologies?
2. How did early forms of thread lifting pave the way for modern minimally invasive facial rejuvenation techniques?

6.2. Types of Thread Lifting

Learning Outcome

1. Describe PDO (polydioxanone) threads
2. Define PLLA (poly-L-lactic acid) threads
3. Explain PCL (polycaprolactone) threads

Thread lifting is now a popular minimally invasive cosmetic procedure to resuscitate the skin by attaining the appearance of a lifted and contoured one. Of all the various thread lifting methods, the most universally applied are PDO threads, poly-L-lactic acid (PLLA) threads, and surgical thread lifts. PDO threads are so popular specifically because of their biocompatibility and natural breakdown by the body over time, stimulating collagen development and firming the skin. Meanwhile, PLLA threads provide a volumizing effect and are most appropriate for patients who need more substantial structural support, e.g., on the cheeks and jawline. Surgical thread lifting, while invasive, has more significant long-term effects compared to non-surgical methods. The choice of thread type is ultimately dependent on the patient individual needs and cosmetic wants, as well as the clinician's experience in their use. The application of different forms of thread lifting technique can significantly enhance the facial aesthetics by mitigating the defects of aging. For instance, PDO threads best fit patients with mild to moderate skin laxity or sagging, as they can easily reposition tissues and restore the facial shape. Conversely, PLLA threads are for patients requiring added volume and firmness, aiding collagen growth to restore youthful plumpness. And, these techniques can even act as great alternatives to traditional facelifts, which, as effective as they are, are more invasive with longer post-treatment recovery times. As dermatological clinics continue to advance, developments in thread lifting are transforming patient choices by expanding the scope of non-surgical treatment for aging signs, thus highlighting an impressive trend towards comprehensive aesthetic treatment regimens (Portilla et al., 2024). Despite their advantages, the disadvantages and potential complications of thread lifting should be noted. Factors , such as the anatomical shape, degree of aging changes, and expected aesthetic outcome must be evaluated to determine appropriateness for treatment. The differential results are occasionally the result of improper procedure or thread selection, emphasizing the importance of practitioner experience. Moreover, even though thread lifting can create dramatic aesthetic improvement, patients must be made aware of possible side effects, including bruising and swelling, with a minimal possibility of thread migration. As the techniques continue to advance, future research will likely render them safer and more efficient, and thread lifting will remain a significant modality in the realm of skin tightening devices (Pourdanesh et al., 2016).

6.2.1. Polydioxanone (PDO) Threads

The growing popularity of non-surgical cosmetic procedures has given rise to more interest in treatments , such as PDO thread lift, which provide skin rejuvenation and tightening with shorter recovery times. The PDO threads, primarily composed of a biocompatible thread, are placed carefully into the subcutaneous tissue to reshape facial contours and provide lifting results. As seen in modern treatments, PDO threads are used to promote collagen production after some time, producing organic results that appeal to both clinicians and patients alike. Their minimally invasive approach contrasts sharply with conventional facelift procedures, which involve lengthy recovery and greater risks. This development in method follows a broader movement within dermatology as focus is being directed towards effective but non-surgical techniques, with the introduction of novel materials like PDO to provide desired aesthetic advantages while maintaining patient safety and comfort (Portilla et al., 2024). While the benefits of PDO thread lifting are significant, one must also remain vigilant regarding the inherent complications of the procedure. Clinical evaluations have documented multiple side effects like swelling, dimpling of the skin, and visibility of threads, which can be a cosmetic limitation. Paresthesia, infection, and thread extrusion are quoted complications on which medical professionals must dwell before recommending PDO threads as a cosmetic treatment. Awareness of risks allows practitioners to prepare for and manage these side effects so that patients are properly informed of what might happen. Additionally, knowledge about complications , such as contour irregularity and incomplete facial paralysis aids practitioners when giving realistic expectations to patients, hence balancing aesthetic objectives with an entire understanding of the technique limitation (Lewandowska et al., 2024). In general, PDO threads represent progress in skin tightening methods that offers an efficient substitute for surgical treatment. With surgeons exploring the application of PDO threads in facial rejuvenation, they must weigh the benefits against the risks of the procedure. An integrative approach involving patient education on side effects, informed consent, and professional acumen will optimize success in procedures. Researching more on the safety and efficacy of PDO threads will ultimately bring new information to maximize techniques and protocols. This ongoing controversy between the cosmetic fraternity also acts to reiterate the requirement to balance safety for patients with concerns for beauty in the ever-evolving landscape of non-surgical cosmetic treatments (Portilla et al., 2024) (Figure 6.5).

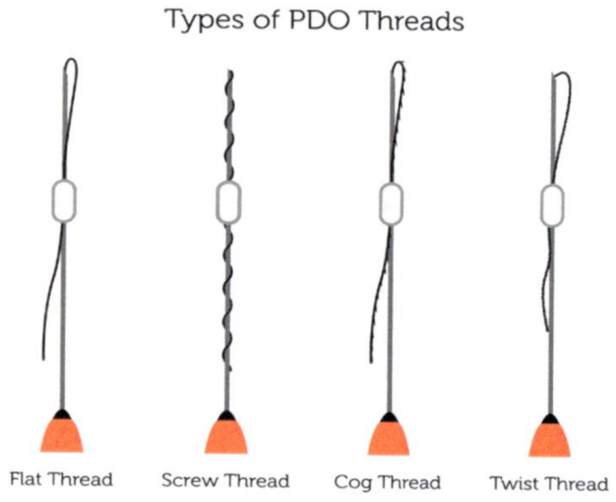

Figure 6.5. Types of PDO (polydioxanone) threads.

Source: https://www.rejuvenceclinic.co.uk/wp-content/uploads/2020/09/PDO-Threads-Types-01.png.

6.2.2. Poly-L-Lactic Acid (PLLA) Threads

As a newer modality in aesthetic medicine, PLLA threads have been a top contender among thread lifting and skin tightening treatments. PLLA is biodegradable and biocompatible, and it stimulates the formation of collagen in the dermis, hence restoring the elasticity and firmness of the skin in the long run. Unlike traditional lifting threads, which are more likely to provide immediate results but may not be lasting ones, PLLA threads encourage gradual rejuvenation by provoking the body's inherent healing processes. This activity renders PLLA threads an attractive choice for patients seeking incremental, natural-looking enhancement without noticeable alterations that can be associated with surgical interventions. PLLA thread application in cosmetic procedures is consistent with growing patient interest in non-invasive, low-downtime treatments. Over time, thinning of subcutaneous tissue and loss of muscle tone enable sagging of the face, which makes people pursue therapies that undo these changes. The use of PLLA threads is also becoming more popular since they offer specific lifting and tightening, which tends to improve the appearance of aging with time (Pourdanesh et al., 2016). Doctors affirm that thread insertion yields better facial contours and texture, for a two-way gain with the integration of both short- and long-term aesthetic enhancement. Thread lifting strategies have evolved tremendously in the past, from more invasive surgical techniques to less invasive methods like PLLA threads.

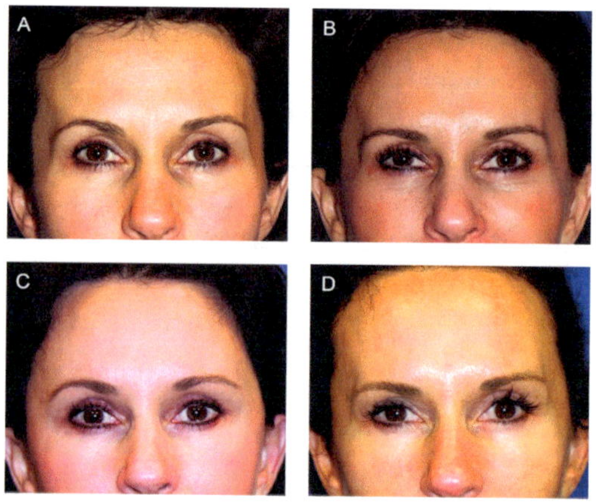

Figure 6.6. Poly-l-lactic acid (PLLA) can effectively restore temporal volume loss with stable improvement. (A) A 45-year-old female patient is shown preoperatively; (B) The patient is shown 2 years after high superficial musculoaponeurotic system (SMAS) facelift and fat injections with temporal hollowing; (C) The patient is shown 4 years after facelift with fat injections and 2 years after PLLA injections in 2 sessions with 1 vial/session concentrated on temporal hollowing; and (D) The patient is shown 7 years after facelift and fat injections and 5 years after PLLA injections.

Source: https://www.researchgate.net/publication/359016337/figure/fig4/AS:11431281097179667@1668488568255/Poly-l-lactic-acid-PLLA-can-effectively-restore-temporal-volume-loss-with-stable.png

Their implementation within the field has transformed the landscape, offering patients a safer alternative to facelifts with comparable results in terms of tightening and rejuvenation of the skin. With increasingly refined technique, familiarity with potential complications becomes essential to ensuring patient safety and satisfaction. Employing and procuring good-quality material and techniques minimizes adverse effects, which are particularly noted in procedural safety reports in other similar fields like laser liposuction (Gold et al., 2021). Thus, in reducing adverse effects by maximizing application technique and encouraging continued research, practitioners will optimize PLLA thread treatments, tailoring them to each patient's needs and optimizing the model of non-surgical facial rejuvenation (Figure 6.6).

6.2.3. Polycaprolactone (PCL) Threads

The use of PCL threads in aesthetic medicine is a paradigm shift in thread lifting and skin tightening procedures. PCL is a biocompatible, biodegradable polymer that has gained wide acceptance due to its favorable mechanical properties and biocompatibility.

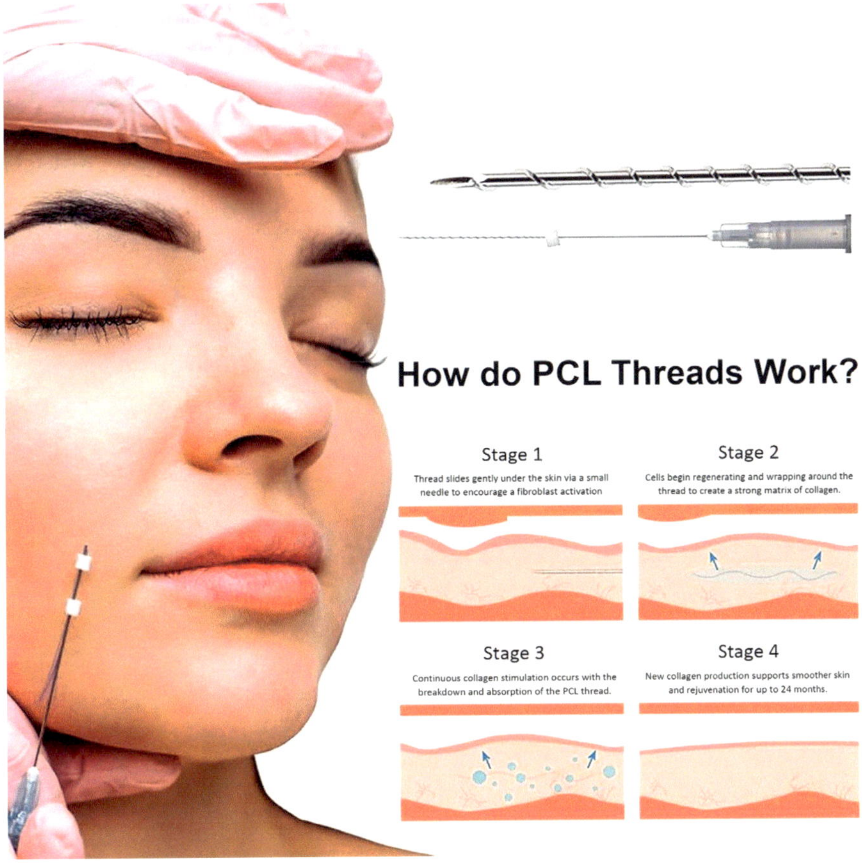

Figure 6.7. How do PCL threads work.

Source: https://m.media-amazon.com/images/I/71TYeuiIc7L._AC_UF1000,1000_QL80_.jpg.

Compared to traditional materials utilized in thread lifting, , such as PDO and PLA, PCL threads maintain their support for longer, as they remain in place for up to two years. Such prolonged action is particularly useful for patients needing spontaneous and gradual lifting effects without the complications associated with more traditional surgical procedures. The application of PCL threads in noninvasive facial rejuvenation treatments is a good substitute for more conventional procedures like surgical facelifts that are often accompanied by longer recovery times and a greater risk of complication (Portilla et al., 2024). In addition to being less risky, PCL threads are also multifunctional. Not only do they provide structural support to dangling skin, but they also stimulate collagen in the neighboring tissues. Such autologous collagen generation is a part of the innate healing mechanisms of the skin and leads to improvement in skin texture and elasticity over time.

Therefore, PCL thread application gives results that can maximize facial aesthetic appeal by making the face appear younger while avoiding the necessity for other interventions. The ability of these threads to integrate well into the dermal layers without causing significant inflammatory responses is a testament to their suitability for long-term aesthetic treatments in aesthetic surgery and dermatology (Akhond et al., 2021). Moreover, the successful application of PCL threads emphasizes the applicability of tailored treatments in aesthetic treatments. Given the patient's anatomy and aging pattern, the practitioners can customize the placement and number of threads for optimal result. Personalization not only ensures patient satisfaction but also enhances the level of care in noninvasive beauty treatments. As the aesthetic climate keeps on changing, the application of PCL threads in therapy sessions is an emerging trend towards less invasive but highly effective procedures for combating the outward symptoms of the aging process. The convergence of novel materials and innovative approaches to therapy holds positive promise for facial rejuvenation in the future, solidifying the role of PCL threads as a key instrument in modern aesthetic medicine (Portilla et al., 2024) (Figure 6.7).

Test Your Knowledge

1. What are the key differences in composition, longevity, and stimulation effects among PDO, PLLA, and PCL threads used in thread lifting procedures?
2. Which thread type is most suitable for patients seeking gradual, long-lasting lifting effects with minimal early swelling?

6.3. Mechanism of Action

Learning Outcome

1. Explain how thread lifting works
2. Discuss about biological response to thread insertion
3. Compare with traditional facelift procedures

Thread lifting and skin tightening procedures mainly consist of the placement of biodegradable sutures into the dermal tissue. The threads create an immediate lift as they mechanically anchor the skin, which is particularly handy around zones that sag. While the threads are being placed, they also stimulate the surrounding tissues and provoke a natural healing reaction. This is not merely refreshing the skin's turgor but also activating collagen over time. The overactivation of fibroblasts enhances collagen and elastin production and consequently the overall firmness and elasticity of the skin.

Thread lifting is therefore counteracting the aging and environmental stresses efficiently with an immediate corrective treatment and a long-term anti-aging approach, tackling effectively the loss of elasticity that results from aging and environmental stresses. Additionally, the substance that is utilized within thread lifts is important for their effectiveness and patient satisfaction. Threads comprised of PDO or PLA are utilized most commonly because they are biocompatible and break down slowly over time within the body. They provide support not only during healing but also minimize the amount of inflammation typically experienced with surgical interventions. The body's response to these threads enhances neovascularization, which is vital for optimal tissue repair and regeneration. Although PDO threads have promising results, however, some findings indicate that outcomes may vary with the specific application technique and the patient's own individual biological responses, indicating the complex nature of human tissue responses to extraneous substances , such as those used in cosmetic operations (Gulbitti et al., 2022). Moreover, the integration of thread lifting techniques into overall tightening schemes underlines the need for the inclusion of various methodologies to provide optimal outcomes. As dermatology evolves, clinicians are increasingly using thread lifting as part of synergistic modalities, including laser and RF treatment.

Together, this is not only enhancing the transient lift effect but also enhancing texture and general skin quality through the promotion of increased collagen remodeling. The combined effect of such techniques takes advantage of the body's own healing powers, thereby maximizing patient benefits while minimizing side effects. The professionals have to remain updated on such developments and assess the patients' needs appropriately to determine the optimal treatment mode, thereby optimizing the solution to skin tightening and facial rejuvenation (Middleton et al., 1985).

6.3.1. How Thread Lifting Works

Thread lifting, a revolutionary process in facial rejuvenation without the need for surgery, is based on placing expert threads under the skin to provide support and elevation to sagging features. These threads are typically made up of biocompatible materials, , such as PDO, that absorb over time, allowing the body enough time to adapt to the changes naturally. The method entails the employment of a long cog thread, which is passed into some layers of the skin, more specifically entering the fascia of the area to be treated in order to provide the best anchorage. In this manner, the threads can hook onto the tissue and form structural support. As a result, not only is the skin lifted but also stimulated to produce collagen, with enhancement of elasticity and texture of the skin, resulting in a smoother appearance, as per recent advances achieved in aesthetic innovations (Kyu-Yi et al., 2024). Thread lifting has the significant aspect of its ability to rejuvenate the face without the invasiveness of traditional surgical procedures. Unlike facelifts involving large incisions and lengthy recovery times, thread lifts involve less invasiveness and, in most instances, can be performed as outpatient surgery. The threading procedure lasts about 30 to 60 minutes, with patients returning to normal activity not long after the procedure. Further, the use of the anchoring technique, where threads are anchored in facial tissues, has the advantage of not just being immediate but also maintaining its effects as the tissues gradually heal and reorganize in the zones where anchor points were made.

This method highlights the utility of thread lifting as a fashionable choice for middle-aged women and men who want to reverse facial aging without making a long-term commitment to invasive surgery (Li et al., 2023). The longevity of thread lifting results varies, although most patients enjoy the effect for one to two years, depending on lifestyle factors and techniques applied. Over time, as the fibers dissolve, the body's natural healing process initiates new collagen growth, tightening the skin and enhancing its appearance. This has a twofold benefit: immediate lifting is paired with long-term skin improvement. The thread lift technique is therefore typically chosen for its ability to rejuvenate the skin and allow for limited downtime, making the procedure an effective addition to the list of skin tightening techniques. As thread lifting continues to evolve, ongoing R&D will likely integrate its efficacy and widen its application areas in aesthetic treatments, further establishing itself as a vital part of non-surgical cosmetic procedures (Kyu-Yi et al., 2024) (Figure 6.8).

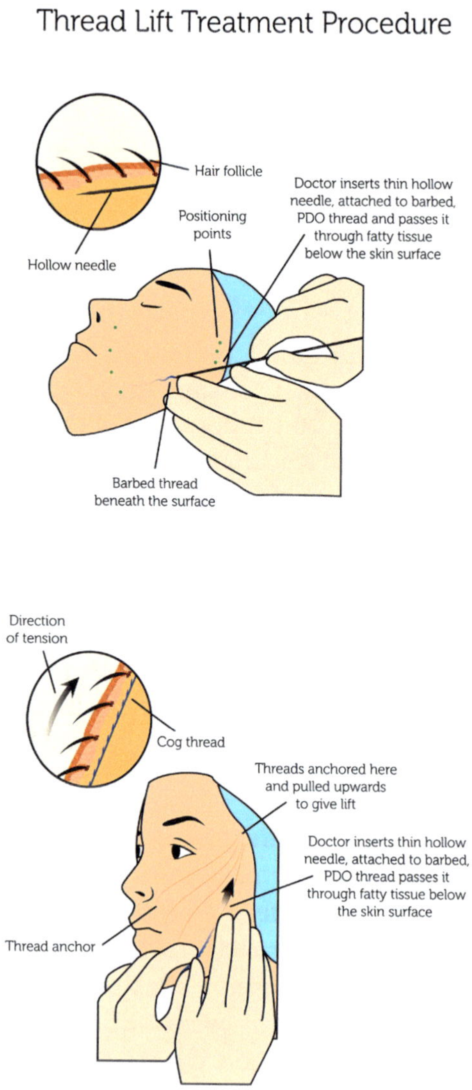

Figure 6.8. Thread lift treatment procedure.

Source: https://www.rejuvenceclinic.co.uk/wp-content/uploads/2020/11/Pdo-Threadlift-Treatment-Procedure-2-01.png.

6.3.2. Biological Response to Thread Insertion

The physiological response to thread implantation, particularly thread lifting and facial skin tightening treatments, is a multi-layered process based on the natural healing mechanism of the body. Upon implantation of threads, usually made of PDO, the immediate response is a retained inflammatory response. This is critical in that it initiates the cascade of events resulting in tissue remodeling. The inflammatory response is employed to initiate migration of many cellular mediators into the insertion site, including fibroblasts involved in collagen formation. This healing response induced by stimulation leads to enhanced elastin and collagen synthesis in the skin, which ultimately leads to the tightening effect and improved texture of skin perceived by patients following such minimal invasive procedures. The biomechanical rationale for these enhancements highlights the popularity of thread lifting as an appropriate intervention against aging (Duncan et al., 2020). As PDO threads eventually biodegrade, they leave a remnant scaffold which prompts continuous collagen production, once more extending the aesthetic benefit beyond the immediate post-procedure timeframe. The hydrolysis degradation of the threads usually occurs in six months, but the created collagen and elastin fibers network lasts much longer after that. Not only does this impact bear witness to the natural regenerative capacity of the organism to react to foreign materials, but it is also indicative of the two-sided action of PDO threads as suspension units for lifting purposes and biostimulators that trigger rejuvenation of the skin. Moreover, the synergistic effects of the simultaneous presence of PDO threads and other treatments, , such as topical exosome therapy, may also further enhance the regenerative process, promoting a whole-system platform for the management of surface aging as well as subcutaneous laxity by a single modality (Duncan et al., 2020). The application of contemporary biomaterials, , such as the application of collagen implants with PDO threads, represents a new and novel area of study that emphasizes the complex biological interaction between host tissue and implanted material. Research has indicated that materials like cross-linked collagen are extremely biocompatible and cause good fibrovascular in-growth and extracellular matrix deposition for maximum reinforcement of the tissue. Such findings are significant, not only because they reaffirm the safety of such novel techniques but also because they underscore the necessity of understanding the host response to both biological and synthetic substances when using therapeutic modalities. By capitalizing on the body's own healing potential with such techniques, practitioners can achieve more long-lasting results with skin tightening and lifting, and thereby illustrate the clinical applicability of biological principles to aesthetic medicine (Figure 6.9).

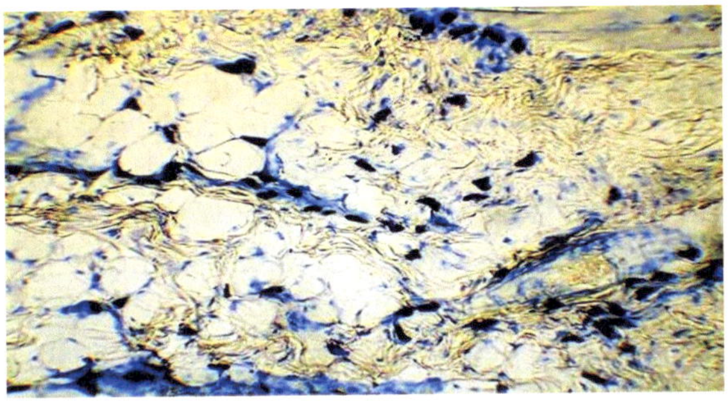

Figure 6.9. Mast cells seen around a PLCL thread 40 days after insertion.

Source: https://www.researchgate.net/publication/348434842/figure/fig2/AS:11431281256205977@1719511425922/Mast-cells-seen-around-a-PLCL-thread-40-days-after-insertion.jpg.

6.3.3. Comparison with Traditional Facelift Procedures

The advent of thread lifting as a tightening method has led to the reconsideration of traditional facelift techniques. Facelifts have traditionally consisted of invasive surgical techniques, which involve long recovery periods and are linked with a multitude of potential complications, including infection and hematoma formation. Traditional facelifts entail deep subcutaneous plane dissection, where reposition of the skin and excision of excess tissue is carried out to create a more youthful appearance. This time-consuming process, while effective, leaves visible scarring and demands a long rehabilitation. Thread lifting presents a less invasive option, utilizing resorbable sutures to lift and tighten sagging skin without the need for massive incisions. This technology not only reduces recovery time but also minimizes the discomfort experienced by the patient, enabling them to get back to their normal lives sooner compared to patients who have undergone conventional facelift surgery (Pourdanesh et al., 2016). In addition to quicker recovery time, thread lifting techniques also provide a safer option compared to conventional facelifts. The latter procedure more often includes general anesthesia and a longer time of surgery, thereby increasing the risk of complications, such as reaction to anesthesia and swelling, which takes longer to subside. Thread lifting, however, is commonly performed under local anesthesia, which reduces the risks involved significantly and gives the patient a more acceptable experience. In addition, since it is minimally invasive, thread lifting tends to create unobtrusive yet meaningful enhancements, which correlate with the modern standards of beauty that prioritize a natural appearance over its extreme transformation. As the world's standards of beauty change, especially in those parts of the world where a naturally elegant look is desired, like South Korea, thread lifting methods might suit such tastes better than conventional facelifts (Marques, 2023). In addition, the availability of thread lifts increases its popularity compared to conventionally performed facelift surgery. Conventionally performed facelifts are commonly viewed as being costly and resource-scarce, which restricts eligibility to many potential clients. Thread lifts, being resource-sparing, can be made available at reasonable costs, making a wider segment of the population eligible for cosmetic interventions. This cosmetic democratization makes thread lifting a suitable option for individuals who desire rejuvenation but without the exorbitant financial or temporal expense associated with traditional surgical treatments. With the beauty world becoming increasingly prone to minimally invasive procedures, thread lifting is one such cutting-edge technology that not only allows skin tightening but also adheres to modern standards of beauty, thereby challenging the rise of conventional facelift surgeries (Pourdanesh et al., 2016).

Test Your Knowledge

1. How does thread lifting achieve skin tightening and lifting effects without surgery?
2. What is the biological response of the skin to thread insertion during a thread lift procedure?

6.4. Skin Tightening Techniques

Learning Outcome

1. Describe RF therapy
2. Understand ultrasound therapy as a non-surgical skin tightening technique
3. Define the laser skin tightening technique

Over the last few years, there has been a high demand for good skin tightening methods, mostly fueled by a need for non-surgical cosmetic procedures. Among the numerous methods, thread lifting has drawn a lot of attention because it serves two purposes: lifting and tightening facial tissues. It entails the insertion of biocompatible threads beneath the skin, which offer structural support while at the same time inducing the growth of collagen. Use of materials , such as polydioxanone in technologies like Smart PDOs™ shows the advancements that are occurring in this field, since the threads promote both short-term and long-term effects on skin tightening and texture. The Cartesian Technique™, involving a planned thread insertion technique, has been demonstrated to enhance lifting effects and facial rejuvenation, with striking improvements in turgidity and wrinkle reduction, proof of the efficacy of the technique as a contemporary treatment for facial aging and loss of elasticity (Gladys et al., 2024). Moreover, the synergy created by combining the methods of threading with other modalities makes them more efficient, thus leading to more complete results. Thread lifting in conjunction with other procedures, i.e., dermal fillers or botulinum toxins, allows practitioners to address multiple aspects of facial aging simultaneously. Besides tightening the skin, this synergy optimizes the global balance of the face, which is critical to derive pleasing cosmetic results. The current trends concentrate on reviving the deeper layers of facial tissues and not merely the resituation of the skin surface. As a result, patients usually enjoy improved collagen remodeling and skin quality, as observed by employing mono and barbed threads, which enhance tissue metabolism and obtain the aspect of a younger face. Researchers continue to examine thread types best suited for multiple treatment goals so that cosmetic wishes can be achieved more effectively (Hong et al., 2024). Lastly, while thread lifting is beneficial in numerous ways, it is not without contention and concern. The debate over how long the lifting effect lasts after thread absorption remains, with focus being called to the need for ongoing scientific research and progress within the specialty. Historically, thread insertions have been compared to fortifying concrete buildings, noting their supportive character against lax skin. However, as with any new modality, practitioners must carefully assess individual patient needs and anatomical responses to achieve the desired outcome. Histological studies suggest threads can elicit fibrotic tissue reactions, thus generating long-term alterations in skin texture, but further study is necessary to validate these findings. Whilst the technology of skin tightening procedures evolves, thread lifting is an upmarket option that testifies to the coming together of science and beauty in contemporary dermatology (Hong et al., 2024).

6.4.1. Radiofrequency Therapy

RF therapy has been among the most prominent techniques in the practice of aesthetic medicine, particularly in relation to thread lifting and skin tightening. RF therapy utilizes the energy of RF to stimulate an increase in collagen and elastin production in the dermis, leading to tightening and rejuvenation of the skin. The non-surgical nature of RF therapy makes it extremely useful for patients who do not wish to be exposed to the potential complications of surgery. As age progresses, intrinsic and extrinsic factors contribute to the breakdown of collagen, which is primarily accountable for the tightness and elasticity of the skin. By erasing these signs of aging, RF therapy can be a highly effective adjunct to thread lifting treatments, enhancing overall treatment outcomes and increasing the length of the procedure. With thread lifting, RF therapy tightens the skin as well as improves its texture and tone by addressing multiple signs of aging simultaneously. Such synergy maximizes patient satisfaction through holistic aesthetic rejuvenation. RF treatments are also tailored, varying in intensity and depth according to target skin types and conditions, which is consonant with the personalized approach that is the hallmark of aesthetic medicine. As also noted in more recent publications, effective planning and sensitivity to the patients' aesthetic goals, regardless of age, are crucial in maximizing the efficacy of treatments.

It is most critical for practitioners because certain demographic factors, age, in turn, as well as patients' ethnic backgrounds, can potentially influence the expected outcomes of aesthetic interventions (Joel et al., 2023). The psychological impact of skin aging can evoke lowered self-esteem and altered self-concept among patients. As highlighted by research, finding effective treatments that enhance patients' emotional health is crucial in aesthetic treatment. RF therapy contributes to this by not only improving patients' appearance but also alleviating the psychological pain associated with visible aging. Besides this, RF combined with thread lifting serves an emerging demand for less invasive approaches to enhancing beauty and mental health. Therefore, the incorporation of RF therapy into treatment regimens is a significant advancement, as it enhances results as per patient expectations for youthful appearance without extensive downtime synonymous with traditional surgery methods (Raslan et al., 2023) (Figure 6.10).

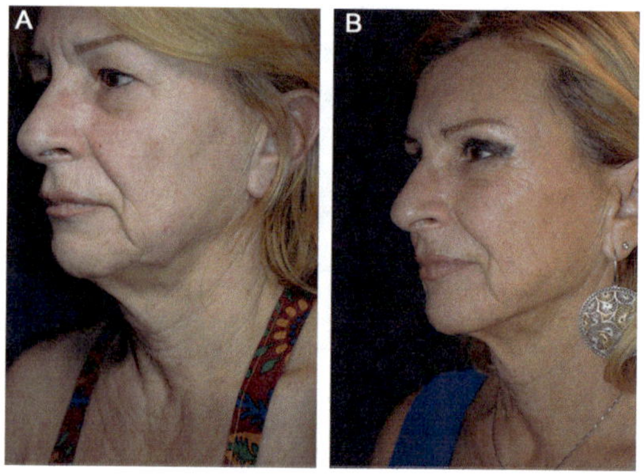

Figure 6.10. Results of radiofrequency-assisted lower face and neck treatment with fractional bipolar radiofrequency. (A) the 64-year-old female patient pretreatment; and (B) results 24 months postoperative.

Source: https://www.researchgate.net/profile/Spero-Theodorou/publication/344431086/figure/fig1/AS:944005743378435@1602079916486/results-of-radiofrequency-assisted-lower-face-and-neck-treatment-with-fractional-bipolar.ppm.

6.4.2. Ultrasound Therapy

Ultrasound therapy has been one of the most significant modalities within the non-surgical variety of skin tightening techniques, providing a novel alternative to traditional surgical procedures. Ultrasound energy is employed to stimulate deep within the skin, thus stimulating collagen and causing a significant enhancement in skin laxity. When skin gets older, it changes its structure as collagen and elastin diminish, which are responsible for its lax nature. By utilizing ultrasound energy, therapists can stimulate cellular rejuvenation, stimulating the natural body response for healing, which tightens the support structure of the skin. The non-surgical treatment addresses the trend towards minimizing patient downtime in achieving optimal aesthetic outcomes. From advocates of ultrasound treatment, its safety and efficacy were quoted, calling it a proven technique for people who need to tighten skin but want the relative dangers of more invasive procedures. Thread lifting is applied in conjunction with ultrasound therapy as a non-surgical dermatologic treatment that can be utilized to augment skin tightening treatments. It involves the strategic placement of resorbable threads within the subcutaneous plane to re-suspend and lift lax tissues. By combining this with ultrasound therapy, practitioners can enhance the overall efficacy of treatments; ultrasound can optimize thread placement by contour mapping the face and optimizing collagen production around the threads, thus further improving lifting. Advances in minimally invasive dermatological treatments—, such as thread lifts—are indicative of a trend towards multi-functional and creative solutions to addressing the multifarious problems of aging skin. As the literature suggests, the integration of these approaches has the possibility of yielding more effective results than either treatment employed separately, indicating the direction toward whole-person anti-aging therapy as outlined in modern-day aesthetic dermatology (Portilla et al., 2024). The global beauty industry has also experienced an increase in the employment of ultrasound treatment, fueled by the increasing popularity in South Korea, renowned for its cutting-edge cosmetic treatments. The drive of culture to achieve a naturally flawless appearance has triggered the demand for less invasive procedures like ultrasound therapy, in keeping with tech- and innovation-fostered Western ideals of beauty. As suggested by recent studies, there is immense potential for the worldwide dissemination of such cosmetic treatments, especially in high-income economies like Switzerland, where minimally invasive procedures are extremely popular and growing rapidly (Marques, 2023). By harnessing technological advancements and advanced techniques, ultrasound treatment is set to stake its position in the global aesthetic market. This innovation reflects an increasing customer desire for treatments that are both effective and safe, a testament to the new complexion of cosmetic dermatology where traditional and innovative techniques come together (Figure 6.11).

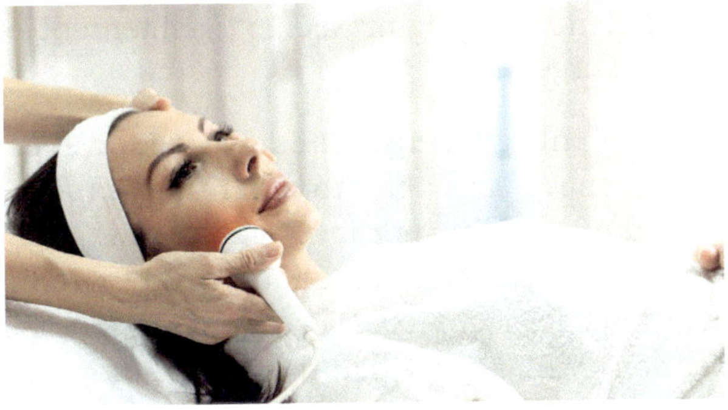

Figure 6.11. Ultrasound skin tightening.

Source: https://www.costhetics.com.au/wp-content/uploads/2013/05/ultrasound_skin_tightening.jpg.

6.4.3. Laser Skin Tightening

The application of laser technology in aesthetic medicine has revolutionized skin tightening procedures with a non-surgical alternative to traditional surgery. Laser skin tightening is based on stimulating collagen production via controlled thermal energy. Specifically, laser application heats the dermal layers below the skin but leaves the epidermis intact, inducing a natural tightening effect over time. This treatment not only enhances the elasticity of skin but also reduces the look of fine lines and wrinkles, targeting many problems associated with aging. Through the lesser invasiveness of this treatment, patients do not have much downtime, which makes it easier for more laser procedure acceptance in the cosmetic improvement field. The continuous development of laser technology enables personalized treatments for individual skin types, hence a one-size-fits-all solution for those seeking rejuvenation without surgery (Kyu-Yi et al., 2024). Additionally, combining laser skin tightening with other non-surgical interventions, , such as thread lifting, is likely to improve aesthetic outcomes. Whereas laser therapy stimulates collagen and firms the skin, thread lifting immediately elevates the support by anchoring the tissue. This combined approach is highly beneficial to clients presenting with initial signs of aging or seeking refinement of earlier surgery.

By integrating these procedures, practitioners are able to offer a complete, three-dimensional approach against skin laxity, ensuring patient satisfaction through long-term appearance. Moreover, advances in laser technology have provided the impetus for new modalities of therapy that are more precise and effective with less discomfort. Consequently, the meeting point of laser skin tightening with procedures like thread lifting is a successful paradigm in contemporary aesthetic medicine, where it is the focus on minimally invasive procedures (Marie-Christen, 2022). Finally, the safety profile of laser skin tightening is a factor in its attraction to patients desiring cosmetic augmentation. Compared to surgery, complications of laser therapy are few and more typically minor side effects , such as redness, swelling, or temporary discomfort. Nevertheless, as in any other cosmetic intervention, proper selection of patients and adherence to treatment modalities are critical to the prevention of preventable complications. The physicians have to conduct proper evaluations in order to identify good candidates for treatment, taking into consideration skin type, intended outcome, and the history of the patient. Educating patients about realistic expectations and potential complications of the procedure encourages a consensus strategy for achieving their aesthetic goals. As there is a growing demand for safe, effective, and non-invasive treatments, laser skin tightening remains a relevant option in the realm of rejuvenation techniques, particularly when combined with other treatments, such as thread lifting (Kyu-Yi et al., 2024) (Figure 6.12).

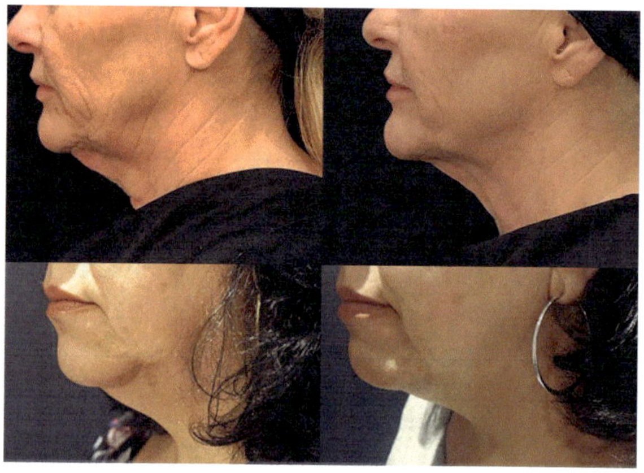

Figure 6.12. Laser skin tightening before and after.

Source: https://www.pulselightclinic.co.uk/wp-content/uploads/2023/08/Laser-Skin-Tightening-Before-And-After.jpg.

Test Your Knowledge

1. How do Radiofrequency (RF), Ultrasound, and Laser skin tightening techniques differ in their method of delivering energy to the skin?
2. Which skin tightening technique is most suitable for targeting deeper tissue layers without affecting the skin surface?

6.5. Benefits of Thread Lifting

Learning Outcome

1. Understand the minimally invasive nature of thread lifting
2. Discuss how thread lifting presents patients with immediate results and a notably reduced recovery time compared to traditional surgical facelifts
3. Evaluate long-lasting effects compared to other methods

With the need for youthfully smooth faces still strong, thread lifting has emerged as a lure to traditional surgical facelifts. It is a minimally invasive procedure with several benefits, the most significant of which is its ability to pull up skin without the extensive postoperative recovery time usually associated with surgical procedures. Unlike a standard facelift involving much dissection and manipulation of the facial tissues, thread lifting uses biodegradable threads inserted under the skin to create a lifting action. Besides the instantaneous effect that it provides, thread lifting also stimulates collagen formation in the long term, which produces a more natural and longer-lasting rejuvenation of youthful skin. The enhancement in techniques of dermal treatments, particularly with materials like PDO and PLA threads, has rendered thread lifting a safe and effective means for restoration, following today's aesthetic standards for minimally invasive interventions that provide remarkable improvements (Portilla et al., 2024). Thread lifting is also noted for its versatility in supporting a range of demographic interests and anatomical variations. This is the best treatment for the individual who desires rejuvenation of various face and neck regions, and it is therefore suitable for various kinds of aging signs , such as sagging cheeks, jawlines, and nasolabial folds. The treatment is suitable for patients who have varying skin types and characteristics of aging, so treatment can be tailored to address structural parameters in addition to individual aesthetic desires. For those nervous about having traditional surgery, due to the fear of cost, recovery, or complications, thread lifting is an appealing compromise. Its minimally invasive nature works into greater social pressures, encouraging minimally invasive cosmetic surgery to enable patients to create desired results with less risk and accelerated return to ordinary living (Pourdanesh et al., 2016).

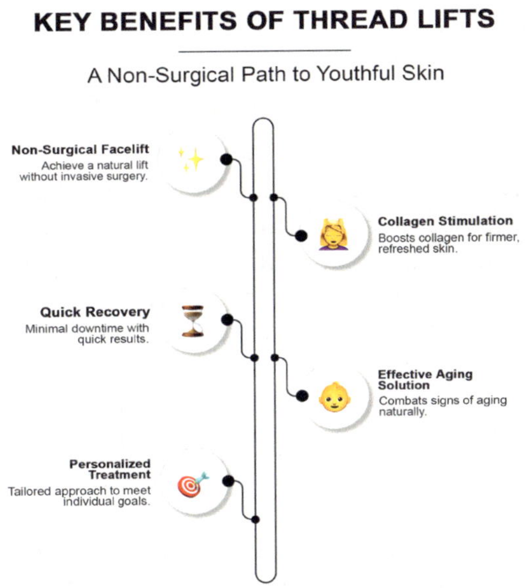

Figure 6.13. Key benefits of thread lift.

Source: https://images.bannerbear.com/direct/4mGpW3zwpg0ZK0AxQw/requests/000/078/031/891/NWlVkgmbMQEZjnxdYZyAqEwDo/96dfb57414db6bb5445f9a05b2c5b82b769120c7.jpg.

Moreover, thread lifting's psychological benefits cannot be ignored. Most individuals report higher levels of self-esteem and better body image after the procedure since it is the small enhancements that can impact perceived beauty and confidence levels significantly. The minimally invasive nature of thread lifting may also eliminate the fear often associated with more invasive procedures, making the experience generally improved. While the patients indulge not only in physical rejuvenation but also in the emotional lift that comes with it, the holistic philosophy of beauty and well-being becomes increasingly appealing. Adding these techniques to cosmetic procedures highlights the trend towards personalized and patient-centric treatment in aesthetic medicine, reasserting the role of thread lifting in bodily transformation and psychological health (Portilla et al., 2024) (Figure 6.13).

6.5.1. Minimally Invasive Nature

The minimally invasive nature of thread lifting has revolutionized aesthetic procedures, with patients achieving dramatic improvement in the look of the skin with reduced danger and time off from work in comparison to traditional surgery. Compared to extensive facelifts that involve lengthy downtime and accompanying complications, thread lifting involves the use of sutures made of biocompatible material to lift and tighten sagging skin naturally. This trailblazing technique triggers collagen production beneath the skin, making the face youthful as time goes on. As dermatology develops further, such less invasive procedures address an increasingly large number of individuals in desperate need of good anti-aging results without the seriousness of surgical complications, highlighting their place in modern aesthetic medicine (Portilla et al., 2024). The appeal of thread lifting is that it can provide remarkable results without sacrificing the natural contour of the face. Where traditional techniques used to result in scarring or unnatural-looking results, newer thread lifting utilizes advanced technology that is crafted to minimize obvious signs of treatment. The use of PDO and PLA threads illustrates this trend with instant lifting, as well as ongoing skin rejuvenation with neocollagenesis. This dual effect minimizes the intrusiveness of the procedure to satisfy patients' requests for natural-looking, subtle outcomes. Furthermore, as cultural aesthetic standards evolve, with heightened demand for minimally invasive treatments that improve but not alter appearance, thread lifting is optimally positioned to meet these demands (Marques, 2023). As the global beauty industry embraces the philosophy of minimally invasive, there are opportunities for growing innovation and adoption of thread lifting treatment across markets. The increasing popularity of such treatments, particularly in countries like South Korea, reflects a significant trend towards beauty treatments that are centered on the client's comfort and satisfaction. With a thriving consumer market eager to experiment with advanced beauty therapies, the world trend towards minimally invasive treatments can benefit from cultural exchange that highlights natural beauty ideals. Through prioritizing safe, efficient, and effective options like thread lifting, practitioners are not only satisfying the needs of patients but also enhancing their provision of services and competing in a constantly evolving aesthetic landscape (Portilla et al., 2024; Marques, 2023).

6.5.2. Immediate Results and Recovery Time

The evolution of thread lifting as a minimally invasive, cosmetic procedure provides patients with immediate satisfaction and remarkably reduced recovery time compared to traditional surgical facelifts. Thread lifting incorporates the placement of biocompatible threads underneath the skin to provide structural support, trigger collagen, and perform slight lifting of facial contours. Patients usually report dramatic improvement in the texture and tightness of their skin immediately after the treatment, which is why it has emerged as a favorite among individuals seeking quick results with little downtime from surgery. The short recovery time is largely because the procedure is local, and since the threads employed are resorbable, weakening the body's healing reaction and hence minimizing post-surgical complications. These characteristics render thread lifting a sought-after choice within the expanding field of beauty treatments for busy individuals. Apart from the straightforward cosmetic benefits, recovery time for thread lifting is significantly less than with traditional surgery methods. Most patients can normally return to their full activity in a day or two after the procedure, which is significantly different from weeks of lost time associated with surgical facelifts. It has been found from research that the least invasive thread lifting has less bruising and swelling, which again leads to a faster recovery process. For instance, research indicates that mild chronic inflammation may be observed close to the threads but is normally self-limiting with a quick return to normalcy of daily functions. This rapid recovery not only enhances patient satisfaction but also fits well with the increasing demand for cosmetic procedures that address contemporary lifestyles and convenience demands. Also, thread lifting effects continue to evolve after the initial treatment due to ongoing collagen generation. Studies confirm that while patients experience immediate lifting results, the full value of skin texture and tightening occurs over an extended timeline, leading to a more enduring effect. Particularly, the integration of the use of aiding technologies , such as RF therapy in combination with thread lifting, has proven promising outcomes in maintaining and fostering these effects. For instance, considerable lifting quantities of millimeters measured in different zones of the face immediately after treatment were seen to persist and even enhance on one-month follow-ups, suggestive of the collagen reaction induced by such treatments. Thus, the twofold advantage of immediate results together with long-term improvement of the skin quality ensures that thread lifting is a central procedure of aesthetic medicine, able to offer immediate gratification as well as long-term benefit, thus being of interest to a heterogeneous group of patients (Kim, 2024; Serov et al., 2024).

6.5.3. Long-Lasting Effects Compared to Other Methods

Among the tools of skin tightening treatments, thread lifting has been a prominent method, primarily due to its long-lasting impacts compared to other prevalent methods , such as facelifts. Thread lifting uses removable sutures to encourage collagen, resulting in a gradual increase in skin elasticity and firmness. This method not only rejuvenates the skin but also gives a subtle lift, and effects remain for a duration of up to 18 months or longer. Facelifts, although good, are likely to require longer recovery and may also result in wide scarring. As a less invasive treatment, thread lifting is appealing to a patient population seeking solutions that deliver without the risks of more invasive treatments, and as such, it stands as a strong option in the wider aesthetic treatment category that both includes surgical and nonsurgical procedures (Portilla et al., 2024). The enduring quality of thread lifting outcomes is also appealing to the growing consumer trend of desiring minimally invasive treatments with natural results, as well. Unlike fillers or chemical peels, improvements achieved with thread lifting are maintained through the natural healing processes of the body. This feature not only meets the aesthetic demands of patients but also addresses the changing beauty standards that support less overt procedures. As noted in current discussions of skin rejuvenation, methods like thread lifting, which involve new technology in the guise of artificial threads, offer a new face to beauty improvement for the modern age. The long-term outcomes from the innovations specifically interest individuals who are ready to commit long-term to their appearance without constantly repeated procedures (Marques, 2023). In looking at the position of thread lifting among broader aesthetic treatments, there is no doubt that this treatment stands in good stead to ride out shifting beauty ideals. The cultural context of beauty, and particularly in territories like South

Korea, has contributed in significant measures to influencing attitudes worldwide and in the adoption of skincare technology. Since there is increasing demand for procedures that fulfill the modern desire for natural appearance with long-lasting effects, the thread lifting technique continues to be a top contender. Its increase in use among the wider aesthetic market fulfills the trend towards delivering efficient, minimally invasive treatments and is comfortable as an option of choice. As global consumers explore such alternatives, the potential for global extension of such approaches underscores the need for ongoing investigation into their efficacy and cultural acceptance among different groups (Portilla et al., 2024) (Figure 6.14).

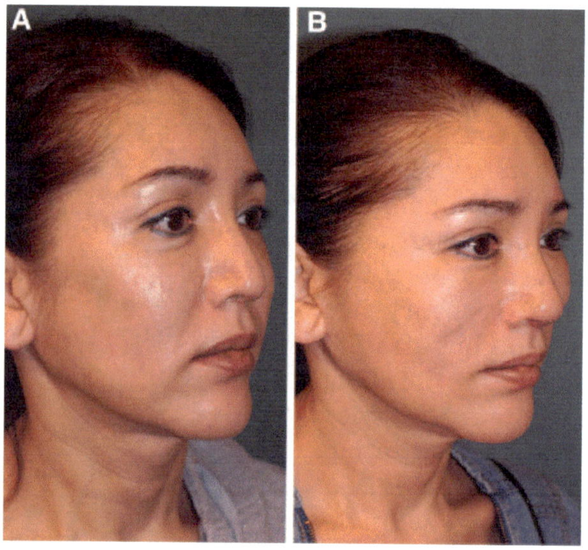

Figure 6.14. Before thread lift (A); and 6 months after thread lift (B).

Source: https://www.researchgate.net/profile/Stamatis-Sapountzis/publication/269715085/figure/fig2/AS:295155509809162@1447381965811/Before-thread-lift-A-and-6-months-after-thread-lift-B-with-REEBORN.png.

Test Your Knowledge

1. How does the minimally invasive nature of thread lifting reduce the risks and downtime associated with facial rejuvenation procedures?
2. What makes thread lifting an attractive option for patients seeking immediate aesthetic improvement with minimal recovery?

6.6. Risks and Considerations

Learning Outcome

1. Describe potential side effects of thread lifting
2. Understand complications associated with skin tightening techniques
3. Explain the importance of choosing qualified practitioners

When thread lifting and skin tightening are options, it is useful to note the risks and factors associated with the treatments. Even though minimally invasive, even these processes can lead to such things as infection, scarring, or allergic reaction to materials within the threads. Further, individuals with certain types of skin or certain health factors may be at more risk for bad outcomes. Patient selection also plays an important role in avoiding such risks since patients with good skin elasticity and correct expectations will exhibit better results. In addition, understanding the facial skeleton anatomy and skin changes caused by aging significantly influences the success of such techniques because improper utilization could lead to unsatisfactory results (Pourdanesh et al., 2016). Additionally, the psychological impacts of undergoing aesthetic treatments must be evaluated attentively. The high expectations of patients regarding the outcome of thread lifting and skin tightening can lead to dissatisfaction when results do not meet such expectations. Educating potential patients on what is achievable with such treatments can help build realistic expectations, ultimately leading to favorable satisfaction levels. Practitioners need to be frank when explaining possible complications and durability of results to patients. For instance, while some treatments may yield immediate results, the sustainability of the same is unclear, and hence it is imperative that patients understand the long-term implications involved in choosing such treatments (Pourdanesh et al., 2016). Secondly, another significant consideration is the intersection of new techniques and traditional processes. This blending of methods, such as thread lifting procedure in conjunction with neck liposuction and application of RF technology, optimizes the process. But where these combined strategies are used, there exist extra risks, including extended recovery periods and the technical difficulty of performing multiple procedures simultaneously. Practitioners should carefully consider the appropriateness of such combinations on a case-by-case basis based on their individual anatomical features and objective preferences. The evolving landscape of aesthetic treatments necessitates ongoing research and clinical evaluation to track safety and satisfaction, underscoring evidence-based practice in the area (Tettamanzi et al., 2024).

6.6.1. Potential Side Effects of Thread Lifting

Thread lifting represents a contemporary alternative for those requiring non-surgical skin rejuvenation. While the procedure is complimented on its relative safety and briefer recovery time compared to traditional surgical facelifts, acknowledgment of the side effects of the technique must be given as well. Commonly reported side effects from patients include swelling, bruising, and transient discomfort at the area of insertion. Temporary numbness or tingling, known as paresthesia, can occur in patients. This can lead to anxiety regarding the outcome of the procedure. The frequency of such side effects is usually heterogeneous based on factors like individual skin type, the method used, and the skill level of the practitioner. Being aware of these potential complications is essential during informed decision-making so that prospective patients can weigh the benefits against the risk of thread lifting (Portilla et al., 2024). In addition to more common side effects, there are also more severe complications that come with it, including extrusion and thread visibility. Threads being visible can be particularly upsetting to patients, as they ruin the aesthetic functions of the procedure. Extrusion is when threads migrate outside through the skin, where further intervention has to be taken to restore the desired appearance. In some cases, the presence of foreign material might trigger an inflammatory response, manifesting as skin dimpling or contour irregularities, detracting from patients' desired transformed appearance. The latter is worthy of explanation through comprehension of the details involved in performing such a consultation with a resultant pre-procedure assessment of all potential risks and realistic expectations of thread lifting (Lewandowska et al., 2024). As the body settles after the procedure, patients must remain aware of signs and symptoms of complications that are bound to occur in the long term. Infections, although quite rare, can compromise the cosmetic results and potentially result in more serious conditions requiring treatment. Similarly, more serious side effects , such as incomplete facial paralysis can occur, although not frequently, and demonstrate the importance of choosing qualified practitioners.

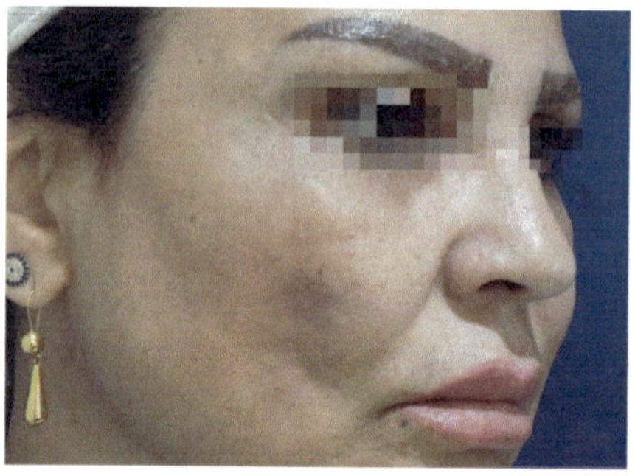

Figure 6.15. Facial dimpling, skin induration, and soft tissue reaction after PDO thread filler to full face.

Source: https://d148x66490prkv.cloudfront.net/hmp_ln/inline-images/Screenshot%202024-02-07%20at%203.14.22%20PM.png.

Awareness of common and severe side effects and initial consultation with a medical practitioner will significantly lower the prospects of adverse effects in the healing process. Lastly, gaining sufficient knowledge of these potential side effects is essential for one wishing to adopt thread lifting in their skin rejuvenation and tightening regimen (Lewandowska et al., 2024; Portilla et al., 2024) (Figure 6.15).

6.6.2. Complications Associated with Skin Tightening Techniques

The quest for improved aesthetically with skin tightening treatments, such as thread lifting, is fraught with great risk and potential complications that must be weighed. One of the primary concerns is with trauma to the underlying tissues when placing threads, which can lead to bruising and swelling, and, in extreme cases, permanent scarring. Moreover, misplacement of threads can result in asymmetry or unnatural contours of the face, which will necessitate subsequent correction procedures. These are the reasons why caution must be exercised in selecting a skilled practitioner who is aware of the complexity of facial anatomy and can appropriately attend to such complications. As seen in the literature, technical complexity embedded within these procedures is generally compounded by other variables , such as aged skin, which naturally undergoes alterations that may have an impact on surgical recovery and results (Pourdanesh et al., 2016). In addition to physical complications of the skin tightening procedures, patients may also experience psychological implications. The cultural influences on appearance can generate unrealistic patient expectations that can result in post-procedure dissatisfaction. That dissatisfaction can occur from complications changing the aesthetic result or from variations in the patient's sense of self subsequent to the procedure. Combining procedures like neck liposuction with emerging technologies, FaceTite RF technology, aims to enhance outcomes; yet, every development has risk factors and complications of its own. It is essential for practitioners who must deal with both the bodily and psychosomatic outcomes of their patients to have an integral grasp of such potential psychological effects (Tettamanzi et al., 2024). Besides, anesthetic complications and infection-related complications are still prevalent risks in the practice of skin tightening treatments. A risk of introducing contamination with pathogen toxins still exists despite the most meticulous technique, leading to post-operative infection and complicating recovery. Sedated or general anesthesia patients are also at risk of inherent complications, , such as respiratory complication or allergic reaction, which demand vigorous pre-operative workup. These medical and aesthetic complications highlight the need for proper extensive patient education on risks entailed in any procedure to improve the skin's appearance. In summary, while skin tightening procedures have promising results, their complication rates require wary and informed management to ensure patient safety and satisfaction (Pourdanesh et al., 2016).

6.6.3. Importance of Choosing Qualified Practitioners

The selection of expert practitioners in thread lifting and skin tightening processes is most important in-patient protection from harm and attainment of the best results. While these processes are regarded as minimally invasive, they require a high level of anatomical knowledge, expertise, and patient-specific factors only an expert practitioner can understand. An expert practitioner by default has the best ability to identify each patient's individualized needs, thereby individualizing treatment protocols for greater efficacy and lesser adverse effects. Further, skilled practitioners who are well-versed in aesthetic treatments are more likely to stay current with new technologies and techniques, allowing for patients to receive the latest, most effective treatment. Without credentials, the risk for substandard results or side effects is significantly higher, thus the need to select practitioners who have had the right training and experience. In addition to creating safety a reality, the art of skilled practitioners weighs heavily on the aesthetic results possible through thread lifting and skin tightening. Aesthetic outcomes rely not only on the technique employed but also on the practitioner's artistic vision and understanding of balance and proportion. When skilled practitioners perform these procedures, they can achieve natural-appearing results consistent with patient expectations. Research shows that practitioners who have high levels of experience and training are in a better position to minimize risks of complications , such as infection and adverse outcomes. High levels of skills are also typically accompanied by patient satisfaction, increasing confidence and enabling good relationships between patient and practitioner. Qualifications must therefore be given priority so that those seeking aesthetic improvements are treated by people who are capable of providing best outcomes responsibly. Lastly, the broader implications of choosing effective practitioners face compliance and regulatory challenges in the aesthetics industry. In recent years, the rising numbers of unqualified practitioners attempting to provide aesthetic treatments have posed problems with patient safety and honesty within the industry. Regulatory bodies have identified a need for practitioners to adhere to established standards of care, which will more likely be adhered to by trained and credentialed practitioners. Further, compliance with relevant laws and ethical guidelines not only protects patients but also adds to the aesthetic industry's overall professionalism. The better-informed patients are about the dangers of non-conformist practitioners, the greater the need for competent professionals will be, thus making it more apparent why rigorous training is obligatory to maintain safety and high standards in the field of thread lifting and skin tightening techniques (Figure 6.16).

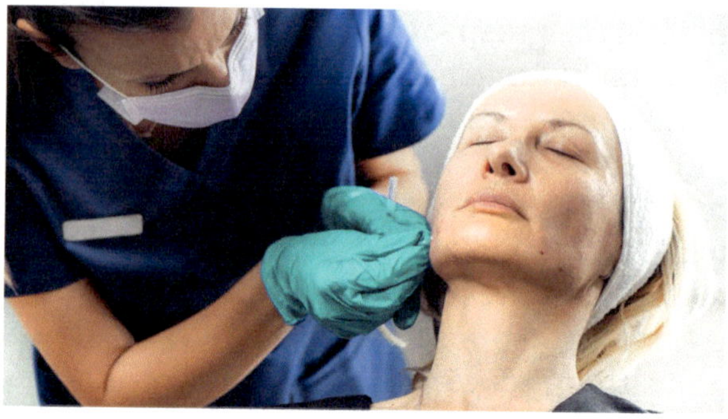

Figure 6.16. Facial thread lift procedure for skin tightening and contouring.

Source: https://i0.wp.com/post.healthline.com/wp-content/uploads/2020/11/Facial_Threads_1296x728-header-1296x729.jpg?w=1155&h=2268.

Test Your Knowledge

1. What are the most common side effects associated with thread lifting?
2. Why is it crucial to choose a qualified and experienced practitioner for thread lifting or skin tightening procedures?

SUMMARY

The revelation of thread lifting and skin tightening techniques reveals a dramatic shift in the approach towards aesthetic enhancement. Contemporary methods stand in complete contrast to the traditional surgical practices, with the focus laid on utilizing minimally invasive procedures that effectively meet the evolving demands of patients seeking youthful appearances without extensive downtime. As described, treatments , such as thread lifts and the use of novel materials , such as PDO threads are a combination of art and innovation in dermatology. They not only yield tangible aesthetic benefits but also meet the demand for more procedures with shorter recovery times and corresponding risks, as reviewed in surgical and noninvasive treatments (Portilla et al., 2024). In addition, the cultural factors that determine aesthetic preferences certainly account for the spread of these methods. The worldwide appreciation for Korean beauty is a case in point in demonstrating the integral role cultural beliefs play in the embrace of certain aesthetic practices. As South Korean innovation in minimally invasive treatments continues to gain popularity across the globe, international expansion becomes ever more evident. Such countries as Switzerland, with more affluent citizens and higher demand for non-surgical treatments, are fertile ground for such innovative approaches to thrive (Marques, 2023). This integration of culture and cosmetic surgery underlines individualizing esthetic services to meet different and evolving consumer demands. Finally, ongoing progress in the field of thread lifting and other tightening modalities is itself a more general trend within the aesthetic industry toward individually tailored treatments that fulfill individual aspirations for beauty. As research continues to show effectiveness and safety for these procedures, practitioners are encouraged to apply knowledge of patient needs to practice. Future studies in this field must take on the dual focus of technical competence and cultural sensitivity, as the new trends in beauty are an integral appreciation of client requirements. Lastly, the commitment to spreading minimally invasive techniques , such as thread lifting, is set to shape the destiny of aesthetic treatment and reaffirm the industry's devotion to innovation and patient welfare.

Thread lifting has emerged as a serious player in the industry of minimally invasive aesthetic procedures, offering a revolutionary answer for facial rejuvenation and skin tightening. Reputed for its ability to offer a natural look without the application of traditional surgical procedures, thread lifting utilizes fine threads, , such as PDO and PLA, to generate collagen stimulation and offer support to the skin. They also stimulate not only the body's natural healing responses but also assist in gradually enhancing the texture and suppleness of the skin. The procedure is a paradigm shift in the practice of anti-aging therapies as it intermixes surgical art with the convenience of non-surgical therapies, and it is an appealing treatment for patients seeking successful rejuvenation with least downtime or recuperation, to fill the current trend in well-tolerated cosmetic procedures (Portilla et al., 2024). In addition to thread lifting, other non-surgical and minimally invasive methods have been popularized, with increased use in the cosmetic industry. The complement of Ultherapy and fat grafting to thread lifting helps further enhance the overall rejuvenating effects of the face. Whereas Ultherapy penetrates deeper layers of the skin by utilizing ultrasound technology, fat grafting offers a means of volumetric restoration in areas where volume is lost with aging. These procedures not only cater to the demands of diverse patients for youthful appearances but also exhibit the combinational effect of different treatments in giving the optimum results. With the dynamic nature of the beauty landscape, blending these modalities demonstrates an inclusive strategy against aging, thus enhancing patient satisfaction through customized solutions addressing the different aspects of dermal changes (Portilla et al., 2024). Moreover, the globalization of cosmetic trends has catapulted minimally invasive treatments, including thread lifts, to the forefront of the cosmetic industry. Increasing popularity of Korean beauty regimens explains this phenomenon, as these procedures align with an appreciation for naturally beautified culture. With South Korea becoming a hub for advanced cosmetic treatments, there is enormous potential for international expansion, particularly in rich economies , such as Switzerland, in which high demand for such technology is present. Globalization not only indicates the competitive technological advantages with which South Korean providers are equipped but also reveals a trend toward embracing more accessible beauty upgrade solutions around the world. It is obvious that the future of cosmetic interventions will remain centered on minimally invasive procedures with maximum results and emphasis on patient satisfaction and convenience.

KEY TERMS FROM THIS CHAPTER

- Aesthetic medicine
- Aesthetic standards
- Beauty standards
- Clinical applicability
- Collagen stimulation
- Cross-linked collagen
- Extracellular matrix deposition
- Facelift surgeries
- Facial cosmetic operations
- Herbal preparations
- Aesthetic rejuvenation
- Anti-aging strategy
- Biodegradable polymer
- Collagen formation
- Collagen synthesis
- Elastic skin
- Extreme transformation
- Facial anatomy
- Facial rejuvenation
- Inflammatory response

CRITICAL THINKING QUESTIONS

1. **Which of the following is the primary purpose of thread lifting?**
   a. To reduce skin pigmentation
   b. To remove wrinkles permanently
   c. To lift sagging skin and stimulate collagen production
   d. To improve skin texture and color

2. **What material are most medical-grade threads used in thread lifting made of?**
   a. Silicone
   b. Polylactic acid
   c. Hyaluronic acid
   d. Polypropylene or PDO (polydioxanone)

3. **How does thread lifting work to improve skin tightness?**
   a. By using heat to shrink the skin
   b. By inserting threads that anchor the skin in place and stimulate collagen production
   c. By using laser technology to melt fat
   d. By removing dead skin cells from the surface

4. **What is one of the most common side effects after a thread lifting procedure?**
   a. Temporary swelling, bruising, and discomfort
   b. Severe skin pigmentation
   c. Permanent scarring
   d. Increased skin elasticity

5. **Which skin tightening technique uses radiofrequency energy to heat the dermis and stimulate collagen production?**
   a. Thread Lifting
   b. Ultherapy
   c. Radiofrequency Microneedling
   d. Thermage

Short Answer Questions

1. What are the most commonly used types of threads in thread lifting procedures, and how do they differ in material and absorption time?
2. Describe the mechanism by which thread lifting achieves skin tightening and lifting effects.
3. List three common indications and three contraindications for thread lifting procedures.
4. What are the possible complications or side effects of thread lifting, and how can they be minimized?
5. Compare and contrast RF and ultrasound-based skin tightening treatments in terms of mechanism, depth of penetration, and expected outcomes.
6. How does collagen remodeling contribute to the effectiveness of non-invasive skin tightening treatments?
7. What factors influence the choice between non-invasive skin tightening methods and surgical options like facelifts?

Answer to Critical Thinking Questions

1. (c); 2. (d); 3. (b); 4. (a); 5. (d)

REFERENCES

1. Akhond, R., & Sharif, A. (2021). Functionality based design of sustainable bio-composite. https://core.ac.uk/download/427504953.pdf (accessed on 11th June 2025).
2. Tettamanzi, M., Muratore, G., Arrica, G., Cuomo, R., Beatrici, E., Ginatempo, I., Trignano, C., Rubino, C., & Trignano, E. (2024). Advancements in Face and Neck Contouring: Integrating Radiofrequency-Assisted Liposuction with FaceTite and Buccal Fat Pad Excision for Facial Slimming. *Aesthetic plastic surgery*, *48*(22), 4667–4674. https://doi.org/10.1007/s00266-024-04245-1(accessed on 11th June 2025).
3. Lewandowska, K., Staniszewska, I., Baran, M., Turczynowicz, M., & Retman, P. (2024). Complications after polydioxanone threads (PDO) for facial lifting - a literature review. *Journal of Education, Health and Sport*, *66*, 50072. https://doi.org/10.12775/JEHS.2024.66.010(accessed on 11th June 2025).
4. Beiu, C., Popa, L. G., Bălăceanu-Gurău, B., Iliescu, C. A., Racoviță, A., Popescu, M., & Mihai, M. M. (2023). Personalization of minimally-invasive aesthetic procedures with the use of ultrasound compared to alternative imaging modalities. *Diagnostics*, *13*, 3512–3512. https://doi.org/10.3390/diagnostics13233512 (accessed on 11th June 2025).
5. Portilla, A. S. P., Portilla, C. S. P., Palacios, G. S. G., Rodríguez, B. S. P., Castillo, S. G. A., Espin, N. E. P., & Pita, G. P. M. (2024). The integration of surgical and dermatological techniques in the treatment of cutaneous aging: multidisciplinary approaches and clinical outcomes - a comprehensive systematic review of current literature. *International Journal of Research in Medical Sciences*, *12*(5), 1659–1667. https://doi.org/10.18203/2320-6012.ijrms20240943 (accessed on 11th June 2025).
6. Christen, M. O. (2022). Collagen stimulators in body applications: A review focused on poly-L-lactic acid (PLLA). *Clinical Cosmetic and Investigational Dermatology*, *15*, 997–1019. https://doi.org/10.2147/ccid.s359813 (accessed on 11th June 2025).
7. Cohen, J. L., Goodman, G., de Almeida, A. T., Jones, D., Carruthers, J., Grimes, P. E., de Maio, M., et al. (2023). Decades of beauty: Achieving aesthetic goals throughout the lifespan. *Journal of Cosmetic Dermatology*, *22*, 2889–2901. https://doi.org/10.1111/jocd.15968 (accessed on 11th June 2025).
8. Duncan, D. I. (2020). Combining PDO threads with exosomes for micro lifting. https://core.ac.uk/download/322580864.pdf (accessed on 11th June 2025).
9. Pourdanesh, F., Esmaeelinejad, M., Jafari, S. M., & Nematollahi, Z. (2016). Facelift: Current Concepts, Techniques, and Principles. InTech. doi: 10.5772/63150 (accessed on 11th June 2025).
10. Gold, M. H., & Robb, C. W. (2021). Complications and solutions for post-operative liposuction deformities. https://core.ac.uk/download/479935968.pdf (accessed on 11th June 2025).
11. Gulbitti, H. A., van der Lei, B., van der Sluis, N., et al. (2022). Lifting the mouth corner: A systematic review of techniques, clinical outcomes, and patient satisfaction. https://core.ac.uk/download/534954693.pdf (accessed on 11th June 2025).
12. Hammond, T. M. (2010). Novel applications of biomaterials in the management of parastomal hernia and anal fistula. https://core.ac.uk/download/30695172.pdf (accessed on 11th June 2025).

13. Hong, G. W., Hu, H., Park, S. Y., Wan, J., & Yi, K. H. (2024). What are the factors that enable thread lifting to last longer? *Cosmetics*, *11*, 42–42. https://doi.org/10.3390/cosmetics11020042 (accessed on 11th June 2025).
14. Hong, G. W., Kim, S. B., Park, S. Y., Wan, J., & Yi, K. H. (2024). Thread lifting materials: A review of its difference in terms of technical and mechanical perspective. *Clinical Cosmetic and Investigational Dermatology*, *17*, 999–1006. https://doi.org/10.2147/ccid.s457352 (accessed on 11th June 2025).
15. Hong, G. W., Kim, S. B., Park, S., Wan, J., & Yi, K. (2024). Characteristics of volumizing, scaffold, lifting cogged thread, and monofilament threads. *Dermatologic Therapy*. https://www.semanticscholar.org/paper/3dd7582c0485b80b9ccb803c5e5bc4cf21c139fe (accessed on 11th June 2025).
16. Kakulapati, V., Rinner, C., Abeykoon, V., Fox, G., Elek, I., Ishaq, A. I., Usman, A., et al. (2023). New trends and challenges in open data. *IntechOpen eBooks*. https://doi.org/10.5772/intechopen.1000267 (accessed on 11th June 2025).
17. Kim, J. (2024). Comparative three-dimensional analysis of facial lifting effects across five aesthetic units following continuous radiation 115-Watt 6.78-MHz monopolar radiofrequency therapy. *Plastic and Reconstructive Surgery Global Open*, *12*. https://www.semanticscholar.org/paper/464dc990e496a4ce72f466f24bf102405a5a0953 (accessed on 11th June 2025).
18. Li, M., Xu, H., Tian, Y., Li, R., & Hao, L. (2023). U-type soft tissue lifting: A new composited technique for reversing lower eyelid and midfacial aging. *Skin Research and Technology*, *29*. https://doi.org/10.1111/srt.13511 (accessed on 11th June 2025).
19. Lipman, K. J., Korman, J., & Nguyen, D. (2024). Addressing the cosmetic resident education gap–A junior cosmetic fellowship program. *Aesthetic Surgery Journal. Open Forum*, *6*. https://www.semanticscholar.org/paper/2c35950ffaf11c6f3133ab0567114f25776ddbdd (accessed on 11th June 2025).
20. Marques, F. M. C. F. (2023). Internationalization of Korean-branded cosmetic procedures and techniques: In-depth market analysis of minimally to non-invasive procedures. A Work Project presented as part of the requirements for the Award of a Master's degree in Management from the Nova School of Business and Economics. https://core.ac.uk/download/614518761.pdf (accessed on 11th June 2025).
21. Middleton, K. G. (1985). The failure of graphite arc-furnace electrodes. https://core.ac.uk/download/16280803.pdf (accessed on 11th June 2025).
22. Raslan, H., El Attar, Y. A., Hegab, D. S., & Doghim, N. N. (2023). Comparison between subcision with carboxytherapy and blunt blade cannula subcision in treatment of acne scars. *International Journal of Dermatology Venereology and Leprosy Sciences*, *6*, 31–39. https://doi.org/10.33545/26649411.2023.v6.i2a.151 (accessed on 11th June 2025).
23. Serov, D. N., & Kruglova, M. S. (2024). Efficiency and safety of thread implantology in the long term: Data from a pathomorphological study. *Medical Alphabet*. https://www.semanticscholar.org/paper/002c3819ec645411c7fa411589467aa683c105ab (accessed on 11th June 2025).
24. Silva, M. I. S. (2023). Internationalization of Korean-branded cosmetic procedures and techniques: In-depth market analysis of facial-invasive procedures. https://core.ac.uk/download/614519077.pdf (accessed on 11th June 2025).

25. Velazco de Maldonado, G. J., Suárez-Vega, D. V., Miller-Kobisher, B., & García-Guevara, V. (2024). Smart PDOs™ and the Cartesian Technique™: A milestone in facial rejuvenation with bioactive scaffolds. *Journal of Cutaneous and Aesthetic Surgery, 17*, 292–306. https://www.semanticscholar.org/paper/2878696fd205346f119721cd4ec3c3fcc1083801 (accessed on 11th June 2025).

26. Yi, K. H., & Oh, S. (2024). Lateral facial thread lifting procedure with temporal anchoring in deep temporal fascia: Anatomical perspectives of superficial temporal artery. *Skin Research and Technology, 30*. https://www.semanticscholar.org/paper/b367b9c82cc5a80d9598009eb4e26ad807c9094b (accessed on 11th June 2025).

27. Yi, K. H., & Park, S. Y. (2024). Marionette lines correction with volumizing threads. *Journal of Cosmetic Dermatology, 23*, 3871–3877. https://doi.org/10.1111/jocd.16490 (accessed on 11th June 2025).

LIPOSUCTION TECHNIQUES

7

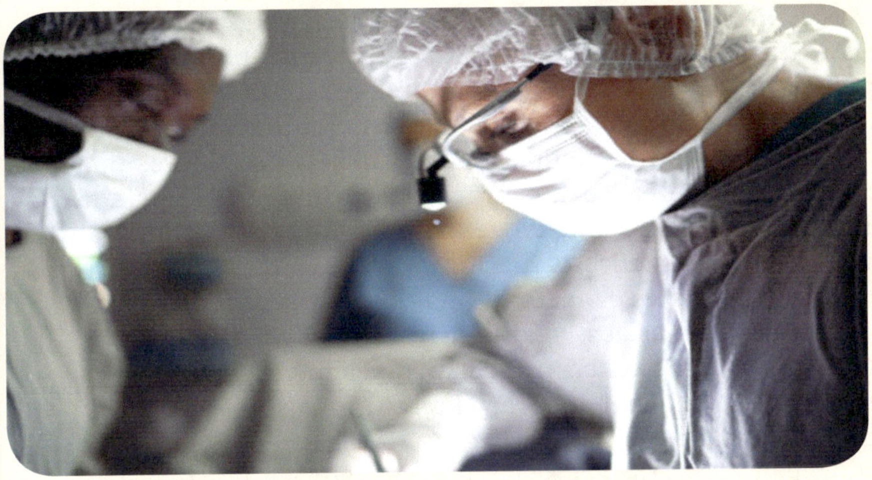

LEARNING OBJECTIVES

After studying this chapter, you will be able to:

1. Describe the types of liposuction procedures
2. Discuss about preoperative thoughts before undergoing liposuction
3. Describe liposuction procedure
4. Care for postoperative care after liposuction
5. Understand the benefits of liposuction
6. Highlight risks and complications

Introduction

Liposuction techniques have gained widespread popularity as cosmetic operations aimed at enhancing the contours and esthetics of the body. The revolution in body contouring is defined by advances that allow surgeons to treat several body areas using minimally invasive procedures. Although driven by aesthetics, liposuction is far from challenge-free, particularly in controlling issues of surgery , such as edema, ecchymosis, and pain. These complications will end up impacting patient recovery and satisfaction, and as such, steps should be taken to ensure that they are averted. This is where the reasons for adopting kinesiotherapy as a management method come into play, an action which constitutes a new approach towards enhancing post-operative outcomes for liposuction procedures as a primary factor worthy of discussion within the field of body contouring techniques (Snla et al., 2023). The application of kinesiotherapy in the post-operative optimization of recovery is an example of an innovative solution that leads to constant belly bandaging for suitable recovery. Clinical treatment through kinesiotherapy is of immense benefit in the resolution of typical post-liposuction complications , such as seromas and chronic edema. Clinical experience with patients undergoing abdominal liposuction records the statistically significant reduction in these complications through the application of the use of daily treatments through kinesiotherapy. Statistical findings of these researches mirror the effectiveness of this technique, with considerable relief from pain and postoperative decrease in edema from the normal recovery process. With each passing day newer techniques of liposuction are being developed, incorporation of adjunctive procedures like kinesiotherapy would enhance the patient's experience in totality through the achievement of aesthetic goals along with better recovery and all-around health outcomes (Snla et al., 2023). Parallel to the development of technologies aimed at maximizing the success of surgery, incorporation of new technologies into regenerative medicine invites reconsideration of how it interrelates with liposuction procedures. Stem cell therapy, and more directly through the use of human pluripotent stem cells and multipotent mesenchymal stem cells, is a technology that could reshape recovery protocols and maximize the potential for tissue regeneration. Exploring the application of stem cells alongside liposuction surgeries might bring about improved recovery, minimized downtime, and higher patient satisfaction. Hence, regenerative treatments in a clinical setup need to be exhaustively studied to determine their feasibility and applicability with conventional methods of liposuction. The collision of these new practice might restructure post-operative recovery procedures as an imposing doorway to further research into aesthetic medicine.

Definition of Liposuction

Liposuction is a surgical method for the extraction of fat from parts of the body and hence contour improvement of the body along with desired aesthetic outcomes. This procedure is extremely appealing to such patients who want localized reduction of fat not responding to conventional weight loss attempts, i.e., exercise and diet. By using suction techniques, the procedure treats various areas of anatomy , such as the abdomen, thighs, hips, buttocks, arms, and neck. Liposuction flexibility allows for both debulking, where increased volumes of fat are removed, and high-definition, where definition and contouring of underlying muscle is attempted. Both are deserving of a place in the Cosmetic Surgery Hall of Fame, with customized patient preferences and safety and effectiveness in implementation. Improvements in liposuction have led to new procedures that advance the procedure to make it safer and more efficient. High-definition liposuction, for instance, is specifically focused on creating clear lines of anatomy and clearer visualization of the muscles, particularly where patients want an increased muscular appearance. As described in contemporary literature, this procedure has been popular because it can sculpt areas , such as the arms and abdomen and, as a result, score high in terms of patient satisfaction. Classical methods of liposuction have been reformulated through the integration of new markings and methods that ensure successful liposculpture to attain patients' expectations. For example, in one recent research, there was evidence that proper pre-operative marking is crucial to the success of high-definition liposuction, highlighting the role of meticulous planning in achieving optimum results (Young et al., 2024). Technological advancement has also refined liposuction procedures, with procedures like VASER-assisted liposuction leading the way. This ultrasonic-guided procedure ensures more precise fat elimination while stimulating skin tightening at the same time, giving rise to smoother lines and fewer complications. The efficacy of VASER liposuction has in recent studies been proven to be especially useful in a number of areas of the body, effectively curing conditions , such as gynecomastia without the necessity of invasive surgical procedures, thus reducing recovery time postoperatively (Nayak, 2025). The ability of these new procedures to be adaptable to the unique requirements of male and female patients serves to further highlight the relevance of liposuction to current aesthetic surgery. Hence, liposuction not only exists to fulfill cosmetic demand but also reflects general trends of surgical advancement towards improved patient satisfaction and results (Figure 7.1).

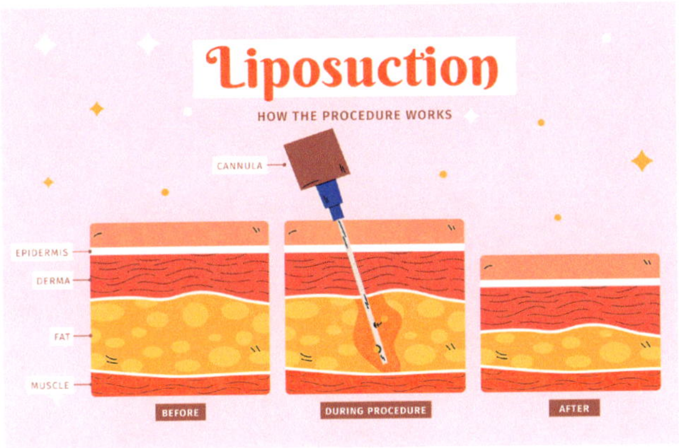

Figure 7.1. Liposuction.

Source: https://handehospital.org/wp-content/uploads/2024/03/25047512_7018457-scaled.jpg.

Historical Background of Liposuction

The history of liposuction traces back to the early 20th century when body contour cosmetic issues were first being treated by surgery. Early procedures were minimal and involved the removal of adipose tissue by invasive means. The procedure left the patient with extensive scarring and postoperative complications. But cosmetic surgery history was forever altered in the late 1970s when Dr. Jeffrey Klein created tumescent liposuction. The method included injecting a fluid that produced localized swelling and anesthesia so that fat could be excised with minimal blood loss and minimal post-procedure pain. Through optimal patient outcome and safety, tumescent liposuction opened the door to the procedure's popularity, becoming one of the most popular body sculpting procedures in cosmetic surgery. As liposuction grew more popular, technology created opportunities for technique and instrument evolution. Evolution in liposuction models brought in the arrival of ultrasound-assisted liposuction (UAL) in the late 1980s, wherein ultrasonic energy was employed to liquefy fat cells so they could be suctioned with ease. Once again, this decreased tissue trauma and further extended the areas of the body that could be addressed with efficacy. With this, in the late 1990s, laser-assisted liposuction (LAL) was developed using laser energy to ablate fat cells irreversibly and also to tighten the skin. All of these technologies not only improved the cosmetic outcome but also made the patient experience less traumatic. The ongoing development of these technologies is a giant historical leap forward in the realm of cosmetic surgery. It has also been brought out in research the significance of managing complications and long-term safety profiles involved in liposuction techniques. While the past history provides evidence of methodology and technological developments, it must be noted with appreciation the evolving clinical scenario in terms of patient safety and patient satisfaction. Critical understanding of the inherent risks involved in various liposuction techniques brings out best practice in the topic. New studies indicate an immediate need for far more than intensified clinical trials and prolonged follow-up assessments to best establish the effects of these methods on patient health and quality of life. This focus on safety and patient outcome continues to be of paramount importance to research and development of liposuction, again underscoring the necessity of informed decision-making by providers and prospective patients in the future.

Importance of Understanding Liposuction Techniques

Both practitioner and patient need to be aware of various methods of liposuction so that they can achieve an optimal cosmetic outcome. Various methods, , such as tumescent, ultrasound, and laser-assisted liposuction (LAL), have varied strengths, weaknesses, and recovery profiles. For instance, tumescent liposuction is most suitable as it is widely regarded as safe and efficient, primarily due to the use of a saline solution that minimizes bleeding and swelling in the process. In contrast, ultrasonic-assisted liposuction can provide greater accuracy and efficiency in the removal of fat deposits. Experts who fully comprehend such techniques are in a stronger position to offer a tailored approach specific to the individual requirements and body of their patients to develop improved overall satisfaction rates and outcomes. Such comprehension is also achieved through studies that indicate certain procedures can be linked to varying degrees of complications, whose impact, in turn, influences patient safety and happiness. Education of the patient regarding liposuction methods is also essential to decision-making. Proper understanding enables patients to participate actively with their caregivers, where they can share their objectives and anxieties. Such patient-surgeon relationship is pivotal in the sense that it allows trust to build and may be followed by more customized surgical treatments. Literature points to the reality that dissatisfaction does exist due to unfulfilled realistic expectations and due to breakdown of communication of technique modalities of the procedure and recovery time. By pointing out the nuances of different liposuction modalities, practitioners are able to set realistic expectations, reduce postoperative tension, and enhance patient satisfaction. This process of learning is required because informed consent decisions result in more harmonious relationships between the patient and the surgeon, which eventually result in better overall outcomes and satisfaction rates for liposuction surgeries. In addition, a educated route of liposuction surgeries can be a key determinant of long-term outcomes as well as future medical complications. Patients who realize the importance of their chosen technique are more likely to adhere to post-operative instructions in a bid to achieve maximum healing and maintenance of results. Definition of lifestyle and hormonal factors also assists in offering realistic maintenance goals.

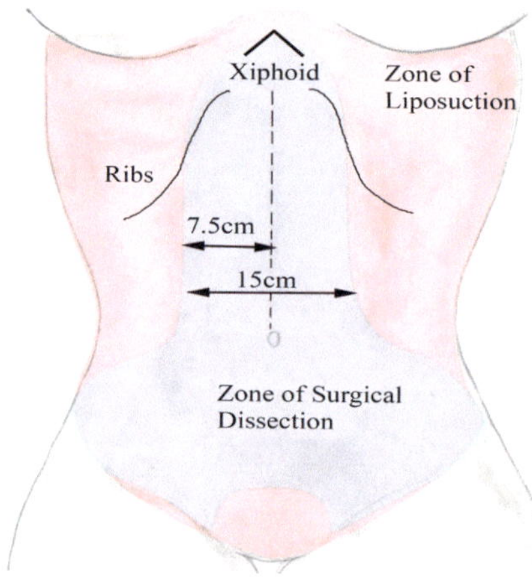

Figure 7.2. Zones of liposuction and zones of dissection for the lipoabdominoplasty technique used in group IV. Liposuction was performed throughout the abdomen, including the epigastric and mesogastric areas. Dissection was limited laterally to 7.5 cm from the midline with an inverted V-pattern at the xiphoid to spare the intercostal arteries.

Source: https://www.researchgate.net/profile/Bianca-Knoll-4/publication/5398765/figure/fig3/AS:667678897348610@1536198462368/Zones-of-liposuction-and-zones-of-dissection-for-the-lipoabdominoplasty-technique-used-in.ppm.

For example, maintenance of body mass index (BMI) following liposuction is crucial because high BMI has been found to increase the complication rate, as evident from corresponding literature. Involving patients in their own treatment process encourages a proactive attitude towards their health, potentially decreasing the likelihood of regret or dissatisfaction post-surgery. Technical competence with liposuction procedures is therefore not only important to maximize short-term cosmetic outcomes but also to guarantee long-term patient well-being and satisfaction (Figure 7.2).

7.1. Types of Liposuction Techniques

Learning Outcome

1. Understand tumescent liposuction technique
2. Describe ultrasonic-assisted liposuction
3. Define laser-assisted liposuction

The branch of liposuction techniques has undergone titanic transformations with the passage of time, and other techniques have been developed to suit various aesthetic requirements. Tumescent liposuction is one such very common technique where a colossal amount of saline solution, typically mixed with adrenaline along with local anaesthetics, is infiltrated into the area to be treated prior to fat extraction. This not only minimizes blood loss but also enhances the comfort level of the patient during surgery. Inducing tumescence makes it easier to remove the fat, with smoother outcomes and decreased risk of complications. As body contouring becomes increasingly in vogue, such sophisticated techniques are being chosen more and more by surgeons with greater respect for patient care and surgical competence, effectively issuing an invitation to make the switch to minimally invasive procedures. The rising need for cosmetic procedures among females indicates the need for such procedures to be new (King et al., 2013). Another interesting development of liposuction is the invention of laser-assisted liposuction (LAL), otherwise referred to as SmartLipo. The procedure applies lasers to liquefy the fat cells initially before suction to ease the suction and encourage skin tightening, an important aspect most patients need. The transmission of laser energy, besides making fat removal more comfortable, reduces the recovery time and risk of bruising. Also, application of the technique is compatible with prevailing aesthetic ideals preferring minimal invasiveness with high-precision effects. Thus, laser liposuction has been preferred by both clinicians and patients and has become popular in cosmetic practice. The history of liposuction surgery continues to be an ongoing pursuit towards increasingly perfectionist methods worthy of patient expectation and overall satisfaction (Nojek et al., 2024). Second, UAL is a new procedure that is predominantly employed in the case of big fat excision areas. The procedure employs the use of ultrasonic energy in liquefying fat cells so that they can be easily removed using suction without inflicting significant trauma on the surrounding tissues. With the use of sonic energy, UAL provides a more extensive removal process, with the advantage of greater fat contouring. UAL is now particularly useful in patients with denser fat deposits or those requiring more body contouring. In addition, minimization of post-operative pain and swelling of UAL makes it more desirable. With the continuous advancement of liposuction as a treatment, all the techniques that have been developed are meant to address various problems and needs, resulting in a well-balanced set of options for possible patients requiring body shaping (Nojek et al., 2024).

7.1.1. Tumescent Liposuction

Tumescent liposuction is a popular body contouring technique that has been extolled for its safety as well as efficacy. Tumescent liposuction is a technique wherein massive volumes of diluted solution of lidocaine, saline, and epinephrine are infused into the fat prior to aspiration. Tumescent fluid not only facilitates fat extraction but also decreases patient discomfort and postoperative edema. By elongating the fat cells, the treatment enhances the precision of the surgeons for accessing targeted areas as well as minimizing blood loss. Epinephrine causes vasoconstriction, which is necessary in order to prevent complications arising from blood loss. Therefore, the outcomes of tumescent liposuction are improved, with patients experiencing faster rates of healing and less bruising than traditional liposuction techniques. Tumescent liposuction has also been found to have the advantage over other therapies, particularly suction-assisted liposuction (SAL) compared to tissue liquefaction liposuction (TLL), a similar but more advanced method. Tumescent methods had a high rate of patient recovery and safety compared to TLL. One study comparing 31 female patients showed that although tumescent and SAL procedures removed the same amount of total fat, tumescent procedures had significantly higher extraction percentages. Most importantly, tumescent procedures had a median fat harvesting time that was 42% shorter than in SAL, and what this means is that tumescent liposuction not only shortens the procedure but also enhances the patient experience by far through reducing patient time under anesthesia as well as lowering postoperative pain (Hunstad et al., 2018). In addition, tumescent liposuction becomes a significant part of the solution of individual problems of beauty, , such as buttock shape, which have been used for centuries to define standards of beauty and attractiveness. The technique allows one to individually change volume and contour personally in not only the buttocks, but in adjacent areas , such as the thighs, and thus it is a handy means of all-around body sculpting. With increased emphasis on achieving proportionate and well-balanced body beauty, tumescent liposuction has become a critical tool of both patients and clinicians. With improving clinician competency, information regarding complex aspects of liposuction techniques, including tumescent techniques, will continue to be an essential standard of delivering acceptable results that are in conformity with clients' sophisticated requests for body sculpting (Miller et al., 2012) (Figure 7.3).

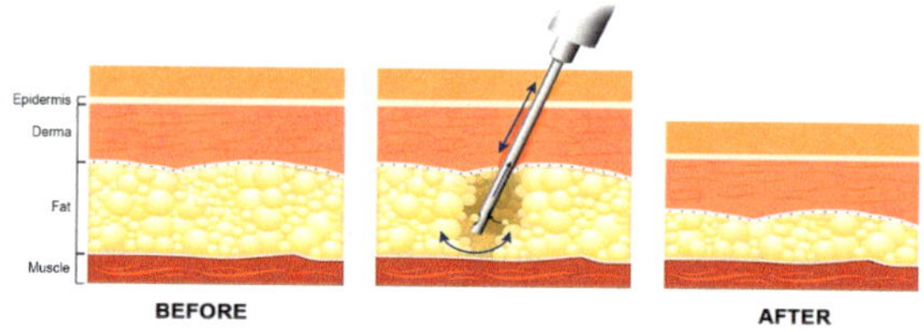

Figure 7.3. Tumescent liposuction.

Source: https://estheticland.com/wp-content/uploads/2023/04/tumescent-lipo.jpg.

7.1.2. Ultrasonic-Assisted Liposuction

Ultrasonic-assisted liposuction, or UAL, is one of the significant advancements in body remodeling techniques, offering a state-of-the-art technique for the selective extraction of fat tissue through the application of ultrasonic energy. The technique involves the application of ultrasonic frequencies, which efficiently make the cells vibrate and melt the fat prior to its suction from the body. This technique not only makes fat removal simpler but also decreases trauma to surrounding tissues, thus causing less bruising and swelling when compared to traditional liposuction techniques. Most significantly, UAL can be particularly beneficial in areas of fibrous fat, , such as the back or male chest tissue, where traditional techniques may struggle to offer the best possible outcomes. These advances underscore the relentless innovation in liposuction methods as clinicians strive to achieve the best results for patients and advance safety (Nojek et al., 2024). One of the overarching themes in liposuction methods evolution is the implementation of innovative technologies for enhancing patient satisfaction and effectiveness. Ultrasonic-assisted liposuction embodies this trend, away from basic fat removal to a more sophisticated regimen that takes into consideration the nuances of patient anatomy as well as variability of adipose tissue. The procedure allies with the growing emphasis on minimally invasive methods, which have been core to optimizing recovery times and reducing procedure-related complications. Besides, UAL's capacity to facilitate fat harvesting for autologous fat transplantation adds another level of versatility with a double benefit of liposuction and subsequent fat implantation. In that sense, the technique is a testament to the changing character of cosmetic surgery, where improvements any procedure must undergo in order to treat patients (Nojek et al., 2024) (Figure 7.4).

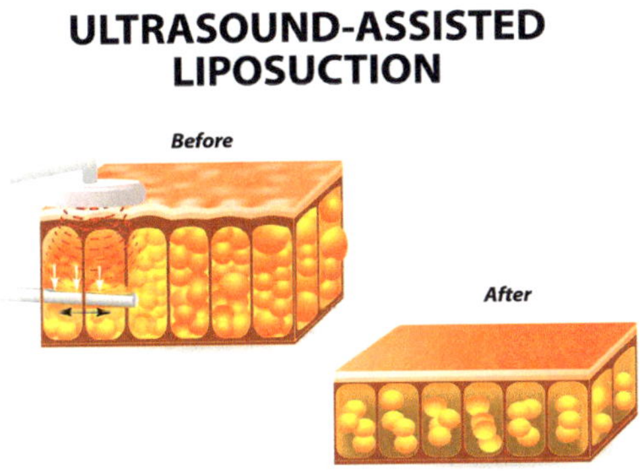

Figure 7.4. Ultrasonic-assisted liposuction.

Source: https://plasticsurgery.in/storage/files/Liposuction-Laser-Ultrasound-Assisted-Lipoplasty-2-1024x746.jpg.jpg.

Despite its advantages, ultrasonic-assisted liposuction is not challenge-free and complication-free and demands a proper understanding of how it is utilized by practitioners. While fat cell liquefaction makes it easier to excise, it is not risk-free, e.g., thermal injury to surrounding tissues if one is not careful. Also, heterogeneity of ultrasonic settings, e.g., frequency, energy levels, can influence patient outcomes to a large extent. Accordingly, technical proficiency and careful technique are most crucial in order to minimize such risks. As the specialty matures, additional research and surgical innovation will naturally continue to refine UAL, both its effectiveness and safety profile. Overall, ultrasonic technology used in liposuction is a part of an overall trend toward enhancing surgical practice in balance with patient benefit and procedural effectiveness (Nojek et al., 2024) (Figure 7.5).

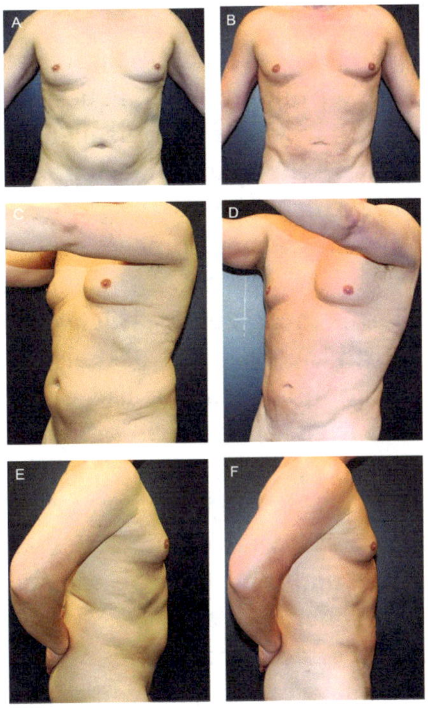

Figure 7.5. A 51-year-old male who underwent ultrasound-assisted liposuction with helium-based plasma technology on abdomen, flanks, chest, and circumferential thighs: (A, B) front view, preoperative and one year postoperative; (C, D) left diagonal view, preoperative and one year postoperative; and (E, F) right side view, preoperative and one year postoperative. Adverse events were not observed.

Source: https://www.researchgate.net/publication/362085751/figure/fig2/AS:11431281090851724@1666213625857/A-51-year-old-male-who-underwent-ultrasound-assisted-liposuction-with-helium-based-plasma.png.

7.1.3. Laser-Assisted Liposuction

LAL has become more popular in recent years as a new way of body contouring, bridging the gap between outdated and new procedures. This procedure employs laser energy in order to liquefy fat before extraction, potentially leading to less trauma for surrounding tissues and may lead to improved recovery for patients. This is a relatively safe procedure that is performed on an outpatient basis.

The procedure involves the implantation of a fine laser fiber into the area in question, where the emitted energy kills fat cells, hence making them easier to eliminate. The benefits of this new technique are many, among which are the abilities to achieve more precise sculpting and contouring of the majority of hardest-to-treat areas, , such as the abdomen, thighs, and under the chin. With the provision of thermal energy, laser liposuction not only focuses on removing fat, but also triggers skin tightening as a result of stimulating collagen, enhancing the whole aesthetic result. Although with the advantage of a superior outcome, laser liposuction is neither risk-free nor complication-free and necessitates a careful consideration of its suitability to each patient. The effectiveness and safety of this procedure may vary significantly based on individual patient factors like body composition, skin elasticity, and underlying conditions.

Evidence confirms that while patients experience high levels of satisfaction due to reduced recovery time and bruising due to laser techniques, in case the procedure is done incorrectly, there are complications , such as burns or alteration in pigmentation. Moreover, the selection of candidates has to be made with precision to yield optimal outcomes; it is crucial that practitioners scrutinize patient history and aesthetic goals before recommending LAL as a solution. This understanding serves to underscore the importance of skilled surgeons who comprehend the nuances of laser technology. With continuous advancements in the technology of liposuction techniques, the comparison of LAL and traditional approaches remains essential to gain an insight into its use in plastic surgery. According to recent publications, including comparative analyses of ultrasonic and laser techniques, the latter tends to result in greater fluid retention and extended recovery periods, whereas laser-assisted approaches result in smoother outcomes with faster recovery (Nojek et al., 2024).

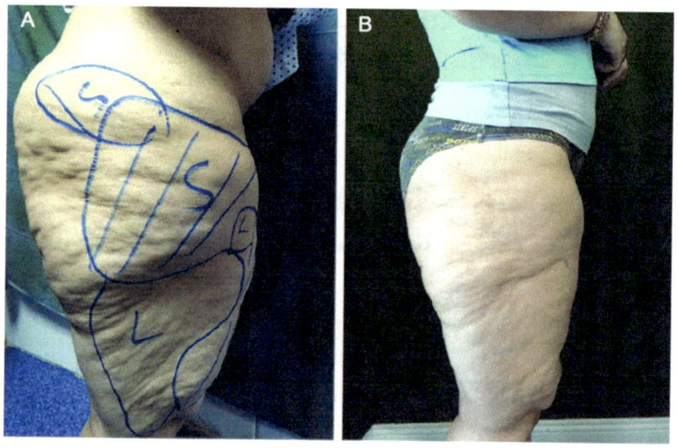

Figure 7.6. A case of thighs laser liposuction: local lipodystrophy with impaired lymphatic drainage: A, Preoperative. B, at 6 months of laser liposuction for the front and lateral sides of the thighs and above knee area. Areas marked by l mean that they were submitted only to laser lipolysis, whereas areas marked with S mean they were submitted to laser lipolysis then liposuction.

Source: https://www.researchgate.net/publication/328071179/figure/fig5/AS:706493611532290@1545452611754/a-case-of-thighs-laser-liposuction-local-lipodystrophy-with-impaired-lymphatic-drainage.png.

Lastly, the application of laser assist compared to traditional liposuction relies upon many different elements including patient wants, prolonged lengths of result, and the key aims of fat removal versus body contouring. In making the decision, clinicians must be familiar with technological advancements in order to offer individualized answers that correspond to patients' desires for improved shape and self-confidence. Thus, laser liposuction is a pioneering tool in the overall range of techniques utilized in liposuction, constantly adapting to shift in the face of evolving aesthetic needs and patient needs (Figure 7.6).

Test Your Knowledge

1. What is the primary purpose of the tumescent solution used in tumescent liposuction?
2. What is a key advantage of LAL over traditional methods?
3. In terms of procedural steps, what typically differentiates tumescent liposuction from the other two methods?

7.2. Preoperative Considerations

Learning Outcome

1. Understand evaluation and selection of patients for liposuction
2. Discuss about risks and complications associated with liposuction
3. Set realistic expectations

Before liposuction, meticulous preoperative considerations are necessary for patient safety and optimization of surgical outcome. It needs an extensive evaluation by the surgeon that includes examination of the patient's medical history, current health status, and customized body contouring goals. This even includes comprehension of the patient's anatomy, as procedures like three-dimensional gluteoplasty have been created to tighten and reshape not only the buttocks but also the surrounding areas like the thighs. Such new procedures require strict preoperative planning to effectively address the patient's aesthetic concerns without aggravating potential complications that are associated with liposuction. Therefore, the initial consultation represents a decisive point in time when patients are finally able to voice their own expectations and permit surgeons to plan a certain strategy that suits personal requirements and anatomical limitations in order to create the foundation for an efficient procedure (Miller et al., 2012). Furthermore, preoperative treatment includes an accurate evaluation of the suitability of the patients for liposuction. Several other factors, such as body mass index (BMI), elasticity of the skin, and overall health, can also significantly influence the outcome of surgery. Being predominantly a body reshaping surgery, it is thus critical that the surgeon discourage prospects with misguided assumptions about its use as a weight loss treatment. This explanation helps establish appropriate expectations and reduces the risk of complications from related medical conditions or wrong patient profiles. Preoperative protocol well delineated can also facilitate identification and management of patients at risk for adverse events, finally resulting in improved safety and patient satisfaction. In this case, adherence to exact preoperative guidelines guarantees that surgeons and patients alike are adequately prepared to perform procedures to follow (Granados-Tinajero et al., 2019). In addition to medical evaluation, patient education on postoperative risks and care is also an essential part of the preoperative process. Liposuction can lead to serious complications, , such as fat embolism or deep vein thrombosis (DVT), unless strict precautions are followed. It is therefore imperative for surgeons to provide appropriate instructions regarding intravenous fluid management, anesthesia technique, and the need to adhere to thromboembolism prophylaxis orders. Moreover, prescribing lifestyle modifications, such as the cessation of smoking or avoidance of medications that interfere with the healing process, can enhance recovery outcomes. Engaging patients in respectful conversations about the risks and benefits of the procedure sets a conducive environment where they can make informed decisions while confirming their readiness for surgery. This process, which is dialogue-centered, ultimately revolves around ensuring holistic preoperative considerations in achieving successful outcomes in liposuction (Granados-Tinajero et al., 2019) (Figure 7.7).

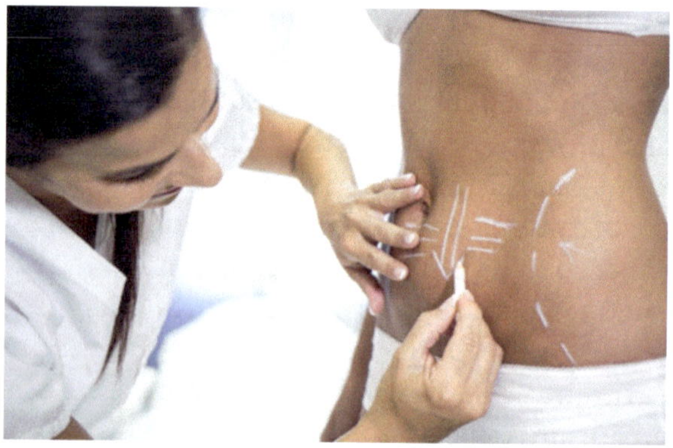

Figure 7.7. Preoperative markings for body contouring surgery.

Source: https://drashishghuge.com/wp-content/uploads/2024/06/Picture1.png.

7.2.1. Patient Evaluation and Selection

Patient selection and evaluation for liposuction are the most important aspect that identifies procedural results and patient satisfaction. Adequate pre-operative evaluation is essential, , such as complete medical history, physical examination, and psychological testing. It assists in identifying contraindications to surgery, such as obesity, unrealistic motivation, or systemic disease. Research suggests a need to establish a patient's reason for seeking liposuction because unrealistic expectations are the cause of dissatisfaction post-surgery. In addition, as argued in Saariniemi. (2011), psychosocial factors have a significant role to play in determining results following surgery, and hence, candidates with stable emotional states are more likely to gain from the surgery. Hence, the medical professionals have to implement a holistic strategy towards the evaluation of patients with a focus on both physical candidacy and psychological readiness to ensure successful surgery results. As part of the range of liposuction operations, the evaluation of a patient's candidacy also involves review of their goals and intended aesthetic objectives. Communication is facilitated, where patients will get to determine their motivation as well as individual objectives towards receiving the procedure. This is important, as certain expectations cannot be met with regard to a person's body type or limitations in liposuction techniques. Clinical practice guidelines also emphasize that the patient is chosen based on the safety and efficacy principles. As an example, previous evidence shows that large-volume liposuction can result in beneficial outcomes in patients with fewer complications, as mentioned by Abd-El-Salam et al. (2009). Finally, agreement on a mutual decision-making process between patient and surgeon will enhance satisfaction and optimize outcomes, and thereby equate surgical goals with realistic outcomes. Further, patient evaluation and selection for liposuction need to take into consideration recovery and satisfaction postoperative variables. Patients, post-operatively, go through various physical changes that can lead to dissatisfaction if not properly addressed or explained before surgery. Surgeons are required to indicate the potential complications and the process of healing, and set a reasonable healing timeline. The outcome of studies, for example, in Saariniemi. (2011), indicates that the preoperative status of a patient, including emotional and psychological hardness, is key to their perception of the postoperative course. By making sure that patients are thoroughly prepared and informed regarding the surgical procedure, healthcare professionals are able to reduce anxiety and optimize recovery, leading to greater satisfaction with the liposuction procedure. This patient-centered approach ultimately increases the safety and efficacy of liposuction procedures (Figure 7.8).

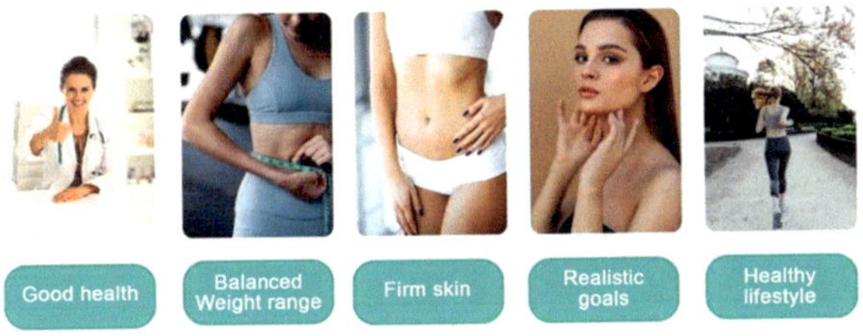

Figure 7.8. Ideal candidates for liposuction.

Source: https://www.drtarekaesthetics.com/wp-content/uploads/2023/08/Liposuction-Meaning--1024x538.jpg.

7.2.2. Risks and Complications

The process of liposuction, while often sought for its possible aesthetic value, carries a range of risks and complications that must be accorded serious consideration by patients. Possibly the most severe of these is the risk of fluid complications, which may result in either hematomas or seromas. These occurrences can require additional medical intervention through the process of drainage in an effort to alleviate associated discomfort as well as prevent the formation of further complications. Also, the complications from the anesthesia are another high-risk factor. During general anesthesia, the patients may have adverse reactions, i.e., respiratory distress, allergic reactions, or even major cardiovascular complications. It is absolutely crucial that the patients go ahead with aggressive consultations with their surgeons so that they have a clear understanding both of the possible risks involved with the surgery and also of the importance of identifying pre-existing medical conditions that could heighten their risks during surgery. Apart from these immediate risks, patients undergoing liposuction are also exposed to potential long-term complications that would affect their post-surgery quality of life. One of which is the likelihood of uneven body contours because of asymmetrical fat removal or fluid retention. Such irregularities can result in further corrective surgeries, thereby creating a cycle of additional medical interventions. Furthermore, a change in skin texture or loose skin may result, particularly among individuals with low skin elasticity. As society's standard of aging further blurs with contemporary society, particularly for women in Brazil, the pursuit of an optimized appearance is frequently preceded by conflicting expectations regarding body image and health outcomes (Edmonds et al., 2014). This points out the importance of setting realistic goals after surgery and also acknowledging that ideal surgery can never be achieved. The psychological effects of liposuction should also be taken into account when assessing risks and complications. Some patients become more anxious or unhappy with their body image even after the surgery, partly because of societal pressures about appearance. The allure of an idealized individual results in patients having unreasonable expectations, and therefore, they are disappointed post-surgery. Patients also grapple with the impact of surgical scars and their influence on their self-esteem. With an evolving cultural view of beauty where body modifications like gluteoplasty are increasingly being sought out for easing sexual appeal (Miller et al., 2012), patients are increasingly seeking it that they are not only provided with information regarding physical side effects but also with discussions regarding emotional wellbeing. Managing such aspects can eventually ensure proper overall knowledge regarding what one can expect from liposuction surgery, enabling improved patient satisfaction and mental health outcomes.

7.2.3. Setting Realistic Expectations

Being realistic is a crucial part of the liposuction process that removes myths and makes patients understand what is possible. Initially, potential patients overestimate what the immediate results of the treatment will be, expecting tremendous body alterations like those normally seen in the media or social media. But it should be stressed that liposuction is not a weight loss surgery, but a body contouring technique with the power to define specific areas by removing localized collections of fat. By setting forth distinctly the limitations as well as the potential of liposuction, surgeons can establish an atmosphere of realistic expectation among their patients so they are psychologically and emotionally prepared for the post-operative state. Also important in creating realistic expectations is the acknowledgment of liposuction's customized aspect. Each patient's anatomy, health, and aspirations are variables in the variations in outcomes. For example, the technique applied, , such as the three-dimensional gluteoplasty (3-DGP) for gluteal augmentation, allows volume, shape, and firmness increase that must be standardized based on the patients' individualized aspirations (Miller et al., 2012). Surgeons need to conduct extensive pre-surgical consultations, discussing potential outcomes and even the need for follow-up interventions to maintain effects over time. Such personalized care helps patients grasp the nuances of the liposuction process, avoiding any chance of being dissatisfied. Additionally, it is necessary to discuss the post-surgical result in the context of realistic expectations. After surgery, recovery varies largely and can determine the ultimate outcome. Patients typically experience swelling and bruising that can conceal the results for weeks or months following the procedure. As demonstrated by recent studies, while complications of large-volume liposuction are typically minor, an understanding of what the likely outcomes are—skin irregularities, seromas, and other minor issues that can arise—is critical (Abd-El-Salam et al., 2009). Thus, intensive communication about the recovery process and timelines to be expected will allow patients to prepare for their rehabilitation with optimism and patience and ultimately reach greater satisfaction with their result.

Test Your Knowledge

1. What are the key factors to assess during patient evaluation and selection for liposuction?
2. What are the most common risks and complications associated with liposuction, and how can patients be counseled about them preoperatively?

7.3. The Liposuction Procedure

Learning Outcome

1. Discuss anesthesia options in the context of liposuction techniques
2. Explain the effectiveness of liposuction techniques
3. Describe the fat removal process

Liposuction is a widely performed cosmetic surgery aimed at removing localized fatty deposits to restore body shape and form. Liposuction is aimed at resistant fat areas that are not responsive to diet and exercise and hence a very popular surgery for both men and women to enhance appearance. Various techniques , such as tumescent liposuction and ultrasound liposuction, have been devised to enhance the procedure. Every method carries different benefits, depending on the patient's desired outcome and the areas of treatment. Having knowledge of the procedural process and advancements in liposuction procedures can help one make informed decisions about body sculpting treatments to employ, hence making the selection of competent professionals that adhere to best practice and safety procedures in such treatments important. The safety and efficacy of liposuction procedures highly depend on the surgeon and the place where the operation is conducted. A consistent assessment of liposuction outcomes demonstrates that if performed by skilled personnel under proper conditions, the outcomes are largely acceptable to patients. The majority of surgeons indicated good results, noting that technical advances and postoperative care are responsible for having fewer complications. However, as per the data, a systematic study is necessary to better interpret the nuances of these procedures and enhance patient satisfaction. For the best results, a judicious pre-operative assessment should be conducted so that the technique can be tailored to each patient's unique anatomical status, hence optimizing the probability of success in the context of desired aesthetic outcomes (Farshad et al., 2018). A key part of liposuction is the significance of patient expectation and the psychological aspect of body image. As patients undergo cosmetic surgery, motivation is often based on cultural values and individual aspirations for beauty and attractiveness. In modern society, physical appearance, as it pertains to body contour, is linked to self-image and identity. Interest in gluteoplasty, emphasizing buttock volume and shape, reflects this cultural emphasis on the body areas of interest. The new methods like three-dimensional gluteoplasty (3-DGP) enhance not just the buttocks but also carve adjacent areas, resulting in a full makeover (Miller et al., 2012). It underscores the need for far-reaching consultations, during which practitioners can frame patient expectations against a realistic surgical outcome to lead to a better post-operative experience and enhanced satisfaction with the result.

7.3.1. Anesthesia Options

Anesthesia options are crucial to discuss in terms of liposuction techniques, both for patient comfort and procedure efficacy. Three principal types of anesthesia are used: local, sedation, and general anesthesia. Local anesthesia, commonly used with tumescent liposuction, is the injection of anesthetic material directly into the affected areas, which removes the pain without rendering the patient unconscious. This method minimizes system side effects and is commonly associated with quicker recovery rates. Alternative sedations may involve a combination of intravenous sedatives with local anesthesia to ensure a sedate condition, restricting awareness and pain. The choice between the two modalities depends on procedure length, patient medical history, and personal choice of the surgeon, illustrating the importance of individualized anesthesia protocols in achieving maximum gain (Miller et al., 2012). General anesthesia is also a popular option for major liposuction procedures, especially when large volumes of fat are to be extracted. General anesthesia comprises the total elimination of consciousness and sensory perception of pain so that more complex surgical motions may be performed and the patients can be assured of lying completely oblivious to the procedure. Nevertheless, patients subjected to general anesthesia need to be closely examined before the procedure to avoid any possible risks involved, including adverse reactions and complications. Vital sign monitoring during the procedure is crucial to treat any untoward event promptly. Further, guidelines for anesthetic management must extend to include dosage principles of local anesthetics because excess infiltration may lead to systemic toxicity, highlighting the need for a balanced and well-supported approach during surgery (Granados-Tinajero et al., 2019).

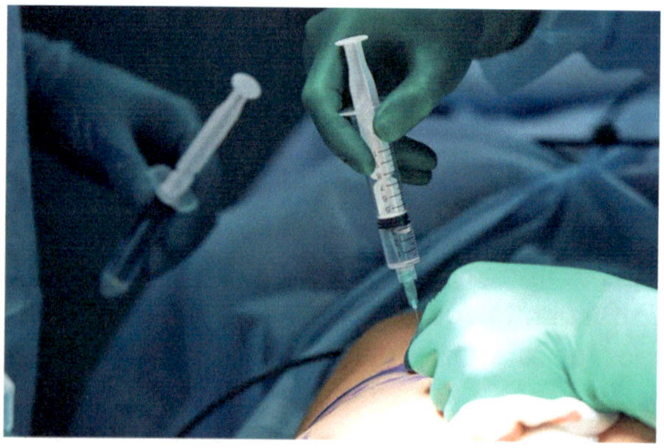

Figure 7.9. Injecting anesthesia before liposuction surgery.

Source: https://restoresdplasticsurgery.com/wp-content/uploads/2024/11/plastic-surgery-with-local-anesthesia-1024x683.jpg.webp.

The issue with anesthesia is not merely with the control of immediate pain but also with potential complications that arise post-surgery. Familiarity with the effects of various types of anesthesia is significant in reducing the risk of potential complications , such as DVT and pulmonary embolism, which remain among the key concerns during and after liposuction. Adherence to strict perioperative protocols will greatly enhance patient safety, as will careful choice of suitable candidates for the procedure. In addition, the minimization of fluid use post-surgery, particularly hydrosaline solution, in recent years is indicative of evolving knowledge about the best means to optimize recovery while minimizing complications. In summary, informed decision-making regarding anesthesia options is critical in not only optimizing the surgical process but also optimizing overall patient outcomes for liposuction procedures (Granados-Tinajero et al., 2019) (Figure 7.9).

7.3.2. Incision Techniques

The success of liposuction techniques relies to a great extent on the incision technology employed while carrying out the procedure. Incisions are critical points of entry through which adipose tissue is removed, and proper handling can make or break the procedure as well as its safety. Earlier techniques used bigger incisions with longer recovery times and more visible scars. While in more recent times, there has been a focus on the employment of smaller, strategically placed incisions that facilitate the process while minimizing the aesthetic impact on the patient's skin. Not only do these new developments help with of improved healing and fewer infections, but also with overall satisfaction on the part of those individuals seeking body contouring with liposuction. Among the numerous incision techniques now employed, the use of tumescent fluid has been the difference-maker. Through the administration of a saline solution with lidocaine and epinephrine injections before incision, surgeons can prevent bleeding and trauma to the tissue around the area. This preparation leads to a more delicate removal of the fat, which ultimately results in smoother contours and fewer complications post-surgery. Furthermore, the use of smaller cannulas in addition to these incisions means that fat extraction is not only effective but also efficient. The transition to such minimally invasive procedures is consistent with the broad trend in aesthetic surgery as well, where safety and patient-oriented protocols have become top of mind, illustrated by advances like UAL procedures. Even with such advances, nevertheless, problems exist within incision procedures themselves, namely the risk for complications. In ultrasound-assisted procedures, utilization of devices , such as VASER®, incisional precision cannot be emphasized enough.

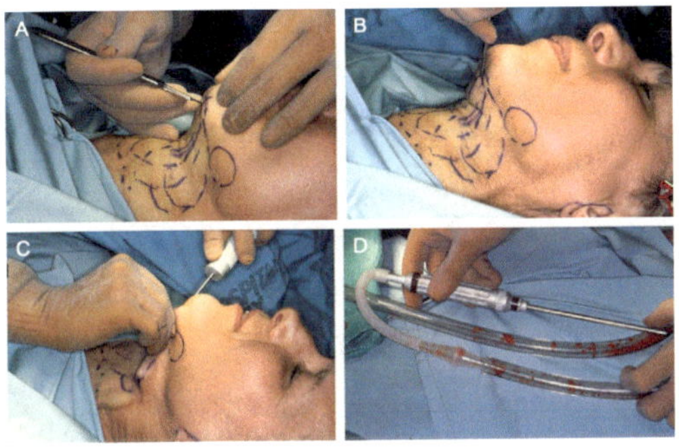

Figure 7.10. (A) A small incision is initially made in the submental line to initiate liposuction; (B) The precise subcutaneous plane is initially created with small scissors; (C) Liposuction is performed with a to-and-fro action of the cannula with gentle manipulation of the cutaneous tissue with the surgeon's opposite hand; and (D) Often significant adipose tissue is removed through this technique.

Source: https://www.researchgate.net/profile/Stephen-Perkins-4/publication/230713552/figure/fig31/AS:718292557778947@1548265699833/A-A-small-incision-is-initially-made-in-the-submental-line-to-initiate-liposuction-B.jpg.

A retrospective review of 1,486 patients undergoing VASER-assisted liposuction noted minor complications of tissue stiffness and transient hyperpigmentation, highlighting the need for meticulous surgical technique and close postoperative follow-up (Kandulu, 2024). In addition, comparison of older and newer methods of creating incisions can offer insightful information regarding the safety and effectiveness of liposuction. Finally, with the advancement of the field, continuous research and comparative studies of incision techniques will be crucial in the development of these techniques towards the best patient outcomes and satisfaction (Figure 7.10).

7.3.3. Fat Removal Process

The development of various fat reduction treatments has transformed the body sculpting environment, particularly within liposuction techniques. Traditional liposuction techniques have been in practice for decades to remove localized fat deposits, offering patients a means to achieve their ideal physique. This invasive treatment involves suctioning fat with a cannula passed beneath the skin. However, with the improvement in body sculpting trends, new practices have emerged that are more patient safety-oriented and result in shorter recoveries. Therefore, there has been a steadfast drive towards less invasive treatments that not only seek to eliminate fat but also enhance skin texture and appearance as a whole, inviting more patients to go for fat removal procedures. New technologies have introduced new methods , such as Ice-Shock Lipolysis, in which acoustic waves are combined with cryolipolysis to treat cellulite and localized fat. The method leverages apoptosis, programmed cell death, to induce gradual disintegration of the fat tissue and, concurrently, improve cellulite-related issues. The efficacy of this dual approach has been corroborated in the form of dramatic clinical outcomes, with measurable reductions in fat thickness and circumference without adverse side effects. These outcomes are paramount for patient groups that may not be optimal candidates for traditional liposuction on account of various aspects of health issues, pointing to the potential of non-surgical fat reduction procedures to effectively cater to a range of requirements in body contouring procedures

(Cataldo et al., 2012). As the practice continues to expand, it is more necessary than ever for surgeons to be acquainted with the multitude of fat reduction procedures at their disposal. With further advances in technology, the lipid aspiratory technique has evolved, including energy-based systems and combination therapies for better results and fewer complications. They now support a customized approach that considers individual patient issues and individualized aesthetic outcomes, making procedural choice aligned with both medical safety and patient desires. As detailed by an international group of renowned surgeons, an understanding of the indications, limitations, and possible complications of various techniques is vital for clinicians to successfully navigate this complex landscape (Miller et al., 2012). By providing a holistic image of the fat removal process, practitioners cannot only optimize results but also enhance the overall patient experience in cosmetic treatments.

Test Your Knowledge

1. What are the different anesthesia options available for liposuction, and how is the choice determined?
2. How are incisions made for liposuction, and what considerations are taken into account when placing them?
3. Describe the process of fat removal during liposuction and the role of the cannula.

7.4. Postoperative Care

Learning Outcome

1. Explain how the recovery timeline following liposuction varies significantly based on the individual's health
2. Manage pain and discomfort
3. Understand the importance of follow-up appointments

Postoperative care of liposuction is also a major component of the overall safety and success of the surgery. After surgery, the patients usually develop swelling and bruising in the regions treated and must have careful monitoring and management. Effective postoperative care is essential to minimize these side effects as well as for optimal recovery. These involve the application of compression stockings, which play a key role in the minimization of swelling and prevention of detachment of the skin from the underlying tissues. In addition, close observation for any signs of complications, , such as infection or improper fluid accumulation, is crucial. Proper education regarding home care practices, including wound care and activity restriction, equips patients with the knowledge to avoid complications and instructs them on the need for follow-up visits to ensure healing. Proper fluid management is another crucial aspect of postoperative care that plays a significant role in patient healing following liposuction. For instance, tranexamic acid (TXA) has been effective for the control of intraoperative and post-procedure bleeding. In a recent study, it was reported that patients who received TXA preoperative and postoperatively had superior hemoglobin levels and fewer instances of transfusion requirement than those receiving it preoperative (Mar et al., 2023). This highlights the importance of applying pharmacological methods alongside routine postoperative care. Minimizing blood loss allows medical professionals to optimize recovery time and patient comfort. As such, including such methods in postoperative care presents a reliable method for optimizing results in liposuction patients. Last but not least, postoperative care is focused on ensuring an uneventful and comfortable recovery while remaining vigilant for complications. Regular follow-up examinations are important to track the healing progress of the patients, to evaluate the aesthetic outcomes, and to handle any issues. Good communication among patients and healthcare providers is important in building trust and promoting compliance with recovery routines. Patient education on realistic expectations and the value of post-surgical care also goes a long way in maximizing overall satisfaction with the outcome. As liposuction techniques evolve, so should the interventions performed during postoperative care to achieve the best possible outcomes for patients (Miller et al., 2012). By addressing these factors first, medical professionals can ensure that liposuction is both safe and effective in body contouring.

7.4.1. Recovery Timeline

The recovery time from liposuction is significant based on the individual's health, the extent of the procedure, and the procedure itself. Swelling, bruising, and pain after surgery are naturally felt by patients, and these are all normal reactions of the body to surgical interventions. The recovery period in the initial phase is a matter of days or a week at most, whereas patients must rest and keep physical activity to a minimum in order to allow the body to settle. The use of compression garments is normally recommended to facilitate recovery and reduce swelling. Secondly, the measurement of personal recovery might be challenging; although some recover adequately to resume light exercise within a week, others might take more time to recover fully. Consequently, the first week is a critical period in the recovery from liposuction, setting the stage for future recuperation. With the progression of weeks after surgery, gradual improvement is likely to be noted. By week two, patients can see significant reduction in bruising and swelling, although some residual effects could persist. Patients can typically return to light physical activity by this point, , such as walking, which aids circulation and promotes healing. Vigorous exercise and high-impact sports, however, are still contraindicated until such time as they are released by a physician, most commonly within the three- to six-week time frame. By now, most patients can resume their gradual return to usual exercise routines. Awareness of this timetable is essential in managing expectations as an accurate estimate of recovery ensures overall satisfaction with the outcome of liposuction. In addition, compliance with the surgeons post-op instructions remains essential in ensuring healing and avoiding complications. Following the first month, patients usually see their bodies taking shape more defined, indicating successful liposuction.

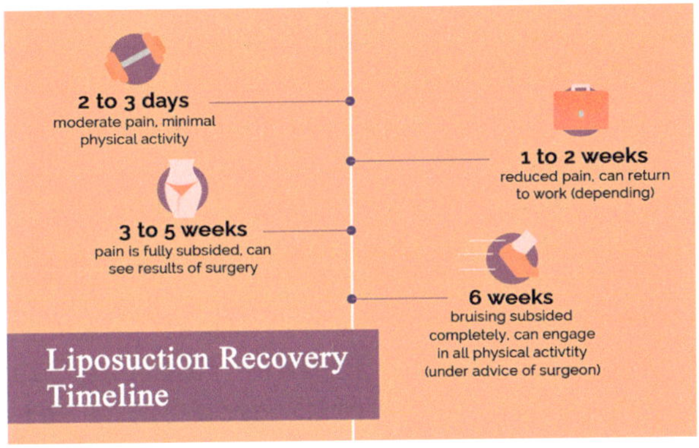

Figure 7.11. Liposuction recovery timeline.

Source: https://davidloh.sg/wp-content/uploads/2020/12/Liposuction-Recovery-Timeline.png.

It is during this time that ultimate results of the surgery are gradually unveiled, but peak results can take several months to be fully realized due to residual swelling. They must be careful about healthful lifestyles, , such as correct diet and physical exercise, so they can achieve the maximum outcome. They also require follow-up visits with their surgical team to confirm that they are healing properly and monitoring for any issues. The healing time hence is not just a matter of physical recovery but also an emotional and mental exercise as patients adapt to new bodies. Keeping an open dialogue with healthcare providers can enhance this process, leading to better outcomes, as highlighted in relevant regulatory discussions of the healthcare system that stress patient autonomy and the need for access to care (Ettinger., 2014Ettinger) (Figure 7.11).

7.4.2. Managing Pain and Discomfort

Effective management of pain and discomfort is a critical component of liposuction that affects outcomes and patient satisfaction. Techniques utilized during the process, , such as tumescent anesthesia, have greatly improved patient comfort. Through the injection of a vasoconstrictor and local anesthetic solution into the area being treated, surgeons can minimize pain at and post-procedure. Aware administration of pain not only enhances comfort but also allows for faster recovery periods, so patients can gain full function sooner. Furthermore, the psychological aspect of pain control cannot be overemphasized, as diminishment of physical pain can lead to improved emotional well-being and satisfaction with results. Strategies addressing both pharmacologic and non-pharmacologic approaches, including preoperative education and counseling, are critical in order for patients to indicate that they feel educated and ready, thus reducing preoperative anxiety and pain perception postoperatively. Postoperative pain management is an ongoing subject of interest and research among liposuction surgeries. Postoperatively, patients experience a number of discomforts, including bruising, swelling, and soreness. Proper recovery process is of paramount importance in facilitating not only physical recovery but also psychological recovery. Management of pain through drugs, for instance, analgesics or anti-inflammatory medication, can efficiently keep one at ease. Furthermore, postoperative procedures may also incorporate guidelines on the use of compression stockings, which assist in keeping swelling under control and provide a favorable environment for recovery. Important also is the recognition of individual patient needs, since an individualized pain management can lead to better outcomes. In studies, well-controlled pain patients also tended to have better psychological recovery and satisfaction with surgical results, affirming the necessity of an integrated pain management approach (Gupta et al., 2017). In addition to pharmacological treatments, there is a need to develop an understanding and treat potential liposuction procedure complications in the alleviation of patient pain. As documented in surgical literature, hematomas, cutaneous necrosis, and infection are potential complications that significantly affect a patient's level of pain and satisfaction.

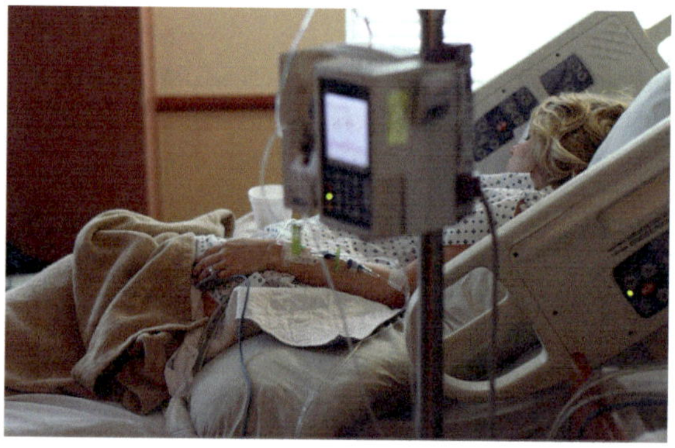

Figure 7.12. Resting after liposuction surgery for relieving pain.

Source: https://i0.wp.com/www.frikosal.net/wp-content/uploads/2023/06/rest.jpg?w=641&ssl=1.

Utilizing stringent preoperative assessment, and tumescent anesthesia, can reduce risks associated with these complications. Identification of warning signs and symptoms of complications enables practitioners and patients to deal with issues in good time, without added discomfort. Also, honest discussions between surgeons on best practice for dealing with complications can enhance general patient safety and satisfaction (Gold et al., 2021). By fostering awareness and preparedness culture, practitioners can effectively reduce discomfort from unexpected happenings and therefore improve patients' overall postoperative outcome after liposuction (Figure 7.12).

7.4.3. Importance of Follow-Up Appointments

The significance of the follow-up visits during liposuction procedures cannot be emphasized. Follow-up visits are essential checkpoints in healing progress, whereby both the surgeon and the patient can assess post-operative outcomes as well as identify any emerging problems. During follow-up, patients can report on their experience with pain control, satisfaction with the result, and complications if occurring. This open avenue of communication fosters reassurance and trust and allows patients to be comforted during the recovery period. Additionally, it allows surgeons to offer personalized advice and interventions capable of optimizing recovery and ultimately providing aesthetic results that meet patient expectations and surgical outcomes. Follow-up appointments are also significant in early complication detection, such as infection, seroma, or asymmetrical contours. Through monitoring of the surgical fields at regular intervals, healthcare providers are in a position to establish prompt interventions with the right interventions to reverse undesired effects, thereby guaranteeing patient happiness and well-being. For example, surgeons can advise on postoperative treatment procedures that can reduce risks, for example, some massage maneuvers or activity level recommendations. The incorporation of an active emphasis into these appointments informs patients about what to look out for, hence enhancing their active involvement in their healing process. Vigilance is particularly relevant in such procedures as liposuction, where patient outcomes are largely contingent on perceptive post-operative care and monitoring. The impact of follow-up visits extends beyond the clinical aspect; it has a significant psychological influence on patient care and outcomes. Many individuals undergo liposuction with the expectation of not only altering their physical appearance but also changing their self-image and body outlook. Hence, follow-up visits provide an opportunity for surgeons to reinforce positive outcomes as well as mitigate any psychological problems that are bound to arise after the surgery, , such as body dysmorphic concerns. Rapport-making during these visits allows for surgeons to gauge the mood of their patients and respond accordingly, if necessary. As seen through recovery priority research, continuous observation and monitoring of patients' recovery processes matter, validating the concept that follow-up consultations are part of an entire strategy in liposuction outcomes (O'Hara et al., 2020; Raheem et al., 2024).

Test Your Knowledge

1. What is the typical recovery timeline after liposuction, and when can patients expect to return to normal activities?
2. What strategies are commonly used to manage pain and discomfort after liposuction?

7.5. Benefits of Liposuction

Learning Outcome

1. Focus on body contouring and aesthetic improvement by liposuction
2. Describe psychological effects and self-esteem
3. Deal with opportunities and challenges for long-term weight management through liposuction

Liposuction is now one of the most popular procedures for cosmetic surgery, and the reason is primarily due to the many benefits of the procedure beyond its aesthetic appeal. Its greatest advantage is how much of a person can get body contouring done and restructure and reform their own body. The transformation can lead to increased self-esteem and confidence in their body, which are vital for one's psychological health. Moreover, the majority of patients make a point to say they have a new enthusiasm for life following the procedure, fully engaging in social activities they previously shunned due to body shape problems. Such psychological improvements tell of how liposuction is not only transforming body looks but can also enhance one's mental state, making it a multi-faceted procedure in treating body image issues. Apart from its aesthetic applications, advancements in liposuction techniques have significantly improved the success of surgery and patient recovery. An excellent example is TLL, where there is a unique technique using pre-heated saline for more convenient fat dislocation, with faster and less invasive outcomes compared to traditional methods. Studies have corroborated that TLL patients experience less swelling, bruising, and tenderness of the treated area than patients who have undergone SAL procedures. TLL has also shown miraculous improvement in the rate of extraction, thus becoming a more sought-after method with surgeons seeking effective means. These developments not only make the process of recovery an excellent one but also cut down on waiting time, which the patients need to wait before resuming normal activities, which is of additional use in occupational and individual life (Hunstad et al., 2018). Beyond cosmetic and healing benefits, liposuction may be an option for some medical conditions related to surplus body fat. For example, liposuction can correct lipomas, lipodystrophy, or localized adiposity that is not amenable to conventional methods of reducing weight.

Moreover, gluteoplasty procedures, intended for buttock shape and firmness adjustment, are increasing. In addition to being an etiology of improved body proportions, the procedure is also a result of evolving aesthetics of beauty that positively accentuate buttocks. The success of these techniques aids in pointing out the versatility of liposuction within the overall domain of cosmetic surgery, with a demand from various populations for both aesthetic and functional improvements (Miller et al., 2012). Taken together, these examples aid in illustrating that liposuction is more than cosmetic surgery; it is a way of overall physical and psychological improvement.

7.5.1. Body Contouring and Aesthetic Improvement

The search for body sculpting and enhancing beauty has gained a lot of pace because the values of beauty in society always change. Out of all the procedures, liposuction is a core procedure that has evolved by leaps and bounds over time. In the beginning, it was created as a quick process of fat tissue pocket excision from localized tissue areas, whereas modern liposuction has reached various techniques that allow the body to be accurately sculpted. This innovation has enabled practitioners to employ liposuction not just as a treatment against fat but as an essential weapon for beauty change. This innovation is part of the larger cosmetic surgery trend towards more natural and proportional effects, thus addressing greater needs for body contouring treatments not only that enhance looks but also express self and confidence. Among the most sought-after examples of body contouring technology is the rising interest in gluteal beauty, particularly if used on three-dimensional gluteoplasty (3-DGP).

The new technique goes beyond simple buttock augmentation; it provides a comprehensive approach to treating the area, including thighs and trochanters. Improvement of the realization of the crucial role of gluteal contours in creating the contours of physical beauty directs towards the importance of those methods which allow volumetric and structural remodeling. As discussed in Blugerman et al. (2011), these treatments address common aesthetic problems and allow patients to achieve their ideal body silhouette. Hence, the incorporation of 3-DGP in the surgeon's repertoire is yet another signal of technological advancement standing the test of changing perceptions of beauty in body sculpting. In addition, refinements in technique for liposuction show a reaction to what modern aesthetics demand like incorporation of minimally invasive technology into newer procedures. As Miller et al., 2012 put it, the multitude of possibilities, whether energy-based devices or combination therapies, is a paradigm change from how practitioners have been dealing with body contouring. This kind of multiaxial system of treatment makes possible treatments tailored to individual patient goals without sacrificing recovery time and complications. Moreover, these advancements demand an even greater respect for the procedural limitations and complications potential, promoting the all-important necessity of expertise at the nuances of body contouring. Thus, the art of liposuction and body contouring becomes more sophisticated, informed by research, innovation, and sheer dedication to aesthetic improvement (Figure 7.13).

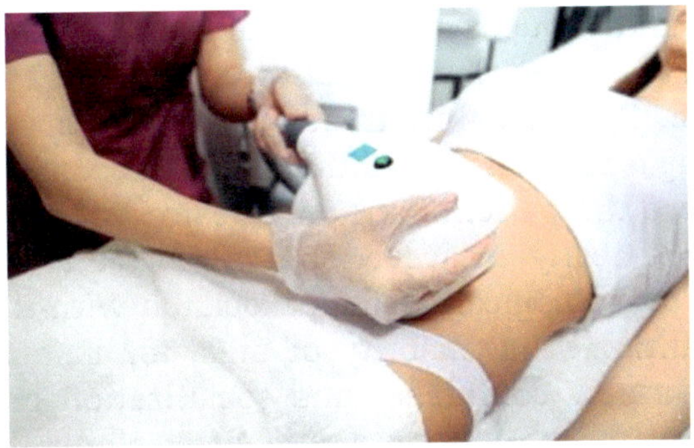

Figure 7.13. Non-invasive body contouring procedure using advanced aesthetic technology.

Source: https://aaams.net/wp-content/uploads/2025/01/non-invasive-bosy-contouring-bigstock-438903635-350x225.jpg.

7.5.2. Psychological Effects and Self-Esteem

The psychoemotional effect of liposuction can also play an extremely strong role in influencing the self-esteem of a patient, with a predisposition to cause dramatic changes in self-image and well-being. Liposuction patients most frequently complain of body image dissatisfaction, which is a result of beauty demands imposed by contemporary society and the condoning of slenderness and beauty of the body. All patients after surgery have improved self-esteem and body image, and this is evidence that liposuction diminishes shame and inferior feelings. For instance, studies have shown that patients of reduction mammaplasty not only get physical gain but also large psychological benefits in the form of decreasing levels of anxiety and depression associated with their ailment. This is in line with broader evidence that surgery can transform an individual's mental health context, highlighting the interconnectedness of body shape and mental state (Saariniemi., 2011). Moreover, the self-esteem boost following liposuction not only stops at individual satisfaction but extends beyond social conduct and interpersonal relationships. Surgery patients become increasingly active in social life and group activities, once they develop a new confidence that they previously did not have. Psychological treatment of one's well-being is touted for conditions like gynecomastia, where the patients not only desire to become aesthetically improved but also don't want the psychological stigma associated with their condition. The majority of men, for instance, feel a new confidence and socialization more completely after surgery, effectively eliminating the weight of shame and social repression through having heavy breasts. These results indicate to what degree successful defeat of physical barriers through procedures , such as liposuction can bestow long-term psychological benefits, thus narrating the overall impact of cosmetic surgery on self-esteem (Gupta et al., 2017). In assessing long-term consequences of liposuction on self-esteem, it is clear that patients' healing relies on individual psychosocial factors before the operation. For instance, patients who have low self-esteem or poor body image may experience an even more dramatic shift than those who already possess their self-esteem at a comparatively high level. The findings of research on surgical procedures are that preoperative psychological assessment is worthwhile, as it offers a chance for tailored intervention, which suits a person's own interests. Improved postoperative self-esteem can lead to long-term quality of life, as the stability of long-term effects demonstrated in patients operated on with breast reduction procedures testifies. This reality points towards the necessity of holistic considerations in deciding suitability for medical procedures, as psychological readiness can even influence surgical outcomes and patient satisfaction (Saariniemi., 2011).

7.5.3. Long-Term Weight Management

Within the sphere of long-term weight management, the addition of liposuction is both desirable and undesirable. Liposuction has been considered a straightforward means of achieving body ideals in contour, but it should be remembered that the long-term weight management is outside the immediacy of surgery. Liposuction removes local supernumerary fat deposits but fails to treat inciting behavior and lifestyle causes of overweight. Therefore, patients who require liposuction must undergo life adjustments after the procedure, including dietetic adjustments and exercise, in an attempt to maintain their results. The necessity for such holism indicates a critical aspect of long-term weight management: results are achieved by balancing mechanisms of surgery with ongoing healthy habits. Moreover, the sociocultural aspect of body image and aging strongly influences long-term weight control strategies. In other cultures, for instance, in Brazil, youthfulness drives many towards cosmetic interventions like liposuction. Individuals have been seen to employ these interventions as a means not only to enhance the appearance of their bodies but also to solve the aging issues and the way they perceive themselves in a youth-worshiping culture. The charm of an optimized aging process can make individuals more reliant on surgical procedures, but this must be balanced against the reality that everybody ages and the quest for eternally youthful years usually undervalues the importance of health quality of life. Hence, the focus must transcend temporary cosmetic changes to encompass long-term health outcomes and overall wellbeing. The success of liposuction as part of long-term weight control can also be noted in patient satisfaction and operation outcome. Liposuction was found to yield satisfactory outcomes if performed by skilled surgeons, boosting the confidence and body image of the patients. But for the procedure to be deemed a success within a composite weight control outcome, follow-up treatment and ongoing patient maintenance need to be instituted. The surgical process is only the initial component; the patient needs to be educated on how to integrate healthier habits, and weight and body composition need to be followed regularly. If this step is not taken, regain in weight after surgery becomes prohibitive magnified. Thus, an understanding of the role of liposuction within a broader vision of control of lifestyle is necessary because it encapsulates the conflict between surgical accomplishment and sustained change, and emphasizes the need for a holistic approach in order to win long-term weight control (Farshad et al., 2018) (Figure 7.14).

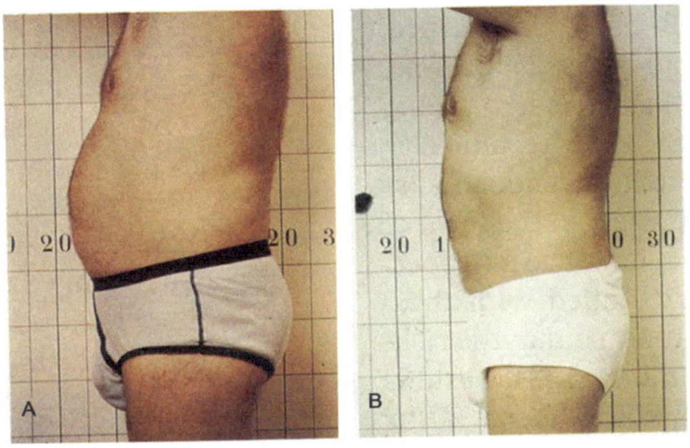

Figure 7.14. A 30-year-old male before (A); and after (B) a weight loss of 17.3 kg.

Source: https://www.researchgate.net/profile/Daniel-Belluscio/publication/19842724/figure/fig4/AS:601612317884431@1520446962217/A-30-year-old-male-before-A-and-after-B-a-weight-loss-of-173-kg-managed-with-the.png.

Test Your Knowledge

1. How does liposuction improve body contour and enhance physical appearance?
2. What psychological benefits can patients experience after successful liposuction?

7.6. Risks and Complications

Learning Outcome

1. Describe common side effects
2. Understand the serious complications associated with liposuction
3. Focus on mitigation strategies in the context of liposuction techniques

Liposuction, while usually envisioned as a rather simple cosmetic procedure, is full of all kinds of liposuction complications and complications that must be thoroughly considered. Bruising, swelling, and infection are some of the frequent liposuction complications arising from the invasive process. Hematomas, i.e., blood clotting outside of blood vessels, leading to painful swelling and swelling of the affected areas, may be created by patients too. More severe complications are seromas, where fluid will form at the site of surgery, and skin necrosis, where there is loss of circulation, leading to death of the skin. These possible results are a demonstration of just how crucial pre-operative consultations are, where patients are left completely informed about what risks are involved with the surgery and can make their own choices with their body and with what they want to achieve. Parallel to the progressive aesthetic merit of varying shapes of the body, particularly buttock enhancement, the methods involved in liposuction must be closely scrutinized for risk factors. The new three-dimensional gluteoplasty (3-DGP), for instance, has the potential to alter the buttocks' volume, shape, and turgidity, as well as the surrounding area, to a great degree. However, technicality and complexity in the procedure render risks-related complications more likely in the form of unbalanced outcomes or asymmetrical shapes. Surgeons have to be highly skilled with their hands and with human anatomy so that the risk-taking is not done during the process. Besides that, cultural values and greater demand for body ideals, particularly in such locations as Brazil, also raise moral issues regarding the outcome of proceeding with such enhancements, possibly on the brink of body dysmorphic problems as individuals are already grappling with social expectations of the body (Edmonds et al., 2014). In addition, liposuction operations not only result in physical complications but also psychological and emotional complications to the individuals. Postoperative dissatisfaction with the result and body image disturbances may lead to heightened anxiety and coping issues. Psychological research reveals that patients develop unrealistic expectations concerning their post-liposuction appearance that might end up leading to disappointment if results are not as expected. This encounter between social norms and the desire for beauty can evoke such feelings, particularly as individuals attempt to gain approval and acceptance by being beautiful (Miller et al., 2012). There must be a recognition on the part of both patients and health professionals that they are working with these psychological elements of liposuction in a way that mental well-being is also taken into account as much as physical outcome, hence the recommendation of an holistic approach to cosmetic surgery.

7.6.1. Common Side Effects

Though liposuction has been deemed a relatively safe cosmetic surgery procedure, prospective patients must be informed of the expected side effects of the different procedures of liposuction. Swelling and bruising are most likely to occur among them as the most common side effects. Patients after surgery may anticipate swelling in the areas treated as a result of tissue disruption involved in removing the fat. Bruising and swelling result from traumatized vessels, and as transient as they are in both cases, it certainly leaves an important effect on how they look postoperatively. Additionally, the extent of bruising and swelling depends on the method of liposuction procedure, volume of fat aspirated, and personal variables , such as healing response and skin flexibility.

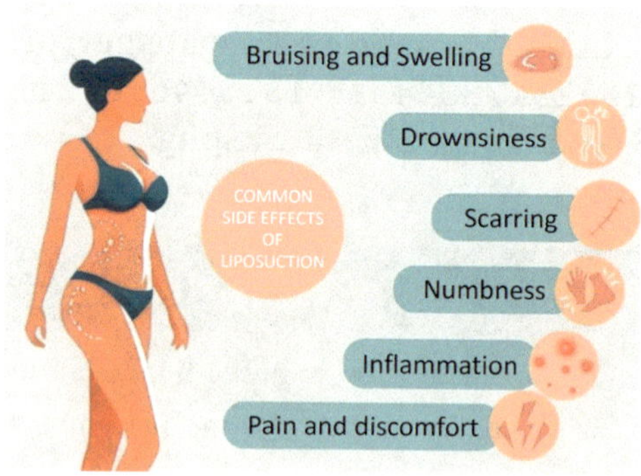

Figure 7.15. Common side effects of liposuction.

Source: https://www.sibelatalay.com.tr/img/blog/liposuction-side-effects.jpg.

Thus, it is essential to identify these side effects to make sufficient recovery time and ultimate outcome expectations. Other common side effects of liposuction are numbness and sensory change over the treated area. These symptoms occur secondary to nerve injury from the procedure. Sensation will typically come back for most patients in a few weeks, but some others have numbness or changed sensitivity, which is frustrating. Second, the technique used can also affect how often such side effects occur because some techniques may kill more nerves than others. Patients must sit down with their practitioners and discuss what they have to offer and thus get a better appreciation of what they are risking. Based on this information, patients are capable of negotiating recovery time with the necessary caution and sensitivity because a more informed decision-making process is established.

With liposuction, infection, fluid accumulation, and asymmetry complications are outcomes with greater medicolegal significance. Infections may be seen after surgery if post-operative management is followed strictly in neglect. Fluid accumulation in the form of seroma may necessitate subsequent interventions, , such as drainage. Asymmetry, which is a risk for every surgery, may lead to dissatisfaction with results. Worst is the more critical side effect, though uncommon, and may result in, for example, DVT and pulmonary embolism. Awareness and education of these side effects are paramount in any type of surgery. Preoperative consultation must incorporate these risks as a means of tailoring each patient's experience so that they will know what to expect when and after the surgery has been done, thereby ensuring a safer overall experience in seeking aesthetic enhancement , such as liposuction (Figure 7.15).

7.6.2. Serious Complications

The background of liposuction procedures cannot be ruled out without being mindful of the serious complications arising during and after the procedure. Liposuction, although immensely popular and commonly considered a cosmetic procedure, is extremely risky, particularly with the removal of massive amounts of fat or in combined surgery. These take the form of complications , such as infection, hematomas, and seromas, or delayed healing or need for further surgical intervention in severe cases. In addition, the cosmetic outcome is marred by contour deformity and disproportion, and as such patient selection and compliance with ideal practices at the time of treatment are a pre-requisite. It should be noted by both practitioner and patient that the possible complications are since this enables informed consent and realistic expectation preoperatively. Among the main causes of serious liposuction complications is that there are risks of adverse events from anesthesia. As liposuction for the majority is performed under general or local anesthesia, patients must accept risks inherent with these modalities. Inadequate monitoring can have catastrophic consequences, including respiratory failure or cardiovascular complications, particularly in medically ill patients. Advances in many liposuction technologies, including ultrasonic and laser-assisted techniques, aim to enhance safety, but more sophisticated technologies do not eliminate anesthetic complications altogether. Therefore, appropriate preoperative evaluation and judicious anesthesia management are critical components in minimizing complications. Such a comprehensive model of care for the patient protects not only patient safety but also the integrity of the aesthetic goals formulated in consultation. Integration of novel methods of liposuction ultimately does not eliminate the risk for major complications like fat embolism syndrome. This rare but potentially fatal complication occurs when fat globules find their way into the circulatory system and obstruct blood vessels. Application of high-energy machines in more recent methods unconsciously contributes to the risk of this complication and thus to the need for closer observation by clinicians during the procedure. Safety protocols in liposuction must be scrutinized periodically and optimized to offset such risks. Greater experience with varying methods helps clinicians better foresee complications and implement steps that enhance the overall welfare of the patient. Lastly, patient awareness and knowledge of the serious complications involved in liposuction operations are the underlying foundation for the establishment of the practice with respect to patient safety and satisfaction in esthetic surgery outcomes.

7.6.3. Mitigation Strategies

Mitigation measures when it comes to liposuction procedures are required to minimize risks of complications and optimize patients' outcomes. Preoperative evaluation, which is evaluating a patient's medical history, BMI, and lifestyle, is a good mitigation measure. Tailoring the liposuction procedure to the specifications of each individual is a good method of reducing risks , such as excess bleeding, infection, or adverse reaction to anesthesia. Besides, the implementation of a multidisciplinary team where physical therapists and nutritionists work alongside surgeons can get the patient better ready for surgery and assist recovery by making patients healthier. These preoperative measures not only make patients safer but also increase patient satisfaction as expectations are satisfied with successful outcomes. During surgery, the implementation of sophisticated surgical techniques is another important mitigation technique. For instance, the method of tumescent liposuction, i.e., infiltration of local anesthetic containing saline solution, has been observed to reduce postoperative bruising and pain to a significant degree. Second, adopting technology-based methods, , such as LAL or ultrasonic-assisted liposuction, allows for improved excision of fat with minimal damage to other tissues. These developments not only contribute to the safety profile of the procedure but can also shorten recovery times, resulting in a more pleasant postoperative experience for the patient. By incorporating these methodologies into practice, surgeons are better positioned to contain risks associated with liposuction procedures and encourage more favorable patient outcomes. Postoperative care is also a critical element of mitigation strategies in liposuction. Compliance with systematic follow-up protocols ensures patients are monitored for complications and their healing progresses as anticipated. Provision of advice on compression stockings, pain management, and a return to physical exercises in a gradual manner can influence healing. Guidance on recognizable indicators of complications, including abnormal swelling or infection, allows patients to seek timely medical treatment if necessary. According to recent reviews, postoperative complications can be minimized efficiently through careful compliance with follow-up appointments and patient education regarding self-care routines (Portilla et al., 2024). Ultimately, the integration of total mitigation techniques into the process of liposuction enhances patient safety as well as aesthetic outcomes and general satisfaction (Douglas et al., 2012).

Test Your Knowledge

1. What are the most common side effects patients may experience after liposuction?
2. What serious complications can occur with liposuction, though rare?

SUMMARY

In concluding the overview of liposuction techniques, the advances in surgical procedures have fundamentally transformed the beauty procedures landscape. TLL is a landmark technique, a milestone that symbolizes not only enhanced efficiency but also superior patient outcomes. As brought out in the comparative review of TLL and SAL, TLL has shown great potential to reduce recovery time and minimize postoperative pain, thus affirming its rising popularity among surgeons as well as patients. The findings point out the ability of TLL to break into body contouring as a disruptor, presenting possibilities for more enhanced practices that prioritize patient well-being as much as they care about aesthetic results. Furthermore, the variability of techniques, , such as the three-dimensional gluteoplasty (3-DGP), also reflects a more discerning appreciation for physical beauty. In allowing the surgeon to alter volume, contour, and firmness not only in the buttocks but also in neighboring tissues, 3-DGP addresses the entire spectrum of the patients' desires for enhancement in their body shape. The emphasis on buttocks as physical beauty and eroticism symbols, as found in contemporary times, also constitutes changing social expectations and personal desires involved with these procedures. Compounding these methods can therefore fulfill personal desires for body sculpting as well as optimize overall satisfaction with surgical outcomes. Finally, the inference derived from the analysis of liposuction techniques is a direction of sight toward the development of better surgical techniques with greater patient satisfaction. As evidenced by the data presented through outcomes on both TLL and the new aspects of 3-DGP, there is a clear movement towards procedures inducing less trauma and an accelerated rate of recovery. Liposuction is increasingly developing as a high-tech specialty with priorities laid on safety, efficiency, and cosmetic gratification. For future practices, how crucial it is to adopt such advanced techniques cannot be overemphasized as they redefine the standards of surgical perfection and redefine cultural attitudes towards body image and beauty. Such a development promises to usher in an era of optimism for patients and practitioners alike who are determined to achieve the most ideal outcomes in cosmetic surgery.

The evolution of liposuction techniques is a technological and surgical innovation that has significantly improved the results in patients. Traditional liposuction, also referred to as suction-assisted lipectomy, involves a cannula to manually break up and vacuum the fat cells. The procedure is linked with high effectiveness in fat reduction but may result in more postoperative discomfort and longer recovery times compared to more modern techniques. More recent technologies , such as ultrasonic and laser liposuction, have introduced novel modalities that seek to minimize invasiveness and optimize recovery. These techniques employ sound waves and laser power, respectively, to vaporize fat before removal, potentially reducing trauma to surrounding tissues and enhancing skin retraction, becoming necessary procedures in cosmetic surgery as such innovations continue enhancing the effectiveness and safety of liposuction procedures (Nojek et al., 2024). Understanding the benefits and limitations inherent in every liposuction technique is vital to practitioners and patients. Ultrasonic liposuction possesses precision and is particularly helpful when treating fibrous fat masses, , such as on the back or male chest. In contrast, however, the risk of thermal destruction of surrounding tissues necessitates masterful handling. Conversely, laser liposuction not only enables fat elimination but also induces collagen formation, which improves the texture of the treated area. Even though such treatments come with numerous advantages, concerns regarding long-term efficacy and complications are issues of ongoing research and controversy. A careful assessment of these treatments, thus, along with patient-specific factors, is essential in the selection of the most suitable procedure for effective results (Saariniemi., 2011). Moreover, realistic expectations as well as patient education play important roles in the choice of liposuction. Patients should be educated not only about what techniques are available but also about how there can be varying outcomes based on physiological as well as psychological factors. For example, patients with pre-existing psychological problems might have varying degrees of satisfaction following the procedure, both based on physical appearance and body image perception. Moreover, given the proven correlation between preoperative psychosocial variables and surgical outcome, treatment planning has an increased level of complexity. As the aesthetic surgery profession continues to evolve, drawing up protocols integrating these elements alongside technological advancements will result in more personalized and efficient treatment, ultimately yielding higher patient satisfaction (Nojek et al., 2024).

KEY TERMS FROM THIS CHAPTER

- Abnormal swelling
- Aging process
- Body shaping
- Fluid management
- Gluteoplasty
- Hemoglobin levels
- High-precision effects
- lidocaine
- Kinesiotherapy
- Laser liposuction
- Aesthetic medicine
- Anesthetic management
- Deep vein thrombosis (DVT)
- Gluteal beauty
- Gluteoplasty procedures
- High-definition liposuction
- Holistic strategy
- Innovative technologies
- Laser energy
- Laser technology

CRITICAL THINKING QUESTIONS

1. **Which of the following liposuction techniques uses high-frequency sound waves to break up fat cells before removal?**
   a. Tumescent liposuction
   b. Laser-assisted liposuction (LAL)
   c. Ultrasound-assisted liposuction (UAL)
   d. Power-assisted liposuction (PAL)
2. **What is the main purpose of the tumescent solution in tumescent liposuction?**
   a. To dissolve fat cells
   b. To hydrate the skin
   c. To accelerate fat metabolism
   d. To minimize blood loss and provide local anesthesia
3. **Which technique uses a vibrating cannula to facilitate fat removal with less manual force?**
   a. SmartLipo
   b. Power-assisted liposuction (PAL)
   c. Tumescent liposuction
   d. Ultrasound-assisted liposuction
4. **Which of the following is considered a minimally invasive liposuction technique that also promotes skin tightening?**
   a. Laser-assisted liposuction (LAL)
   b. Traditional liposuction
   c. Water-assisted liposuction (WAL)
   d. Dry liposuction
5. **What distinguishes water-assisted liposuction (WAL) from other liposuction techniques?**
   a. Use of a vibrating cannula
   b. No use of anesthesia
   c. Use of a pressurized stream of saline to dislodge fat
   d. Use of a laser to melt fat

Short Answer Questions

1. What are the key differences between traditional (suction-assisted) liposuction and tumescent liposuction in terms of technique and safety?
2. How does ultrasound-assisted liposuction (UAL) differ from power-assisted liposuction (PAL), and what are the primary indications for each?
3. Describe the purpose and composition of the tumescent solution used in liposuction procedures. What roles do each of the components play?
4. What are the advantages and potential complications associated with laser-assisted liposuction (LAL)?
5. In what scenarios is high-definition liposuction preferred, and what unique techniques does it employ to enhance muscle definition?
6. List and explain at least three common complications or risks associated with liposuction, regardless of the technique used.
7. What are the main anatomical considerations a surgeon must evaluate before performing liposuction in areas , such as the abdomen, thighs, or neck?

Answer to Critical Thinking Questions

1. (c); 2. (d); 3. (b); 4. (a); 5. (c)

REFERENCES

1. Abd-El-Salam, A. E. R., Abd-Elsayed, A. A., El-Oteify, M., et al. (2009). Safety and benefits of large-volume liposuction: A single center experience. https://core.ac.uk/download/pdf/8267968.pdf (accessed on 11th June 2025).

2. https://core.ac.uk/download/299809007.pdf Hunstad, J. P., Godek, C. P., Van Natta, B. W., Kortesis, B. G., Bharti, G., Crantford, J. C., Daniels, M. A., & Andrew, M. S. (2018). A Multicenter, Prospective, Randomized, Contralateral Study of Tissue Liquefaction Liposuction vs Suction-Assisted Liposuction. *Aesthetic surgery journal*, *38*(9), 980–989. https://doi.org/10.1093/asj/sjy001 (accessed on 11th June 2025).

3. Anwar, A. I., Lu, L., Plaisance, C. J., Daniel, C. P., Flanagan, C. J., Wenger, D. M., McGregor, D., et al. (2024). Fluoroquinolones: Neurological complications and side effects in clinical practice. *Cureus*, *16*. https://www.semanticscholar.org/paper/2a8c20013a494af2fa118736c2bace96a106cfb0 (accessed on 11th June 2025).

4. Bayter Marín, J. E., Cárdenas Camarena, L., & Hoyos, A. (2023). Effectiveness of tranexamic acid in the postoperative period in body contour surgery: Randomized clinical trial. https://core.ac.uk/download/641681320.pdf (accessed on 11th June 2025).

5. Nojek, P., Pawlik, W., Zimonczyk, M., Zawół, M., Błaszczyński, G., & Nowotarska, A. (2024). Comparison of Different Techniques: Ultrasonic, Laser, and Traditional Liposuction with a Discussion on New Directions and the Future of Liposuction Techniques. *Journal of Education, Health and Sport*, *71*, 55957. https://doi.org/10.12775/JEHS.2024.71.55957(accessed on 11th June 2025).

6. Granados-Tinajero, S., Buenrostro-Vásquez, C., Cárdenas-Maytorena, C., & Contreras-López, M. (2019). Anesthesia Management for Large-Volume Liposuction. IntechOpen. doi: 10.5772/intechopen.83630 (accessed on 11th June 2025).

7. Portilla, A. S. P., Portilla, C. S. P., Palacios, G. S. G., Rodríguez, B. S. P., Castillo, S. G. A., Espin, N. E. P., & Pita, G. P. M. (2024). The integration of surgical and dermatological techniques in the treatment of cutaneous aging: multidisciplinary approaches and clinical outcomes - a comprehensive systematic review of current literature. *International Journal of Research in Medical Sciences*, *12*(5), 1659–1667. https://doi.org/10.18203/2320-6012.ijrms20240943 (accessed on 11th June 2025).

8. Cataldo, C., D'Andrea, F., De Francesco, F., Ferraro, G. A., Nicoletti, G., & Rossano, F. (2012). Synergistic effects of cryolipolysis and shock waves for noninvasive body contouring. https://core.ac.uk/download/pdf/55147261.pdf (accessed on 11th June 2025).

9. Ciancio, F., Ciccarelli, F., Cuccaro, C., et al. (2024). Experience in post-bariatric abdominoplasty for patients with significant weight loss: A prospective study. https://core.ac.uk/download/622823823.pdf (accessed on 11th June 2025).

10. Daley, A., & Griffiths, E. A. (2025). Advancements in liver retraction techniques for laparoscopic gastrectomy. *World Journal of Gastrointestinal Surgery*, *17*. https://www.semanticscholar.org/paper/505b799cd0dc3241e01bcfc7d869cba41270b20a (accessed on 11th June 2025).

11. Duncan, D. I. (2022). Enhanced liposuction. https://core.ac.uk/download/534904133.pdf (accessed on 11th June 2025).

12. Edmonds, A. (2014). Surgery-for-life: Aging, sexual fitness and self-management in Brazil. https://core.ac.uk/download/28979727.pdf (accessed on 11th June 2025).

13. Ettinger, J. A. (2014). Seeking common ground in the abortion regulation debate. https://core.ac.uk/download/268217901.pdf (accessed on 11th June 2025).

14. Farshad, M., Koehler, C., Kuenzi, W., Scholz, et al. (2018). Clinical outcome and long-term follow-up after liposuction procedures. https://core.ac.uk/download/159150388.pdf (accessed on 11th June 2025).

15. Gold, M. H., & Robb, C. W. (2021). Complications and solutions for post-operative liposuction deformities. https://core.ac.uk/download/479935968.pdf (accessed on 11th June 2025).

16. Goutman, S. A., Savelieff, M. G., Sakowski, S. A., & Feldman, E. L. (2019). Stem cell treatments for amyotrophic lateral sclerosis: A critical overview of early phase trials. *Expert Opinion on Investigational Drugs*, *28*, 525–543. https://doi.org/10.1080/13543784.2019.1627324 (accessed on 11th June 2025).

17. Gupta, S., Mehta, J., Nakade, D. V., Shahane, et al. (2017). Gynecomastia: Our surgical experience using liposuction and minimal invasive surgical excision and its psychological benefits to young patients. https://core.ac.uk/download/543135985.pdf (accessed on 11th June 2025).

18. Hoang, D. M., Pham, P. T., Bach, T. Q., Ngo, A. T., Nguyen, Q. T., Phan, T. K. T., Giang, N. H., et al. (2022). Stem cell-based therapy for human diseases. *Signal Transduction and Targeted Therapy*, *7*. https://doi.org/10.1038/s41392-022-01134-4 (accessed on 11th June 2025).

19. Kandulu, H. (2024). Evaluation of postoperative complications in VASER®-assisted liposuction: A retrospective study of 1,486 cases. *Namık Kemal Tıp Dergisi*. https://www.semanticscholar.org/paper/41f52d3bb24e3bf06e78fc20d422177633f9b545 (accessed on 11th June 2025).

20. King, K. K., Merianos, A. L., & Vidourek, R. A. (2013). Medicalization of female beauty: A content analysis of cosmetic procedures. https://core.ac.uk/download/51087636.pdf (accessed on 11th June 2025).

21. Lawand, J. J., Hantouly, A. T., Bouri, F., Muneer, M., Farooq, A., & Hagert, E. (2024). Complications and side effects of wide-awake local anesthesia no tourniquet (WALANT) in upper limb surgery: A systematic review and meta-analysis. *International Orthopedics*, *48*, 1257–1269. https://www.semanticscholar.org/paper/1e79f1053bfe6a85c83a6b9d54305d72b3fa788d (accessed on 11th June 2025).

22. Luisa, S. N. L. A., Araujo-López, A., Cardona-Ochoa, P., Pacheco, V. H. R., Paez, Y. A. C., Leon-Serna, R. R. D., Rios Lara-Y, L. R. L., et al. (2023). Abdominal liposuction post-surgical management controlled with kinesiotherapy. *Journal of Surgery Open Access*, *9*. https://doi.org/10.16966/2470-0991.271 (accessed on 11th June 2025).

23. Miller, D. L., Smith, N. B., Bailey, M. R., Czarnota, G. J., Hynynen, K., Makin, I. R., & Bioeffects Committee of the American Institute of Ultrasound in Medicine (2012). Overview of therapeutic ultrasound applications and safety considerations. *Journal of ultrasound in medicine : official journal of the American Institute of Ultrasound in Medicine*, *31*(4), 623–634. https://doi.org/10.7863/jum.2012.31.4.623 (accessed on 11th June 2025).

24. Nayak, S. K. (2025). Body contouring using VASER liposuction: Retrospective analysis of 175 consecutive cases at a single centre. *International Journal of Aesthetic Plastic Surgery*, *1*, 63–69. https://www.semanticscholar.org/paper/265ea9652ee20cfbeb2f5eee8207870118d8afeb (accessed on 11th June 2025).

25. O'Hara, N., Kringos, D., Slobogean, G., Degani, Y., & Klazinga, N. (2020). Patients place more of an emphasis on physical recovery than return to work or financial recovery. *Clinical Orthopedics and Related Research*, *479*, 1333–1343. https://www.semanticscholar.org/paper/47bea679abb2da45d3f3941205ba005a43b4acd6 (accessed on 11th June 2025).

26. Pereira, A. C., Ramos, B., Reis, A. C., & Cunha, M. V. (2020). Non-tuberculous mycobacteria: Molecular and physiological bases of virulence and adaptation to ecological niches. *Microorganisms*, *8*, 1380–1380. https://doi.org/10.3390/microorganisms8091380 (accessed on 11th June 2025).

27. Raheem, O., Venishetty, N., Areti, A., Kalidoss, S., & Kocjanic, E. (2024). (178) Glandular resurfacing with buccal mucosa graft for superficial glans penile cancer: Surgical technique. *The Journal of Sexual Medicine*. https://www.semanticscholar.org/paper/da7c67ebdc32824286cceb1bb2e6fcf52cbb393b (accessed on 11th June 2025).

28. Saariniemi, K. (2011). The effects of reduction mammaplasty. https://core.ac.uk/download/14920859.pdf (accessed on 11th June 2025).

29. Young, S., & Lowery, C. (2024). High-definition liposuction contouring of the arms in males and females. *The American Journal of Cosmetic Surgery*, *41*, 269–273. https://www.semanticscholar.org/paper/1febc569d43e48ee2ffe02ef6eb5dec2248e1273 (accessed on 11th June 2025).

VASCULAR LESIONS AND COSMETIC TREATMENTS

8

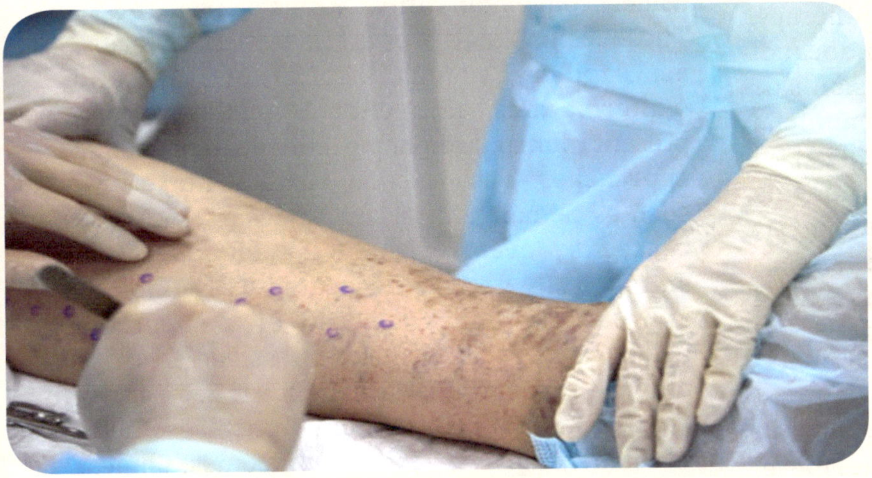

LEARNING OBJECTIVES

After studying this chapter, you will be able to:

1. Explain the vascular lesion classification
2. Discuss risk factors and causes
3. Understand diagnosis of vascular lesions
4. Explain the cosmetic implications of vascular lesions
5. Provide an overview of treatments cosmetically
6. Emphasize efficacy and safety of treatments

Introduction

The study of vascular lesions and their corresponding cosmetic therapy has gained widespread interest in the fields of dermatology and aesthetic medicine. Vascular lesions, a wide variety of abnormal vascular structures ranging from hemangiomas, varicosities, to glomuvenous malformations, have the potential to significantly impact the quality of life of an afflicted patient. Lesions can manifest as discolored patches or papules on the skin, with a tendency to induce psychological morbidity due to concomitant cosmetic dissatisfaction. With a better understanding of skin pathology and health, contemporary therapy has become advanced with increased methods of symptomatic alleviation and cosmetic renewal. Modern developments in the area offer new techniques that not only tend to correct the physical manifestations of vascular lesions but also tend to correct the emotional implications of their visibility in social life, thus this topic is an indispensable need for integrative dermatological practice (Boffa et al., 2004).

New modalities , such as sclerotherapy, laser, and electrosurgery are now frontiers in the treatment of vascular lesions, testifying to an expansion of the continuum of less invasive procedures with efficient interventions with lower levels of recovery. These procedures allow the clinician to treat individual vascular anomalies without disrupting the integrity of the surrounding tissue structure, thereby resulting in optimum cosmetic outcomes. For instance, the glomuvenous malformations study demonstrates the effectiveness of sclerotherapy, where chemical compounds like polidocanol have been used to effectively lower lesion size and improve cosmetic appearance with minimal severe adverse effects (Aranha et al., 2019). In addition, the evolution of sophisticated imaging technologies and genetics maximizes diagnosis and treatment planning for complicated vascular lesions, promoting a more individualized regimen consistent with current medical practice.

Thus, technological advance coupled with clinical expertise is a paradigm shift in vascular lesion management. Furthermore, the research of vascular lesions is entwined with universal problems in medical ethics and cultural perceptions of beauty that raise problematic questions about the accessibility of treatments and psychological therapy for patients. Perception of the conditions by society can influence not only patients' choices of whether or not to undergo therapy on cosmetic grounds but also the way medical practitioners approach such issues. With greater awareness of the physiological and psychological morbidity that accompanies vascular lesions, it becomes more essential that dermatologists embrace an interdisciplinary model of their management, with a focus on total care that includes physical and psychological health issues in patients. With the inclusion of the aesthetic factor within medical knowledge, specialists can create better patient advantages aesthetically and psychologically and thus emphasize the supreme need for further research and communication in this crucial area of dermatology (Boffa et al., 2004).

Definition of Vascular Lesions

Vascular lesions refer to blood vessel lesions and are caused by a broad array of causative mechanisms. They can be categorized into two main categories: vascular tumors and vascular malformations. Vascular malformations are usually congenital, with abnormal vessel growth. These lesions may present in numerous forms, i.e., capillary, venous, arterial, or lymphatic malformations, each with a specific clinical presentation and requiring individual diagnostic approaches. The vascular tumors, however, , such as hemangiomas and angiosarcomas, are caused by overgrowth of the blood vessels and typically need to be treated with different approaches. Understanding of the correct definition and classification of vascular lesions is crucial in cosmetic treatment, for it determines the selection of proper therapeutic procedures to further improve aesthetic outcomes. Clinical presentation may be quite disparate in vascular lesions, thus impacting their diagnosis as well as treatment. Symptoms may be heterogeneous based on the type and anatomical site of vascular lesions, ranging from skin color, edema, or functional impairment. These adjectives carry severe social and psychological effects on the victims, with most of them being pressured into receiving cosmetic therapy. For example, port-wine stains, which are malformations of the capillaries, may cause embarrassment and render one vulnerable to cosmetic alteration. Patients with extensive venous malformations may also have complications to be addressed. Thus, cosmetic therapy has evolved to address such complications, and various types of therapy are provided that range from laser therapy to minimally invasive procedures. Evaluation of the therapies, along with their effectiveness and safety, is crucial in ensuring optimal patient results in the case of vascular lesions. The latest innovation in vascular lesion diagnosis and therapy emphasizes the relationship between patient satisfaction, diagnosis, and treatment. Improved classification has increased diagnostic accuracy, and as a result, this serves as a guide for individualized therapeutic intervention. Malformations of blood vessels, which have been the subject of recent research, have been confronted with rare challenges in management due to complexity as well as variability in presentation (Inês et al., 2018). For instance, whereas some of the lesions can be treated with non-surgical treatment methods, others would require more invasive treatment strategies, , such as surgery, among the strategies (Geiger et al., 2021). Thus, the use of an evidence-based plan is useful in the practice of these interventions to keep practitioners abreast of the efficacy of different intervention modalities. Finally, educating people about the nuances of vascular lesions and their management fosters improved relationships between patients and healthcare providers. It encourages improved communication and improved clinical outcomes in cosmetic treatment (Figure 8.1).

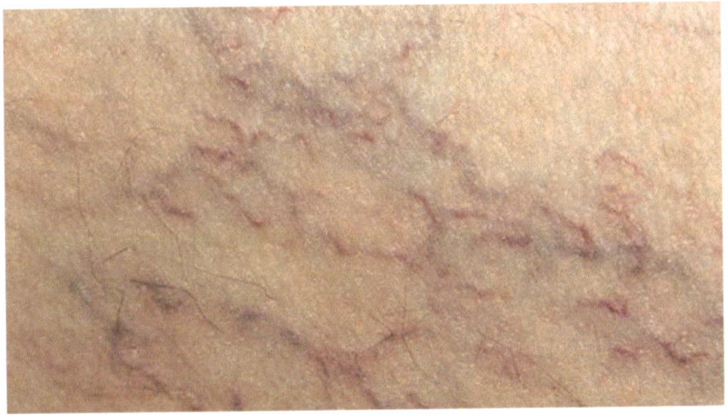

Figure 8.1. Vascular lesions.

Source: https://www.sydney-plasticsurgery.com.au/wp-content/uploads/2020/09/Screenshot_20200909-160645_Chrome.jpg.

Importance of Cosmetic Treatments

Recent years have seen the importance of cosmetic surgery reach the front page of aesthetic medicine, as it has in the news. Advanced technology has made several treatments available to address issues , such as vascular lesions, which may have an adverse impact on a patient's looks and mentality. Cosmetic treatments not only make the cosmetic appearance of the lesions simpler but also pave the way for higher levels of self-esteem and confidence in patients. By making vascular lesions less apparent through treatments , such as laser treatments, which have proven to be highly effective, cosmetic treatments play an essential role in contributing to mental, as well as physical, beauty. The development of treatments like the flash-lamp pulsed-dye laser (FPDL) is proof of how advanced treatments can make remarkable enhancements in patient satisfaction as well as quality of life in general and thus mark the role of cosmetic therapy in society (Clementi et al., 2024). Secondly, the application of accurate diagnostic machines, i.e., handheld ultrasound, has brought a huge difference to the cosmetic therapy sector. By precise imaging of vascular lesions and concurrent disease, physicians can tailor their therapies to the individual patient's specific anatomical features, allowing them to attain optimal results. By the use of high-frequency linear array transducers to image fat deposits and the tissue beneath, doctors are able to make informed decisions regarding the most appropriate therapies. These individually prescribed treatments not only optimize the effectiveness of procedures but also integrate the cosmetic treatment's safety record. When patients are planning interventions, having the ability to make comprehensive analyses improves practitioners' credibility with clients, subsequently supporting compliance with aesthetic medicine. This intersection of technology and individualized care highlights the growing dominance of cosmetic interventions in fixing not just aesthetic concerns but also individualized requirements (Gon et al., 2024). The commonality of cosmetic treatment across the world and the validity of such in modern society points towards a cultural transformation towards an appreciation of physical appearance and mental health. Patients now view such treatments not just as luxuries but as valid ways of contributing to their overall health. With improved education and knowledge of available treatments, more patients request interventions for vascular lesions and other skin conditions. The psycho-emotional benefit of feeling safe about one's looks cannot be overemphasized, as enhanced self-esteem is usually paired with enhanced socialization and improved psychological well-being. Since aesthetic treatments get more complex every year, they focus on creating a good environment in which people feel confident to experiment with solutions that meet their own concept of beauty. Social validation also legitimates the professional activity of aesthetic therapies as a part of integral treatment, making general health, beauty, and acceptance discourse richer.

8.1. Types of Vascular Lesions

Learning Outcome

1. Describe capillary malformations
2. Understand venous malformations
3. Explain arteriovenous malformations

The spectrum of vascular lesions encompasses a broad spectrum of abnormalities, classically divided into two broad categories: vascular malformations and vascular tumors. Vascular malformations include infantile hemangiomas, whose onset of growth starts early in infancy and may cause functional or cosmetic disability if they appear on the face or other exposed surfaces. Although the majority of infantile hemangiomas regress spontaneously during childhood, those that will not regress will require treatment, especially if they are cosmetic deformities or compressing a vital function. As opposed to vascular malformations, a dilation of a blood vessel, vein, or lymphatics, like capillary malformations, tends to remain stable or increase in size relative to the patient. Therefore, examination of the lesions is warranted; some of them, like the capillary malformations, potentially suggesting the presence of secondary syndromic disorders for which workup and potential treatment programs need to be entertained, as described in later literature (Diociaiuti et al., 2021). Another important group of vascular lesions is the angiokeratomas, benign vascular tumors consisting of telangiectasias and hyperkeratosis. These angiokeratomas are extremely frequent in the genitalia and limbs and of diverse colors from pink to dusky red with age and variety. From the literature, the most frequent among the angiokeratomas is the Fordyce angiokeratoma, predominantly in males and confined to the scrotum. Histopathological study is characterized by classical findings of hyperkeratosis and dilated blood vessels of the dermis that reveal their benign nature. While largely steering clear of symptoms, the lesions should be observed for change with time or potential cosmetic interventions. Treatments like diathermy have been found to be of benefit in treating solitary angiokeratomas, offering an avenue for alleviating patient anxiety regarding cosmetic outcome (Sharquie et al., 2021). Differential diagnosis of these vascular lesions is of utmost significance not only for their cosmetic significance but also for syndromic relevance that can develop. As a matter of example, complex malformations that encompass those with PIK3CA-related overgrowth syndromes will likely possess a complex relationship with systemic disturbance and may need to be treated by more than one specialty for best results. Klippel-Trenaunay syndrome is just one indication of the vascular disease's complexity. Further, adequate characterization of these lesions will enable early intervention, which will avoid significant complications, particularly those affecting airway obstruction. Vascular lesion classification is continuously updated based on investigations into the genetic basis of vascular lesions, their pathogenic mechanisms, and contribution to clinicians' expertise (Diociaiuti et al., 2021). Therefore, the evolving nature of vascular lesion types in turn demonstrates the importance of smart treatment paradigms that always prioritize both functional and esthetic considerations in the treatment of patients.

8.1.1. Capillary Malformations

Capillary malformations, also referred to as port-wine stains, are a prevalent kind of vascular lesions that are almost entirely present at birth. Malformations occur due to the abnormal development of the capillaries with consequential ongoing capillary dilation in the lesion on the skin. Presentation is generally in the form of flat, red or pinkish-colored lesions that become darker over time and are most commonly localized on the face or other extremities. Though mostly asymptomatic and benign, these vascular lesions can cause cosmetic distress of significant severity in the affected patients. Psychological stigma is severe in the face of obvious lesions and affects the patient's sense of self-esteem, leading to stigmatization and low self-esteem, thus the need for efficient cosmetic treatments. The introduction of therapeutic modalities for capillary malformations has changed the treatment strategy. Above all, laser therapy has evolved as a hallmark treatment modality in the form of using specific wavelengths to selectively target and coagulate the pathologic vessels without any damage to the normal surrounding tissue. The procedure is based on selective photothermolysis, in which the laser light is absorbed by the hemoglobin in the vessels and promotes progressive malformation disappearance. Furthermore, technology has improved efficacy rates and safety profiles, with fewer side effects from treatment compared to traditional methods. As encouraging as that sounds, the outcome depends upon lesion size and depth and other factors, and thus treatment planning has to be individualized to optimize outcome. The combination with laser has encouraged greater use of sclerotherapy as a good choice for capillary malformations, especially those that are complicated in nature. It is a minimally invasive technique that includes the injection of sclerosing agents that induce fibrosis of the enlarged vessels, making the visibility greatly reducing visibility. Electrochemical sclerotherapy with bleomycin, a chemotherapeutic agent, has been found to optimize the effectiveness of treatment through enhanced penetration into tissues and selectivity for malformations (Ciofani et al., 2025). These innovative technologies augur a greater appreciation of the need for multidisciplinary treatments in the management of vascular anomalies. Hence, ongoing studies continue to analyze the long-term efficacy and safety of such treatments, underscoring the necessity of a multidisciplinary therapeutic regimen for patients of capillary malformation (Raja et al., 2024) (Figure 8.2).

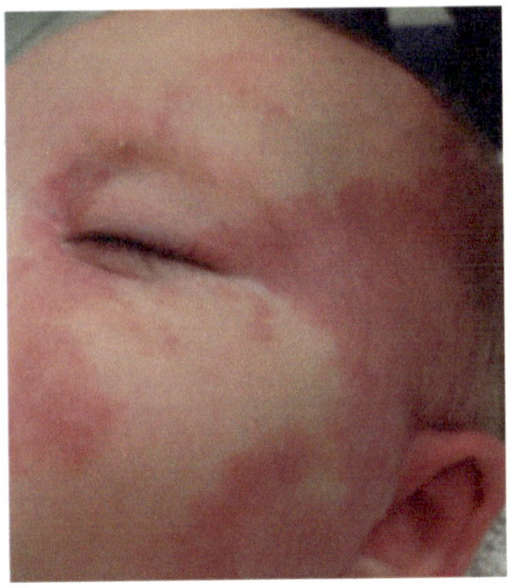

Figure 8.2. Capillary malformation (port wine stain) of the left face in infant.

Source: https://www.researchgate.net/profile/Gresham-Richter/publication/225050773/figure/fig4/AS:302674642784257@1449174666050/Capillary-malformation-port-wine-stain-of-the-left-face-in-infant.png.

8.1.2. Venous Malformations

The specialty of vascular medicine is fraught with a myriad of challenges, particularly venous malformations, which, by definition, are low-flow vascular anomalies. They are characterized by an abnormality of the venous system with dilated venous channels that can have both aesthetically and functionally deleterious effects. Though most often diagnosed in children, venous malformations are capable of causing chronic pain, cosmetic deformity, or even life-threatening complications if they invade essential structures. With vascular anomalies of other kinds, the very nature of venous malformations usually mandates a multidisciplinary management strategy aimed at functional as well as cosmetic rehabilitation of the patient. Through the greater understanding that comes from understanding the effect of such lesions, clinicians can better apply individually specific treatment to counter the individual challenge in each instance. Advances in treatment methods have also resulted in more options becoming available for treating venous malformations. One especially notable technique is electrochemical sclerotherapy with bleomycin (BEST), where electric impulses are utilized to enhance the therapeutic effect of bleomycin, a chemotherapeutic sclerosant. This therapy has become popular because it does not require surgery and has less opportunity to develop complications than other treatment modalities , such as ethanol sclerotherapy or surgery. Clinical experience indicates that BEST can significantly decrease the size of the lesion and its related symptoms, thereby enabling rapid recovery along with reduced side effects. With ongoing progress in treatment modalities, it is also more critical to evaluate the safety and efficacy of new modalities for cosmetic veneer formation and symptom management of venous malformations and patient quality of life (Ciofani et al., 2025). Coincident with these therapy advances in treatment have been imaging modality advances, e.g., photoacoustic microscopy, which have transformed diagnostic potential in venous malformations. This photoacoustic imaging technique takes advantage of tissue optical properties to provide improved contrast and spatial resolution compared to standard techniques like ultrasonography. Photoacoustic microscopy has been beneficial, particularly in vascular abnormalities architecture visualization and characterization. A case series of pediatric subjects highlighted the benefit of vessel caliber and length measurement, key parameters in grading the venous malformation size. These imaging modalities not only improve diagnostic potential but are able to allow real-time evaluation of treatment efficacy, guiding clinicians toward making evidence-based decisions about therapeutic options and outcomes in prognosis (Tay et al., 2024) (Figure 8.3).

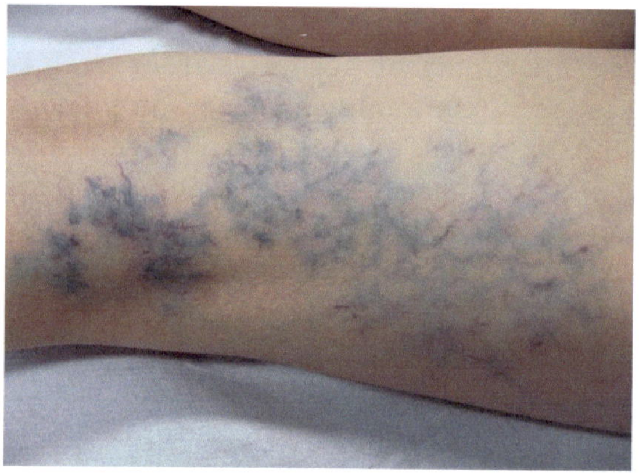

Figure 8.3. A venous malformation is present on the right leg of this 12-year-old boy.

Source: https://www.compva.com/fileadmin/images/wissenschaftliche-artikel/1-5-venoese-malformation/1-5-03-venoese-malformation-bein.jpg.

8.1.3. Arteriovenous Malformations

Arteriovenous malformations (AVMs) are a more complex type of vascular lesion, with anomalous vascular connections between arteries and veins, bypassing the capillary bed. They can occur in most parts of the body, including the brain, and can lead to serious complications, , such as hemorrhage or neurological damage. Where AVMs are symptomatic, the treatments can be highly variable, often in reference to size, location, and grade of the lesion. A Spetzler-Martin grading system is a standard classification system for surgeons to use in determining proper therapeutic intervention. A diagnosis of AVM will tend to elicit a thorough examination of the various treatment options, including surgical excision, embolization, and radiosurgery, tailored specifically to each patient's unique situation, thus ensuring a comprehensive approach to treating these potentially life-threatening conditions (Figure 8.4).

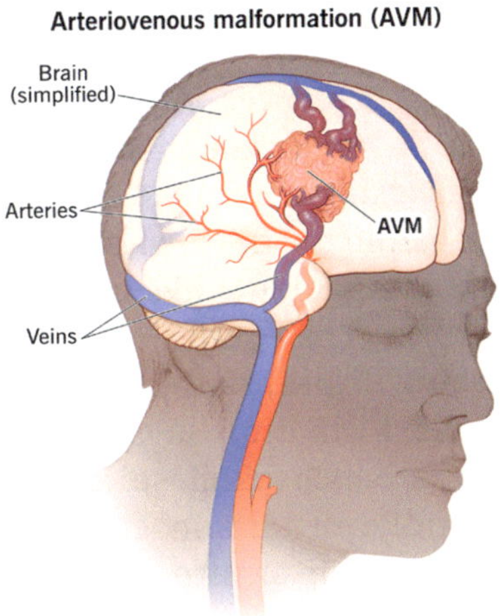

Figure 8.4. Arteriovenous malformation.

Source: https://my.clevelandclinic.org/-/scassets/images/org/health/articles/16755-arteriovenous-malformation-avm.

New innovations in embolic agents have improved the efficacy and safety of treatment for AVM. The CLARIDAD clinical trial was performed on the novel liquid embolic agent ihtObtura that showed marvelous success in neurovascular embolization of AVMs, dural arteriovenous fistulas, and hypervascular tumors. The agent enables occlusion of the vascular structure as a whole with significant improvement of anatomical visualization during intervention and overall treatment effectiveness. Interestingly, the study referenced a 99% therapeutic efficacy in catheterizations, noting the precision and reliability of this procedure. Moreover, the minimal loss in radiopacity also bodes well for the effectiveness of ihtObtura as a promising drug for the treatment of vascular lesions, and it could be a game-changer agent in the market.

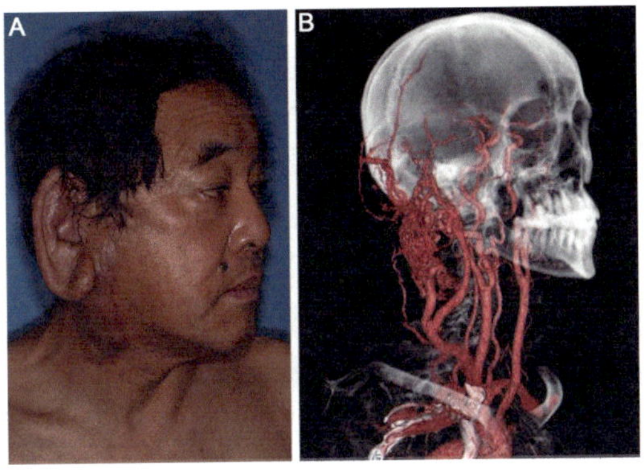

Figure 8.5. Arteriovenous malformation (AVM) of the head and neck. A, preoperative photograph of the AVM involving the right temporoauricular and neck. The lesion showed rapid enlargement. B, preoperative enhanced computed tomography showing a large AVM.

Source: https://www.researchgate.net/publication/350366530/figure/fig1/AS:1007098116706309@1617122310983/Arteriovenous-malformation-AVM-of-the-head-and-neck-A-preoperative-photograph-of-the.ppm.

Thus, such innovation promises a brighter future in terms of improved procedures for those suffering from AVMs, resulting in improved patient prognosis and quality of life. While treatment of AVMs has evolved to include newer techniques, understanding the genetic underpinnings and associated conditions is still significant. One such traditional example is hereditary hemorrhagic telangiectasia (HHT), a genetic disorder that predisposes individuals to vascular malformations, including cerebral

AVMs. Surgical intervention for AVMs in patients with HHT was reported to be successful with minimal rates of complications in systematic reviews. Complete eradication is often achievable with a brief hospital course, a reflection of the potential for successful management in this high-risk group. As ongoing research continues to educate us further regarding AVMs and related conditions, it also points toward the importance of individualized treatment plans that consider both the genetic and clinical histories. These findings will be vital in advancing the treatment of AVMs and achieving optimal cosmetic and functional outcomes in patients, thus highlighting the need to integrate medical data with cosmetic therapy in the management of vascular lesions (Frantzias et al., 2024; Llíbre-Guerra et al., 2024) (Figure 8.5).

Test Your Knowledge

1. What are the key clinical differences between capillary malformations and venous malformations?
2. Which type of vascular malformation is most likely to cause complications?

8.2. Causes and Risk Factors

Learning Outcome

1. Discuss genetic predisposition in the development and manifestation of various vascular lesions
2. Explain how vascular lesions are profoundly influenced by environmental factors
- Describe the role of hormonal changes in the development and exacerbation of vascular lesions

The pathogenesis of vascular lesions depends on a plethora of determinants which can be generally categorized into genetic, environmental, and lifestyle determinants. A history of vascular disorders in the family can predispose a person to the risk, and in certain inherited syndromes, the blood vessel structure and function can be impaired, leading to abnormal growth or lesions. In addition, environmental factors , such as exposure to toxins or ultraviolet light may exacerbate pre-existing vascular issues, ultimately resulting in lesion formation. The union of these environmental and genetic variables helps to demonstrate the intricacy of vascular health and the need for ongoing research to ascertain the full spectrum of causes associated with vascular lesions. Lifestyle components are highly responsible for the formation of vascular lesions, including diet, physical activity, and smoking habits. The intake of saturated fats, refined carbohydrates, and processed foods is related to the formation of such diseases as atherosclerosis, which manifests itself as vascular lesions. Secondly, physical inactivity is a proven risk factor, since physical exercise guarantees blood circulation and may be responsible for the prevention of lesion formation. In contrast, smoking entails the introduction of toxic substances into the blood flow, which not only detrimentally affects the vascular endothelium but also promotes inflammation and thrombosis. It is therefore crucial to grasp these lifestyle aspects to facilitate prevention and optimal management of vascular lesions, in favor of the necessity for public health policy to promote healthier lifestyles. Comorbidities also significantly enhance the risk of vascular lesion development, and obesity and diabetes are prime candidates. In diabetes, hyperglycemia that is long-standing can lead to endothelial dysfunction, making blood vessels susceptible to damage and lesion development. Obesity is also associated with systemic inflammation and changes in lipid metabolism, both of which enhance vascular-related health issues. Available evidence confirms that the immune system remains to be discovered in this regard, with natural killer (NK) cells influencing vascular homeostasis and responding to obesity cues (Palano et al., 2022). The relationship between the conditions and how they influence vascular function supports the necessity of holistic treatment and prevention measures, with the improved understanding of the multifactorial evolution of vascular lesions.

8.2.1. Genetic Predisposition

Genetic predisposition plays a central role in the pathogenesis of most vascular lesions and their consequent presentation and management. They are predisposed to occur with hereditary characteristics, as seen in glomuvenous malformations. That there are sporadic and familial cases indicates the presence of a genetic factor, since some patients inherit pathogenic mutations that predispose them to the formation of these vascular malformations. Identification of these genetic factors offers an improved understanding of the pathophysiology, thereby maximizing treatment modalities. With the progression of modern genetics, it uncovers intricate relationships between clinical expression and genetic alterations, underlining the importance of incorporating genetic analysis in the management of vascular lesions, ultimately directing cosmetic treatment strategies and improving patient results (Boffa et al., 2004). In cosmetic therapy for vascular lesions, genetic predisposition can direct clinicians with regard to the most appropriate therapeutic approach. For instance, glomuvenous malformation patients will need different measures according to their genetic structure. Surgical interventions, as much as they are suitable for solitary lesions, prove difficult in multiple or familial cases. Recent studies have reported that therapies , such as sclerotherapy may offer significant cosmetic advantages, especially if guided by profound insight into the genetic cause of the lesions. Knowledge of the specific mutations involved could direct practitioners to customized therapies that maximize efficacy with minimized side effects, exemplifying the intersection of genetic science and clinical dermatology (Aranha et al., 2019). Furthermore, identification of genetic susceptibility both enhances the efficacy of treatment and the patient's overall comfort. Patients who understand the genetic origin of their vascular lesions feel reassured that their condition is not solely the result of environmental factors. Such an awareness can ensure greater compliance with therapeutic regimens and encourage active care measures. Besides, as dermatology evolves, using genetic information in cosmetic treatments can lead to more patient-specific care. It targets both the cosmetic and the medical treatments, such that aesthetically pleasing results are obtained in the patients while their conditions' genetic components are addressed. Ultimately, developing an overarching understanding of genetic predisposition will be most important in determining how to improve therapeutic modalities in vascular lesions and their cosmetic consequences (Boffa et al., 2004).

8.2.2. Environmental Influences

Vascular lesions are quite susceptible to external factors, which can amplify their incidence and influence the effectiveness of cosmetic treatments. Of these, ultraviolet (UV) light is a primary causative agent in skin damage and vascular disease. Chronic exposure to UV light can lead to changes in the structure and function of the skin and eventually have vessels become more conspicuous and susceptible to lesions. In addition, environmental pollutants , such as particulate and chemical matter can induce inflammatory mechanisms that amplify underlying vascular disease. These considerations add to the many factors contributing to skin aging and lesion formation, where both intrinsic and extrinsic mechanisms are involved, further emphasizing the value of thorough assessment and tailored treatment protocols. As such, familiarity with these environmental issues takes on extreme significance when comparing the efficacy of cosmetic treatment modalities for improving the appearance of vascular lesions. Another environmental factor that influences vascular lesions is lifestyle, particularly eating, smoking, and stress control behaviors. Poor diet, which leads to obesity and chronic inflammation, can exacerbate vascular diseases , such as rosacea, thereby requiring dedicated cosmetic treatments for improvement. On the contrary, a healthy diet rich in antioxidants will enhance vascular health and potentially retard the formation of lesions. Furthermore, smoking is also known to cause significant adverse effects on vascularity and cosmetic appearance of the skin, and hence, it is a significant factor in evaluating treatment outcomes. The interaction between lifestyle modification and appropriate cosmetic procedures yields measurable patient satisfaction and quality-of-life enhancement. Therefore, therapists should integrate discussion regarding lifestyle change into their vascular lesion treatment planning and identify the interconnectedness of these environmental factors. The role of weather conditions, temperature, and humidity also greatly contributes to the impact on vascular lesions and treatment. Extreme temperatures are likely to produce vascular responses, e.g., vasodilation or vasoconstriction, and make vascular lesions more visible. As an illustration, cold will lead to blood vessels constricting, whereas in warm and humid environments, they will become dilated, aggravating conditions , such as rosacea. Understanding these environmental variables allows clinicians to prescribe efficient skincare regimens and cosmetic therapies appropriate to certain patient needs. In addition, seasonally based fluctuations in UV exposure necessitate adaptive treatment approaches to mitigate the altered conditions impacting skin health. By incorporating these variables into treatment protocols for vascular lesions, healthcare professionals can maximize the effectiveness of interventions and promote better skin health through the long term, as a consequence of which patient outcomes are maximized (Figure 8.6).

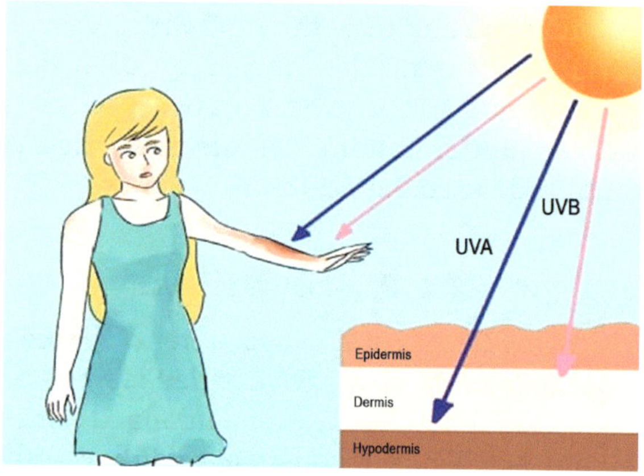

Figure 8.6. Ultraviolet (UV) radiation: a significant contributor to skin damage and vascular abnormalities.

Source: https://treatcancer.com/wp-content/uploads/2022/06/670px-Understand-the-Effects-of-Different-UV-Rays-Step-1-450x338-1.jpg.

8.2.3. Hormonal Changes

Hormonal changes play a central role in the pathogenesis and exacerbation of vascular lesions, which typically take place in young people as well as in older adults. Hormonal changes, particularly during stages , such as puberty, pregnancy, and menopause, are likely to exert a significant impact on the vascular system. These changes may predispose to the formation of many vascular lesions, including telangiectasias and port-wine stains, as visible engorged capillaries, which may cause both cosmetic problems and psychological distress to the patients. Identifying the dermal hormonal mechanisms is critical to both dermatologists and aesthetic practitioners in planning effective therapy for the treatment of such lesions. By realizing the function of hormones, clinicians can tailor interventions not just to improve the look of the lesions but also to consider the overall hormonal status of the patients to prevent recurrence or further complications. Progress in the arena of cosmetic procedures has increasingly included evidence-based care tailored to the unique requirements of the hormonal changes. For instance, laser therapy, , such as the FPDL, has been well-documented to be an effective modality for the treatment of hemoglobin-bearing vascular lesions. Research evidence assessing the effectiveness of FPDL has shown that an extremely high rate of patients showed excellent clearance of lesions following treatment, testifying to the effectiveness of focused interventions in cosmetic dermatology (Clementi et al., 2024). These technological advances, besides providing a solution to the cosmetic impact of hormonal changes, highlight the significance of knowing the hormonal composition of a patient. Such an understanding enables practitioners to optimize the treatment results through personalized care that deals with individualized hormonal factors. Further, the long-pulse alexandrite laser is also another significant advance in the treatment of vascular lesions, particularly those influenced by hormonal changes. This laser system has worked on the basis of selective absorption by melanin and hemoglobin, thus usable on various vascular and pigmented lesions. With ongoing research indicating advancements in this area, practitioners can utilize the long-pulse alexandrite laser more optimally to treat conditions exacerbated by hormonal fluctuations (Chen et al., 2023). With greater knowledge of how hormones impact vascular lesions, practitioners must be ever cautious in their treatment strategy to ensure safety and efficacy. The blending of hormonal insight and state-of-the-art pictorial treatment method positions cosmetic dermatology as able to address the physical and psychological elements of vascular lesions, treating the malady whole while providing total care for victims of the condition (Figure 8.7).

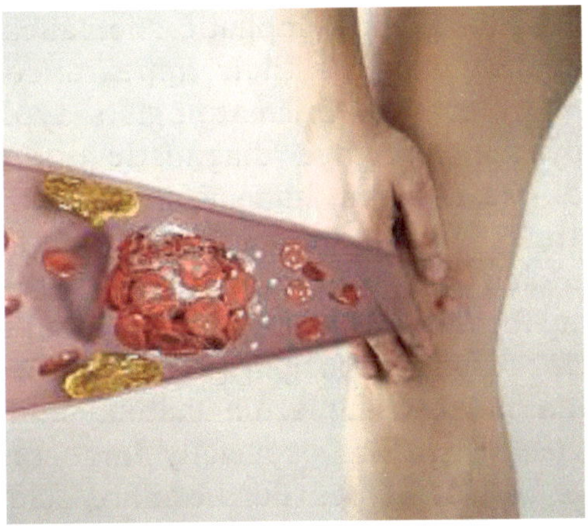

Figure 8.7. Illustration of deep vein thrombosis (DVT) in the lower limb.

Source: https://encrypted-tbn0.gstatic.com/images?q=tbn:ANd9GcSNM2JHWEmGo6R3_qpev8wFqzsjs7CX6seoEw&s.

Test Your Knowledge

1. Which genetic mutation is most commonly associated with vascular lesions?
2. Can environmental factors trigger the development or worsening of vascular lesions?

8.3. Diagnosis of Vascular Lesions

Learning Outcome

1. Explain the importance of clinical examination in the assessment and treatment planning for vascular lesions
2. Describe imaging techniques
3. Define biopsy procedures

Vascular lesion diagnosis entails a certain degree of familiarity with their multifaceted presentations and pathophysiology. Vascular lesions, , such as hemangiomas, venous malformations, and lymphatic anomalies, can significantly vary in their appearance and clinical relevance. Dermatologists typically employ the combined diagnostic output of clinical presentation, imaging modalities, and sometimes histopathological examination to define such lesions appropriately. Non-surgical imaging techniques like Doppler ultrasound and magnetic resonance imaging (MRI) are especially essential in assessing lesion anatomy and flow patterns, which are especially important to resolve between types. Furthermore, scientific advances in dermatology continue to narrow down diagnostic approaches, paving the way for more powerful surveillance and management regimens that coexist with evolving aesthetic and health agendas within dermatology (Boffa et al., 2004). Categorization of vascular lesions hitherto has been the most difficult due to nomenclature and treatment variabilities. Accurate diagnosis is not only necessary for effective treatment but also for reassurance and patient education. The most common vascular lesions, e.g., capillary malformations and arteriovenous malformations, need to be thought over carefully to plan their treatment modalities. Early diagnosis reduces the chances of complications and improves the quality of cosmetic outcomes, and thus it is essential for practitioners to be knowledgeable about available classification systems. The overlap of multidisciplinary approaches, with contributions from surgical, dermatological, and interventional radiology specialties, ensures maximum diagnostic precision. This collaborative model enables healthcare clinicians to develop comprehensive treatment plans for treating the medical and aesthetic concerns of vascular lesions (Davidson et al., 2015). The use of advanced diagnostic techniques is supplemented with the increasing number of cosmetic treatments accessible for the cosmetic concerns of vascular lesions. For instance, laser therapy is now a prime non-surgical option, designing specifically to target the vascular targets without tissue-destructive damage in the proximity. The integration of diagnostic imaging and therapeutic treatment allows for treatments to be tailored that are patient-specific in their features and preferences. Additionally, advances in pharmaceutical technology further expand the range of interventions available, providing patients with maximum minimal morbidity while optimizing aesthetic results. As dermatology progresses, prioritization of refining finer diagnostic methods is poised to advance therapies for improving clinical efficacy and aesthetic satisfaction in those with vascular lesions (Boffa et al., 2004).

8.3.1. Clinical Examination

Clinical examination is also the backbone for vascular lesions evaluation and treatment planning in cosmetic dermatology. Apart from the close visual inspection of the lesions, it also entails a thorough patient history and symptom assessment. The clinicians must remain sharply aware of the characteristics of various vascular lesions, which are hemangiomas, telangiectasias, and varicose veins. Understanding the clinical presentation allows for differentiation between benign lesions and those needing investigation or intervention. Such complete assessment is necessary because improper diagnosis results in suboptimal treatment and complications. The clinician must also ascertain the psychological impact of these lesions on patients as vascular lesions have a profound effect on self-esteem and quality of life. A detailed strategy is thus required during clinical examination to formulate the best treatment plans for patients seeking cosmetic treatment. Since the broad armamentarium of vascular lesion treatments on offer makes it difficult to decide on the best intervention without a clinical examination, this should be the guiding principle for the selection of the best intervention. Laser treatment, sclerotherapy, and PDT are just some of the treatments commonly employed in cosmetic practice with specific indications and contraindications following examination. As an example, laser therapy can be highly effective in superficial vascular lesions due to specificity for targeting hemoglobin in blood vessels. In comparison, PDT, with great success in most clinical trials, offers a new approach using photosensitizers to produce reactive oxygen species that can destroy vascular structures (Demian et al., 2017). Clinicians must be current with new treatments and adapt examination protocols accordingly, such that treatment is in line with up-to-date evidence-based practice but individualized to every patient's unique presentation and preferences. Moreover, the integration of clinical guidelines into the examination is essential in optimizing patient care in cosmetic dermatology. The ESC Guidelines stress the importance of structured practice in exercising clinical judgment and treating patients, particularly in the case of vascular health (Habib et al., 2015). The guidelines may serve as a guide to clinicians on how to ensure that they are not only evaluating vascular lesions correctly but also considering the broader implications of treatment. For instance, an understanding of the systemic impact of certain vascular conditions can influence the choice of cosmetic therapy, i.e., routine monitoring for potential sequelae. By adhering to established protocols and staying vigilant in clinical assessment, practitioners can optimize their results and foster an effective collaboration with patients, one that entails mutual decision-making within the cosmetic therapy process (Figure 8.8).

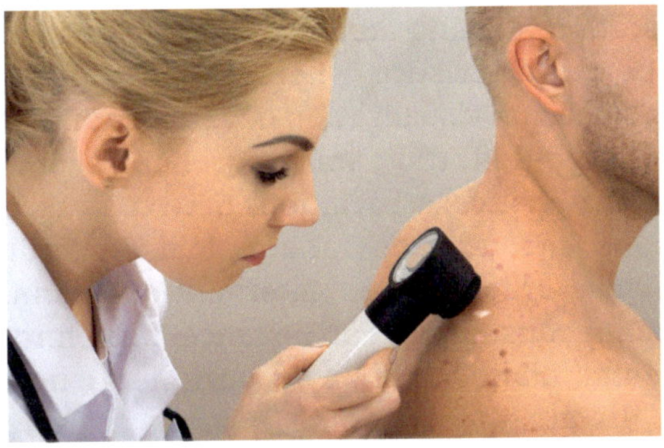

Figure 8.8. Clinical examination of assessment for vascular lesions.

Source: https://www.outsourcestrategies.com/wp-content/uploads/2019/10/dermatology-medical-billing-and-coding-key-considerations-for-success.jpg.

8.3.2. Imaging Techniques

Enhanced imaging techniques form the basis of the diagnosis and therapy of vascular lesions and contribute significantly to cosmetic treatment efficacy. Various modalities , such as ultrasound, MRI, and computed tomography (CT) provide essential information regarding the anatomy, flow, and vascular anatomy of the lesions. Ultrasound, specifically, is a non-invasive real-time imaging modality that allows clinicians to assess vascular malformation hemodynamics for a more accurate diagnosis and personalized treatment plan. Through the proper determination of lesion size and extent, ultrasound allows for the delivery of next-generation therapeutic strategies, which enhance patient outcomes. This confluence of treatment and imaging modalities emphasizes the imperative for an integrated approach to vascular lesion management in the field of cosmetics, allowing practitioners to deliver interventions that are both clinically effective and aesthetically ideal. Access to advanced imaging modalities has significantly enhanced our knowledge about vascular lesions and surrounding anatomy in the last few years," Imaging modalities , such as MRI, are high-resolution imaging methods that delineate soft tissue characteristics, whereas CT angiography offers optimal visualization of vascular anatomy. Such high-definition imaging enables one to recognize critical associations between vascular lesions and adjacent anatomical structures, which is crucial when intervention planning is being considered. For instance, proximity of vascular malformations to peripheral nerves can dictate the style and type of treatment, as has been determined in studies that have explored ultrasound-guided microwave ablation techniques for treatment of such lesions. Therefore, the incorporation of state-of-the-art imaging technologies into procedural interventions not only allows for accurate diagnoses but also prevents complications during procedural interventions, thereby improving the safety profile of cosmetic procedures. Furthermore, the evolving landscape of imaging technologies continues to influence and refine treatment paradigms for vascular lesions. Imaging technologies , such as hydrodissection, employed in ultrasound-guided microwave ablation, are a prime example of how imaging can be utilized to protect vital structures in such a way that cosmetic procedures yield optimal results without compromising adjacent tissues. The ability to image and guide complex vascular networks in real time is revolutionary, particularly as it makes interventions more specific. As highlighted in recent studies, the safety of treatment and efficacy of treatment are significantly improved with precise imaging, with patients subsequently achieving high satisfaction rates. Through vigilant monitoring of imaging information, therapists are able to quantify therapy outcomes and organize follow-ups, ultimately enhancing the process of patients with vascular lesions during cosmetic therapy (Wang et al., 2024; Ciofani et al., 2025) (Figure 8.9).

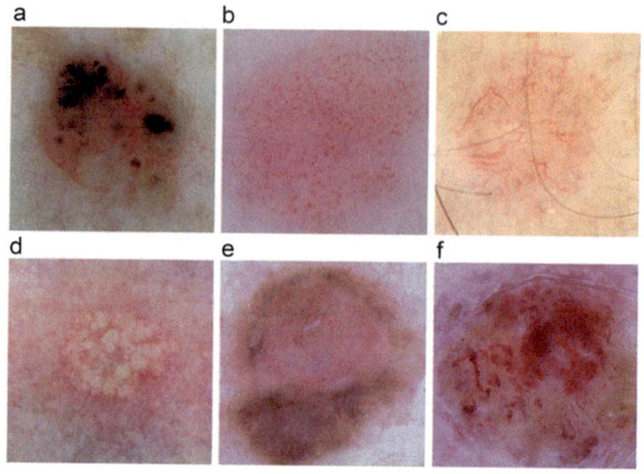

Figure 8.9. Examples of vascular structures seen in dermoscopic images of skin lesions: a linear b dotted c hairpin d linear crown e arborizing f polymorphous vessels. Some of these structures give very specific diagnostic clues as in (d) the presence of crown vessels (linear straight) distributed on the periphery of the lesion surrounded by yellowish globular structures is a specific marker for sebaceous hyperplasia.

Source: https://www.researchgate.net/publication/322341299/figure/fig1/AS:961825160052761@1606328396832/Examples-of-vascular-structures-seen-in-dermoscopic-images-of-skin-lesions-a-linear-b.gif.

8.3.3. Biopsy Procedures

Biopsy procedures are valuable in the diagnostic evaluation of vascular lesions, particularly in the distinction between neoplastic and non-neoplastic vascular lesions, as well as between benign and malignant neoplasms. Biopsy procedures allow for direct analysis of tissue specimens, by which the pathologist can assess cellular architecture and direct the appropriate therapy. In vascular lesions, a biopsy procedure can be helpful in the distinction between hemangiomas and more sinister lesions, including angiosarcomas, which may require aggressive management. Varying techniques, including excisional, incisional, and needle biopsies, are utilized, and the choice of these generally depends on the size of lesions, their location, and clinical suspicion of malignancy. The inclusion of advanced imaging modalities, , such as optical coherence tomography (OCT), serves to guide these biopsies, improving diagnostic yield and expanding the scope of available treatment for superficial vascular tumors, which leads to improved cosmetic outcome in cosmetic procedures (Giral et al., 2023). Besides, minimally invasive biopsies are more sought after for the treatment of vascular lesions due to their lower morbidity. Traditional surgical biopsies, as invasive, can cause severe scarring or complications and are therefore particularly undesirable in cosmetic applications. Techniques , such as fine needle aspiration (FNA) and core needle biopsy not only minimize tissue disturbance but also enable rapid diagnosis. With the developments in imaging and anesthesia, these can be performed on an outpatient basis, which improves a lot in patient satisfaction and experience. The potential to utilize laser therapies like laser-assisted biopsy is also enhanced with the trend towards more cosmetic procedures, providing a modality for real-time intervention with the added benefit of sparing overlying healthy tissue. This approach not only improves cosmetics in patients but also reduces the possibility of complications from more aggressive treatments (Barile et al., 2018). Biopsy serves a function more than diagnosis; it profoundly affects treatment protocols for vascular lesions. Successful biopsies can inform clinicians regarding the disease's extent, something relevant in particular to cosmetic treatment planning. Once a diagnosis has been confirmed, a variety of treatment modalities like laser therapy, cryosurgery, and sclerotherapy can be tailored according to the findings on biopsy. For instance, where basal cell carcinoma is found, as has been discussed in the literature, non-surgical approaches could be employed in an attempt to produce the most favorable cosmetic outcome while ensuring oncological clearance. The synergy between accurate biopsy analysis and subsequent cosmetic treatment protocols ultimately enriches the therapeutic scene of patients with vascular lesions, and thereby assists in more individualized and aesthetically rewarding outcomes in vascular lesion therapy (Giral et al., 2023) (Figure 8.10).

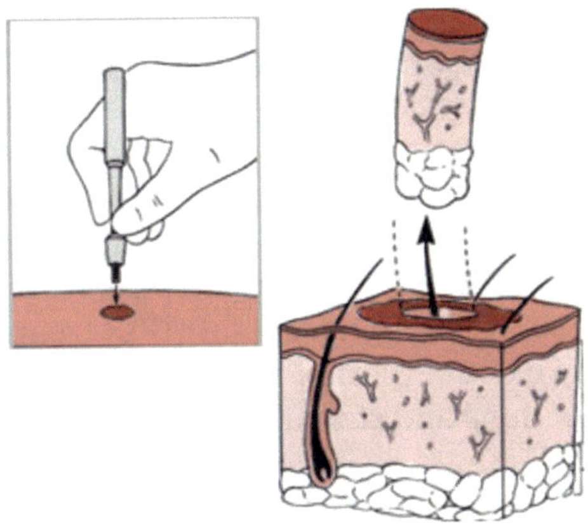

Figure 8.10. Skin biopsy.

Source: https://www.fvhospital.com/wp-content/uploads/2020/03/sinh-thiet-da-2.jpg.

Test Your Knowledge

1. What clinical features help differentiate a capillary malformation from other vascular lesions?
2. Which imaging modality is most appropriate for evaluating the extent and flow characteristics of a vascular lesion?

8.4. Cosmetic Implications of Vascular Lesions

Learning Outcome

1. Understand the psychological impact on patients
2. Describe the social stigma surrounding vascular lesions
3. Explain the importance of early intervention

The aesthetic impact of vascular lesions is also widespread, extending beyond matters of appearance. Spider veins and hemangiomas, and other vascular lesions, tend to cause visits for correction because they are noticeable. Their influence on self-esteem and social interactions is a powerful consideration that has fueled demand for cosmetic correction with the aim of enhancing appearance. With growing demands for non-surgical cosmetic procedures, practitioners have been eager to employ advanced technologies involving non-ionizing radiation (NIR) to provide effective outcomes. Laser and intense pulsed light (IPL) treatments can be particularly used to target such vascular imperfections and stimulate rejuvenation of the skin with minimal side effects. Although some aesthetic enhancement may be achievable at once, long-term effects and the likelihood of side effects remain research areas and a subject of concern for the field of dermatologic aesthetic practice (International Commission on Non-Ionizing Radiation Protection, 2020). With injectable procedures gaining strong ground in the realm of aesthetics, hyaluronic acid (HA) dermal fillers have become center stage, particularly in patients that want to reverse the appearance of vascular lesions. Even as these fillers are touted for their facial structure support and tightening of the skin, they too are not completely risk-free. Vascular occlusion is a severe adverse effect of HA injectables in the event that the filler inadvertently obstructs blood vessels, which leads to severe outcomes, including necrosis of the tissue. Therefore, clinician education and awareness of vascular occlusion hazards are essential in performing such procedures. There are new quality improvement (QI) initiatives focusing on ensuring the enhancement of clinician knowledge and proficiency in treating complications. Through systematic educational intervention, practitioners are better able to prepare for, recognize, and handle vascular occlusion incidents, ultimately promoting improved patient outcomes and safety (Sanders et al., 2024). The creation of combined treatment modalities for vascular lesions serves as a testament to the healthcare profession's commitment to patient-centered practice. Technological innovations in treatments, including combination therapies that integrate laser treatments with injectable fillers, hold promising avenues for maximizing cosmetic results while addressing underlying vascular conditions. With new methods and technology becoming available, regulation is required to ensure their safety and efficacy. The International Commission on Non-Ionizing Radiation Protection (ICNIRP) also emphasizes stringent standards of application of NIR devices. Additionally, ongoing studies on adverse effects and rates of complications need to be carried out to assess the full scope of effects in patient populations, particularly where higher-risk individuals are present. The industry's proactive response to regulation and training of clinicians serves to shore up the columns of effective, safe, and aesthetically satisfying treatments for vascular lesions in the cosmetic field (International Commission on Non-Ionizing Radiation Protection, 2020).

8.4.1. Psychological Impact on Patients

Perceptibility of vascular lesions can do a great deal in influencing the psychological health of a person. Patients normally develop embarrassment and anxiety when confronted with disfigurement of the skin, as societal beauty standards normally come with unblemished skin. These emotions normally cause social withdrawal, lower self-esteem, and ultimately the development of depression. Secondarily, if vascular lesions present more as less severe illnesses, , such as those with similar presentations (e.g., hemangiomas), fear and apprehension about the health status can result from incorrect diagnosis. The psychological distress generated by these lesions underscores the necessity of accurate diagnostic methods, which can allay fear of potential malignancy and its impact on overall well-being. Therefore, even the cosmetic treatments of the emotional effects of vascular lesions are most important in providing comprehensive care that minimizes both physical and mental consequences. The cosmetic treatments for vascular lesions, although often wanted for their cosmetic effects, have the ability to also prevent psychological consequences. Successful treatment can lead to dramatic enhancements in patients' perceptions of themselves and how they relate to others, enabling them to return to social environments that might otherwise have been avoided. Cosmetic patients often report improved self-esteem and less anxiety following treatment as evidence of the close relationship between bodily looks and mental health. Thus, medical professionals need to take both the physical and psychological impacts of cosmetic treatment of vascular lesions into account. Encouraging a holistic approach that acknowledges the psychological impact, medical professionals can better treat and satisfy patients. Additionally, individualized psychological support is essential in treating vascular lesions, particularly among patients with severe lesions or complex treatments. Integration of psychological counseling in a holistic treatment regimen can provide patients with coping measures to help them deal with the emotional workload of their conditions. Therapy sessions or support groups, for example, can enable individuals to share their experiences and build resilience against societal pressure regarding appearance. Incorporating patient education on the types of their condition, as defined in pathology literature on conditions , such as rosacea and their psychological impact, serves to promote understanding and acceptance. This multidisciplinary approach, in addition to attempting to enhance the efficacy of cosmetic therapy, prompts patients experiencing complications related to vascular lesions to be in better spirits, ultimately leading to a better therapeutic outcome.

8.4.2. Social Stigma and Perception

Social stigmatization of vascular lesions has significant impacts on individuals treatment choices and emotional well-being. A majority of individuals with apparent vascular disorders—, such as port-wine stains or hemangiomas, are exposed to social judgment that may lead to shame or inadequacy. This social judgment usually stems from historical fallacious beliefs linking physical appearance and inner value or character. Therefore, the sufferers may avoid public interaction or decline medical treatment because they are afraid of being ridiculed or stigmatized. The stigma could be particularly pronounced in children, who may be bullied or shunned due to how they look. Resolving these with awareness and education is very crucial in eliminating the myths that exist with vascular lesions and building a less prejudiced attitude towards individuals who access cosmetic procedures. Attitudes towards cosmetic treatment of vascular lesions also play a central part in how one is going to engage with one's healthcare decisions. Certain patients will think treatments, anything from excision to laser therapy, are cosmetic, prioritizing appearance over serious health concerns. Therefore, such an attitude might deter patients from getting the option that can have the most impact on one's quality of life. The combination of perceived efficacy and stigma can create even more stress or unwillingness to undergo treatment, as patients combat societal beauty and normalcy standards. Cultural differences in what constitutes a cosmetic intervention complicate this even more. Natural appearances are preferred in other cultures, and others have beauty norms, which exert additional pressure on those with vascular lesions to conform to specific expectations, as observed in patient recovery and empowerment studies (Chukwu & Mankila, 2018). Physicians, particularly dermatologists, enjoy the unique privilege of countering stigma and myths surrounding vascular lesions through empathetic care and education. Effective communication and patient education play a key role in the removal of myths over such conditions and their treatment. Dermatology nurses and specialists need to play a key role in establishing a facilitative setting that will ensure open discussion of patients' issues and treatment requests. By highlighting the health significance of skin and also the psychological advantages of cosmetic procedures, practitioners can enable patients to make educated choices that are in line with their individual needs and values. Such positive interactions not only restore confidence among the providers and patients but also assist in reducing stigma against vascular lesions, evolving towards a more tolerant practice of cosmetic treatments and leading individuals to gain access to care that they are entitled to (Lai et al., 2018) (Figure 8.11).

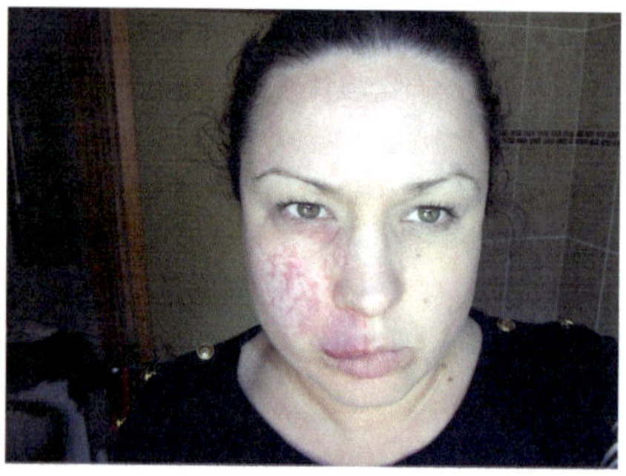

Figure 8.11. Facial port-wine stain birthmark in an adult patient.

Source: https://www.birthmarksupportgroup.org.uk/media/22036/beth-higgins_1.jpg.

8.4.3. Importance of Early Intervention

Early treatment of vascular lesions is of greatest significance for optimal patient outcomes in cosmetic situations in which physical appearance directly influences self-esteem and quality of life. Research has shown that treatment at an early point can lead to improved aesthetic results and less complications. For instance, early patients with hypertrophic scars are treated using procedures like IPL in conjunction with a fractional erbium laser and achieve far better outcomes than those treated with conventional therapies after the healing process is advanced. Such interventions introduced early can potentially prevent the formation of more severe scarring and hence emphasize the clinical importance of treating early after trauma (Dai et al., 2024). Such an aggressive approach not only enhances the cosmetic outcome of scars but also accelerates healing, giving patients with visible vascular lesions psychological and emotional comfort. In complex cases, , such as scalp AVMs, the need for urgent treatment becomes more significant because of a potential risk for serious complications and aesthetic loss. AVMs in the scalp require early intervention and treatment because late treatment poses a risk of hemorrhage and widespread cosmetic deformity. An example case of one young female patient serves to demonstrate this, where endovascular embolization followed by surgical resection gave a definitive solution to the vascular anomaly. Timely diagnosis with the assistance of advanced imaging techniques allowed the medical professionals to create an appropriate and effective treatment strategy, indicating the importance of having a multidisciplinary team for treating such conditions (Haq et al., 2024). By addressing the issue at the initial stage, medical professionals maintained not only the patient's physical well-being but also her confidence and mental health. The combined results of various studies confirm that early intervention is most effective in curbing the psychosocial consequences incurred due to vascular lesions. Patients with such lesions are likely to experience not only physical disabilities but also emotional distress regarding their appearance. Active treatment can minimize the severity and duration of such consequences, thereby protecting patients' mental health. Additionally, the significant improvements in patients after receiving early intervention procedures, , such as reduced visibility of scars and better skin texture, also go towards reinforcing their sense of self-image. The implications of early intervention, thus, extend beyond the physical level, with a further focus on healthcare systems being able to ensure their patients receive early diagnosis and treatment protocols for vascular lesions. This combined understanding enhances both clinical practice and the quality of life of those affected, promoting a healthier arena for emotional and physical recovery (Figure 8.12).

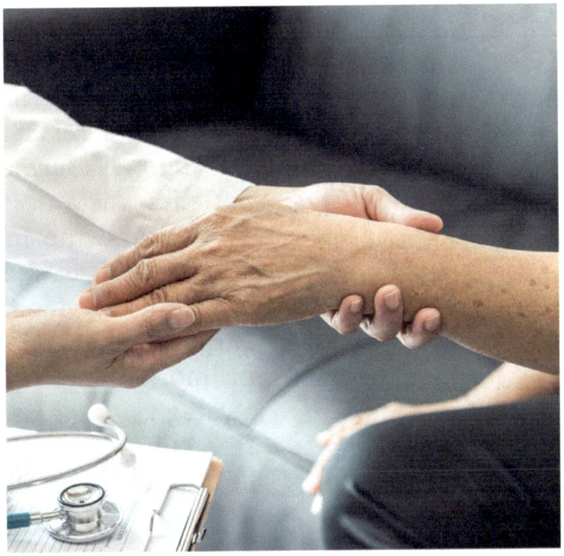

Figure 8.12. Early intervention in the treatment of vascular lesions.

Source: https://ysm-res.cloudinary.com/image/upload/ar_1:1,c_fill,dpr_3.0,f_auto,g_faces:auto,q_auto:eco,w_500/v1/yms/prod/deebeebf-4c05-4bd7-9b2a-5f5491996ec5.

Test Your Knowledge

1. How do vascular lesions influence a patient's self-esteem and body image?
2. What role does societal perception and stigma play in shaping the experiences of individuals with visible vascular lesions?

8.5. Overview of Cosmetic Treatments

Learning Outcome

1. Define laser therapy
2. Explain sclerotherapy
3. Describe surgical options

The cosmetic treatment market has grown significantly, goaded by the new technology and increasing societal pressure to be good-looking. Among the gamut of treatments on offer, lasers have turned out to be a choice favorite with their non-surgical or highly minimally invasive intervention that guarantees specific treatment. With different wavelengths, the machines treat different skin imperfections like disorders of pigmentation, vascular lesions, and scars. Reflectance confocal microscopy (RCM) is a key tool in this area that provides dermatologists with information regarding skin morphology without invasive manipulation. RCM is applied even in sensitive areas , such as the face, with extensive observation of post-laser procedure changes. RCMs unique ability to gain information about the epidermis and dermis supports the effectiveness of laser treatments, thus making it a critical element of contemporary cosmetic treatment practice (Cassalia et al., 2024). In treating vascular lesions most specifically, cosmetic treatments have been revolutionary to patients, physically and emotionally. There are a variety of modalities, , such as laser treatments, sclerotherapy, and other state-of-the-art treatments, each tailored to the type and severity of the lesion. Laser treatment, in turn, employs precise wavelengths that target and destroy targeted blood vessels without damaging surrounding tissue. Such precision decreases downtime and accelerates recovery, and it's an extremely popular choice among most patients. Further, the synergy of laser therapy with complementary treatments, such as injectable fillers, has proven to be an emerging therapeutic method, particularly in localized scleroderma. Synergies among these treatments can result in effective improvement in atrophy and loss of volume of the skin, demonstrating the dynamic development of cosmetic procedures (Cassalia et al., 2024). The increasing sophistication of cosmetic procedures calls for ongoing research and clinical investigation to optimize treatment results and advance techniques. Evidence-based practice is on the rise in cosmetic dermatology, with systematic reviews outlining the success of various methods. One of the ways that using injectable fillers along with laser therapy represents how the use of several modalities together will result in improved overall outcomes for complex dermatological conditions among patients. Also, as the concept of skin biology evolves and the individual factors influencing response to treatment evolve, the employment of individualized methods of treatment in cosmetic surgery grows more significant. Through the promotion of technical applications and clinical strategies progresses, the cosmetic industry can treat more vascular lesions and improve the lives of millions (Cassalia et al., 2024).

8.5.1. Laser Therapy

Laser therapy has been a revolutionary advancement in the treatment of vascular lesions, particularly for tufted angioma (TA) and port wine stains (PWS). These benign malformations and tumors may represent considerable aesthetic issues, often leading to psychological distress for patients. Pulsed dye laser (PDL) technology is increasingly recognized for its ability to selectively target hemoglobin in these vascular lesions, causing the destruction of dilated capillaries with minimal trauma to surrounding tissues. The vascular selectivity is capable of delivering noteworthy improvements in color and texture of lesions along with improvement in cosmetic outcomes in treated patients. In a case of a 15-year-old girl with TA, PDL demonstrated remarkable reductions in redness and associated pain of the lesions after several sessions, again emphasizing the effectiveness of such conditions in practical treatment (Dwiyana et al., 2023). The effectiveness of laser therapy is not only confined to tufted angiomas but also exhibits hopeful results for individuals with more prevalent vascular malformations like PWS. Flashlamp-pumped dye lasers (FPDL) have long been the gold standard for PWS treatment, but newer laser technology is always under study for greater effectiveness. The PhotoDerm VL is one device in this category, being a broad-spectrum, non-coherent high-intensity pulsed light source. It has shown promise in current research, with at least a 50% improvement cosmetically in the look of the PWS in patients treated with this system. Patient satisfaction is typically in line with psychological relief following noticeable improvements because these congenital vascular malformations can produce significant social distress. The risk of complications from the PhotoDerm VL remains low, though, and therefore represents a viable alternative to traditional laser therapy (Cliff et al., 1999). With continued development of laser therapy, its ongoing mechanisms and effects represent key areas of study for optimal treatment protocols in vascular lesions. Comparative analysis of different laser modalities, e.g., FPDL and PhotoDerm VL, is required to determine the optimal therapeutic regimens for particular patient profiles. Skin type, lesion maturity, and personal tolerance to treatment are among the factors that should be taken into account to customize laser therapies appropriately. With the refinement of these techniques, physicians can enhance the quality of patients' quality of life with vascular lesions in a way that allows for more optimal cosmetic results and lower emotional distress. Ultimately, laser treatment is not only marked by technological advancement but also by its capacity to combat the battle of the treatment of vascular lesions for cosmetic dermatology (Figure 8.13).

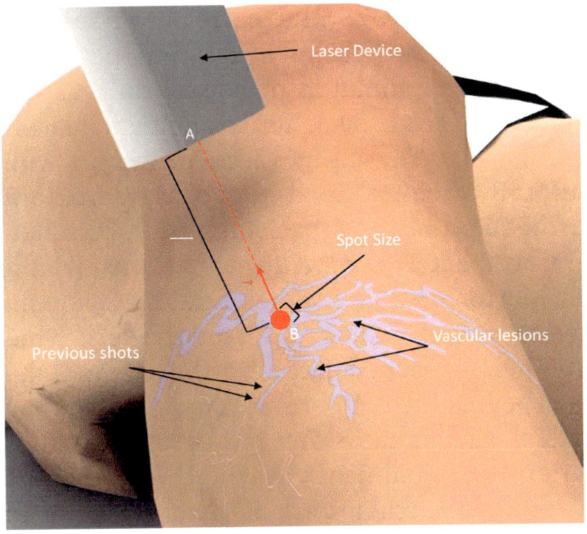

Figure 8.13. Laser treatment representation.

Source: Oliveira B, Morais P, Torres HR, Baptista AL, Fonseca JC, Vilaça JL. Characterization of the Workspace and Limits of Operation of Laser Treatments for Vascular Lesions of the Lower Limbs. *Sensors*. 2022; 22(19):7481. https://doi.org/10.3390/s22197481

8.5.2. Sclerotherapy

Sclerotherapy is a primary treatment mechanism of vascular lesion control, particularly with low-flow vascular malformations (LFVMs). LFVMs have slow-flow blood vessels and can appear in various manifestations of venous and lymphatic defects. Sclerotherapy involves the injection of a sclerosing agent into the targeted vessels, leading to destruction of the endothelium, obliteration of the vessels, and eventual fibrosis. In particular, the inclusion of electrochemical sclerotherapy with bleomycin (BEST) has made the traditional methods more efficient through the use of electrical pulses, with which the bleomycin can penetrate target tissue better. This new technique has proven to be exceptionally effective in the treatment of LFVM, where it can reduce the size of the lesion and relieve symptoms that come with the condition, basing its importance on vascular lesion treatment as a minimal procedure over surgical excision

(Ciofani et al., 2025). In the realm of cosmetic surgery, sclerotherapy has found particular use in the elimination of superficial vascular malformations , such as telangiectasias and spider veins. These tiny vascular lesions, while generally benign, tend to be a bothersome cosmetic problem for patients seeking cosmetic improvement. Sclerotherapy entails the injection of hypertonic saline or other available sclerosing agents directly into the dilated vessels, which are then absorbed later by the body. It has been evidenced by research to have high patient satisfaction rates post-treatment with patients predominantly having high clearance of lesions. Further, with its shorter recovery time and fewer complications compared to other traditional methods, sclerotherapy is a highly desirable choice for those unwilling to consider more invasive procedures. All these points speak to the success of sclerotherapy in enhancing the aesthetic result and the patient's self-worth (Clementi et al., 2024). Improvements in sclerotherapy materials and technique have expanded its application and success. While traditional sclerosing agents like ethanol remain effective, new agents and techniques like the BEST of the above demonstrate the expansion of the specialties. Improved application of the sclerotherapy technique can minimize side effects and maximize patient outcomes significantly. Emerging research still seeks to optimize treatment regimens, with each patient being treated according to specialized care to attain maximum results with least risk. Despite its promising results, specialists must remain vigilant for the complexities surrounding various vascular lesions, keeping in mind individualized approaches to each illness. With growing evidence through ongoing clinical studies and trials, the position of sclerotherapy as a first-line treatment for vascular lesions is further established within cosmetic dermatology with the promise of effective measures to deal with both health and aesthetic interventions (Ciofani et al., 2025) (Figure 8.14).

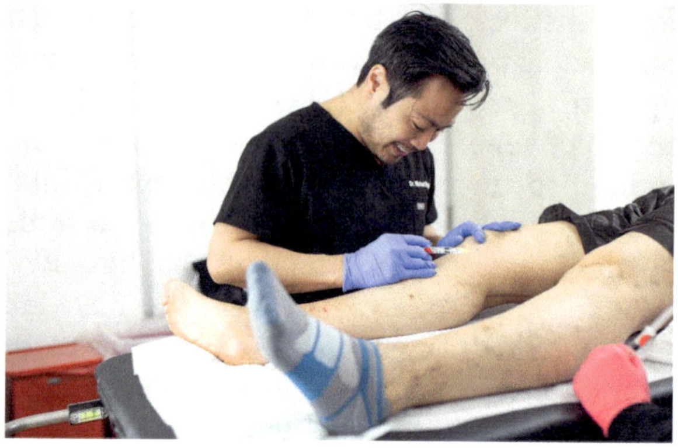

Figure 8.14. Sclerotherapy treatment.

Source: https://www.veintreatmentclinic.com/wp-content/uploads/2019/04/IMG_7321.jpg.

8.5.3. Surgical Options

Surgical options for the treatment of vascular lesions encompass a range of procedures designed to address both cosmetic and medical concerns. Surgical excision is one of the most common forms of treatment, particularly for lesions with a risk of developing complications or malignancy. Alternatively, treatments , such as laser therapy offer a less traumatic alternative, destroying blood vessels while minimizing damage to surrounding tissues. This differentiation is pertinent because patients typically require interventions that not only enhance cosmetic appeal but also maintain skin integrity. The success of these interventions is largely dependent on the specific nature of the vascular lesion, including size, location, and depth. The practitioner must understand the nuances of these treatment modalities in order to provide effective care appropriate for each patient's individual requirements. The increasing prevalence of vascular lesions has prompted the development of sophisticated surgical techniques, thus enhancing patient outcomes. For instance, advancements in laser technology have revolutionized treatment of disorders , such as hemangiomas and spider veins. The technologies enable practitioners to achieve significant reduction of vascular lesions with little downtime in comparison to the traditional excisional procedures. Secondly, pre- and post-procedural integration is fundamental in maximizing the outcomes of surgical procedures. All-encompassing protocols of care, as quoted in current literature, are of prime importance in overall success and satisfaction rates of aesthetic procedures. Counseling patients regarding these postoperative procedures guarantees avoidance of complications and facilitates a team-driven healthcare pathway for maximum results (Dhawan et al., 2022). Moreover, the choice of surgical treatment in many cases also relies on a careful weighing of lesions characteristics in tandem with patient preference. For congenital melanocytic nevi, for example, both surgery and laser treatments have become standard interventions. Decision making is complicated, however, by the absence of explicit evidence-based recommendations regarding when to use one intervention over the other. Studies contrasting the functional effect of treatments indicate their different implications for the quality of life among pediatric patients, which may not always be captured in cosmetic outcomes. As further comprehensive models of treatment selection are sought by the medical community, both procedural effects and their long-term psychosocial ramifications must still be appreciated (Lai et al., 2018).

Test Your Knowledge

1. What type of laser is commonly used to treat vascular lesions?
2. What are surgical options available for treating vascular lesions?

8.6. Efficacy and Safety of Treatments

Learning Outcome

1. Explain the success rates of various treatments
2. Describe potential side effects of treatment of vascular lesions
3. Understand long-term outcomes of vascular lesions treatment

The safety and effectiveness of vascular lesion treatments continue to remain important issues for both practitioners and patients in the cosmetic dermatology practice. The use of non-ionizing radiation (NIR) devices has opened up options for the treatment of various skin disorders, including vascular lesions. The treatments have proven effective with great improvement in patient comfort and appearance. Common applications of N. I. R. technology are epilation, skin rejuvenation, and the elimination of vascular lesions, hence demonstrating their diverse utility in aesthetic therapies. However, while many studies best document the efficacy of such treatments, such studies often fail to report on potential adverse side effects. By overlooking the safety profile, health professionals risk subjecting patients to risks that might have been prevented through prudent consideration and oversight, as explained in data aggregated from various studies and case reports (International Commission on Non-Ionizing Radiation Protection, 2020). In evaluating the safety of NIR treatments, proper attention should be paid to the side effects documented in various studies. The common side effects of the form of temporary pain, erythema, and swelling are typically mild; however, there could be rare and severe complications like blistering, scarring, and color change, which could occur. The severe outcomes underline the necessity of acquiring a complete understanding of patients' histories, particularly in dark-complexioned, high sun-exposure, or those on photosensitizing medications. The restricted evidence on the safety of such treatments during pregnancy complicates the risk assessment picture further. Variations in regulation between countries also complicate protective measures, since, unlike in similar safety measures used for these devices as medical devices in different regions, the treatment is often different for patients. Hence, randomized controlled trials are needed, which would go a long way towards addressing the issue of safety (International Commission on Non-Ionizing Radiation Protection, 2020). Novel minimally invasive techniques with an emphasis on the treatment of thyroid nodules are representative of the evolving nature of therapeutic intervention in cosmetic medicine. It has been reported in guidelines that such procedures have been remarkably useful in reducing nodules and relieving accompanying symptoms with an impressive safety record and minimal complication rate. The shift towards such less invasive treatments is not only an indication of advances in medical science but also a reaction to patient preferences for less risky treatments. Although differences exist depending on the types of nodules and involved conditions, overall outcomes suggest that less invasive techniques provide viable options for those unwilling to turn to more traditional surgical intervention. Because of this, the commitment to ongoing research and development of these new types of treatment holds potential to further increase the overall effectiveness and safety of vascular lesion treatment in cosmetic procedures.

8.6.1. Success Rates of Various Treatments

The success rate of various treatments for vascular lesions greatly influences patient outcomes and the overall efficacy of cosmetic procedures. Recent studies have indicated that endovascular therapies, , such as the use of interwoven nitinol stents, have positive results for conditions , such as common femoral artery (CFA) lesions. Technical success was an overwhelming 100% in a cohort study involving 20 patients. Moreover, cumulative primary patency rates were appreciable at 93.3% at one- and two-years post-treatment, proving the efficacy of the intervention in treating arterial occlusions (Suwanruangsri et al., 2024). These findings reflect the importance of selecting effective treatment modalities that enhance both functional and cosmetic results in patients seeking cosmetic improvements involving vascular lesions. On the contrary, other devices , such as the WRAPSODY endoprosthesis, have proved to be suitable alternatives for patients with complications related to arteriovenous access circuits. In a cohort of 15 cases, the WRAPSODY had a 100% technical success and no device-related adverse events were observed at follow-up. Notably, primary patency of the target lesion was maintained at an impressive 100% during the initial twelve months, showcasing its effectiveness in preventing complications that can detract from access circuit function (Richard et al., 2024). The robustness of the WRAPSODY device directs attention towards long-term success, thus rendering it a reliable solution for difficult anatomies prevalent in cosmetic vascular interventions. Overall, differential success rates between the treatments validate the need for personalized therapy about the patient profile and diagnosis. As shown in the outcome with both the interwoven nitinol stent and the WRAPSODY endoprosthesis, procedural success not only enhances cosmetic results but also yields long-term enhancements in quality of life in patients. As medical technology advances, the study of numerous treatment options for vascular lesions will remain an integral aspect in maximizing therapeutic outcomes and patient satisfaction in cosmetic therapy. Continued tracking of success rates will allow healthcare providers to make well-informed choices on proper intervention strategies, ultimately tilting towards patients with vascular cosmetic requirements (Figure 8.15).

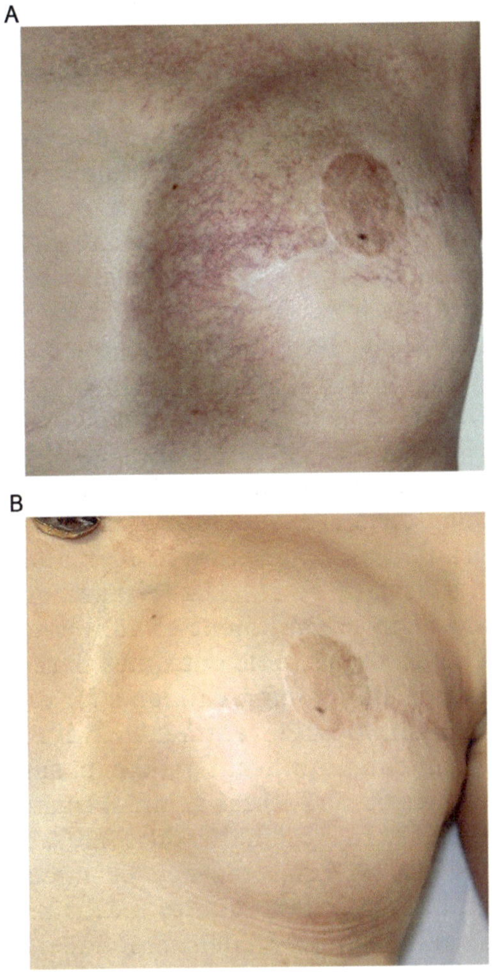

Figure 8.15. Example of results obtained after two sessions of vascular laser and two sessions of fractional non-ablative laser.

Source: https://www.researchgate.net/publication/320820800/figure/fig2/AS:11431281256185297@1719510465628/Example-of-results-obtained-after-two-sessions-of-vascular-laser-and-two-sessions-of.jpg.

8.6.2. Potential Side Effects

Treatment of vascular lesions through cosmetic procedures, while successful, is not without certain probable side effects. The most frequent types of treatment are laser therapy, sclerotherapy, and IPL, each of which can cause reactions that, although largely temporary in nature, have the potential to influence patient satisfaction. Redness, swelling, bruising, and changes in skin pigmentation are most frequently observed as reactions to these procedures. Specifically, laser therapies can cause erythema and edema, which typically resolve in several days but are cause for concern to patients. Familiarity with these possible side effects is important, as it aids in managing patient expectations and facilitating informed decision-making about treatment modalities. Side effects indicate the need for practitioners to be familiar with the technology employed, as well as the identification of the variety of side effects it can produce in the healing process. Moreover, secondary effects of cosmetic procedures on vascular lesions can lead to complications beyond the first procedure. For instance, too much use of sclerotherapy has the potential to result in skin necrosis, while laser treatments can result in scarring or persistent hyperpigmentation among darker-skinned patients. These complications can necessitate additional treatments, further contributing to patient concern over their original vascular lesions. It is even more crucial to consider the predisposing skin disease that can cause patients to have adverse effects, particularly with the newer dermatologic therapies and their burgeoning presence in clinical practice. Serial advances in dermatological science, as thrilling as they make new treatment possibilities, also require an appropriate familiarity with the disadvantages of their effect on the skin (Boffa et al., 2004). Monitoring such problems enables practitioners to manage them effectively, hence ensuring patient health as well as cosmetic outcomes. On the basis of these findings, practitioners must employ a judicious but not inadequate approach in the area of cosmetic treatments of vascular lesions. Adding pre-treatment assessments can aid in the identification of patients who may be at higher risk for side effects, so appropriate treatment protocols that minimize side effects can be ordered. Additionally, educating patients on the important components of post-treatment care, , such as sun protection and moisturizing, is essential to maximize healing and minimize associated side effects. Stress on communication can lead to greater trust and encourage early reporting of abnormal symptoms by the patients, allowing for early interventions. With dermatology continuing to evolve with new treatment methods, the identification, handling, and reducing the potential side effects of cosmetic procedures will be essential to ensure patient safety and satisfaction (Cantisani et al., 2014). In doing this, clinicians are not only able to enhance esthetic results but can also aid in creating a positive treatment experience.

8.6.3. Long-Term Outcomes

Treatment of vascular lesions with cosmetic treatments has now come to enjoy increased interest after the promising long-term outcomes with these methods. Non-melanoma skin cancers (NMSCs), which are a significant public health problem, may be efficiently treated with a variety of cosmetic treatment modalities. Photodynamic therapy (PDT) has been established to achieve excellent cosmetic results while having successful treatment of superficial lesions at their initial stages. By inhibiting DNA damage and allowing healing, the therapies not only arrest cancer development but also offer long-term healing in the complexion of the skin. The effectiveness lasting so long in such treatments helps to emphasize the dual role of such therapies as prevention and cure, eventually enhancing patients' quality of life (Cantisani et al., 2014). In addition to vascular lesion treatment, combined treatment involving laser therapy and injectable fillers holds great promise for long-term outcomes in localized scleroderma (LS). Fractional CO_2 laser therapy used in combination with hyaluronic acid fillers has been shown to effectively enhance skin texture and volume, cosmetic appearance, and functional capacity of involved tissues. The long-term outcome of these combined therapies can lead to extensive tissue remodeling and long-term aesthetic enhancement, which is substantiated by patient response. The synergistic strategy not only may improve immediate visual outcomes but also can deliver long-term psychological benefit, hence favoring an enhanced quality of life for patients with LS to manage. Thus, awareness of these long-term consequences is crucial to the maximization of patient care in dermatological clinics (Cassalia et al., 2024). Furthermore, the long-term commitment to follow-up and maintenance of cosmetic outcomes is required for patients undergoing treatments for vascular lesions. Supportive treatment and regular follow-ups can significantly help ensure the maintenance of the success of initial treatments. For instance, the cosmetic outcome accrued with the use of laser therapy or injectables can diminish over time due to mechanisms of natural skin aging or environmental factors. Having such a comprehensive post-treatment protocol in place that includes preventive interventions and periodic follow-ups, then, becomes essential to the achievement of maximum duration of treatment effect. Continual patient education regarding skincare and lifestyle change optimizes maintenance of aesthetic gain. Lastly, this integrated approach not only facilitates the long-term sustainability of the therapeutic effects but also empowers patients by reinforcing their active participation in ongoing skin management.

Test Your Knowledge

1. What are the comparative success rates of commonly used treatments for vascular lesions, , such as laser therapy, sclerotherapy, and surgical excision?
2. What are the most common short-term and long-term side effects associated with treatments for vascular lesions?

SUMMARY

The study of vascular lesions and their aesthetic treatment brings an in-depth understanding of the complex balance of medical necessity and aesthetic concern. Vascular lesions, ranging from simple birthmarks to more complicated expressions, often necessitate a combined pattern with therapeutic and aesthetic interventions. The individual characteristics of such lesions, , such as their severity, subtype, and impact on a patient's quality of life, highlight the necessity of individualized treatment regimens. Demonstrated by advances in modern medicine, treatments like laser therapy and sclerotherapy are very effective in minimizing the visibility of vascular lesions, hence improving patients' self-esteem and social performance. The positive impacts of these treatments reinforce the principle that cosmetic treatments must be perceived not only as superficial additions but as key components of holistic healthcare dedicated to maximizing overall well-being. The recent interest in nanomedicine and novel delivery systems has opened new avenues for the therapy of vascular lesions. With the employment of nanoparticles and nanoscale materials, researchers aim to enhance precision in reaching affected areas with fewer systemic consequences. The developing field has tremendous potential for revolutionizing the traditional methods of cosmetic therapies with the capability to address vascular lesions. As highlighted in recent studies, integrating nanotechnology with traditional healing methods can synergistically lead to more potent drugs and improved patient outcomes. As such, these technologies can render cosmetic care an integral part of patient management regimens, offering the psychological advantages that accompany improved appearance in addition to good medical treatment. The dual focus on aesthetic enhancement and clinical outcome is a positive addition to the therapeutic landscape for vascular lesions. Lastly, the intersection of vascular lesion therapy and its beauty effects is a testament to a vision of patient treatment that cares about body and psyche alike. The current state of bespoke therapies, particularly those based on strength through green nanotechnology and targeted drug delivery, signals a new era in therapy for such conditions. Due to the acquisition of a more profound understanding of the biological nuances of vascular lesions and due to developments in novel forms of treatment, the clinician is in a position to offer customized and efficient solutions. Not only does this enhance cosmetic appearance but also overall well-being, thus further endorsing the relevance of integrated care in modern medicine. As we continue in the challenging field, ongoing research and cooperation will be the way to respond to both the aesthetic and therapeutic needs of those patients affected by vascular lesions, as a means to offer a complete and compassionate healthcare experience to each patient.

A comprehension of vascular lesions is essential to the development of cosmetic procedures that can increase aesthetic outcomes. Vascular lesions, from a variety of conditions like hemangiomas and varicosities, can have an extreme physical as well as psychological impact on patients. The selection of available treatment possibilities ranges from less invasive treatments like laser therapy to more severe surgery. The success of such treatments largely relies on the accurate diagnosis of the severity and nature of the vascular lesion and mandates competent evaluation by healthcare providers. Further, greater patient satisfaction could be due to the practitioner's ability to accurately inform the patient of the benefits and limitations of the treatment, and such a patient-centered cosmetic dermatology and vascular medicine practice is therefore indicated. Aside from diagnostic challenges, the treatment of vascular lesions requires clinical management within an interdisciplinary context, in certain instances involving dermatologists, vascular surgeons, and cosmetic physicians. The team context may achieve the best result of treatment while offering patients a greater understanding of their disease and potential treatments. Evidence shows that patient outcome improves when the treatments are optimally individualized to meet their respective conditions and circumstances and taking into consideration , such as the nature of the lesion and the patient's overall condition. For instance, vascular lesions that are caused by chronic illness, for instance, venous ulcers, require special treatment protocols to achieve successful healing and cosmetic results. Therefore, the merging of a number of specialties not only leads to enhanced therapeutic results but also highlights the significance of ongoing education and training on novel cosmetic treatments regarding vascular pathologies. Socioeconomic impacts of vascular lesions, particularly venous ulcers, highlight the fact that adequate research on causes and mechanisms of such pathologies must be conducted in order to manage them properly. Research has shown that venous ulcer patients experience major quality of life impairment in the form of protracted healing times and recurring bouts, which can also be reflected in economic loss. For instance, the prevalence of chronic venous insufficiency (CVI) and complications like venous ulcers is an area that emphasizes carrying out research to enhance nursing practice and treatment interventions. As established in ongoing research, high levels of nursing intervention are crucial in the management of such ulcers because proper care enhances both healing rates and the patient outcome as a whole. Addressing the challenge that is vascular lesions, either cosmetically or medically, yields improved care pathways and improved patient experiences in managing these recalcitrant conditions.

KEY TERMS FROM THIS CHAPTER

- Blood vessels
- Computed tomography (CT)
- Fine needle aspiration (FNA)
- Genetic analysis
- Genetic predisposition
- Hemangiomas
- Hormonal fluctuations
- Hypervascular tumors
- Inherited syndromes
- Long-pulse alexandrite laser
- Capillary malformations
- Cosmetic dissatisfaction
- Genetic alterations
- Genetic disorder
- Glomuvenous malformations
- Hereditary hemorrhagic telangiectasia
- Hyperkeratosis
- Imaging modalities
- Lesion formation
- Low-flow vascular malformations

CRITICAL THINKING QUESTIONS

1. **Which of the following vascular lesions is most commonly treated with pulsed dye laser (PDL)?**
   a. Spider angioma
   b. Port-wine stain
   c. Cherry angioma
   d. Hemangioma
2. **What is the primary chromophore targeted in laser treatment of vascular lesions?**
   a. Melanin
   b. Water
   c. Hemoglobin
   d. Keratin
3. **What is a potential side effect of laser treatment for vascular lesions?**
   a. Acneiform eruption
   b. Hyperpigmentation or hypopigmentation
   c. Hair loss
   d. Sebaceous gland hyperplasia
4. **Laser therapy for vascular lesions primarily works by:**
   a. Heating and coagulating blood vessels
   b. Stimulating collagen production
   c. Reducing pigmentation in the skin
   d. Exfoliating the skin surface
9. **What is the main principle behind sclerotherapy as a treatment for vascular lesions?**
   a. Freezing and destroying the blood vessel
   b. Using intense heat to vaporize the blood vessels
   c. Applying a chemical peel to remove superficial vessels
   d. Injecting a substance that causes the blood vessel to collapse and fade

Short Answer Questions

1. What are the common types of vascular lesions seen in dermatology, and how do they differ in appearance and clinical significance?
2. How do congenital vascular malformations differ from vascular tumors in terms of pathophysiology and clinical behavior?
3. Which imaging modalities are most useful in evaluating deeper or complex vascular lesions and why?
4. What are the potential complications of untreated or improperly managed vascular lesions in pediatric patients?
5. What is the mechanism of action of pulsed dye laser (PDL) in treating vascular lesions like port-wine stains and telangiectasias?
6. What are the most common side effects and contraindications associated with laser treatments for vascular lesions?

Answer to Critical Thinking Questions

1. (b); 2. (c); 3. (b); 4. (a); 5. (d)

REFERENCES

1. Cassalia, F., Federico, S., Danese, A., Franceschin, L., Amato, S., Gratteri, F., Battilotti, C., Caroppo, F., Zappia, E., Bennardo, L., Belloni Fortina, A., & Nisticò, S. P. (2024). Advances in the Management of Localized Scleroderma: A Systematic Review of Laser Therapy and Injectable Filler Approaches. *Journal of personalized medicine*, *14*(8), 872. https://doi.org/10.3390/jpm14080872 (accessed on 11th June 2025).
2. Aranha, J., Gil, F., & Ortiz, S. (2019). Escleroterapia no tratamento de malformações glomuvenosas cutâneas disseminadas familiares: Relato de caso. https://core.ac.uk/download/322632762.pdf (accessed on 11th June 2025).
3. Barile, A., Quarchioni, S., Bruno, F., Ierardi, A. M., Arrigoni, F., Giordano, A. V., Carducci, S., Varrassi, M., Carrafiello, G., Caranci, F., Splendiani, A., Di Cesare, E., & Masciocchi, C. (2018). Interventional radiology of the thyroid gland: critical review and state of the art. *Gland surgery*, *7*(2), 132–146. https://doi.org/10.21037/gs.2017.11.17 (accessed on 11th June 2025).
4. Belloni Fortina, A., Bolzon, A., Caroppo, F., et al. (2025). Congenital dermatofibrosarcoma protuberans—An update on the ongoing diagnostic challenges. https://core.ac.uk/download/654524189.pdf (accessed on 11th June 2025).
5. Boffa, M. J. (2004). *Dermatology*. https://core.ac.uk/download/46601884.pdf (accessed on 11th June 2025).
6. Bond, R. G., Arasu, R., Jantzen, T. M., & Alley, R. P. (2024). Patency rates following treatment with the WRAPSODY™ Cell-Impermeable Endoprosthesis for recalcitrant renal access circuit dysfunction: Results from a tertiary Australian center. *Vascular*. https://www.semanticscholar.org/paper/cf7ad25578cc8b7499ee7ad7f0d36c2e01f7595b (accessed on 11th June 2025).
7. Carqueja, I. M., Sousa, J., & Mansilha, A. (2018). Vascular malformations: Classification, diagnosis and treatment. *International Angiology*, *37*. https://doi.org/10.23736/s0392-9590.18.03961-5 (accessed on 11th June 2025).
8. Chen, C., & Ke, Y. (2023). Applications of long-pulse Alexandrite laser in cosmetic dermatology: A review. *Clinical, Cosmetic and Investigational Dermatology*, *16*, 3349–3357. https://www.semanticscholar.org/paper/f46af7cae0c035667f692658e1e8e310144e8b23 (accessed on 11th June 2025).
9. Chukwu, R., & Mankila, J. (2018). Dermatology nurses' job description: Literature review. Bachelor's thesis Degree programme in Nursing PNURSS15 2018. https://core.ac.uk/download/161432240.pdf (accessed on 11th June 2025).
10. Cifuentes-González, C., Rojas-Carabali, W., Olate Pérez, Á., Carvalho, E., Valenzuela, F., Miguel-Escuder, L., Ormaechea, M. S., et al. (2023). Risk factors for recurrences and visual impairment in patients with ocular toxoplasmosis: A systematic review and meta-analysis. *PLOS ONE*, *18*. https://www.semanticscholar.org/paper/0a41f5ab97edfc475e00eaf5051941af874f2b16 (accessed on 11th June 2025).
11. Ciofani, L., Massi, I., Baldazzi, G., Antonacci, N., & Tessari, M. (2025). Electrochemical sclerotherapy with bleomycin for the treatment of low-flow vascular malformations: A comprehensive review. *Veins and Lymphatics*. https://www.semanticscholar.org/paper/9f5203ea658d7fe4ab244d3003ebc3940b892b15 (accessed on 11th June 2025).

12. Clementi, A., Cannarozzo, G., Amato, S., Zappia, E., Bennardo, L., Michelini, S., Morini, C., et al. (2024). Dye laser applications in cosmetic dermatology: Efficacy and safety in treating vascular lesions and scars. *Cosmetics*. https://www.semanticscholar.org/paper/d267a3ad2303f021d12094baa208aed4235ac1a1 (accessed on 11th June 2025).

13. Cliff, S., & Misch, K. (1999). Treatment of mature port wine stains with the Protoderms VL. *Journal of Cutaneous Laser Therapy*, *1*(2), 101–104. https://www.semanticscholar.org/paper/a0605ec1ed9e34428beacfe2edb4c61057222b56 (accessed on 11th June 2025).

14. da Silva, D. C., Budó, M. L., Schimith, M. D., Rizzatti, S. J. S., Durgante, V. L., & Robaina, M. L. (2013). Issues addressed on venous ulcer in theses and dissertation of nursing. *Journal of Nursing Ufpe Online*, *7*, 6671–6677. https://www.semanticscholar.org/paper/ff681b5cd1bf8433e15d1256388d44a33c24eace (accessed on 11th June 2025).

15. Dai, Q., Cheng, L., & Wang, C. (2024). The effectiveness of early treatment with intense pulsed light combined with fractional erbium laser in preventing post-traumatic hypertrophic scar formation. *The Journal of Craniofacial Surgery*, *36*, e342–e345. https://www.semanticscholar.org/paper/f3fa47bb14ec9b270a2f3d588827395a72bf37e4 (accessed on 11th June 2025).

16. Davidson, J., & Ford, K. (2015). Paediatric surgery: A core surgical trainee's guide to vascular malformations in children. https://core.ac.uk/download/336578222.pdf (accessed on 11th June 2025).

17. Dhawan, S., Kandhari, R., Madnani, N., et al. (2022). Expert opinion on pre and post procedure care in aesthetic dermatology. https://core.ac.uk/download/539912253.pdf (accessed on 11th June 2025).

18. Diociaiuti, A., Paolantonio, G., Zama, M., Alaggio, R., Carnevale, C., Conforti, A., Cesario, C., et al. (2021). Vascular birthmarks as a clue for complex and syndromic vascular anomalies. *Frontiers in Pediatrics*, *9*. https://www.semanticscholar.org/paper/0ebc51a31f1d66e88fb946e3c061ca544e356936 (accessed on 11th June 2025).

19. Dwiyana, R., Lestari, E. R., Effendi, R. M. R. A., Gondokaryono, S. P., Diana, I. A., Usman, H., Suhada, K. U., et al. (2023). Effectiveness of pulsed dye laser treatment in tufted angioma: A promising intervention. *Clinical, Cosmetic and Investigational Dermatology*, *16*, 2885–2891. https://www.semanticscholar.org/paper/d177fa9db48642085f4c8858505108ffd0c63d26 (accessed on 11th June 2025).

20. Feitosa, R. G. F., Pedroso, J. C. M., & Neto, M. S. (2024). The importance of portable ultrasound in neck fat assessment and treatment. *Journal of Dermatology & Cosmetology*. https://www.semanticscholar.org/paper/2c5d9a3e3b12c527bcd47e9fa6d88ce9f3e71056 (accessed on 11th June 2025).

21. Fernández-Varela-Gómez, F., Sandoval-García, A., Cabrera-Rios, V., et al. (2024). Signs of skin aging: A review. https://core.ac.uk/download/613230159.pdf (accessed on 11th June 2025).

22. Frantzias, J., Bagley, J. H., & Steinberg, G. K. (2024). Surgical treatment of brain arteriovenous malformations in patients with hereditary hemorrhagic telangiectasia: A single-center experience. *Journal of Neurosurgery*. https://www.semanticscholar.org/paper/43622f95f2ae9393023dd8ceec7e42a096f23e8b (accessed on 11th June 2025).

23. Furlepa, N., Jedlikowska, W., & Sieradocha, K. (2024). The role of inflammatory pathways in the development of rosacea. https://core.ac.uk/download/636386008.pdf (accessed on 11th June 2025).

24. Geiger, J. L., Ismaila, N., Beadle, B. M., Caudell, J. J., Chau, N. G., Deschler, D. G., Glastonbury, C. M., et al. (2021). Management of salivary gland malignancy: ASCO guideline. *Journal of Clinical Oncology*, *39*, 1909–1941. https://doi.org/10.1200/jco.21.00449 (accessed on 11th June 2025).

25. Gonçalves, M. M. B. M., & Pina, M. E. S. R. T. (2017). Dermo cosmetic care for rosacea. https://doi.org/10.1590/s2175-97902017000400182(accessed on 11th June 2025).

26. Habib, G., Lancellotti, P., Antunes, M. J., Bongiorni, M. G., Casalta, J. P., Del Zotti, F., Dulgheru, R., et al. (2015). 2015 ESC guidelines for the management of infective endocarditis. *European Heart Journal*, *36*, 3075–3128. https://doi.org/10.1093/eurheartj/ehv319 (accessed on 11th June 2025).

27. Haq, K., Waqas, M. A., Akhter, S., Cardona, J. J., Scalia, G., Umana, G., & Chaurasia, B. (2024). Surgical resection of a rare scalp arteriovenous malformation: A case report. *Annals of Medicine and Surgery*, *86*, 6805–6809. https://www.semanticscholar.org/paper/ae5680d20e8e42a8b6bc2537490e3d3e350ecad0 (accessed on 11th June 2025).

28. International Commission on Non-Ionizing Radiation Protection. (2020). Intended human exposure to non-ionizing radiation for cosmetic purposes. https://core.ac.uk/download/552405446.pdf (accessed on 11th June 2025).

29. Lai, Y. (2018). Comparing congenital melanocytic nevus treatment effect on children's health-related quality of life. https://core.ac.uk/download/475688229.pdf (accessed on 11th June 2025).

30. Llíbre-Guerra, J. C., Guimaraens, L., Kadziolka, K. B., Siddiqui, A., Chapot, R., & Gil, A. (2024). ihtObtura: A novel liquid embolic agent with post-embolization radiopacity loss, in endovascular treatment of brain arteriovenous malformations, dural arteriovenous fistulas, and tumors: CLARIDAD trial. *Journal of Neurointerventional Surgery*, *17*. https://www.semanticscholar.org/paper/2192e8488d65d6556371c91665ff4ef470e73faa (accessed on 11th June 2025).

31. Palacio Giral, A. (2023). Optical coherence tomography-assisted 1064nm Nd:YAG laser therapy of superficial and nodular basal cell carcinomas with ≤1mm tumor thickness. https://core.ac.uk/download/618185853.pdf (accessed on 11th June 2025).

32. Palano, M., Cucchiara, M., Gallazzi, M., Riccio, F., Mortara, L., Gensini, G., Spinetti, G., et al. (2022). When a friend becomes your enemy: Natural killer cells in atherosclerosis and atherosclerosis-associated risk factors. *Frontiers in Immunology*, *12*. https://www.semanticscholar.org/paper/d73d706222430adb8eb3f1825b8a8a14ebef2d03 (accessed on 11th June 2025).

33. Patra, J. K., Das, G., Fraceto, L. F., Campos, E. V. R., Rodriguez-Torres, M. P., Acosta-Torres, L. S., Díaz-Torres, L. A., et al. (2018). Nano based drug delivery systems: Recent developments and future prospects. *Journal of Nanobiotechnology*, *16*. https://doi.org/10.1186/s12951-018-0392-8 (accessed on 11th June 2025).

34. Radcliffe, R., Liu, S. Y., Cook, V., Hurcombe, S., & Divers, T. (2022). Interpreting abdominal fluid in colic horses: Understanding and applying peritoneal fluid evidence. *Journal of Veterinary Emergency and Critical Care*, *32*(S1), 81–96. https://www.semanticscholar.org/paper/e043fe5d71d00c793e6cf68f69f46a966197d370 (accessed on 11th June 2025).

35. Raja, J., Williams, D., & Oser, R. (2024). Primer on embolic agents and sclerosants for the treatment of vascular malformations. *Seminars in Interventional Radiology*, *41*, 370–375. https://www.semanticscholar.org/paper/eceb0ec69e6b0ef77f86b80236452c1be88f71f9 (accessed on 11th June 2025).

36. Sanders, G. (2024). A bundle of care for prevention, early recognition, and treatment of hyaluronic acid dermal filler associated vascular occlusion. https://core.ac.uk/download/616423550.pdf (accessed on 11th June 2025).

37. Sharquie, K., & Jabbar, R. I. (2021). Classification and clinical evaluation of the types of angiokeratoma. *Our Dermatology Online*. https://www.semanticscholar.org/paper/1a9ccba520428d438d0505e0092cd763e92f9f5d (accessed on 11th June 2025).

38. Suwanruangsri, V., Bokerd, S., Chanchitsopon, V., & Jowcharoen, S. (2024). Endovascular treatment with interwoven nitinol stent for common femoral artery lesions: 2-year outcomes of a single center experience. *Vascular*, *33*, 19–25. https://www.semanticscholar.org/paper/48abd51f6647f6de20fae6cfeab6d308f5d8857e (accessed on 11th June 2025).

39. Tay, C. J., Koh, M. J. A., Toh, L. H. W., Wee, L., Su, B., Tan, L. S., & Tey, H. (2024). Photoacoustic microscopy offers a new perspective on imaging of vascular anomalies: A case series of venous malformations. *Journal of Vascular Anomalies*. https://www.semanticscholar.org/paper/13736c4a6569f8b2ed6fe6b80d1920f18e9cee66 (accessed on 11th June 2025).

40. van Straten, D., Mashayekhi, V., de Bruijn, H., Oliveira, S., & Robinson, D. J. (2017). Oncologic photodynamic therapy: Basic principles, current clinical status and future directions. *Cancers*, *9*, 19–19. https://doi.org/10.3390/cancers9020019 (accessed on 11th June 2025).

41. Waks, A. G., & Winer, E. P. (2019). Breast cancer treatment. *JAMA*, *321*, 288–288. https://doi.org/10.1001/jama.2018.19323 (accessed on 11th June 2025).

42. Wang, L., Lu, M., Min, Z., Liang, Y., Wang, S. S., & Li, J. (2024). Microwave ablation with hydro dissection used for the treatment of vascular malformations: Effectiveness and safety study. *Frontiers in Oncology*, *14*. https://www.semanticscholar.org/paper/7b27ba6f0f3c749c7b06e9bd337bc4ff8bcb0fe3 (accessed on 11th June 2025).

CELLULITE AND STRETCH MARKS MANAGEMENT

9

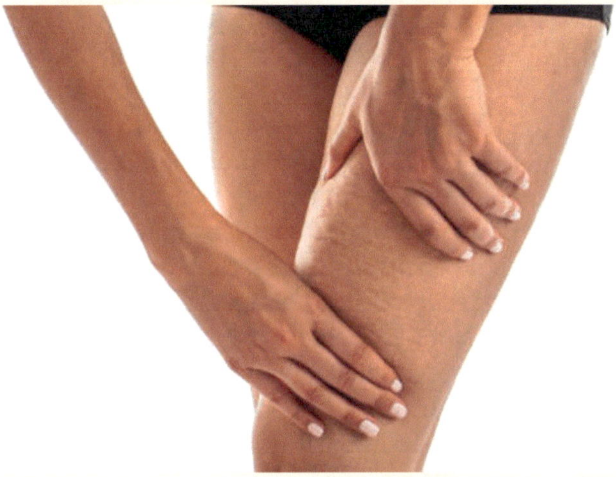

LEARNING OBJECTIVES

After studying this chapter, you will be able to:

1. Understand cellulite and stretch marks
2. Describe traditional treatment options for cellulite and stretch marks
3. Explain advanced treatment options for cellulite and stretch marks

Introduction

The increasing popularity of cosmetic procedures has further accentuated the need for effective treatment of conditions , such as cellulite and stretch marks in the field of cosmetic dermatology. Both conditions are ubiquitous across a variety of populations and often have considerable impacts on individuals' body image and self-esteem. Cellulite, or the dimpled look, is mostly a female problem, while striae, or stretch marks, take place when the skin is suddenly undergoing an alteration due to conditions like pregnancy, weight loss or gain, or hormonal changes. With patients seeking methods to enhance their physical looks without subjecting themselves to aggressive surgeries, the landscape of cosmetic dermatology has evolved to encompass a variety of treatment options. This summary attempts to explore the latest advances in treating cellulite and stretch marks, as well as the contribution of non-invasive technologies and objectively evaluating the efficacy of treatment through clinical examination. To address the problems concerning cellulite and stretch marks, contemporary cosmetic dermatology relies on the synergy between cutting-edge technology and evidence-based practice. Techniques like ultrasound imaging and 3D skin analysis have become essential aids for clinicians, with the help of which they can determine the maturity and type of stretch marks. The use of these technologies not only augments diagnostic precision but also helps guide treatment (Bleve et al., 2011). For example, research has shown that high-frequency ultrasound is able to detect the structural makeup of striae and hence make way for individualized therapeutic strategies. This degree of specificity in treatment has resulted in promising outcomes for patients who wish to enhance these disorders, as testified by a high trend toward personalized care in contemporary dermatology clinics. Furthermore, studies on non-surgical aesthetic treatments have boosted the treatment of skin disorders like stretch marks and cellulite. Technologies, including injectables, laser treatments, and radiofrequency (RF), have transformed body contouring and skin texture improvement methods to offer alternatives to surgical procedures (Andronache et al., 2019). These technologies not only carry less risk and quicker healing times but also align with the growing consumer preference for minimally invasive treatment. With ongoing efforts to find best practices in managing cellulite and stretch marks, it is important for dermatologists to be current with the latest developments and treatment modalities in order to keep pace with patient needs and optimize aesthetic outcomes. This introduction serves as the basis for a comprehensive discussion of evolving techniques in cosmetic dermatology.

Definition of Cellulite and Stretch Marks

The definition of cellulite has radically changed in the face of differing scientific concepts about its etiology and definition. Cellulite, now better referred to as gynoid lipodystrophy," is essentially characterized by structural, biochemical, and inflammatory subcutaneous tissue alterations leading to skin irregularities , such as dimpling (Atamoros et al., 2018). With an estimated prevalence reported to be impacting up to 90% of women, particularly from puberty, it not only presents cosmetic concerns but also affects the quality of life among those impacted. The lack of a commonly accepted classification reflects the complexity of the condition, thus the diversity of terms employed, , such as lipodystrophy and edematofibrosclerotic panniculitis (EFP). These secondary identifiers underscore the numerous different morphological and pathophysiological effects associated with cellulite and mirror the necessity of a more holistic approach to cosmetic dermatology (Terranova et al., 2006). Comparatively, stretch marks or striae are scars on the dermis that occur when the skin undergoes sudden stretching due to factors , such as puberty, pregnancy, or rapid weight changes. These lesions will most often begin as erythematous or purplish marks, which later become thinner to a lighter hue, more evident on certain skin types (Atamoros et al., 2018). Stretch marks are the consequence of collagen fiber tearing within the dermis, which is triggered by hormonal changes that affect skin elasticity and firmness. In contrast to cellulite, which is largely a female issue, stretch marks can involve both males and females, but continue to be more common in females. Their multifactorial etiology and unique biological processes require integrated treatment strategies taking into account the unique patient factors in the practice of cosmetic dermatology (Terranova et al., 2006). The management of stretch marks and cellulite in cosmetic dermatology is an area of growing interest, reflecting the common desire for therapeutic interventions of value. Practitioners are presented with the challenges of the sheer volume of anecdotal therapies and lack of standardized treatment protocols, leading to patients being inclined to embrace untried or empirical therapies, which can produce less than satisfactory outcomes (Atamoros et al.,

2018). Effective interventions must incorporate evidence-based practice from thorough research as well as consensus from experts. Various treatment methods, , such as topical therapies, minimally invasive therapies, and lifestyle modification, are undergoing ongoing study. Critical evaluation of these treatments forms the basis of enhanced clinical decision-making such that practitioners can develop individualized strategies that address the unique needs of their patients to deliver the optimal outcomes in the treatment of cellulite and stretch marks (Terranova et al., 2006) (Figure 9.1).

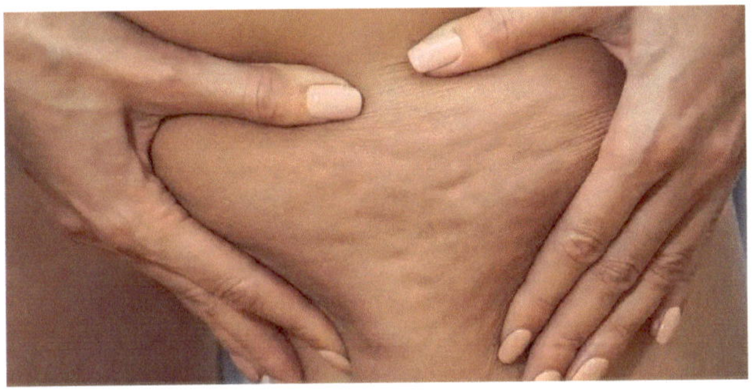

Figure 9.1. Visible cellulite on the thigh region.

Source: https://www.beatxp.com/blog/wp-content/uploads/2023/07/what-is-cellulite-symptoms-and-treatment.jpg.

Prevalence and Significance in Cosmetic Dermatology

Cellulite and stretch marks share a commonality in the field of cosmetic dermatology that is a growing concern for both practitioners and patients. They primarily appear in women, and studies have indicated that nearly 90% of women experience cellulite at least once during their lifetime, mainly following puberty. Stretch marks, or striae, also develop in a considerable percentage of individuals, with figures as high as 80% in pregnant individuals or those with sudden weight fluctuations. Such a preponderance of diseases presents an urgent need for the advancement of effective management in the cosmetic dermatology area, highlighting the necessity for research and development of treatment modalities. It is crucial to comprehend the etiologic factors underlying the development of these cosmetic conditions, , such as hormonal and genetic factors, so that customized treatment modalities may be developed to optimize patient satisfaction and self-esteem. The significance of cellulite and stretch marks extends beyond their cosmetic appearance, as they tend to have psychological implications for the patients concerned. Research has demonstrated that both disorders have been linked to feelings of inadequacy, body dissatisfaction, and poorer quality of life. The linkage serves as a reminder that it is important to address not just the cosmetic disorder, but also the psychological and emotional wellbeing of the patient in question. Incorporating psychological assessment into treatment planning can provide a more integrated approach to the treatment, allowing dermatologists to better address these multifaceted concerns. As underscored by quality of life and body satisfaction studies among pregnant women, the prevalence of such conditions as fibroedemageloide (FEG) may not always play a critical role in their self-perception; however, the overall physical attractiveness and psychological effect cannot be overlooked in seeking better management techniques (Nascimento, 2019). Evolutions in cellulite and stretch marks treatment modalities continue to characterize the field of cosmetic dermatology. Treatments , such as microneedling and laser therapy have been found to be effective treatments, demonstrating their efficacy in reducing the appearance of both conditions as well as stimulating collagen turnover. A sample study on microneedling demonstrated its use to improve atrophic acne scars, which is a basis for a similar mechanism in the use of stretch marks and cellulite (Sivaranjani, 2019). With the ever-growing popularity of these modalities, clinicians must keep abreast of the up-to-date literature and emerging technologies to offer evidence-based care to their patients. Furthermore, patient education about realistic treatment outcomes and the importance of lifestyle changes, diet and exercise, for instance, can also be beneficial in maximizing the effectiveness of these treatments, generating greater patient satisfaction and a higher quality of life among those who are receiving cosmetic dermatologic therapy.

9.1. Understanding Cellulite

Learning Outcome

1. Explain the causes and contributing factors of cellulite
2. Describe types of cellulite
3. Understand the psychological impact on individuals.

Cellulite is a syndrome of multifaceted skin disorder characterized by a puckered look of the skin, which is most commonly found on the thighs, buttocks, and abdomen. The syndrome is the product of the elaborate interface between septae, or fibrous connective tissue, and subcutaneous fat layers. As the fat cells increase in size due to changes in hormone levels and genetics, they are squeezed against the adjacent tissues. This squeezing causes the puckering of the skin. Interestingly, cellulite is not only a cosmetic issue; more importantly, it usually denotes underlying physiological changes that can be reflective of the overall health of individuals. It is therefore important to know these mechanisms so that optimal management in cosmetic dermatology can be achieved not only for the cosmetic treatment of cellulite but also keeping in view its significance on the health and well-being of individuals. The most recent findings in the realm of cosmeceuticals unveiled the potential of substances isolated from marine algae to facilitate the management of cellulite. Bioactive-rich in nature, these substances have been found to promote skin health through a variety of mechanisms. As an illustration, their antimicrobial and anti-inflammatory effects are held accountable for overall improvement in the skin matrix and can potentially reduce the appearance of cellulite. Use of these algal preparations is aptly in consonance with a new wave in cosmetic dermatology towards products that are both therapeutic as well as aesthetically pleasing. As explained in recent literature, the use of such cosmeceuticals can revolutionize the treatment protocols for practitioners by enabling them to employ a new arsenal to fight the multi-factorial etiology of cellulites (Haresh et al., 2024).

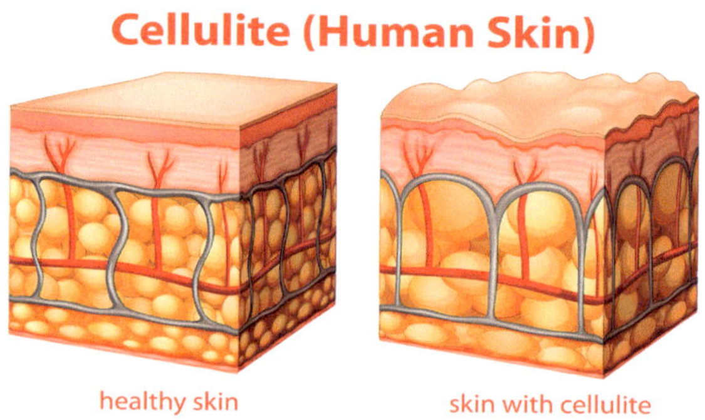

Figure 9.2. Normal skin versus skin with cellulite.

Source: https://www.researchgate.net/profile/Mona-Arafa-5/publication/344513508/figure/fig1/AS:948641430773760@1603185150005/Normal-skin-versus-skin-with-cellulite-Designed-by-Freepik.png.

Together with regional treatments, non-invasive modalities like photobiomodulation (PBM) are gaining popularity as valuable therapeutic options in cellulite. PBM uses distinctive wavelengths of light to energize cellular processes, induce tissue repair, and enhance blood flow in areas where cellulite is present. Such an effect also targets the cellular signaling pathways that govern collagen production and lipid metabolism, which contribute to the smoothing of skin texture and firmness. The simplicity that PBM is not invasive, with minimal side effects, makes it a desirable option in cosmetic dermatology. While continued research continues to validate the efficacy of PBM for the treatment of skin diseases, its role in the therapy of cellulite receives more limelight, offering promise to the sufferers who desire to minimize the appearance of cellulite while maintaining security and comfort during the treatment process (María et al., 2024) (Figure 9.2).

9.1.1. Causes and Contributing Factors

The etiology and pathogenic causes of cellulite and stretch marks are multifactorial, consisting of a multitude of biological and environmental variables. One of the leading hypotheses is that cellulite is generated by edema caused by overactive hydrophilicity of the intercellular matrix, interfering with tissue structure and function. This postulate proposes that fluid buildup in connective tissue may exacerbate the dimpled character of cellulite and that it is most common in women due to discrete anatomical variations in subcutaneous fat content in men and women. A microcirculatory homeostatic shift captured in the word EFP highlights the role of vascular changes in the adipose tissue. These evolving perceptions demonstrate the need for continuous research to reconcile these varied theories and an increased understanding of cellulites pathophysiology (Terranova et al., 2006). Stretch marks, as compared to cellulite, are significantly distinct in their causality and appearance, developing primarily as a result of rapid skin alterations due to hormonal changes, genetics, and body tension. These stretch marks most commonly occur following weight gain, pregnancy, or growth spurts, in which the skin is stretched beyond its elastic limits. The accompanying hormonal shifts in the state of pregnancy can noticeably relax the framework of the connective tissue of the skin, making it more susceptible to tearing and subsequent scarring. Genetic considerations, thus, worsen matters; individuals with positive family histories of stretch marks have a higher proclivity for developing these alterations in the skin. This bio-unique process needs special management strategies to mitigate the physical and psychological impacts of stretch marks (Boshoff, 2016) (Figure 9.3).

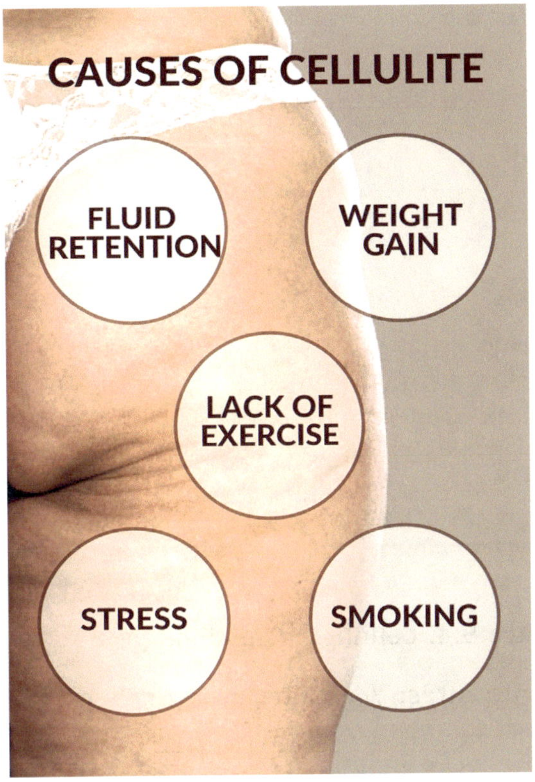

Figure 9.3. Causes of cellulite.

Source: https://i0.wp.com/www.mirrorfriendly.com/wp-content/uploads/2018/01/mirror_friendly_causes_of_cellulite.jpg?fit=800%2C1200&ssl=1.

In addition to inherent biological factors, several lifestyle elements also contribute to the development of cellulite and stretch marks. Dietary lifestyles that feature large amounts of sugar and processed foods increase inflammation, thereby weakening skin health and producing cellulite. Sedentary lifestyles also contribute by decreasing lymphatic drainage as well as deranging circulation, which are necessary for a healthy structure of the skin. Besides this, smoking and excessive sunlight can damage elastin and collagen fibers of the skin to make an individual more susceptible to developing stretch marks and cellulite. Altering these life-style variables with proper nutrients, exercise, and protective measures against skin impairment might be an all-inclusive treatment strategy in the cosmetic dermatology situation (Terranova et al., 2006; Boshoff, 2016) (Figure 9.4).

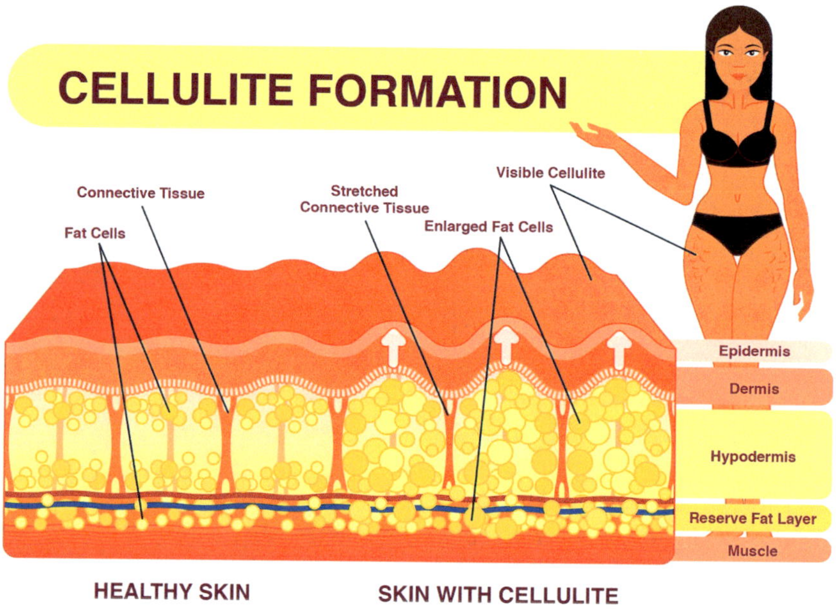

Figure 9.4. Cellulite formation.

Source: https://celluliteslayer.com/wp-content/uploads/cellulite-on-thighs-and-bum-07.png.

9.1.2. Types of Cellulite

It is paramount to identify cellulite forms in treating it effectively under the scope of cosmetic dermatology. Cellulite exists in three primary types: soft, hard, and edematous cellulite. Soft cellulite, often described as lumpy or dimpled appearance of the skin, is more likely to affect those who have a higher percentage of body fat. It is more prevalent in women and is accounted for by genetics and hormonal variation. Hard cellulite is a harder, less pliable texture and can be seen in individuals with lower body fat percentages. This case shows how even individuals with lower body fat are not immune to cellulite. The third type, edematous cellulite, occurs when there's over-retention of water that causes puffiness and redness, typically due to inadequate lymphatic drainage or circulatory processes, pointing to the significance of specialized treatment procedures addressing the respective type of cellulite illustrated. The treatments for every type of cellulite require sensitivity towards the underlying causes and character. For instance, the treatment of soft cellulite may include fat reduction and tightening of the skin with procedures like liposuction or non-invasive therapy like RF. Hard cellulite can be treated by circulating and collagen-stimulating treatments , such as massage or laser therapy. Edematous cellulite, which is seen with water retention, often responds well to lymphatic drainage massages or compression therapy that decreases swelling and improves overall skin texture. Each of these individual therapies demonstrates the merit of procedure tailoring to the category of cellulite. Treated in such a manner, practitioners can maximize patient outcomes and thereby enhance overall effectiveness of cellulite treatment regimes in clinical practice. In the face of the new science of cosmetic dermatology, developments have driven the additional exploration of new treatments for cellulite. The application of nanotechnology in dermatological treatment, particularly in the delivery of nanopharmaceuticals and nanocosmeceuticals, provides a highly promising solution to repairing the structural integrity of the skin and its appearance. Quoted in one study, topical use of such new formulations can be utilized for rejuvenation of aged skin by stimulating collagen production and elasticity, essential to reverse the effect of cellulite (Souto et al., 2020). Further, an understanding of the multifactorial etiology of cellulite can be utilized to design integrated treatment protocols that combine lifestyle modification with cosmetic interventions. This combined strategy, with treatment and prevention in equilibrium, is imperative in enhancing the patient satisfaction and outcome, a significant future prospect for managing cellulite in the cosmetic dermatology industry (Figure 9.5).

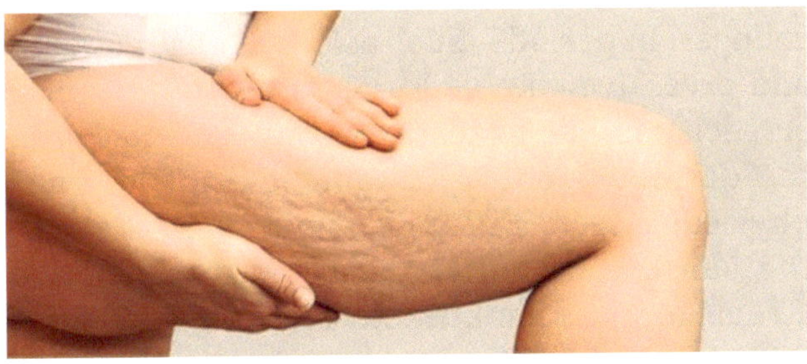

Figure 9.5. Edematous cellulite.

Source: https://cdn.shopify.com/s/files/1/0030/9408/5745/files/edemateus_480x480.jpg?v=1648897487.

9.1.3. Psychological Impact on Individuals

Psychological impacts of stretch marks and cellulite are not restricted to the physical looks of these conditions, as they catastrophically shatter an individual's self-concept and body image. Because the condition is universally associated with beauty standards, victims end up having negative body perception, which adds to anxiety and depression. The sense of inadequacy is exacerbated by the viewing of idealized images on social media sites, where flawless skin prevails. Even more, individuals will compare themselves to these posed, idealistic images and ultimately internalize their worthlessness. As such, the pursuit of cosmetic dermatology solutions becomes not only a quest for the improvement of the body, but a necessary return to mental wellness and self-acceptance. Furthermore, the body positivity movement has emerged as a counter-narrative to the conventional constructs of beauty as an effort to promote all body types, including those with cellulite and stretch marks. While advocating for acceptance and self-love, however, an investigation of how body positive individuals navigate their experiences online is also crucial. Even in empowering environments, one finds a paradox where it is possible to be nauseated by non-normative bodies through internalized societal norms. Based on body positive-related research, such a paradox may be undermining of psychological progress for individuals working through their own problems, so much so that it calls for a balanced approach that respects both psychological healing and acceptance of the body. This highlights the imperative to construct constructive environments within which current norms of beauty are challenged and inner worth of the individual is fostered. Ultimately, the psychological impact of skin diseases like cellulite and stretch marks too often includes not only personal misery but also more social impact. Individuals withdraw from social interactions, lest they be stigmatized or mocked for their bodies' parts, and this creates isolation and further exacerbates mental disorder. As identified in aesthetic medical tourism studies, there are multiple risks that surround the sector of beauty treatments; of which psychological risks form a subset. These high-order factors are significant to comprehend because they merge physical safety with psychological stability. Overall management protocols in cosmetic dermatology should thus focus on meeting these psychological needs in addition to physical treatment, allowing for an integrated approach to health that recognizes the interconnected nature of body and mind in the context of beauty (Figure 9.6).

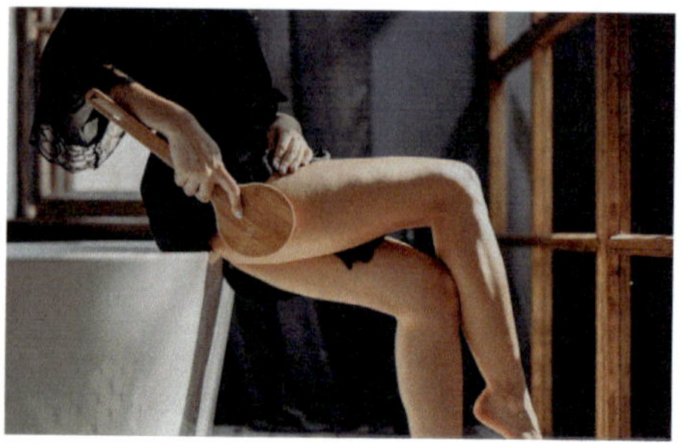

Figure 9.6. Dry brushing technique for cellulite management.

Source: https://www.soup.io/wp-content/uploads/2024/02/Cellulite-on-Legs-What-Is-It-1024x683.png.

Test Your Knowledge

1. What are the different types of cellulite, and how can they be classified based on their appearance or severity?
2. What are the main causes of cellulite, and how do factors , such as genetics, hormones, and lifestyle contribute to its development?
3. How do emotional and psychological factors influence the way individuals perceive and react to cellulite?

9.2. Understanding Stretch Marks

Learning Outcome

1. Describe the causes and contributing factors of stretch marks
2. Explain the stages of stretch mark development
3. Describe the psychological impact on individuals

Stretch marks, or striae, are universal dermal disturbances resulting from sudden skin stretching. Stretch marks usually manifest as linear scars that are usually various colors, red to purple, with lighter tones towards the end.

The etiology of stretch marks is multifactorial and has contributory factors like genes, hormonal variation, and drastic body weight changes. In periods , such as pregnancy, puberty, and excessive gain or loss of weight, the skin's elasticity is put to test, creating microtears in the dermis. Such a phenomenon not just has physical effects but psychological as well, in the sense that individuals come to perceive stretch marks as unattractive lesions, which can influence self-esteem and body image. The body positive social media movement has emerged in opposition to shame of skin imperfections like stretch marks. As women embrace body positivity, they take social sites to redefine expectations about beauty and acceptance. The movement is also confronted with contradictions as some members pursue dominant ideals of unblemished skin simultaneously. The battle between appreciating diverse bodies and upholding traditional standards of beauty shows that while social media has the ability to design empowering spaces, it will also solidify their self-judgments. Evidence shows that female viewers, even when they engage in body positivity, are able to create visceral disgust for non-normative bodies, thus showing the sophistication in the social seeing of skin abnormalities , such as stretch marks (Cwynar-Horta et al., 2016). In cosmetic dermatology, therapists and clinicians are examining various treatment modalities to manage stretch marks effectively.

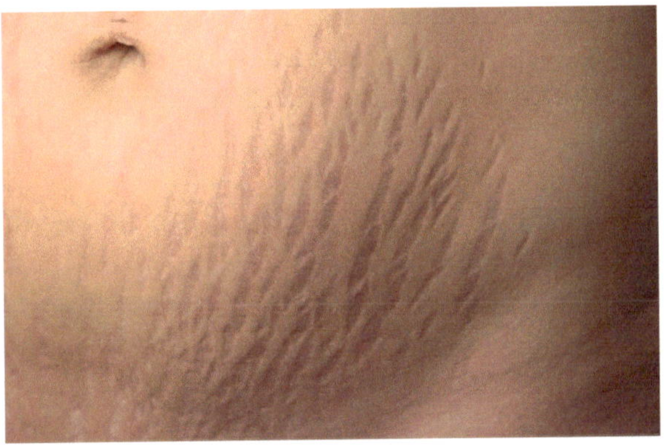

Figure 9.7. Stretch marks.

Source: https://assets.nhs.uk/nhsuk-cms/images/A_0119_stretch_mark_white_skin_abdo_F6XPNA_U.max-600x600.jpg.

Treatment modalities , such as laser therapy, microdermabrasion, and topical retinoids have been viewed to be effective in minimizing the appearance of such scars. Within the wealth of treatments, Mesotherapy Eporex has been proposed as a possibility for decreasing scars, especially in a postoperative environment, as shown by studies analyzing its effect after surgical procedures like bilateral mammary reduction (Boshoff, 2016). Promising as these methods may be, scientific evidence remains a main concern in establishing their role in clinical practice. Continued advancement in research and technology will surely better the treatment and understanding of stretch marks so that individuals can have healthier skin in addition to improved self-esteem (Figure 9.7).

9.2.1. Causes and Contributing Factors

The etiopathogenesis of cellulites is still a mystery, largely because the theories explaining its causes and predisposing factors have been conflicting. Many hypotheses have come up in attempts to explain the causation of cellulite, with specific emphasis on microcirculation and fluid trapping. One of the postulates has been that an excess of hydrophilia in the intercellular matrix causes the interstitial edema that is responsible for the appearance of cellulite on the skin surface as dimpling. Another perspective considers microcirculatory alterations at the level of the regions, described by the term EFP, suggesting an alteration of the delivery of nutrients and elimination of waste products in the dermal layer. These various interpretations highlight the complexity of cellulite as a phenomenon requiring further research to explain the variations between current studies (Terranova et al., 2006). Additionally, the structural differences between the male and female subcutaneous tissue have been described as key players in the high incidence of cellulite in women. The characteristic hormonal climate among women gives rise to the patterns of fat distribution that make them susceptible to cellulite development. In women, fatty tissue tends to be more vertically arranged, a predisposition that could make it easier to create the puckering effect characteristic of cellulite. Such anatomical structure, and hormonal influences , such as estrogen, is in accord with the hypothesis that biological sex is also a significant element in the etiology of cellulite. Evidence shows that awareness of these underlying variables is key to proper management plans since treatments may need to compensate for the unique structures and biological processes differentially impacted by sex (Terranova et al., 2006). Apart from physiological conditions, habits of life and hereditary factors also play an important role in management and appearance of both cellulite and stretch marks. Excessive stress and poor dietary intake can be causative factors that act as accelerators of conditions to deranged collagen and elastin production which will have a direct impact on the resilience and elasticity of skin. Aside from these, genetic factors can influence a person's predisposition to forming cellulite or stretch marks, and a hereditary history might be a marker for such conditions. The newly found aesthetic treatments, including Mesotherapy Eporex, is a potential route of treatment to address post-op scarring but awaits scientific evidence of its effectiveness in managing conditions , such as stretch marks and cellulite. Understanding all these causes in depth is crucial for creating specific interventions in cosmetic dermatology (Figure 9.8).

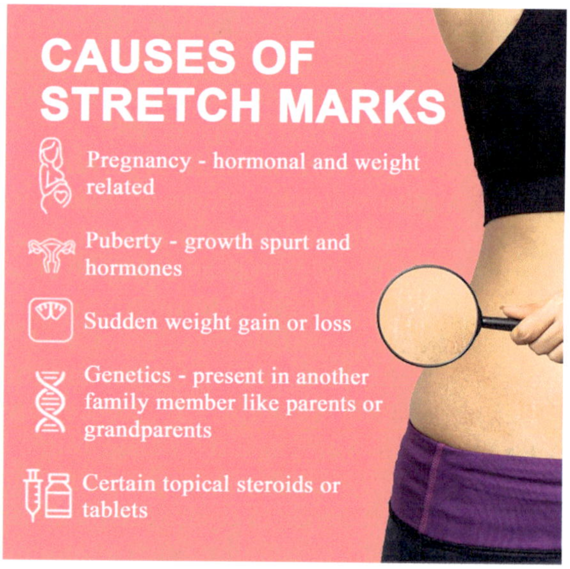
CAUSES OF STRETCH MARKS
Pregnancy - hormonal and weight related
Puberty - growth spurt and hormones
Sudden weight gain or loss
Genetics - present in another family member like parents or grandparents
Certain topical steroids or tablets

Figure 9.8. Causes of stretch marks.

Source: https://img.bebeautiful.in/www-bebeautiful-in/An-expert-guide-to-dealing-with-stretch-marks-in-teenagers_1_0.jpg?w=300.

9.2.2. Stages of Stretch Marks Development

The development of stretch marks, which are officially known as striae, is in certain phases and begins with striae rubra, or red stretch marks. These initial marks are characterized as being raised and pink in hue, indicating that there is new collagen production occurring and a rise in blood vessels to this area of the skin. During this stage, stretch marks are most responsive to treatment because the skin is still pliable and the dermal changes can be reversed. Treatment of striae rubra is particularly necessary because treatment at this stage can lead to more satisfactory results in terms of appearance and depth of the lesions. Research has indicated that intervention measures at the early stage, including topical interventions and laser therapy, work best at this phase because they seek to enhance collagen remodeling and minimize vascularization (Bleve et al., 2011). Over time, striae rubra matures into striae alba, or white stretch marks, as there is a significant transformation in the texture and look of the skin. These changed marks are also described as flatter, lighter, and less elevated, which suggests loss of blood flow and formation of collagen in the dermal layer. At this juncture, the possibilities of widespread improvement with therapies are reduced significantly due to the developed status of the skin changes and the challenge of stimulating regeneration in an area deficient in vascularity. Despite this, some treatments , such as microneedling and advanced laser treatment have been found to have minimal efficacy in rejuvenating the affected regions, although the improvement is not as dramatic as with early stages. Therefore, understanding the evolution of morphology during the striae rubra to striae alba process is key in planning proper care in cosmetic dermatology (Terranova et al., 2006). The journey of stretch marks through the phases highlights the need for early treatment and wise treatment decisions. Proper management calls for a good understanding of the unique features of each growth phase and the treatment modalities that can be used accordingly. Advanced diagnostic aids like high-frequency ultrasound and 3D imaging have to be used by clinicians to evaluate the type and maturity of stretch marks. Such objective assessments not only enhance treatment planning but also form a basis for measuring therapeutic efficacy over the long term, as reflected in more recent studies. Furthermore, discussion concerning the psychosocial impact of stretch marks, especially in females, underscores the need for individualized treatment strategies addressing both the physical and psychological aspects of this entity, eventually resulting in increased patient satisfaction in cosmetic dermatology (Bleve et al., 2011) (Figure 9.9).

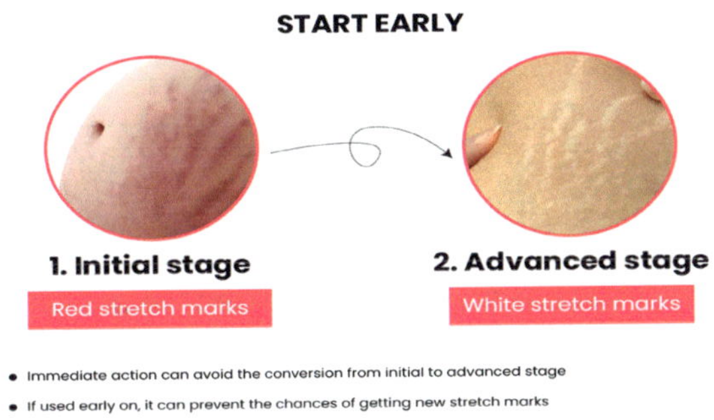

Figure 9.9. Stages of stretch marks.

Source: https://m.media-amazon.com/images/S/aplus-media-library-service-media/0ddbf1d3-547d-4107-9300-b4d61f82df20.__CR0,0,970,600_PT0_SX970_V1___.jpg.

9.2.3. Psychological Impact on Individuals

The psychological impact of stretch marks and cellulite on individuals cannot be overstated since these are common dermatologic issues that have significant emotional impairment. Most individuals, particularly women, feel embarrassed and ashamed about their appearance, and this usually diminishes their self-esteem as well as increases an unfavorable self-image. This is further contributed to by societal beliefs regarding beauty, which emphasize flawless skin, creating unrealistic expectations for most individuals. Thus, the patients of such conditions will be susceptible to various forms of anxiety and depression, thereby modifying their quality of life. The effect of stretch marks and cellulite is not just confined to the appearance of the skin, suggesting a far-reaching correlation between physical condition and mental health, highlighting the role of proper management in cosmetic dermatology to alleviate psychological suffering. Combating the psychological concerns raised by cellulite and stretch marks involves an integrated approach that spans both physical and psychological aspects of health. Current studies report the success of non-surgical dermatological treatments, , such as the application of seaweed mud, proven to improve the texture of the skin and reduce the perceived severity of cellulite. These procedures not only enhance the cosmetic appeal but also assist in improving patient satisfaction and psychological outcomes. When patients notice noticeable changes in their skin, they feel more confident and experience a body satisfaction. Therefore, cosmetic dermatology not only has to mind the body modifications but also the advantageous psychological impacts that accompany the success of treatment, thus encouraging a complete patient care approach (Amuso et al., 2024). Besides, the practice of medical tourism with the non-surgical beauty procedure has an even more powerful influence on the psychological landscape of the individuals who undergo treatment for cellulite and stretch marks. Because patients travel across borders to undergo aesthetic improvement, they perceive varying perceptions of risk, including psychological and social risk of undergoing treatment in another country. Clinicians and patients alike must understand these risks because they can have an impact on making treatment choices. Through the identification of these variables, practitioners will be able to better counsel patients regarding the psychological implications of their choices, thus improving the overall impact of treatment plans. In the end, incorporation of psychological support into the model of aesthetic medical tourism provides a feasible method of optimizing patient results and satisfaction in this burgeoning industry (Simpattanawong, 2016).

Test Your Knowledge

1. What are the primary causes of stretch marks?
2. How do stretch marks develop over time, and what are the different stages of their appearance and progression?
3. What psychological effects can stretch marks have on individuals?

9.3. Traditional Treatment Options for Cellulite

Learning Outcome

1. Understand topical treatments and their effectiveness
2. Explain massage and physical therapies
3. Focus on lifestyle changes and their role

The management of cellulite with traditional interventions has been greatly improved over the years, spurred primarily by advancements in cosmetic dermatology. Topical interventions rank high among these interventions, and they consist of creams and lotions that reportedly reduce the appearance of cellulite. Caffeine and retinol are two of the most frequently used ingredients with the aim of improving skin texture and firmness. However, the effectiveness of these treatments is often inconsistent, therefore casting suspicion on dermatologic practitioners. In the majority of cases, although such topical creams and applications will provide temporary results, they do not provide significant long-term changes in fat composition or skin type. The shortcomings of these procedures open up the search for more invasive methods, as practitioners strive to meet patient expectations of long-term results. Another beneficial treatment choice for cellulite is massage, which has been observed to be potentially beneficial in helping lymphatic drainage and improving circulation in affected areas. Treatments , such as endermologie, a mechanical massage with a machine used to manipulate the skin, have been shown to firm tissues as well as to reduce the surface roughness of the skin. Whereas patient satisfaction is typically self-assessed, the time-dependent nature of these outcomes should be remembered. Clinics also prefer to pair these massage therapies with lifestyle therapy , such as diet and exercise, which form an integral part of integrated cellulite therapy. Long-term outcomes, however, are contingent upon regular sessions, with some patients falling into a vicious circle of continued treatment that is both time-consuming and expensive. Liposuction has also been a more permanent method of decreasing cellulite, particularly in cases involving localized fat deposits. As a cosmetic fat removal surgery, better techniques have delivered a more sculpted appearance that can treat the uneven skin texture of cellulite. Minimally invasive methods have driven the practice towards greater safety and possibility among the population. Still, the process is not hazard-free and fraught with potential sequelae, as described in the literature on the removal of adipose tissue (Terranova et al., 2006). Adding to patient attitudes are also body image attitudes in society, which are increasingly influenced by social media and internet forums, where airbrushed images of toned skin fuel unrealistic expectations and make cultural beauty standards real (Cwynar-Horta et al., 2016).

9.3.1. Topical Treatments and Their Effectiveness

The growing popularity of cosmetic dermatology has been the impetus for a quest for a variety of topical treatments to address such afflictions as cellulite and stretch marks. There are now a variety of products, from creams and gels to serums, that claim to enhance the texture of skin and reduce the appearance of these afflictions. Yet the quality of such topical treatments tends to be unpredictable, particularly because of formulation differences and individual subjects' physiological reactions. Clinical tests show that most of these treatments yield weak evidence to back claims, as evidenced by an absence of systemic approval and risk of side effects. This insufficiency can lead to disappointment of the patients as well as disbelief regarding the impact of topical treatments on cellulite management, which may indicate the necessity of rigorous investigation and qualification of such products in clinical settings. One of the most impressive topical treatments is seaweed mud treatment, which has been quite effective in managing cellulite characteristics. A sixty-woman study of the application of seaweed mud over four weeks demonstrated remarkable improvement in skin elasticity, hydration, and structural tissue of cellulitic tissues. Microscopic results in biopsies had improved dermal organization, reduced inflammation, and collagen deposition, which collectively suggest a beneficial therapeutic result (Amuso et al., 2024). Furthermore, participant questionnaires in regard to satisfaction demonstrated enhanced comfort and lower body circumferences, underlining the integral benefits of this topical intervention. These observations suggest that with scientific verification, the topical interventions can offer significant improvement in the management of cellulite and may result in greater patient satisfaction.

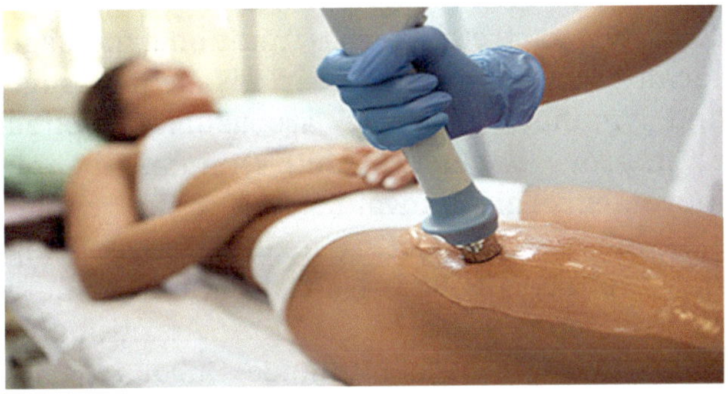

Figure 9.10. Cellulite treatment with gel.

Source: https://images.ctfassets.net/1ny4yoiyrqia/568OTlGi8NlZ2T6UKE7OHx/a0a16845f0016492e35c90514c0fba56/cellulite-acoustic-wave-therapy.jpg.

In contrast to the positive outcomes attributed to some topical modalities, the overall aesthetic environment of cellulite treatments is not free from obstacles. Many topical treatments currently on the market have limited scientific backing and are mostly anecdotal, which only helps to add to user frustration. Such a treatment is applied by the patient without an understanding of the multifactorial condition of cellulite, something that isn't solely cosmetic in nature but involves structural, inflammatory, and biochemical alterations to subcutaneous tissue (Atamoros et al., 2018). This complexity underscores the necessity of a critical selection of treatments with the awareness of dermatological consultation and evidence-based practice that measures patient expectations with feasible outcomes. Ongoing evaluation of topical treatments, particularly those with favorable results, is necessary to advance standards of care in the management of cellulite in cosmetic dermatology (Figure 9.10).

9.3.2. Massage and Physical Therapies

In the area of cosmetic dermatology, there is a high potential for physical treatments and massage in the management of conditions like cellulite and stretch marks. Traditional massage techniques, , such as deep tissue massage and lymphatic drainage, are usually applied to improve circulation and stimulate lymph movement. This is advantageous to the general skin look by eliminating toxins and reducing the retention of fluid, which could contribute to the appearance of cellulite. Additionally, these therapies can minimize fibrous tissue that typically exacerbates the appearance of cellulite. The use of massage in conjunction with other aesthetic treatments offers an integrated approach that might optimize desired outcomes while inducing patient relaxation and wellness, particularly critical in cosmetic therapy. In addition to the traditional massage therapies, newer physical treatments , such as ultrasound and RF therapy are taking on increasing significance in the treatment of cellulite and stretch marks. These modalities release energy to stimulate collagen synthesis, improve the elasticity of the skin, and improve texture. For instance, ultrasound therapy is reported to induce destruction of fat cells and increase dermal thickness, thus improving the texture of the skin overall. These therapies are often used in conjunction with traditional massage to provide maximum effectiveness, creating a synergistic effect that can create sudden improvements in the texture of the skin with repeated usage. As cosmetic dermatologists continue to look for new modes of treatment, the role of physical therapies becomes more and more crucial for the best cellulite and stretch marks treatment. Besides, there is a growing interest in the application of mesotherapy as an additional therapy in this case. Mesotherapy is the injection of various active ingredients into the mesoderm, which is the layer of connective tissue and fat found in the skin. The technique has been of interest because, aside from treating cellulite, it can also treat post-operative scarring, which is a worry for many in their quest for cosmetic treatments. Even if anecdotal evidence for the efficacy of mesotherapy in these areas is great, scientific rigor to attest to its efficacy, particularly in its use in correcting scarring from surgery, needs to be in place. With advancements in science, potential according to mesotherapy and how it can be integrated with conventional therapies can greatly reshape treatment paradigms in addressing cellulite and stretch marks within cosmetic dermatology (Boshoff, 2016). In addition, the establishment of other non-surgical approaches, as the research shown in literature like also indicates the importance of an integrative approach to body contouring and facial rejuvenation strategies (Figure 9.11).

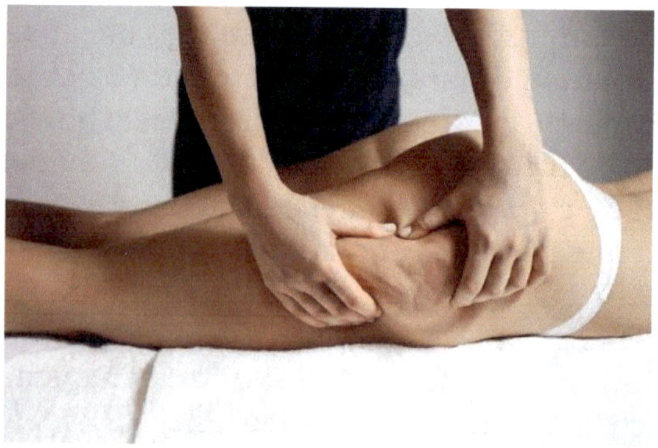

Figure 9.11. Massage therapies for managing cellulite conditions.

Source: https://celluliteslayer.com/wp-content/uploads/AdobeStock_259189522-2048x1367-1-580x400-4.webp.

9.3.3. Lifestyle Changes and Their Role

To counteract the problems associated with cellulite and stretch marks, the treatment approach must be multidisciplinary in scope, involving medical therapy as well as radical adjustments in lifestyle. Understanding of the structural, inflammatory, and biochemical alterations involved in the conditions , such as lipodystrophy, also known as cellulite, illustrates the nature of the conditions. Interestingly, the condition occurs in a significant percentage of women, sometimes even starting at puberty, and has the ability to significantly impact their quality of life. Hence, incorporating lifestyle changes like a healthy diet, routine exercise, and proper hydration can go a long way to enhance the appearance of the skin as well as overall health. Application of these adaptations not only assists in counteracting the effects of cellulite but also instills a proactive approach towards the health of the skin, thus underlining the relationship between everyday habits and efficacy of cosmetic dermatological treatments (Atamoros et al., 2018). Physical exercise, particularly strength training and aerobic, has also been shown to enhance the elasticity of the skin and circulation, which are vital factors in the management of cellulite and stretch marks. Exercise, when performed on a regular basis, can help to reduce body fat as well as build muscle tone, which can subsequently aid in the uniform distribution of subcutaneous fat and help lessen the appearance of cellulite. Furthermore, exercise-assisted weight regulation is in line with dietary methods intended to reverse the inflammatory mechanisms linked to both. In this case, lifestyle changes emerge as effective complements to clinical procedures and surgery being provided in cosmetic dermatology, further testifying to the idea that personal habits of self-care are key to determining treatment outcomes (Boshoff, 2016). For this reason, adherence to a disciplined lifestyle becomes essential to those seeking to effectively treat these dermatological conditions. Also, stress control and proper relaxation are often overlooked but crucial elements of an integrated program for the treatment of cellulite and stretch marks. Stress can increase skin issues through hormone disturbance and inflammatory pathways, and thus stress-reducing activities like mindfulness, yoga, or meditation can work very well. Similarly, proper rest benefits the repair processes of the body, promoting skin regeneration and perhaps reducing the frequency of stretch marks. Understanding that these lifestyle changes can be beneficial not only to dermatological health but overall emotional health, identifies their worth as part of an overall treatment plan. Taking on a lifestyle of physical, mental, and emotional well-being allows individuals to highly accomplish more attractive skin as well as a sense of empowerment and satisfaction with their own personal care routine (Atamoros et al., 2018).

Test Your Knowledge

1. What types of topical treatments are commonly used for cellulite, and how effective are they in reducing its appearance?
2. How do massage techniques and physical therapies work in the treatment of cellulite, and what results can be realistically expected?

9.4. Advanced Treatment Options for Cellulite

Learning Outcome

1. Describe laser therapy and its mechanisms
2. Define radiofrequency treatments
3. Deal with surgical options and their outcomes

The development of cosmetic dermatology has witnessed the launch of many new treatment modalities targeted at cellulite, a condition that affects many women. Of these treatment options, hypertonic sodium chloride creams have emerged as very promising. In a recent article, the mechanism of action of hypertonic cream with high levels of sodium chloride was depicted in terms of how it significantly reduces thigh circumference and enhances water retention that accompany cellulite formation.

The effect is primarily a result of osmosis, whose function is to pull off stored fluid between fat cells, hence minimizing inflammation and improving overall skin appearance. The results revealed a statistically significant reduction in thigh circumference for the hypertonic cream group compared to the placebo group, reflecting the treatments potential efficacy and safety in treating this challenging cosmetic concern (Azzella et al., 2024). Outside of topical treatments, manual subcision has gained popularity as an established remedy for combatting cellulite dimpling. The technique involves precise cutting of fibrous septa responsible for the skin's lumpy appearance. Using a specifically designed class IIA medical device known as Celluerase, the practitioner can create visible improvement in skin smoothness and elasticity. In a multi-center observational study of 200 female patients, objective medical measurement and subjective assessment of the patient also both demonstrated significant improvements in the cosmetic outcome, with an average improvement score of 8.1 and 7.8, respectively. This means that manual subcision is not only effective for early cosmetic improvement but also provides patient satisfaction, and therefore it is a good option for treatment of cellulite (Tunay et al., 2018). While both manual subcision and hypertonic cream individually possess advantages, a need arises to consider the vast range of cutting-edge treatment modalities available for cellulite. Minimally invasive procedures , such as laser therapy, ultrasound therapy, and RF therapy have also joined the fray as important players in the field of aesthetics. Such treatments act by inducing collagen production, stimulating lymphatic circulation, and correcting skin texture. Thus, the association of these novel treatments could provide more integral results, addressing the complex nature of cellulite. Last but not least, the treatment must be personalized to patient needs and desires, taking into account the intensity of cellulite and the expected result, in order to offer an overall treatment of cellulite in cosmetic dermatology.

9.4.1. Laser Therapy and Its Mechanisms

The application of laser therapy in cosmetic dermatology has come under much attention for its efficiency in treating conditions like cellulite and stretch marks. Laser therapy uses specific wavelengths of light to reach the deeper layers of skin, which helps in remodeling the collagen and elastin.

This is all needed to enhance the skin's texture and elasticity. For instance, the application of laser energy creates therapeutic heat damage to specific tissues, causing a healing response. Subsequently, the fibroblasts in the dermis are activated to produce new collagen, resulting in a more flexible and elastic skin appearance. Moreover, differential absorption of laser light by various chromophores present in the skin allows multifunctional applications, varying from reducing the appearance of stretch marks to managing more conspicuous cellulite features effectively. Moreover, research shows that laser treatment provides a cutting-edge method for treating cellulite as it stimulates enhanced blood circulation and lymphatic drainage. Such microcirculatory enhancements are essential since they reduce localized fat accumulations and enhance skin tone. The non-surgical, low-down-time quality of laser treatment makes it a highly desirable treatment for those patients who want to decrease the visual impact of cellulite and stretch marks.

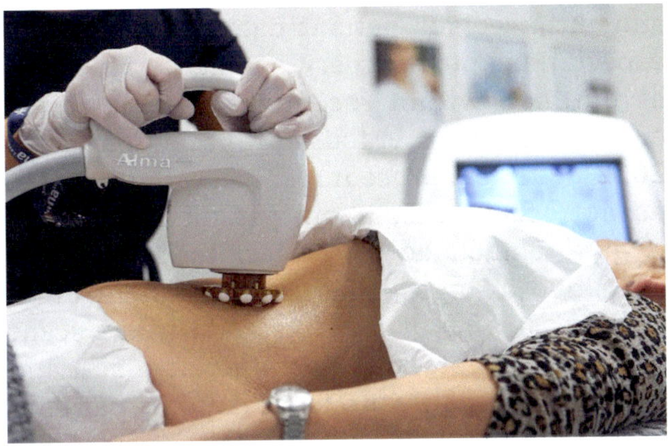

Figure 9.12. Laser therapy.

Source: https://ddclinical.com/wp-content/uploads/2019/10/DSCF9470.jpg.

Aside from surface cosmetics, other laser therapies, including fractional laser resurfacing, address deeper structural restructuring of the dermal matrix instead of the epidermis, treating the underlying pathophysiology of the skin condition. Tailoring treatment parameters to suit individual skin types enhances its efficacy, and laser therapy is a viable choice in cosmetic dermatology for treating skin concerns. Of specific interest is its synergistic combination with complementary therapies like carboxytherapy, since this could enhance outcomes in the treatment of cellulite. Carboxytherapy utilizes carbon dioxide in stimulating microcirculation and collagen generation, which has synergistic effects with the application of laser modalities. This holistic approach aligns with newer studies affirming the merit of multi-mode treatment regimens in realizing maximum gains from cosmetic procedures (Amuso et al., 2024). As research continues to refine and validate these methods, synergistic approaches that incorporate laser treatments with supportive treatments like carboxytherapy may redefine best practices in cellulite and stretch mark treatment. Last but not least, awareness of the mechanisms behind such therapies enhances the dermatologist's arsenal, improving patient satisfaction and overall effectiveness. Laser therapy, in conjunction with a holistic treatment regimen, is an example of a modern evidence-based practice for aesthetic dermatology (Borysiuk et al., 2021) (Figure 9.12).

9.4.2. Radiofrequency Treatments

The increasing demand for effective, noninvasive methods for cosmetology has worked significantly to change the situation for stretch marks and cellulite treatment in dermatology. Among the many approaches, RF treatments have become favored since they can improve the texture of the skin without undergoing surgery. RF treatments accomplish this by delivering energy to the dermal layers and inducing the synthesis of collagen and remodeling tissue.

It results in better skin elasticity, reduced appearance of cellulite, and better stretch marks over time. RF technologies have been seen to induce a noticeable difference in the quality of the skin, as per research, and are thus an attractive option for people seeking body sculpting treatments without the risks of the conventional, invasive treatments. With the application of RF power, common cosmetological problems may be treated quickly and effectively by dermatologists, hence illustrating the critical role of the treatment in contemporary cosmetic dermatology clinics. Combination therapies with other modalities, i.e., HIFEM therapy, have also yielded good results, particularly for those patients with challenging skin conditions. The synergistic effect of these multi-modalities is astounding; while HIFEM addresses muscle laxity and abdominoplasty, simultaneously RF enhances the aesthetic value by addressing superficial dermal layers. Such dual phenomenon not only optimizes fat reduction but also addresses skin tone and texture overall, a multi-dimensional approach to body contouring. In addition, these combinations become increasingly relevant in the context of escalating patient demand for reduced-recovery-time, non-surgical treatments.

As highlighted in more recent literature, strategic integration of RF with other novel technologies can potentially realize maximum aesthetic results, offering a solution to the extensive scope of patient concerns directed towards cellulite and stretch marks treatment (Chilukuri et al., 2022). Enhanced non-surgical esthetic procedures, particularly RF procedures, emphasize the continuous growth of cosmetic dermatology.

As documented, RF has several benefits over traditional injectables or surgeries that make it more popular. The key benefits are reduced levels of pain, fewer side effects, and shorter recovery periods compared to procedures like liposuction. Also, as body sculpting techniques become increasingly popular, it is crucial that practitioners remain current with the latest advancements in RF technology and use these observations to optimize patient outcomes. Lastly, effective treatment of cellulite and stretch marks relies on a balanced comprehension of the applications of RF and how these may be merged with various cosmetic treatments, providing a framework for delivering high-quality care and patient satisfaction (Andronache et al., 2019).

9.4.3. Surgical Options and Their Outcomes

Surgical operations are an important branch of cosmetic dermatology when addressing issues , such as stretch marks and cellulite. Liposuction is one such operation that has turned into a top fat-reduction treatment for body curves. What was initially just a fat-removal surgery has developed into a highly sophisticated method involving various minimally invasive and non-invasive methods. Expert surgeons now use a range of methods, often in combination with the application of energy-based instruments and customized combination therapies in an attempt to optimize patient result. The constraints of these interventions, , such as complications and the need for patient data on reasonable expectations post-surgery, should be accepted, as outlined within recent in-depth analyses of the different methods of liposuction (N/A, 2022). Surgical procedures, being therapeutic, do not occur in isolation; patient satisfaction is quite embedded in the facilitation of post-operative changes, like scarring and wound healing. By way of example, data from recent research indicate that post-operative scarring remains a significant issue among patients undergoing mammary reduction surgery. While this procedure can be of visually appealing benefit to those women who wish to eliminate the physical and emotional discomfort of large breasts, the reality of scarring will deter some possible candidates from undergoing the surgery. Therefore, there is also growing interest in adjunct treatments, , such as Mesotherapy Eporex, which has been studied for its potential to make scars look better as well as to treat cellulite and skin tightening. However, scientific proof of its efficacy in postoperative interventions is still absent today, which calls for research in the field (Boshoff, 2016). Not only does the efficacy of surgical interventions in cosmetic dermatology rely on the techniques applied but also on the subsequent management and treatment modality implemented post-intervention. The integration of newer adjunctive treatments with surgery can enhance overall patient satisfaction and reduce the incidence of post-surgical complications. As the field of cosmetic dermatology continues to evolve, outcomes reported by patients will become increasingly prevalent, offering insight into the effectiveness of different modalities in the treatment of stretch marks and cellulite. As such, then, it would appear that a multidisciplinary approach to encompass surgical dexterity, education of the patient, and novel therapies holds out the best possible results, irrespective of complexity, toward tailored care strategies and improved quality of life for patients with the dilemmas of body image concerns.

Test Your Knowledge

1. How does laser therapy work to reduce the appearance of cellulite?
2. What are radiofrequency treatments for cellulite, and how do they stimulate collagen production and skin tightening to improve skin texture?

9.5. Traditional Treatment Options for Stretch Marks

Learning Outcome

1. Describe topical treatments and their effectiveness
2. Discuss chemical peels and microdermabrasion for stretch marks
3. Focus on lifestyle changes and their role

Typical conventional therapies for stretch marks, familiar in cosmetic dermatology, primarily include topicals, laser treatment, and surgery. Topicals are generally in the form of creams and oils said to boost skin elasticity and moisture. Such ingredients as hyaluronic acid, retinoids, and vitamin E are commonly used due to their purported potential to stimulate skin renewal and provide the appearance of current marks. Although some research suggests that such products can yield modest gains, they are often limited in their effectiveness and cannot be relied on to be uniformly effective across individuals, and thus stronger treatments for overall management of stretch marks are needed. Besides topical treatments, laser therapy has also gained popularity due to its capacity to treat stretch marks by stimulating collagen synthesis and remodeling of the skin. There are various laser modalities that include fractional laser and pulsed dye laser (PDL) therapy, which target the deeper skin layers without inflicting much damage on the surface. As per research, the lasers are able to reduce the appearance of new and old stretch marks considerably by inducing the body's natural healing process. It is important that clinicians gauge individual patient needs and skin types so as to correctly tailor laser treatments, based on the reality that both the size of the stretch marks and also the patients complexion may play a role in successful treatment. Surgical interventions, being more invasive, are also an available means by which to treat old stretch marks, particularly where conservative interventions have failed. Surgical treatments like abdominoplasty are capable of removing excess skin and all but remove stretch marks from visibility. Procedural treatments, however, are disadvantageous in their scarring nature, a factor that discourages many patients from taking treatment; post-surgery complications could arise that would make the recovery process more difficult and lead to additional aesthetic problems. Observing this, studies continue to examine adjunct therapies, , such as Mesotherapy Eporex interventions, targeted towards the aesthetic look of scars resulting from surgical interventions and thus a potential avenue for women wishing to improve their overall result from surgical interventions (Boshoff, 2016).

9.5.1. Topical Treatments and Their Effectiveness

Topical treatment has been the area of concern in the management of cellulite and stretch marks in cosmetic dermatology. Non-surgical treatments are extremely popular because they offer patients an escape from surgical interventions, which are more risky and demand longer periods of recuperation. They have creams, gels, and masks available for their claimed abilities to enhance the texture, elasticity, and complexion of the skin. They generally contain active ingredients , such as caffeine, retinoids, and plant extracts, which are reported to stimulate circulation, enhance the production of collagen, and reduce fat cell size. Although there is anecdotal evidence to support their effectiveness, rigorous clinical trials would be needed to establish efficacy. The complexity of skin biology suggests outcomes are likely to be variable, based on individual skin type and preparation applied. Research has begun examining specific topical regimens, , such as the use of seaweed mud, which in recent studies has been reported to generate promising results. Four weeks' treatment of sixty women with seaweed mud on a controlled trial led to enhanced skin elasticity, hydration, and structural arrangement of cellulite-affected tissues. Findings included a notable reduction in cellulite severity, as well as scores of patient satisfaction reflecting a positive response to the treatment outcome. These findings are indicative of the potential for natural agents applied topically as treatment for the common condition of cellulite. Such microscopic examination also highlighted these claims with the documentation of extensive dermal reorganization in association with enhanced collagen synthesis and decreased inflammation from the treatment program. This suggests that a few of the topical treatments can be well-established by science, which contributes to their application in cosmetic treatments. Although promising results are associated with some of the topical therapies, the overall treatment efficacy of such treatment remains questionable. Most of these products still lack robust clinical warrants, and patients apply empirical or unsupported treatment without awareness of the biologic mechanisms. Such a scenario can lead to patient frustration and discontent, as emphasized by findings that imply a significant portion of treatment, though strongly desired, for the most part, does not meet expectations. Hence, further exhaustive research is needed to confront the array of modalities presented, weigh their actual efficacy, and establish best-practice regimen standards for their uses in aesthetic dermatology. This synthesis of current literature attempts to offer a better avenue for patients desiring effective solution alternatives for cellulite and stretch marks so that they can better make informed decisions regarding their dermatologic health. Furthermore, it emphasizes the importance of giving precedence to scientifically backed treatments in order to optimize patient satisfaction and overall treatment outcomes (Figure 9.13).

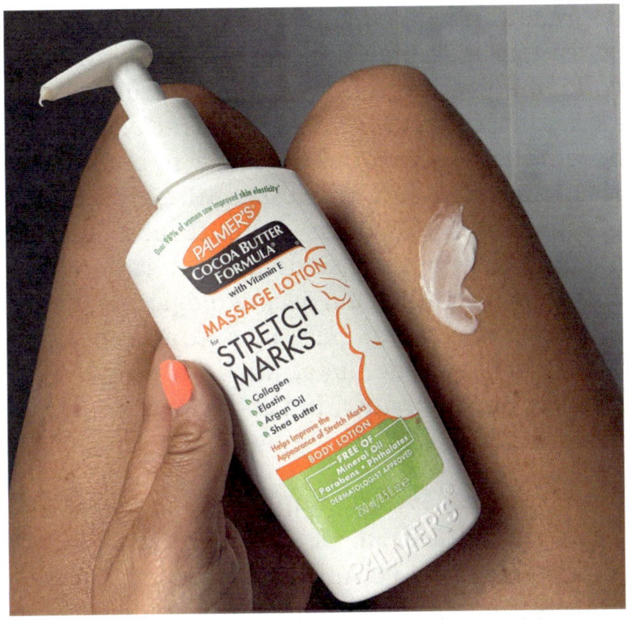

Figure 9.13. Application of stretch mark lotion for skin hydration and elasticity.

Source: https://hips.hearstapps.com/vader-prod.s3.amazonaws.com/1723144973-img-2677-66b51afae2055.jpg?crop=1.00xw:0.751xh;0,0.199xh&resize=980:*.

9.5.2. Chemical Peels and Microdermabrasion

Both chemical peels and microdermabrasion are gaining more application in cosmetic dermatology for the management of skin imperfections , such as cellulite and stretch marks. Chemical peels are applied by putting down a solution that strips away the outer layers of the skin, addressing conditions , such as textured skin and hyperpigmentation. This therapy can induce collagen synthesis and rejuvenate the skin, actually erasing most varieties of stretch marks by leveling the skin's texture. Multiple different chemical peels with shallow, medium, or deep levels of exfoliation allow dermatologists to tailor procedures to suit the specific patient's skin type and severity of condition. According to recent studies, these personalized treatments increase the level of patient satisfaction and experience, thus making chemical peels an effective option in the regenerative treatments of skin texture, , such as cellulite-related issues (Sivaranjani, 2019). Microdermabrasion is another non-surgical treatment, which complements chemical peels with its physical exfoliative method that enhances the overall look of the skin. Using a minimally abrasive device, microdermabrasion exfoliates the surface layer of dead skin cells in an orderly fashion, provoking deeper layers without causing harm to the epidermis. It is most beneficial for individuals with early onset aging and dermatological disorders like stretch marks because it evens out the texture and promotes a balanced skin surface. Clinical impressions have revealed microdermabrasion to induce observable tightening of skin firmness and elasticity, which are critical factors for the treatment of cellulite.

Notably, patients are satisfied with the treatments' minimal downtime and compatibility with daily skincare regimens, with it being a favorite among patients when coupled with other dermatological treatments (Simpattanawong, 2016). Moreover, microdermabrasion as well as chemical peels are equally powerful tools of natural skin care, particularly for the treatment of cosmetic problems like stretch marks and cellulite.

The combination plan of applying both these methods simultaneously can result in synergistic effects, optimizing the look and feel of the skin as well as reducing the risk factor of side effects compared to more aggressive treatments. Recent studies have shown that patients receiving the combined therapy of chemical peels and microdermabrasion have higher satisfaction levels, primarily due to the enhanced results achieved through the use of the two treatments in combination in treatment regimens. Through detailed assessment and the implementation of customized treatment protocols, dermatologists can improve results for patients seeking to improve their skin condition. These advancements in such non-surgical techniques not only indicate the continued growth of the field of cosmetic dermatology but also give patients alternative solutions to treat skin imperfections to the best effect (Sivaranjani, 2019) (Figure 9.14).

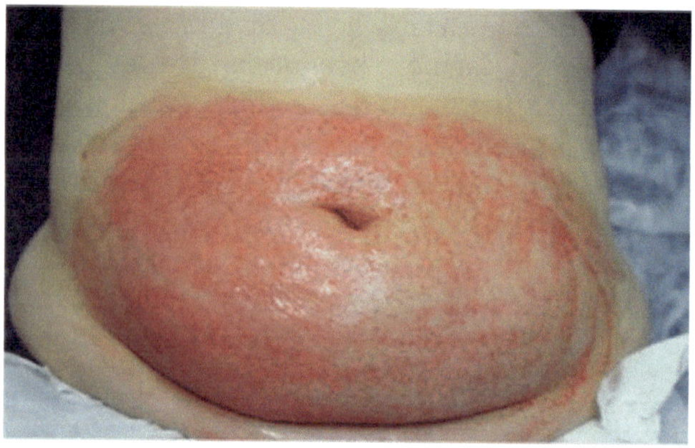

Figure 9.14. Microneedling. Microneedling was performed in conjunction with 20% ascorbic acid applied using a sterilized disposable brush before each microneedling pass. The endpoint was mild bleeding (after approximately 20 passes).

Source: https://www.researchgate.net/publication/320069867/figure/fig2/AS:546739003957248@1507364144359/microneedling-microneedling-was-performed-in-conjunction-with-20-ascorbic-acid-applied.png.

9.5.3. Lifestyle Changes and Their Role

Stretch mark and cellulite management in cosmetic dermatology is a multi-faceted process with lifestyle adjustment as the central function. One aspect of this method is the adoption of an equalized diet that is antioxidants and essential nutrient-supplemented, which favors good skin. Dietary intervention has tangible impacts on the elastic capacity of the skin and general complexion of the skin, combating the degradation that occurs with age. Daily intake of fruits, vegetables, and healthy fats promotes collagen production, which is essential for skin tautness. Additionally, hydration cannot be emphasized enough because it boosts the elasticity of the skin and lessens the appearance of blemishes , such as cellulite and stretch marks. Therefore, these dietary alterations not only improve individual dermatologic conditions but are an integral part of a comprehensive theory of health, demonstrating the remarkable synergy between nutrition and skin appearance in dermatology.

Exercise is an important adjunct to dietary modification, as an integral part of the management of cellulite and striae. Regular exercise promotes blood flow, which helps carry oxygen and nutrients to the skin cells, potentially making skin rejuvenation and elasticity more robust. Aerobic exercise, , such as running and swimming, has the specific effect of thinning layers of body fat, thus smoothing out the appearance of cellulite as it improves skin overall consistency. Resistance exercise is also beneficial in enhancing muscle tone, and this can minimize the prominence of stretch marks by redistributing fat and providing a more advantageous contour.

Moreover, physical activity is accountable for hormonal equilibrium and stress reduction, both of which favorably affect skin health and overall well-being. These alterations are indicative of how a positive attitude towards cosmetic dermatology necessitates that physical and cosmetic alterations are not mutually exclusive. Psychosocial factors, including mental health and stress management, are increasingly recognized as part of managing conditions , such as cellulite and stretch marks. Stress has the ability to cause harm to the skin's health by stimulating inflammatory mechanisms and speeding up the aging process, leading to fiber breakdown of collagen and elastin, as witnessed in Mohiuddin (2019). Thus, the incorporation of lifestyle changes that include mindfulness therapies , such as meditation and yoga can be immensely beneficial in counteracting stress levels and providing healthier skin. The role of relaxation techniques and self-care routines not only provides a more youthful glow to the face but also enhances individuals' overall health. Thus, lifestyle modifications that address physical and psychological dimensions create a complete model for the treatment of cellulite and stretch marks in the specialty of cosmetic dermatology and, in the long run, benefiting patients' skin and self-confidence.

Test Your Knowledge

1. What types of topical treatments are commonly used for stretch marks?
2. How do procedures like chemical peels and microdermabrasion help improve the texture and color of stretch marks?

9.6. Advanced Treatment Options for Stretch Marks

Learning Outcome

1. Explain laser therapy and its mechanisms
2. Describe microneedling and its benefits
3. Understand surgical options and their outcomes

Cosmetic dermatology has advanced highly in treatments for stretch marks, such that now patients have a variety of treatment options. The primary aim is to minimize the appearance of skin imperfections using treatments that restore the production of collagen and elastin. Techniques , such as laser therapy, employing focused light to rejuvenate the texture of the skin, are popular because they can reduce color and volume disparities present in stretch marks. Chemical peels, which consist of varying acid combinations, can also be used to regenerate the skin, making the surface of the skin smoother and even. These new treatments are generally debated in comprehensive clinical guidelines, emphasizing their effectiveness when given as standalone therapies or used as combination therapy with other treatments to manage patient-specific conditions better, to offer a general approach to the management of stretch marks in cosmetic dermatology (Sivaranjani, 2019). Mesotherapy is another new treatment modality that has been emphasized for the management of stretch marks. In this procedure, active substances are injected directly into the mesodermal layer of the skin, thus triggering local metabolism and boosting the elasticity of the skin. Research indicates that active molecules are capable of triggering collagen synthesis and imparting an overall improvement in the texture of the affected region. While traditionally used to treat cosmetic problems like cellulite and localized adiposities, the potential of mesotherapies in the treatment of stretch marks is an area of increasing research interest among dermatologists. Although there remain few empirical validations of its efficacy for this specific application, preliminary findings are encouraging. As shown in studies of other surgical procedures—, such as reduction of breasts, management of surgical scars continues to be of the highest priority, illustrating the demand for cosmetic solutions , such as Mesotherapy to provide (Boshoff, 2016). The use of combination treatments in managing stretch marks is increasingly well understood by dermatologists. By way of the synergistic outcome of multiple treatment modalities used together, practitioners are able to more effectively tailor interventions to patient-specific variables. As one example, a combined treatment strategy of both laser therapy and topical retinoids can yield enhanced overall results by interchanging deep tissue reconstruction with surface skin improvement. This integrative approach does not merely address its immediate cosmetic function but is also interested in the long-term well-being of the skin. Besides, it proves the evolving knowledge base of cosmetic dermatology; the methods are becoming more holistic and patient-specific, with a focus on obtaining maximum patient satisfaction. With more research being made available on these new methods, it is expected that guidelines for treating stretch marks will continue to evolve, thereby yielding better outcomes for those seeking effective solutions in this regard (Sivaranjani, 2019).

9.6.1. Laser Therapy and Its Mechanisms

The advent of laser therapy has significantly transformed cosmetic dermatology, particularly in the management of conditions like cellulite and stretch marks. The new treatment process uses the principle of light energy to provide a variety of varied dermatological impacts. By applying specific light wavelengths, laser therapy can penetrate further into the skin and initiate biological responses that result in enhanced collagen production, improvement of color tone, as well as general rejuvenation of the skin. Depending on the laser that is used, a variety of amounts of heat can be introduced into the dermal tissues, leading to an elective injury that triggers the body's natural response to healing. Thus, this procedure not only stimulates remodeling of the injured skin but also minimizes the visibility of superficial skin imperfections , such as cellulite and stretch marks. As it pertains to the treatment of cellulite, laser therapy can help stimulate lymphatic flow and microcirculation, critical in eliminating patterns of fibrous connective tissue responsible for skin dimpling. Upon relaxation of these bands of fibrous tissue, along with attendant fat cells, patients often find a significant smoothness of the skin. Evidence has demonstrated that laser treatments can minimize the appearance of cellulite through fibroblast stimulation and improved blood flow, leading to a healthier dermis and improved structural support of the skin. Furthermore, since laser treatments are not surgeries, they are preferable for patients who seek effective treatments without endangering the risks of surgeries and hence improving overall patient satisfaction in a clinical practice. In addition, pairing laser therapy with other procedures, e.g., carboxytherapy, might maximize outcomes and improve the efficacy of treatment. Carboxytherapy involves carbon dioxide administration to induce physiological effects that help in treating skin looseness and local fat accumulations. The synergy provides an improved method of addressing not just the dermal layer but also touching on systemic causes of cellulite severity (Borysiuk et al., 2021). The synergistic action of such therapies can not only lead to cosmetic improvement but also lead to dramatic improvements in skin elasticity and hydration, essential to long-term management of conditions like cellulite and stretch marks. The intersection of technologies in cosmetic dermatology ultimately leads practitioners towards more individualized treatment protocols, ensuring that patients receive detailed, comprehensive care tailored to their individual skin conditions (Figure 9.15).

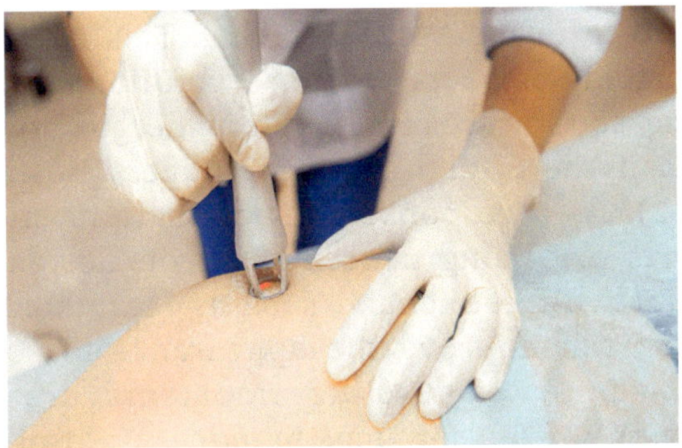

Figure 9.15. Laser stretch mark removal treatment.

Source: https://sdbotox.com/wp-content/uploads/2017/10/Untitled-design-2.png.

9.6.2. Microneedling and Its Benefits

Microneedling is a highly revered procedure in cosmetic dermatology, and one that is particularly useful for the treatment of stretch marks and cellulite. It is a highly minimally invasive procedure where tiny needles are applied to create microscopic wounds in the skin, which stimulates the body's own healing process and collagen as well as elastin formation. The controlled trauma produced by the needles enables numerous reparative processes, providing the skin with improved texture and elasticity. The advantages are conclusive in the correction of dermal atrophy of both cellulite and stretch marks, making microneedling a vital component of comprehensive skin management programs. The advantages of microneedling extend beyond mere cosmetic benefits; they include psychological improvement among patients. Studies reveal that patients who have received microneedling typically demonstrate high rates of satisfaction following observable results and minimized scarring. The long-term rise in collagen density not only improves the health of the skin, but it can also increase the level of a patient's quality of life, particularly in those who experience self-esteem issues associated with stretch marks or cellulite. Moreover, the minimally invasive nature of the procedure is part of its appeal since, on average, it involves a minimal amount of downtime and bearable side effects that align with patients interest in less invasive types of cosmetic treatment.

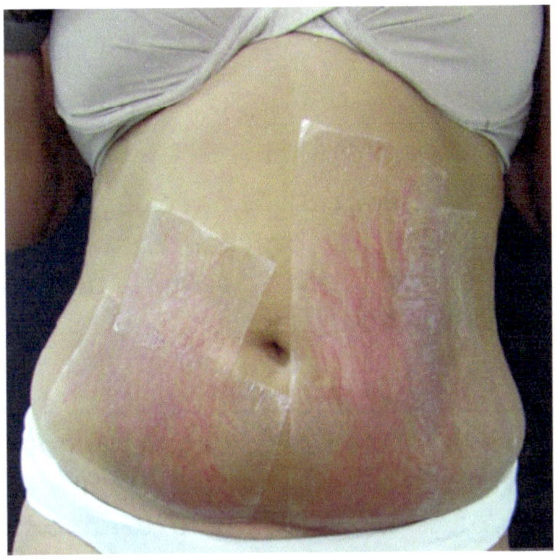

Figure 9.16. Demonstration of the expected endpoint after microneedling and how the plastic film should be placed.

Source: https://www.researchgate.net/profile/Marisa-Cunha-3/publication/370547782/figure/fig1/AS:11431281156011900@1683306856552/Demonstration-of-the-expected-endpoint-after-microneedling-and-how-the-plastic-film.png.

Moreover, microneedling is often seen to be a hands-on treatment option that will complement other cosmetic treatments nicely. By enhancing the skin's ability to absorb, microneedling can then be applied synergistically with topical treatments, enhancing their efficacy. Such synergy is valuable in treating conditions like stretch marks and acne scars, where modalities combined can produce an improved outcome. As cosmetic dermatology evolves, microneedling stands out for its significant contribution toward transforming patient care, with solutions that are effective and sensible. The advances in microneedling technique, like the use of automated equipment, also enhance its application and efficiency to allow dermatologists to personalize treatment for individual skin conditions, thereby optimizing outcome in the management of cellulite and stretch marks (Sivaranjani et al., 2019) (Figure 9.16).

9.6.3. Surgical Options and Their Outcomes

The area of cosmetic dermatology presents a variety of surgical procedures that address beauty concerns , such as cellulite and stretch marks. Liposuction, among them, has gained even wider popularity as a less surgical method for localized fat reduction deposits. Initially designed as a basic operation, modern liposuction is performed by sophisticated procedures that not only aspire to remove fat but also improve body shaping in general (Sivaranjani, 2019). Though the procedure works in body aesthetics, one should also point out limitations and complications of liposuction, including post-operative scarring and healing times. The surgeons should carefully evaluate candidates in order to properly meet expectations and results to facilitate patient satisfaction in the management of conditions like cellulite. In addition to fat reshaping procedures, operations , such as mammary reduction have significant implications on womens body perception, in the majority of instances, repairing issues exacerbated by both stretch marks and cellulite. While the physical pain of excess tissue is mitigated by such operations, they also introduce their own complication, largely linked to post-surgical scarring. This scarring negatively impacts women's emotional well-being, so they are reluctant to undergo surgery even if there might be advantages (Boshoff, 2016). As a response to such matters, more efforts are being concentrated on designing adjunctive treatments, , such as Mesotherapy, which can improve the appearance of scars post-surgery. These developments are an example of multi-modal practice of cosmetic surgery, whereby surgical in addition to non-surgical procedures support one another in order to provide maximum benefit to the patient. The integration of the various surgical techniques involved in cosmetic dermatology supports the necessity of custom treatment protocols formulated based on patient-specific demands. Outcomes may significantly vary with the selected surgery, the expertise of the practitioner, and patient factors , such as skin type and healing capacity. Thus, it is imperative that practitioners are up to date with the latest advancements in technique and technology and demand from patients (Sivaranjani, 2019). Also, research into new modalities, like Mesotherapy, aims to enhance aesthetic results and manage complications as a result of surgical treatments, and thus hold out an exciting horizon in treating cellulite and stretch marks. With the advancing branch of science, the joining of surgical and non-surgical therapy is sure to introduce more comprehensive solutions for individuals who wish to experience improvement in their dermatological problems.

Test Your Knowledge

1. How does laser therapy work to reduce the appearance of stretch marks?
2. What is microneedling, and how does it promote collagen production and skin regeneration to improve the texture and appearance of stretch marks?

SUMMARY

The management of cellulite and stretch marks in dermatologic cosmetics practice underscores the importance of refining treatment modalities directed at both efficacy and patient satisfaction. Today's patients are more informed about the range of alternatives, ranging from invasive procedures to non-invasive topical therapy. The recent research into treatments, , such as seaweed mud packs, holds good news for non-surgical treatments that not only improve the cosmetic appearance of the areas involved but also enhance tissue elasticity and moisturization. Primary results, , such as the return of dermal organization and patient satisfaction, indicate the potential of those procedures that satisfy today's need for safe yet effective cosmetic treatments (Amuso et al., 2024). Additionally, the societal context in which body image is found plays a role in addressing concerns like cellulite and stretch marks. Platforms like Instagram facilitate a body-positive culture that goes against traditional ideas of beauty and promotes freedom among women. However, such platforms also have a doubled narrative where the embrace of various shapes can sometimes coexist with existing society stigmas surrounding non-normative appearances. This nuanced interaction means that while acceptability has been promoted, the medical field must also watch out for the psychological impacts exercised by cultural standards on patients with the problem of cellulite and stretch marks (Cwynar-Horta et al., 2016). Lastly, the relationship of clinical efficacy and acceptability presents a complex scenario in aesthetic dermatology. While researchers work on identifying effective treatments, the sector needs to campaign for wider definitions of beauty that embrace all body types. This holistic approach not only fosters a more inclusive conversation but also brings treatment practices in line with changing patient needs and psychological well-being. Therefore, the future of treating cellulite and stretch marks needs to merge clinical advances with action aimed at encouraging self-acceptance and resisting common beauty ideals to usher in a gentler atmosphere in cosmetic dermatology.

The complexities of cellulite and stretch mark treatment have been an issue of cosmetic dermatology that has stemmed from the physical as well as the psychological nature of these skin conditions. Cellulite, characterized by pitting of the skin common in women, has come under varying interpretations regarding its etiology. The existing literature shows that there is a lack of agreement regarding the nomenclature and basic nature of cellulite, and the use of terms , such as panniculopathy and lipodystrophy interchangeably in scientific literature (Terranova et al., 2006). This lack of understanding emphasizes the necessity for further study to more clearly define the histopathologic characteristics and etiological factors like genetics, hormones, and lifestyle that make individuals more susceptible to this disease, presenting data towards more efficient management. The intractability of the cure for stretch marks, or striae, introduces another degree of difficulty to the field of dermatologic aesthetics. Stretch marks only occur after acute tension of the skin, most often due to hormonal changes or growth. Traditionally, the treatment options ranged from superficial treatments to advanced interventions like laser therapy. Amongst them, Mesotherapy has become popular, which is predominantly recognized for its application in improving skin texture and elasticity, and it also looks very promising in the management of scars following surgical procedures like mammary reduction (Boshoff, 2016). However, the lack of firm scientific evidence for the treatments upholds the importance of cautious analysis of current methodologies and how effective they are to ensure an evidence-based consideration towards the optimization of patient outcomes in cellulite and stretch mark treatment. Therefore, mastering the intricacies of cellulite and stretch marks requires a comprehensive understanding of their physiopathology and effective management procedures. The counter-theories to the causative agents of cellulite highlight the intricacies in dermatological research in the need for an integrated response to treatment based on the particular requirements of the individual patient. The production of novel solutions , such as Mesotherapy, reflects the continued effort towards optimizing aesthetic results, yet empirical data in order to support claims of efficacy (Terranova et al., 2006; Boshoff, 2016). As the field grows, it will become increasingly important to gain cooperation between the clinicians and researchers so that valid interventions may be created, which address both the physical presentation and psychological impact of common skin diseases.

KEY TERMS FROM THIS CHAPTER

- 3D imaging
- Bilateral mammary reduction
- Cell size
- Cellulite management
- Collagen-stimulating treatments
- Dermatological treatment
- Edematous cellulite
- Etiopathogenesis
- Fibroedemageloide (FEG)
- High-frequency ultrasound
- Anatomical structure
- Carboxytherapy
- Cellulite
- Collagen fibers
- Cosmetic dermatologic therapy
- Edematofibrosclerotic panniculitis (EFP)
- Environmental variables
- Fatty tissue
- HIFEM therapy
- Lymphatic drainage

CRITICAL THINKING QUESTIONS

1. **Which of the following treatments is commonly used to improve the appearance of cellulite?**
   a. Retinoids
   b. Cryotherapy
   c. Radiofrequency therapy
   d. Oral antibiotics
2. **What is the primary cause of stretch marks (striae)?**
   a. Bacterial infection
   b. Hormonal imbalance and skin stretching
   c. Poor hygiene
   d. Allergic reaction
3. **Which topical ingredient is often recommended for improving the appearance of stretch marks?**
   a. Benzoyl peroxide
   b. Tretinoin
   c. Coal tar
   d. Salicylic acid
4. **Which stage of stretch marks is most responsive to treatment?**
   a. Mature white striae (striae alba)
   b. Scabbed-over stretch marks
   c. Newly formed red or purple striae (striae rubra)
   d. None of the above
5. **Which of the following non-invasive procedures is often used to treat both cellulite and stretch marks?**
   a. Microdermabrasion
   b. Liposuction
   c. Botox injections
   d. Laser therapy

Short Answer Questions

1. What is cellulite, and what causes it to form beneath the skin?
2. Which lifestyle changes can help reduce the appearance of cellulite?
3. Name two non-invasive treatments commonly used to manage cellulite.
4. What causes stretch marks to form on the skin?
5. Which ingredients are commonly found in topical treatments for reducing stretch marks?
6. At what stage of development are stretch marks most responsive to treatment?

Answer to Critical Thinking Questions

1.(c) 2.(b) 3.(b) 4.(c) 5.(d)

REFERENCES

1. Pérez Atamoros, F. M., Alcalá Pérez, D., Asz Sigall, D., Ávila Romay, A. A., Barba Gastelum, J. A., de la Peña Salcedo, J. A., Escalante Salgado, P. E., Gallardo Palacios, G. J., Guerrero-Gonzalez, G. A., Morales De la Cerda, R., Ponce Olivera, R. M., Rossano Soriano, F., Solís Tinoco, E., & Welsh Hernández, E. C. (2018). Evidence-based treatment for gynoid lipodystrophy: A review of the recent literature. *Journal of cosmetic dermatology, 17*(6), 977–983. https://doi.org/10.1111/jocd.12555 (accessed on 11th June 2025).
2. Amuso, D., Medoro, A., Scapagnini, G., Gambacorta, A., Davinelli, S., Iorio, E. L., Bonetti, L. R., & Sbarbati, A. (2024). A pilot study on the efficacy of a seaweed mud application in the treatment of cellulite. *Journal of cosmetic dermatology, 23*(6), 2181–2189. https://doi.org/10.1111/jocd.16268(accessed on 11th June 2025).
3. Andronache, L. F., Balalau, C., Hainarosie, R., et al. (2019). Modern concepts in non-surgical esthetics; a review. https://core.ac.uk/download/232440314.pdf (accessed on 11th June 2025).
4. Azzella, G., Bianchi, L., Campione, E., et al. (2024). Clinical and ultrasound efficacy of topical hypertonic cream (Jovita Osmocell®) in the treatment of cellulite: A prospective, monocentric, double-blind, placebo-controlled study. https://core.ac.uk/download/621399164.pdf (accessed on 11th June 2025).
5. Bagherani, N., Smoller, B. R., Tavoosidana, G., Ghanadan, A., Wollina, U., & Lotti, T. (2023). An overview of the role of carboxytherapy in dermatology. *Journal of Cosmetic Dermatology, 22*, 2399–2407. https://doi.org/10.1111/jocd.15741 (accessed on 11th June 2025).
6. Bayrakci Tunay, B., Boraldi, E., Caruso, D., Chang, H., Croce, M. A., de Godoy, J. M. P., de Godoy, M. F. G., et al. (2018). Treatment of dimpling from cellulite. https://core.ac.uk/download/217583732.pdf (accessed on 11th June 2025).
7. Terranova, F., Berardesca, E., & Maibach, H. (2006). Cellulite: nature and aetiopathogenesis. *International journal of cosmetic science, 28*(3), 157–167. https://doi.org/10.1111/j.1467-2494.2006.00316.x(accessed on 11th June 2025).
8. Bleve, M., Capra, P., Pavanetto, F., et al. (2011). Ultrasound and 3D skin imaging: Methods to evaluate efficacy of *striae distensile* treatment. https://core.ac.uk/download/pdf/8655842.pdf (accessed on 11th June 2025).
9. Borysiuk, I., Drogovoz, S., Kalko, K., et al. (2021). The versatility of carboxytherapy in pathogenic therapy. https://core.ac.uk/download/491071775.pdf (accessed on 11th June 2025).
10. Boshoff, T. M. (2016). Mesotherapy Eporex treatments on post-operative mammary reduction scarring. https://core.ac.uk/download/222967500.pdf (accessed on 11th June 2025).
11. Chilukuri, S., Duncan, D. I., Hoffmann, K., et al. (2022). Non-invasive alternatives for liposuction. https://core.ac.uk/download/492702817.pdf (accessed on 11th June 2025).
12. Souto, E. B., Fernandes, A. R., Martins-Gomes, C., Coutinho, T. E., Durazzo, A., Lucarini, M., Souto, S. B., Silva, A. M., & Santini, A. (2020). Nanomaterials for Skin Delivery of Cosmeceuticals and Pharmaceuticals. *Applied Sciences, 10*(5), 1594. https://doi.org/10.3390/app10051594 (accessed on 11th June 2025).
13. Cwynar-Horta, J. C. (2016). Documenting femininity: Body-positivity and female empowerment on Instagram. https://core.ac.uk/download/77106923.pdf (accessed on 11th June 2025).

14. Duncan, D. I. (2022). Enhanced liposuction. https://core.ac.uk/download/534904133.pdf (accessed on 11th June 2025).

15. Hernández-Bule, M. L., Naharro-Rodríguez, J., Bacci, S., & Fernández-Guarino, M. (2024). Unlocking the power of light on the skin: A comprehensive review on photo biomodulation. *International Journal of Molecular Sciences*, *25*, 4483–4483. https://doi.org/10.3390/ijms25084483 (accessed on 11th June 2025).

16. Kalasariya, H. S., Maya-Ramírez, C. E., Cotas, J., & Pereira, L. (2024). Cosmeceutical significance of seaweed: A focus on carbohydrates and peptides in skin applications. *Phycology*, *4*, 276–313. https://doi.org/10.3390/phycology4020015 (accessed on 11th June 2025).

17. Mohiuddin, A. K. (2019). Skin aging & modern age anti-aging strategies. *International Journal of Clinical Dermatology & Research*. https://doi.org/10.19070/2332-2977-1900052 (accessed on 11th June 2025).

18. Nascimento, V. F. N. do. (2019). *Principis afecções dermatological facias e corporals em gestates residents na citadel de Santa Cruz/RN*. https://core.ac.uk/download/635089708.pdf (accessed on 11th June 2025).

19. Simpattanawong, D. (2016). *Non-invasive aesthetic medical tourism in Bangkok : a qualitative analysis of stakeholder risk. https://doi.org/10.24384/C7Q9-Q433* (accessed on 11th June 2025).

20. Sivaranjani, J. (2019). *Percutaneous Collagen Induction in the Treatment of Atrophic Acne Scars using an Automated Microneedling Device: A Novel Approach* (Doctoral dissertation, Stanley Medical College, Chennai).(accessed on 11th June 2025).

PSYCHODERMATOLOGY AND BODY DYSMORPHIC DISORDER

10

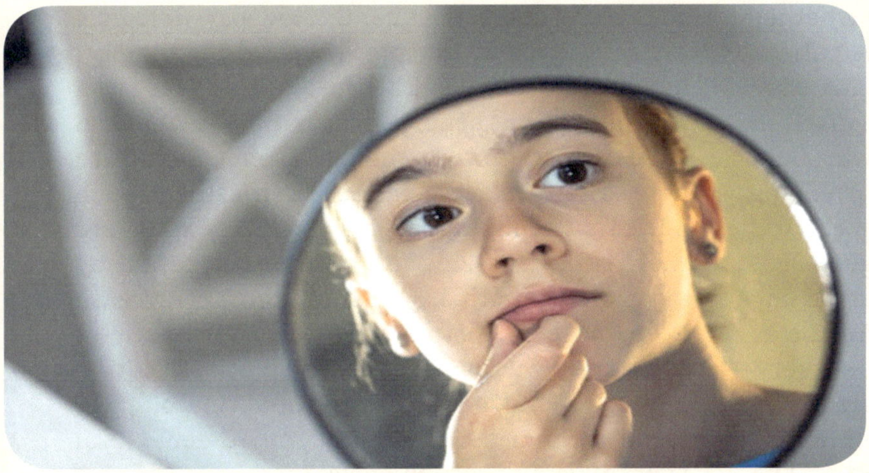

LEARNING OBJECTIVES

After studying this chapter, you will be able to:

1. Understand the historical context surrounding psychodermatology and body dysmorphic disorder (BDD)
2. Describe the psychological aspects of body dysmorphic disorder
3. Focus on dermatological manifestations and psychological well-being within psychodermatology
4. Explain the treatment of body dysmorphic disorder (BDD)
5. Define the role of healthcare professionals in the recognition and treatment of psychodermatological conditions
6. Deal with current research trends in the psychodermatology field

Introduction

The crossover between psychological illness and skin illness has resulted in psychodermatology, an area of study that explores how psychological conditions can express themselves as dermatological issues. BDD is one of the most prominent cases to be found in this area, where a disabling preoccupation with perceived flaws in appearance leads to repetitive actions aimed at correcting said flaws. This condition not only affects mental health but also significantly affects how patients relate to healthcare systems, particularly those who receive cosmetic procedures as a solution to their discomfort. Literature indicates that BDD individuals have a complex relationship with cosmetic surgery, one that isn't necessarily followed by the alleviation of the underlying psychological aspects and therefore demands scrutiny of motives and outcomes involving elective surgical intervention (Juodikis et al., 2024). Literature indicates alarming statistics regarding the connection between BDD and cosmetic surgery, further elevating risks for the subject undergoing aesthetic enhancement. BDD patients tend to undergo aesthetic procedures even with heightened postoperative risks and general dissatisfaction with results. Studies indicate that up to 60.6% of BDD patients have undergone comparable surgical procedures before, only to become dissatisfied afterward (Juodikis et al., 2024). The complexity of BDD treatment is underscored by a gap in the literature that limits the way psychological health is affected by plastic surgery. Against this backdrop, there is a critical need to redefine the criteria for whether or not surgery can be warranted in this patient population to emphasize mental health over skin correction. Surgeons are highly engaged in the management of BDD, but their awareness and training regarding psychological problems are uneven. A recent study emphasizes that even though the majority of plastic surgeons are cognizant of the symptoms of BDD, hardly any of them refer to mental health professionals as a routine measure before carrying out surgery. It is an ethical concern and emphasizes the need for improved education and guidelines for cosmetic operators immediately. The challenges are compounded by potential aggressive acts on the part of patients with BDD, which can interfere with the clinician-patient relationship. As plastic surgeons deal with more individuals with BDD, there is a need to develop comprehensive assessment protocols incorporating psychological screenings to make sure patients are given the full picture of their physical as well as their mental health.

Definition of Psychodermatology

Psychodermatology is an interdisciplinary practice that brings together concepts of both dermatology and psychiatry, focusing on the complex interaction between skin and mental states. The specialty addresses the way psychological disorders manifest themselves as cutaneous disorders, as well as the recognition that dermatologic disease can exacerbate mental illness. Psychodermatology is best utilized in the explanation of disorders , such as BDD, where the patient may become excessively concerned with imperfections in their body, often with significantly compromised social and occupational functioning. The importance of this subdiscipline is that it puts the point of comprehensiveness across, noting the importance of dermatologists and mental health professionals colliding to provide complete patient care. This convergence offers a clearer picture of how skin diseases can affect emotional well-being and consequently, how psychological distress leads to or aggravates dermatological disorders (Patel, 2022). In addition, research has shown that acne, psoriasis, and eczema can have catastrophic psychological effects , such as depression, anxiety, and poor self-esteem. Such patients usually undergo a vicious cycle where their skin problems are further worsened by psychological stress, causing them to increase even more in distress and unhappiness with their body. Such a feedback loop of correlation highlights the need for psychodermatological treatments in the form of cognitive-behavioral therapies and other psychiatric treatments to break such a cycle. It's worth noting this dynamic in considering the treatment approach for patients who present with skin problems, especially those with BDD. Multidisciplinary collaboration can facilitate better outcomes through addressing both physical and emotional conditions of the patient (Patel, 2022). Psychodermatology bears more than just treatment; it has a great impact on raising public awareness of the psychological consequences of skin disorders. Healthcare and the general public can be taught about the psychological aspects of dermatologic issues to develop a more empathetic and holistic understanding of health-related issues. Public education campaigns can encourage early treatment and appropriate mental health interventions alongside dermatologic treatment, particularly in those at risk for BDD. With increased study into psychodermatology, there is potential for groundbreaking methods of treatment that can address the needs of patients with the combination of skin pathology and psychological distress. Through learning and sharing the interconnected nature of skin health and mental health, the topic of psychodermatology paves the way for improved patient-centered ways of healthcare (Patel, 2022) (Figure 10.1).

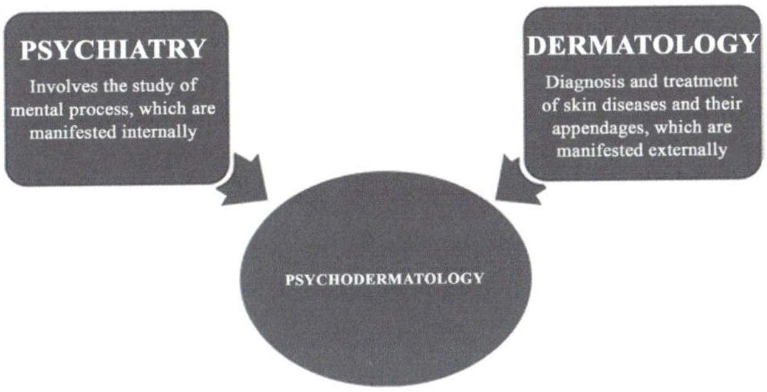

Figure 10.1. Psychodermatology.

Source: https://www.medicaljournals.se/acta/content_files/files/web/4665-web-resources/image/9936.png.

Overview of Body Dysmorphic Disorder (BDD)

BDD is a severe mental disorder that involves a preoccupation with imagined defects of appearance, which are generally nonexistent or minor. BDD typically emerges in late adolescence or early adulthood and nearly always affects adolescents and young adults in the teens and twentysomething age groups. Those with BDD will typically develop a ritual act , such as repetitive checking of themselves in mirrors, picking at the skin, or repeatedly seeking reassurance of their appearance. The cognitive distortions of BDD have been linked to significant emotional distress, most importantly disrupting daily functioning and impairing quality of life. Such pervasive appearance preoccupation may be a barrier to social relationships, such that individuals are likely to have difficulty sustaining relationships or identifying vocational undertakings, and might also co-occur with other mental disorders, including depression and anxiety, complicating treatment. Evidence attests to the profound psychosocial impact of BDD, consistent with its dermatological effects. Impacted individuals can experience disturbance in self-esteem and general well-being, leading to global anxiety, depression, and suicidal tendencies. Societal stigma regarding mental illness, particularly appearance-based, exacerbates feelings of isolation and heightens symptoms. Treatment of BDD is likely to have to be multimodal, , such as the application of cognitive-behavioral therapy (CBT) coupled with medications , such as selective serotonin reuptake inhibitors (SSRIs). Unfortunately, as particular treatment methods are not highly regarded, the majority of those who suffer remain untreated or misdiagnosed, a sign of health crisis that should receive more research and exposure within both the psychology and dermatology fields. Also, the intricate interaction between BDD and skin conditions cannot be exaggerated, as ailments like acne weigh significantly upon the manifestations of BDD. Acne, prevalent in nearly 80% of individuals between 11 and 30 years of age, has been found to have very significant correlations with reductions in psychosocial functioning, wherein up to 85% of adolescents experience negative psychological ramifications associated with this skin condition. Such effects include increased depression, anxiety, and low self-esteem, showing the importance of treating the psychosocial effect of skin diseases in practice. The integration of dermatological treatment with psychological care can be highly effective. By establishing a system where both physical and psychological realms are diagnosed and treated simultaneously, medical practitioners can make an enormous impact in the lives of BDD patients, aware that the complications resulting from such disorders run much deeper than cosmetically observable, as evidenced by the recurring necessity of combined psychodermatological treatment (Massoud et al., 2022; Patel, 2022) (Figure 10.1).

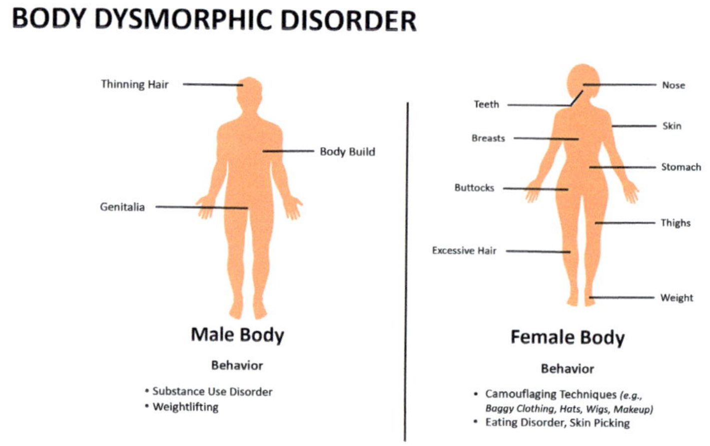

Figure 10.2. Body dysmorphic disorder (BDD).

Source: https://www.collidu.com/media/catalog/product/img1/8/6/867d555b5af799832e3db74c0082f6326cfd527800d6d863554d38fbb3ed5f57/body-dysmorphic-disorder-slide2.png.

Importance of the Connection Between Psychodermatology and BDD

The psychodermatology link to BDD is central to establishing the psychological factors influencing skin-related issues. Psychodermatology speaks to the relation between dermatological conditions and psychological well-being. In individuals with BDD, the perceived flaws most frequently occur on the skin, hence offering a multifaceted relationship where emotional suffering is increased. These patients are usually found to have compulsive behavior about their appearance, which in turn gives rise to or worsens skin conditions , such as eczema or acne. It is hence very important to treat both the psychological and the skin aspect for not only effective treatment but also to improve overall quality of life in such individuals. The integration of psychodermatology in treatment protocols allows practitioners to identify and manage the multifaceted nature of BDD, advocating for a holistic approach that treats both mind and body. In addition, the implementation of therapeutic interventions grounded in psychodermatology can produce seismic changes in the management of BDD. CBT and psychopharmacological treatments are fundamental components, as these seek to modify maladaptive thought patterns and behaviors towards body image. Research shows that these treatment models can decrease the disabling symptoms of BDD effectively while enhancing emotional and social functioning among patients. Clinicians have clinically reported that an integrative model, with psychodermatological principles included, results in better outcomes, primarily by forming stronger therapeutic alliances. In this study, clinicians and patients alike preferred treatment approaches that combine educational psychology with dermatological management, as they highlighted the need for such collaborative treatment models in successfully treating BDD. The incorporation of qualitative data in conceptualizing treatment for BDD underlines the need to sustain psychodermatological rapport. Recent studies indicate that while the existing treatment models are beneficial, there remain gaps in the best practice knowledge of treating BDD. For instance, clinician feedback indicated dissatisfaction with existing treatments and calls for more competence to address the psychological issues related to skin perception impairment. Patient experiences also promote the need for emotional support and empathy, emphasizing the strength of an effective therapeutic relationship. It becomes apparent that deepening the overlap between psychodermatology and BDD not only requires an enhanced assessment of current treatments but also determination towards additional research in confluence with patient requirements, thereby streamlining therapeutic procedures and enhancing aggregate effectiveness in treating this complicated disorder (Govender, 2021; Brun et al., 2024).

10.1. Historical Context

Learning Outcome

1. Understand the evolution of psychodermatology as a field
2. Describe historical perspectives on body dysmorphic disorder
3. Focus on key studies that shaped the understanding of BDD

The historical context of BDD and psychodermatology illustrates a deep shift in the understanding of the interconnectedness of psychological and dermatological health. Initially, the field of psychodermatology emerged as a response to recognizing that skin diseases are psychologically based, and skin conditions like eczema and psoriasis were linked to stress and tension. This recognition provided an entry point for research on BDD, a psychiatric disorder involving preoccupation with actual or perceived imperfections of appearance. The placement of BDD in the Diagnostic and Statistical Manual of Mental Disorders (DSM) has provided legitimacy to this connection, underscoring the need to treat both psychological and dermatologic aspects. As paradigms of mental illness evolved, clinicians began to consider how underlying psychiatric illness could exacerbate skin disease and thus established the foundation for integrative treatment approaches to both areas. With the establishment of the discussion of BDD, an additional examination of associated disorders , such as muscle dysmorphia, unveiled the complex dynamics of body image disturbance. Muscle dysmorphia, one of the BDDs, is characterized by a preoccupation with bodily imperfections in body-image dimensions of muscle size and definition. The preoccupation generally results in the compulsion of individuals towards ill health, which includes the misuse of anabolic steroids as well as PEDs, in trying to gain an ideal body. This history of the issue is critical, as societal pressures as well as societal representations of the ideal body have rendered the pressures more salient for this individual, particularly males. Moreover, the intersection of psychological and physiological elements reveals how hormonal and neural transformations contribute to muscle dysmorphia addiction cycles.

These results emphasize the importance of a comprehensive view of psychosocial as well as physiological dimensions of body image disorders, requiring personalized treatments. Increased awareness of the intricate relationship between psychological health and dermatological disorders created a need for interdisciplinary models of treatment in psychodermatology. In the past, therapy for BDD and co-occurring skin disease had been piecemeal, to the extent of treating only the dermatologic or psychiatric aspect. More recently, an integrative approach of cognitive-behavioral therapy and pharmacotherapy combined with dermatologic treatment is encouraged. The shift has been brought about by research emphasizing the need for holistic models that take into account the neuroendocrine effects of conditions like muscle dysmorphia. By acknowledging the fact that drug abuse-induced hormonal imbalance is the cause of widespread changes in brain function and mood disorders, practitioners are in a better position now to design personalized treatment plans. These multidisciplinary strategies are most essential in addressing the complex dimension of BDD and how this affects individuals' lives, which is a significant breakthrough in the historical pathway of both psychodermatology and mental healthcare (Bassetti et al., 2024; Metin, 2024).

10.1.1. Evolution of Psychodermatology as a Field

The evolution of psychodermatology as a specialty has been greatly influenced by expanding awareness of the interplay between psychological and dermatologic states. Defined initially in terms of bridging the psychosomatic link implicit in numerous skin diseases, psychodermatology now treats a broad range of psychological processes that impact the skin. The field draws on the fields of dermatology, psychiatry, and psychology to address the intricate overlaps of mental illness and skin disease—like depression, anxiety, and BDD. The more that is understood about these associations, the more mental health professionals have come to integrate more multidisciplinary and integrative treatment, moving beyond older models to encompass treatments targeting both the psychological and physical basis of skin disease. BDD, in the language of psychodermatology, is a striking example of the influence of psychological processes on dermatological awareness and management. BDD is characterized by a repetitive preoccupation with actual or perceived flaws of appearance, which compels individuals to seek out repetitive cosmetic procedures or engage in self-damaging acts. The frequency of the disorders—projected at a high of 2% of the general population, highlights the importance of proper treatment (Safitri et al., 2025). In addition, the majority of individuals with BDD encounter barriers to psychological therapy, including stigmatization and insufficient awareness among health practitioners of the complexity of BDDs. This constitutes a core challenge to psychodermatology that calls for continued research, education, and the creation of fine-tuned treatments tailored to BDD. The impetus to create new treatment protocols in psychodermatology is also fueled by emerging evidence on the therapeutic benefit of mindfulness-based interventions. With clinical data further substantiating the case for the benefits of mindfulness for disorders like BDD, eating disorders and social anxiety disorder, a body of data is emerging to support its application in enhancing mental health outcomes among individuals with BDD (Safitri et al., 2025). Mindfulness techniques operate to promote acceptance, reduce anxiety, and create more positive body image awareness, representing a promising adjunct to traditional treatment methods. As psychodermatology continues to evolve, the integration of such new therapies is a reflection of a broader movement toward personalized treatment that addresses both dermatological and mental health needs, representing a more holistic treatment paradigm for addressing those suffering from the two-part pathology of psychodermatological disorders.

10.1.2. Historical Perspectives on Body Dysmorphic Disorder

Historical conceptualization of BDD has evolved by leaps and bounds from the last century, from being vague and ambulatory notions of perceived ugliness to being recognized as a psychiatric disorder. Initially described in the early 20th century, BDD-type symptoms were previously noted with more concrete psychological illnesses, wherein patients would make strong complaints against their appearance without classically fitting into such. It was this generality that helped fuel the misdiagnosis of so many patients who actually had severe self-image disturbances, with less-than-optimal treatment and results. With increased awareness in the latter half of the 20th century, the medical community came to acknowledge BDD as a discrete disorder that paved the way for more refined diagnostic criteria that went a long way in guiding the treatment options and the research efforts in this condition today. The intersection of the sociocultural factors and BDD has also been significant, so that it can be understood historically. Various research works have also indicated how cultural and media beauty standards, which are socially constructed, have instilled more self-consciousness about appearance in individuals. With the research on habits like skin bleaching, whose roots can be traced back to colorism and discrimination of darker-skinned individuals, researchers have demonstrated the underlying motivations behind individuals engaging in dangerous habits for the sake of society's approval. Consumers of substances applied for skin bleaching, for instance, normally complain about self-esteem problems, noting the adverse psychological effect that such pressures from society have on individuals with BDD. These results emphasize that BDD is not merely one psychological disorder but a construct highly intertwined with cultural beauty and acceptance standards (Al-Sarraf,, 2022). When treatment of BDD is considered, it is historical perspectives that come into consideration, with rich contributions to the present clinical practices. In one that assessed adherence to National Institute for Health and Clinical Excellence (NICE) guidelines for BDD treatment, there was a lack of identification and use of evidence-based treatment. While there were some positive outcomes in favor of CBT and medication treatment, the majority of patients reported persistent symptoms and dissatisfaction with treatment efficacy. This discrepancy highlights the historical absence of a clear understanding of BDD among clinicians, which has resulted in inadequate care and a need for improved training and resources to meet patient needs more effectively. The importance of developing a strong therapeutic alliance between practitioners and patients cannot be overstated, as it has a significant impact on treatment outcomes and ongoing care for those afflicted with this disabling disorder (Govender, 2021) (Figure 10.3).

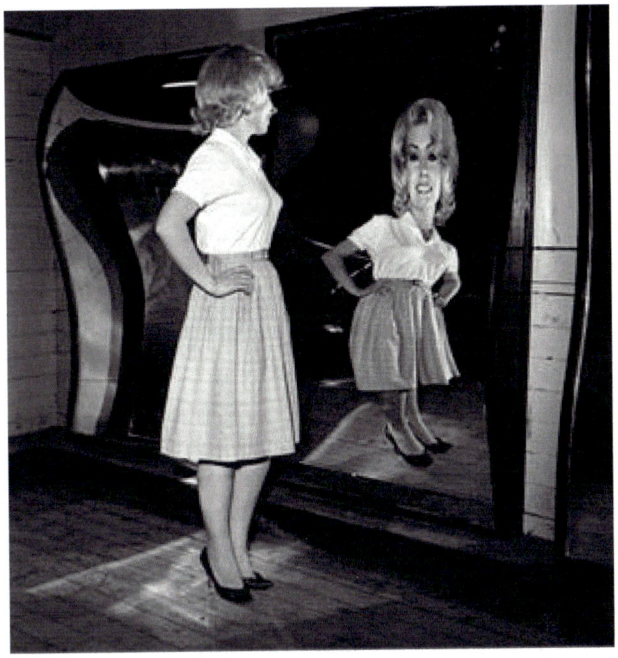

Figure 10.3. Distorted self-perception metaphor in body dysmorphic disorder (BDD).

Source: https://images.squarespace-cdn.com/content/v1/5b38a93c50a54fdfbd2c2593/1530447559338-KXHRVOISGK51LKDLD3IG/071205_BodyDysmorphia_vl-vertical.jpg.

10.1.3. Key Studies that Shaped the Understanding of BDD

Evolution of understanding concerning BDD has been heavily influenced by classical studies that describe the complex interplay between psychological and dermatological mechanisms. One such early study highlighted that various main psychiatric disorders, of which BDD is one, express via dermatological symptomatology, which indicates the secondary character of such skin changes as self-dehydrated responses to internal psychological distress. Such recognition is crucial, particularly in dermatological settings where patients are likely to deny the psychiatric origin of their symptoms, hence making it difficult for successful intervention plans. Through its focus on highlighting the fact that skin alterations are manifestations of inherent psychopathology, the study emphasizes how dermatologists should adopt a supportive and empathetic approach. Establishing trust can permit referral for psychiatric evaluation, which in turn can be a response to the intricate nature of BDD and its treatment (Basta-Juzba et al., 2015). In the discussion of BDD, some studies have also proceeded to elucidate the implications of atopic dermatitis in children, discovering a frightening correlation with other mental illnesses. One QI project aimed at enhancing knowledge of healthcare providers regarding body image impairment in such a population found that children with atopic dermatitis showed higher risk factors for BDD and other mental illnesses. Even though education was being done, the study showed a subtle difference in the level of knowledge among healthcare providers, thereby establishing a massive need for specialist training. This serves to reinforce the need for mental illness screening within dermatology, where early diagnosis could lead to improved health outcomes. These findings serve to underscore the central role that clinicians can play in bridging the gap between dermatological disease and its psychological consequences (Sanchez., 2023). Further research has underscored the multi-faceted nature of BDD, where its etiology becomes inextricably linked to both genetic and environmental factors. Family patterns of BDD have been researched to show that genetic weaknesses can be transferred by such predispositions, and therefore, the importance of an overall perspective towards the condition. Further, the sociocultural milieu, specifically about standards of beauty and media representation, has also been a key factor in shaping individuals' perceptions of their bodies, further making the disorder complex. As researchers unmute these layers, the more it is seen that the comprehension of BDD in its entirety does not just signify a focus on clinical symptoms but also an exploration of psychological, family, and social factors. With such an interdisciplinary methodology, psychology and psychodermatology can advance toward leaving symptom-oriented treatments behind and approaching interventions for individuals with BDD more effectively.

Test Your Knowledge

1. How did psychodermatology emerge as a distinct interdisciplinary field, and what were the key milestones in its historical development?
2. Which historical figures or early clinicians first documented cases resembling Body Dysmorphic Disorder?

10.2. Psychological Aspects of Body Dysmorphic Disorder

Learning Outcome

1. Describe common psychological symptoms associated with BDD
2. Explain the role of self-esteem and body image
3. Understand the impact of societal standards on BDD

The psychological aspects of BDD play a critical role in the comprehension of the disorder's impact on individuals. Essentially, BDD is characterized by a preoccupation with perceived flaws in appearance, which are often nonexistent or minimal. This preoccupation is strong enough to result in significant social and occupational impairment as individuals withdraw from social contacts due to their faulty perception of self. This psychological distress can result in comorbid conditions , such as depression and anxiety, increasing a person's state of hopelessness and loneliness. With the person struggling with his or her imperfect body perception, they will seek out too many cosmetic procedures or engage in activities that are meant to cover up the imperfections perceived, which actually increases their psychological difficulty and illustrates the close connection between psychological well-being and body perception. Observing the role played by dermatological symptoms of BDD reveals an intricate interaction between dermatological and psychological problems. BDD patients can develop body complaints , such as picking at skin or excessive grooming behavior that results in skin damage or irritation. The self-induced dermatological issues are able to cause repetitive referrals to dermatologists, but the psychiatry-related aspect is typically not addressed. This disconnect underscores the necessity of an interdisciplinary approach to BDD, with dermatologists, psychiatrists, and psychologists collaborating to provide integrated treatment. The alleviation of both the psychological suffering and the resulting skin findings can lead to more effective treatment regimens which address the patient's psychological health as well as their physical symptomatology, ultimately providing a better global understanding of the disease (Ader et al., 2017). Further, empathy towards the patient with BDD is also required for effective management. The skin practitioners are typically the first to encounter patients suffering from this condition, but they need to appreciate that BDD skin changes are typically self-induced and rooted in endogenous psychiatric issues (Basta-Juzba et al., 2015). By ensuring they have a nurturing environment, medical practitioners are able to establish trust and get patients to start dealing with mental health care, which is essential for effective treatment. Early intervention should be centered on comprehending the psychological complexity of each patient, exploring their perceptions through open dialogue, and coaxing them towards investigating the psychological bases of their issues. This gradual approach not only assists in alleviating skin issues but also tackles the overall psychological aspects of BDD, culminating in recovery and improved quality of life in individuals.

10.2.1. Common Psychological Symptoms Associated with BDD

BDD typically manifests as obsessive worry about real or imagined flaws in the appearance of one's own body, which can be minor or nonexistent. Such all-consuming worry may lead to a lot of psychological distress, often compounding into symptoms of depression and anxiety. Individuals with BDD tend to feel worthless for being perceived as unworthy of social interaction or intimacy by their appearance. This self-concept not only influences their everyday lives but also creates a cycle of social avoidance and increased anxiety as they fear judgment. Added to the psychological handicap of body dissatisfaction, these symptoms can lower a person's quality of life overall and cause them to be seen in both dermatology and psychiatry, as successful treatment is essential for remission from these disabling psychological symptoms. Furthermore, BDD has also been linked closely with obsessive-compulsive behavior, where the individual may exhibit compulsive appearance checking or appearance grooming behavior. The behaviors may include frequent mirror checking, asking others for reassurance about how they look, or even not going out to social gatherings in order to escape possible evaluation. The pathological need to rectify perceived flaws may find the individual spending a significant amount of time on these rituals, further decompensating daily functioning and contributing to compromised overall life satisfaction. Proper healthcare collaboration is underscored by the association, as correction of psychological aspects in dermatologic management remains necessary for best management. Research indicates that while dermatologists might find themselves frequently with patients who exhibit BDD symptoms, they tend to lack proper training to recognize the psychiatric aspects of their patients' disorder, hence complicating the process of treatment (Osman et al., 2017). While examining the psychological symptoms of BDD, it is also important to examine the impact of comorbid psychiatric disorders. Studies identify that BDD patients may have a higher prevalence of social anxiety disorder, major depressive disorder, and other mood disorders. Treatment for this multi-dimensional presentation needs to be multi-dimensional as well and should integrate psychodermatology with traditional psychiatric therapy. There needs to be close coordination between the dermatologists and the mental health professionals, as reflected in the published literature that reports skin illnesses, i.e., acne, as having the potential to exacerbate BDD symptomatology (Czernecka et al., 2020). Understanding these associations is key in creating effective treatment programs, leading ultimately to greater outcomes in both skin and psychological health. Addressing the dermatologic and psychological aspects allows clinicians to facilitate a more holistic process, ultimately producing an improvement in quality of life for patients with this complex disorder (Figure 10.4).

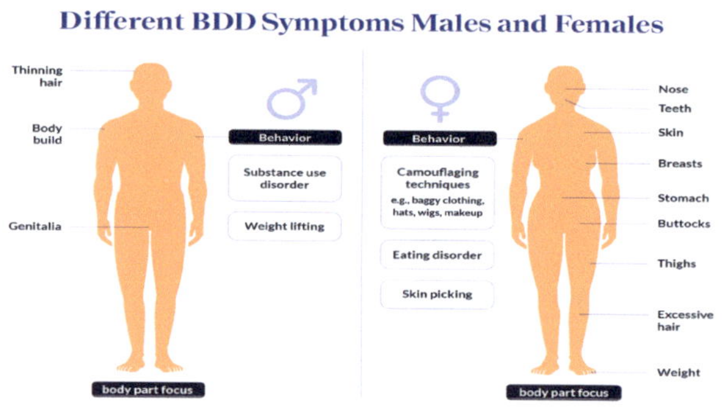

Figure 10.4. Different BDD symptoms males and females.

Source: https://images.ctfassets.net/ld5gan8tjh6b/5EUGynNlCIVcHVKKTIt2B4/5ee53aa1f527822c0b940580c3bc6d7d/Different_BDD_symptoms_males_and_females.png.

10.2.2. The Role of Self-Esteem and Body Image

Body image and self-esteem are very interrelated constructs that have a significant influence on mental health, most specifically in BDD. Individuals with negative body image are prone to have inaccurate perceptions of their own physical appearance and thus poor levels of self-esteem. Research indicates that low levels of self-esteem can escalate dissatisfaction with the body, precipitating or exacerbating disorders , such as BDD. These individuals tend to get preoccupied with appearing imperfect, which leads to compulsive behavior attempting to transform or camouflage their appearance. As such, maintaining positive self-esteem and a healthy body image is essential since it serves as a defense against BDD and other associated disorders. Formation of a positive self-concept gives people the necessary strength to withstand social pressures, especially those that propagate via social media and social expectations, which tend to exacerbate feelings of inferiority in vulnerable populations. The evolving nature of social media has had a tremendous impact on how young adults perceive body image and self-esteem. Sites full of idealized images usually foster unachievable beauty, which consequently skews users' self-perceptions and leads to higher BDD rates. Lamba (2025) observes that the link between body image, self-esteem, and predisposition to BDD is significant, such that higher self-esteem is associated with lower dysmorphic tendencies.

Quantitative analysis indicated societal comparisons breed negative self-judgments among adolescents, particularly when confronted with influencers as role models for setting beauty standards. This increased exposure can lead to severe self-esteem issues, creating a self-reinforcing cycle where body image discontent nurtures low self-esteem. Thus, these pressures from outside are at the core of mental health interventions aiming to promote self-acceptance and reduce the incidence of BDD among young people. Moreover, the empirical research on the body image-self-esteem connection has existential implications for the development of preventative measures against BDD. The study conducted by Safitri et al. (2025) provides an outline of how approximately 47.5% of the explanation of BDD tendencies among adolescents is attributed to body image and self-esteem, with the identification of the significance of such variables in mental health outcomes. Notably, the contributions of body image were larger than those of self-esteem, which showed that mental attitudes towards the way one looks are a central factor in the development of BDD. This calls for specially developed education programs that enhance media literacy at the same time while promoting better body image perceptions and improved self-perception. By doing so, the stakeholders can not only reduce the risk of BDD but also enhance overall psychological health in adolescents who are battling through the pressures of contemporary beauty ideals (Figure 10.5).

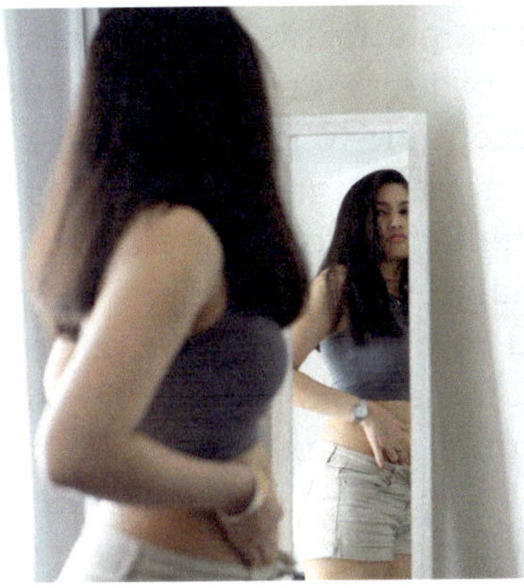

Figure 10.5. Negative body image perception associated with body dysmorphic disorder (BDD).

Source: https://discoverymood.com/wp-content/uploads/2019/08/Body-Dysmorphia-1200x800.jpg.

10.2.3. Impact of Societal Standards on BDD

The widespread influence of social standards over personal beliefs and what is considered beautiful is a significant contributing factor in the development and sustenance of BDD. Social standards of beauty, typically disseminated through the media, social media, and cultural stories, promote unattainable ideals that many attempt to conform to. This ongoing pursuit of an unattainable ideal fosters an even more intense sense of discontentment with one's body since those afflicted with BDD tend to see themselves as flawed or monstrous in the face of objective assurances to the contrary. Internalization of such societal ideals can therefore lead to heightened emotional suffering, bringing about maladaptive coping strategies, social isolation, and inhibited functioning.

These dynamics underscore the significance of increased awareness and critical analysis of beauty standards in social discourse to mitigate their ill effects on mental well-being, particularly BDD, and its accompanying psychosocial impacts. Further, the role of internet spaces and social networking platforms exacerbates the ill effects of social beauty standards on vulnerable individuals susceptible to BDD. Visual-centered platforms promote a narrow definition of beauty, has a tendency to idolize certain body shapes and facial features and demonize others. The users tend to be subjected to images that depict unrealistic models of reality, with the eventual outcome of unhealthy comparison and feelings of inadequacy. As painted by more recent scholarship, individuals who are engaged in beauty-focused internet forums are likely to recount an increased motivation to adapt to these standards, expressed in exaggerated behavior typical of BDD, , such as excessive grooming or an obsession with so-called imperfections. Such interactions between users in virtual spaces reinforce negative body image and reduce self-esteem, emphasizing the importance of interventions addressing not only personal treatment but also societal forces on standards of beauty (Brun et al., 2024). It is also essential to detect the cultural dimensions of body image and BDD because societies propagate various standards of beauty affecting individuals in distinctive ways. In other societies, light skin is valued, and this has generated practice of whitening the skin, which can be extremely unhealthy (Al-Sarraf,, 2022). Sociocultural factors, including colorism and bias, intersect with symptoms of body dysmorphic, adding further depth to the BDD profile. Individuals may be subject to pressure to adhere to prevailing standards of beauty, and these can have adverse consequences for mental health and physical disease. This kind of comprehension of BDD will need to be complex that recognizes the diverse cultural narratives regarding beauty and promotes inclusivity and acceptance. By opening the conversation of BDD and body image and mapping the intersectionality of social norms, we are able to allow for improved support for individuals struggling with BDD and facilitate environments in favor of positive self-perception and acceptance.

Test Your Knowledge

1. What are the most common psychological symptoms associated with Body Dysmorphic Disorder?
2. How does low self-esteem contribute to the development and maintenance of BDD symptoms

10.3. Dermatological Manifestations

Learning Outcome

1. Describe common skin conditions linked to BDD
2. Understand the psychosomatic relationship between mind and skin
3. Focus on studies illustrating dermatological symptoms in BDD patients

The intricate interplay between dermatological manifestations and psychological well-being is the main focus of psychodermatology, especially in the case of BDD patients. Individuals with BDD are usually found to exhibit intense preoccupation with actual or perceived flaws in their looks that lead to severe psychological distress along with compulsive behavior directed towards rectifying these illusory flaws. These expressions are not superficial; they can worsen the psychological distress these patients undergo, leading to a cycle where distress is physically expressed, which in turn makes them more obsessed with their appearance. Here, the need for dermatologists to look beyond the skin is crucial, that is, to comprehend the emotional and psychodynamic dimensions of skin disease in patients who come with dermatological presentations likely related to their internal psychological status (Poot et al., 2007). Developments in psychodermatology reflect an increase in the perceived need for specialized education in addressing such intricate patient profiles. The evolving educational models provided by bodies of learning like the European Academy of Dermatology and Venereology are marked by a comprehensive approach to psychodermatology, an integration of dermatological expertise and psychological awareness (Gieler et al., 2019). The training aims to equip dermatologists and related health professionals with the skills for diagnosing and treating emotional problems manifested through skin conditions. Familiarity with psychosomatic interactions and experience with specific presentations, , such as self-mutilating skin lesions or anxiety-related dermatologic symptomatology, enhances the clinician's capacity to tailor interventions to these patients' unique needs. Moreover, the occurrence of alexithymia, a symptomatology of not being able to perceive or express one's own feelings, has a propensity to complicate the clinical presentation in dermatologically symptomatic patients. This barrier can disrupt communication between physician and patient, thus raising levels of frustration as well as misinterpretation of the reaction to treatment. This is why psychodermatological consultation is becoming more the rule, with emphasis on the comprehensive understanding of the mind-body interface (Poot et al., 2007). By creating an environment where patients feel heard and nurtured, professionals can develop more effective treatment plans that address the psychological, in addition to the dermatologic needs of care. Not only does this integrative approach calm the manifestations of BDD, but it also allows for a more profound healing process, enabling patients to navigate their emotional landscape alongside their physical condition.

10.3.1. Common Skin Conditions Linked to BDD

BDD is characterized by preoccupation with perceived defects in appearance that cause a preoccupation and individuals feel the need to seek repetitive attempts to "correct" perceived blemishes. The preoccupation presents itself in numerous forms, typically as skin disturbances , such as acne, scarring, and disorders of pigmentation. These flaws are seen by those who have BDD as much worse or more noticeable than they really are, and this results in more psychological distress and social isolation. For instance, a person may have pimples but worry only about one zit being an overwhelming source of shame and resort to compulsions , such as excessive skin picking or excessive purchase of skincare products in hopes of finding a solution to it. Such habits not only exacerbate existing skin illness but can also create new dermatological illnesses, highlighting the complicated interconnection among psychological and dermatological health in psychodermatology (Poot et al., 2007). Furthermore, eczema and psoriasis are frequently characterized in patients with BDD. These inflammatory cutaneous disorders have concrete visible characteristics that again amplify insufficiency and self-consciousness. The recurring nature of BDD will exacerbate these illnesses, as stress and anxiety are known causes of flare-up. Exacerbation makes patients fixate on the looks of their skins, believing that all they require is treatment to cure their mental anguish. Unfortunately, this focus takes away from coping mechanisms that address the condition of the skin and the psychological factors behind them. The majority of patients misinterpret symptoms of their skin condition as personal failures, and this, in turn, heightens their body dysmorphic concerns, hence demonstrating how widespread skin diseases are likely to complicate the cycle of BDD and its associated psychological impact (da Novaes et al., 2018). Acquaintance with clinical significance of BDD calls for an integrated treatment that intervenes simultaneously in both dermatology and psychology. Psychodermatologic integrated models of care emphasize the need for practitioners to be vigilant for warning signs of BDD in skin-presenting patients. Effective management includes collaboration between dermatologists and mental health workers to assist in addressing the complexity of the disorder. By initiating discussion between the two professions, clinicians can offer treatment programs that not only heal the skin disorders but also attempt to deconstruct the resulting cognitive distortions of BDD. This concurrent treatment is significant, as not only does it improve patients dermatological health but also constructs sustained psychological resilience, ultimately leading to substantial improvements in quality of life for those afflicted with both BDD and associated skin issues (Poot et al., 2007) (Figure 10.6).

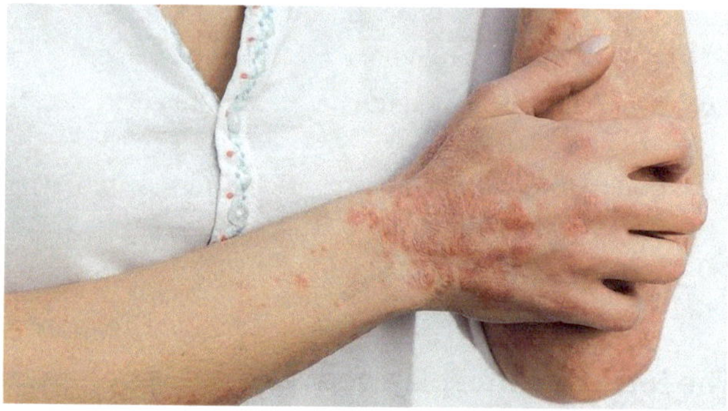

Figure 10.6. Chronic skin inflammation.

Source: https://assets.technologynetworks.com/production/dynamic/images/content/346379/chronic-skin-inflammation-molecular-mechanisms-identified-346379-960x540.jpg?cb=11141844.

10.3.2. The Psychosomatic Relationship Between Mind and Skin

The intricate relationship between the skin and the mind is a central theme of psychodermatology, highlighting how psychological disorders manifest themselves physically as diseases of the skin. Studies have confirmed that rosacea, atopic dermatitis, acne vulgaris, and psoriasis usually occur together with psychiatric illnesses , such as anxiety and depression. For instance, stressors in rosacea enhance body symptoms through the activation of neurobiological pathways that also impinge on mood regulation. This case demonstrates the dual role of psychological health as both a determinant on skin integrity and in the overall sense of well-being. The interactive impact of these systems indicates the necessity for comprehensive treatment approaches that combine dermatologic and psychotherapies, especially among patients in whom the skin disease has an impact on the mental status (Mar et al., 2023). Moving further to the psychosomatic link, it is evident that chronic cutaneous diseases may be implicated in BDD or morbid preoccupation with perceived defects in physical appearance. BDD patients tend to report heightened sensitivity to their appearance, prompting compulsive behavior to check or hide perceived defects. This mounting preoccupation can yield an affective burden that exacerbates dermatologic conditions, creating a cycle of cause and effect in which both psychiatric distress and skin pathology are mutually reinforcing. The implications for treatment are far-reaching; clinicians need not only to treat the open evidence of skin disease but also the intercurrent mental illness that can perpetuate them.

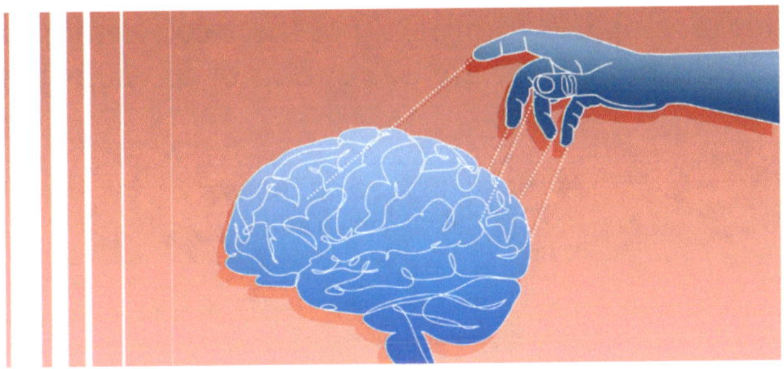

Figure 10.7. Mind and skin connection.

Source: https://media.licdn.com/dms/image/v2/D5612AQFtcbNJ_PQI7w/article-cover_image-shrink_720_1280/article-cover_image-shrink_720_1280/0/1690563187626?e=2147483647&v=beta&t=nr0O0daX4bhb0U9FMW7rONf1oYBFd0Nl5llclCkKwck.

An intricate, biopsychosocial approach that integrates dermatologic care with psychological treatment is needed to effectively cure individuals who have BDD (Rodríguez-Cerdeira et al., 2011). In addition, the establishment of psychodermatology as an official specialty indicates the growing recognition of this mind-skin connection among specialties. Current advancements have led to societies that cater exclusively to promoting multidisciplinary therapeutic practices among dermatologists, psychiatrists, and psychologists. Interdisciplinary communication plays a critical role in developing individualized practices taking into consideration the psychological impact of skin disease on patients. In particular, with the development of psychodermatology, more work is needed to better explain the mechanisms responsible for linking psychological well-being to skin health. This could minimize the treatment gap and possibly discover new interventions that address both the mental and physical results in patients with chronic skin disease (Rodríguez-Cerdeira et al., 2011) (Figure 10.7).

10.3.3. Studies Illustrating Dermatological Symptoms in BDD Patients

The intersection of BDD and dermatological illness would most likely present in dramatic form, , such as case studies that embody the internal angst that lies behind external presentation. One such example was the case of a patient who suffered from melasma, a face condition that features brown patches brought on by sun exposure or hormonal changes. This patient was profoundly preoccupied with their skin, perceiving their condition as a gross disfigurement that required inordinate cosmetic intervention. These case histories illustrate how intense BDD can amplify the emotional significance of dermatologic symptoms, so patients become overwrought and socially reclusive, coddling their perceived defects. The overlap of BDD and melasma suggests the ways in which a dermatologic condition can be distressing and also one form of manifestation of more profound psychological issues, again highlighting the use of multifaceted treatment approaches in psychodermatology, especially with complicated mentally in-need patients (Zhu et al., 2024). In disorders like acne vulgaris, self-image impact is likewise disastrous. Acne, as inflammatory skin lesions, becomes the focal point for individuals who are suffering from

BDD. A thorough case study analysis about a young adult who had severe acne provides us with an understanding of how the physical condition resulted in excessive concern about imagined defects and maladaptive body image. The patient was quite socially anxious and exhibited avoidance behavior due to their preoccupation with the appearance of their skin. This clinical observation is in accord with more extensive evidence that reports high rates of BDD in patients presenting with dermatological issues, pointing out that psychological distress is often an complicating factor in the presentation of skin disorders (Li et al., 2024). All such complications in these case presentations point to the necessity for integrative assessments that address both the emotional and physical aspects of care. In addition, ailments like psoriasis carry a unique double burden for BDD patients. Psoriasis, characterized by red, scaly lesions on the skin, is likely to cause embarrassment and social stigma. A case study presented a patient whose exacerbations of psoriasis worsened their symptoms of BDD, prompting them to seek multiple treatments in vain. The interaction between their external manifestations and deranged self-perception created a cycle of psychic distress that was hard to break. This case presents a poignant illustration of the manner in which dermatological manifestations can affect one's quality of life and psychological well-being. Moreover, it emphasizes the necessity of an integration of psychological care and dermatological management to further promote patient outcomes, as patients with BDD may require intervention with specialized treatments addressing the complexity of their concomitant conditions (Li et al., 2024; Zhu et al., 2024).

Test Your Knowledge

1. What are the most commonly reported skin-related concerns in individuals with Body Dysmorphic Disorder?
2. How does the psychosomatic relationship between the mind and skin manifest in individuals with BDD?

10.4. Treatment Approaches

Learning Outcome

1. Describe psychological therapies for BDD
2. Focus on dermatological treatments and their effectiveness
3. Understand integrative approaches combining both fields

Treatment of BDD is a multifaceted process that incorporates psychotherapy, pharmacotherapy, and novel alternative treatments tailored to the individual's requirements. Cognitive behavior therapy (CBT) is proven to be the most effective psychotherapeutic treatment for BDD, allowing patients to change distorted appearance-related cognitions and reduce compulsive behaviors of the disorder. Furthermore, recent advancements in machine learning have also placed special emphasis on treatment credibility as a good predictor of the intervention outcome, where findings suggest that treatment credibility outweighs traditional markers , such as initial symptom severity. This finding allows clinicians to better tailor their treatment by focusing on boosting patients belief in administered treatments. These tailored interventions are important in fostering patient activation and improving overall treatment compliance, ultimately towards greater psychological improvement and well-being for individuals affected by BDD (Costilla-Reyes et al., 2025). Pharmacological interventions, particularly SSRIs, have been found to be moderately effective at alleviating BDD symptoms but fall short of providing complete relief. While useful, however, most BDD patients do not want to seek medication due to concerns about dependence or stigma surrounding mental health treatment. Mental health professionals thus need to be sensitive to barriers to seeking care and try to create an open and non-judgmental communication space. Early detection of BDD by professionals would improve the accessibility as well as the effectiveness of treatment quite noticeably. In addition, the introduction of mindfulness-based therapies is in the pipeline as an effective adjunctive therapy since studies posit their potential to minimize similarities in symptomatology of associated disorders , such as social anxiety disorder and obsessive-compulsive disorder. Clinicians can treat BDD more effectively and its complex presentations through expanding the treatment repertoire (Safitri et al., 2025). Lastly, incorporating mindfulness strategies into treatment programs provides a novel way of approaching the core symptoms of BDD, possibly not fully captured by more traditional interventions. Mindfulness enhances mindfulness, reduces anxiety, and fosters an attitude of non-judgment of one's own physical appearance, all of which are necessary for patients dealing with the unavoidable negative self-perception of BDD. Clinical reports indicate that these treatments are effective in bringing about changes in body image disturbance and cognitive rigidity, two of the most salient aspects of the disorder. As physicians consider these complementary therapies, they must also consider the benefits of a total holistic approach, , such as psychological support and emotional validation for victims of BDD. Lastly, the intersection of advanced treatment options will better treat BDD with patients having advanced care tailored to their unique needs and situations (Safitri et al., 2025) (Figure 10.8).

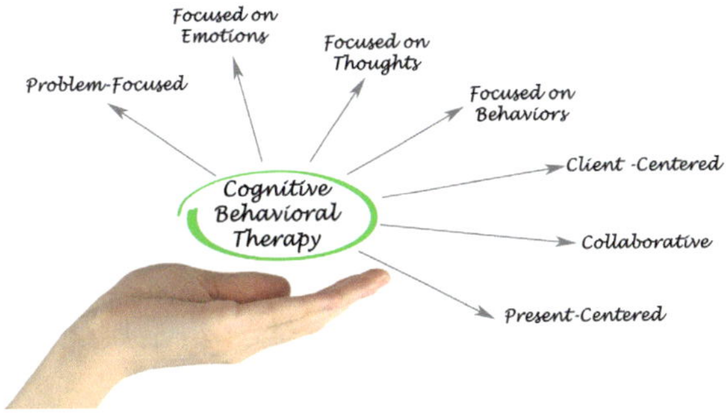

Figure 10.8. Cognitive behavioral therapy (CBT).

Source: https://cdn.myrx.in/contents/articles/1199817512IMG.png.

10.4.1. Psychological Therapies for BDD

Treatment of BDD often involves a multidisciplinary treatment, best with psychological treatments that address the cognitive and affective symptoms of the disorder. CBT is usually regarded as the first-line treatment of BDD. Through challenging and restructuring mistaken beliefs about appearance, CBT allows patients to confront and ultimately alter maladaptive thoughts. This mode of treatment encourages patients to confront their obsessions about perceived flaws and strengthens healthy coping mechanisms. Also, the inclusion of exposure and response prevention measures in CBT helps lower symptoms by exposing patients to gradually threatening body image situations and inhibiting their compulsive behaviors. The value of psychological therapies extends beyond symptom relief; they also contribute to enhancing patients' overall psychological well-being, and for these reasons, there is a need for further study in this field to enhance the effectiveness and accessibility of treatments. Researchers have, in a review of the literature, highlighted the serious psychological consequences of BDD, particularly for those with skin diseases , such as acne, psoriasis, and vitiligo. The fact that BDD often co-exists with these dermatological disorders illustrates the need for treatments that address both the psychological issue and the dermatological symptoms concurrently. The convergence of psychodermatological therapies, an integration of dermatological treatment with interventions for psychology, has proven to significantly improve the outcome of treatment. For example, individuals with readily apparent skin defects can benefit from treatments that not only serve to improve their appearance but also alleviate the psychological distress associated with BDD. By acknowledging the mutually dependent nature of the relationship between dermatological disease and mental health, practitioners can optimize their intervention to the individual's needs in a way that will enable total well-being, ultimately leading to improved quality of life for individuals who are afflicted by BDD (Li et al., 2024). Furthermore, the specific complexities of BDD necessitate an extension of current knowledge of psychological treatments beyond the norm. Future research must explore novel models of therapy that encompass mindfulness-based therapies and acceptance and commitment therapy (ACT), both of which have shown promise for the treatment of many psychological disorders. Mindfulness will allow the patients to cultivate a non-judgmental acceptance of their feelings and thoughts and be capable of living more present in the moment rather than ruminating on perceived physical flaws. Similarly, ACT encourages acceptance of the individual's thoughts while sustaining values-based action, hence encouraging resilience when dealing with distress. With increasing emphasis on the development of integrated treatment plans, these novel treatments can be useful additions to existing psychological therapies for BDD, complementing patient treatment and maximizing therapeutic yield. Blending these approaches can also yield new information concerning the psychosocial aspects of BDD, once more pointing to the critical intersection of dermatology and psychology in practice (Li et al., 2024) (Figure 10.9).

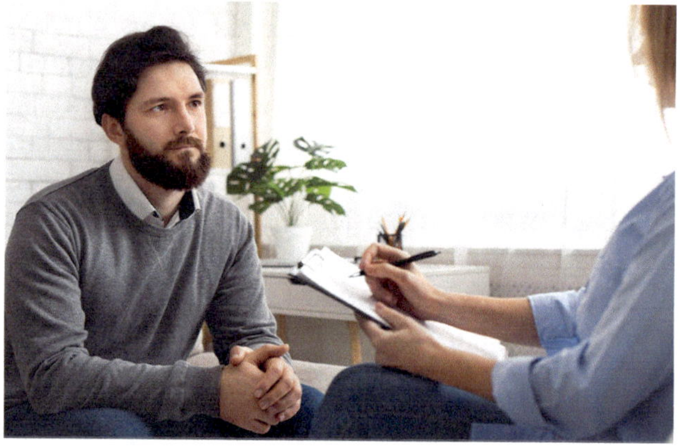

Figure 10.9. Psychological treatment.

Source: https://firstcityrecoverycenter.com/wp-content/uploads/2025/03/mRx9G8g2qGgXCPwmyL_56QPi197o4lPNEDeaRqiUtqw-1.jpg.

10.4.2. Dermatological Treatments and Their Effectiveness

The intersection of dermatology and psychiatry has created increasing interest in the treatment of conditions that are psychologically derived, particularly when it comes to BDD. Dermatologic interventions may be become critical among patients with BDD, wherein imperfections in the skin magnify psychological misery. Traditional dermatologic treatment, , such as topical or systemic medication, laser therapy, and surgical correction, may reduce symptom-based skin distress transiently. However, their effectiveness can be undermined where the underlying psychological problems are not treated. On some occasions, the treatments may unconsciously reinforce patients' focus on their skin conditions, further exacerbating their distress rather than alleviating it. Accordingly, it is essential for dermatologists to collaborate with mental health professionals in an effort to have a holistic approach, acknowledging that successful treatment is usually more than treating the physical symptoms (Benea et al., 2015). The complex interplay of psychological processes and skin disease necessitates an integrated model of treatment. Psychodermatology aims to emphasize the significance of how mental illness, , such as anxiety and depression, can manifest in skin disease. The strategy is to promote the collaborative action of dermatologists, psychiatrists, and psychologists to offer improved treatment outcomes for psychocologically-influenced conditions. For example, psychodermatological therapies that include the utilization of cognitive-behavioral methods can effectively treat compulsive actions, , such as skin picking, which is commonly present in BDD. Such integrated methods are easier for patients to better understand their conditions and to cope with the psychological and dermatological components of their concerns. The integration of dermatological interventions with psychological therapy is significant in the development of better overall health outcomes and in enhancing the quality of patients' lives (Ader et al., 2017). Moreover, research on the efficacy of dermal therapies under psychodermatology reveals not just the necessity to treat the physical symptoms but also the psychological ones that underlie these disorders. The twofold role of mental and cutaneous health is elucidated in patients who may see their emotional state largely determined by how their skin looks such that it creates an anxiety-distress cycle. Therefore, effective treatment must involve careful assessment of the psychologic underpinnings of dermatologic illness. Such an emphasis underscores the importance of education of the patient regarding treatment modalities and setting realistic expectations. If healthcare providers understand and appreciate the holistic nature of cutaneous disease enmeshed with BDD, they can treat patients more effectively on the path to health. Lastly, an integrative practice style has a better opportunity to provide long-term psychological and dermatological well-being (Benea et al., 2015).

10.4.3. Integrative Approaches Combining Both Fields

Integrative psychodermatology and BDD share a high potential for enhancing patient outcomes with an integrated understanding of the interaction between psychological and dermatological conditions. Present treatments tend to target dermatologic symptoms or psychological distress in isolation and usually fail to yield sufficient outcomes. But an integrative approach considers two-way influence of mental illnesses and skin disorders as well as how they feed into one another. As research indicates, BDD patients can become increasingly preoccupied with perceived physical imperfections, adopt maladaptive habits, and aggravate their skin issues (Costilla-Reyes et al., 2025). By combining treatment approaches of the two specialties—, such as dermatologic therapies, cognitive-behavioral therapy, and mindfulness strategies, health practitioners can devise personalized treatment plans that more appropriately address both sets of needs. This wide-ranging view is a step towards conceptualizing holistic patient care, ultimately improving psychological and physical health outcomes. Furthermore, growing evidence also supports the effectiveness of mindfulness-based interventions as a key component of integrated treatment regimens. Mindfulness allows more interoceptive awareness and encourages the individual to become an honest observer of their thoughts and feelings, and this is helpful for individuals with BDD (Safitri et al., 2025). The application of mindfulness techniques in therapy has the potential to decrease the intensity of negative thinking and self-criticizing behavior typical in BDD. Second, given that mindfulness interventions have been shown to have promising effects in related disorders , such as social anxiety and eating disorders, their use in treating BDD holds the potential for psychodermatology innovation. Finally, this integrative model also necessitates the interrelatedness of mental and physical health, which enables clinicians to borrow from evidence-based practices that consider the multifaceted expressions of body image disturbance. Lastly, integration of technological advances into treatment modalities is one of the large possibilities to optimize the treatment of BDD under the umbrella of psychodermatology. The application of digital intervention, , such as teletherapy or mobile applications focused on mindfulness and symptom tracking, has the potential to maximize outreach and availability for patients who would otherwise be precluded from treatment (Costilla-Reyes et al., 2025). The barriers to care, including lack of awareness among health practitioners and stigma related to mental illness, can be overcome using novel approaches that successfully leverage technology. Through the delivery of support and resources through online platforms, clinicians can successfully target individuals with BDD, enhance treatment adherence, and ultimately realize better therapeutic outcomes. The marriage of advanced technology and clinical expertise is the integrative process that will typify transforming the treatment paradigm in psychodermatology and managing the complex needs of individuals with BDD.

Test Your Knowledge

1. What are the most effective psychological therapies for Body Dysmorphic Disorder?
2. How do dermatological interventions impact individuals with BDD?

10.5. Role of Healthcare Professionals

Learning Outcome

1. Explain the importance of interdisciplinary collaboration
2. Understand the importance of training and awareness for dermatologists and psychologists
3. Describe the strategies for effective patient communication

Healthcare professionals have a key role to play in detection and treatment of psychodermatological disorders, and most particularly in the case of BDD. Their specific position makes them uniquely able to reconcile the often disparate disciplines of dermatology and mental health. To illustrate, dermatologists would usually be best placed to make first contact with patients whose symptoms are on the skin and potentially the outcome is psychological in nature. This initial encounter underscores the importance of dermatologists possessing the ability to identify mental health risk associated with skin diseases, including atopic dermatitis. As noted by Sanchez. (2023), poor mental health screening among pediatric patients with dermatology disorders indicates a pressing need for greater training and sensitivity among clinicians to obtain improved patient outcomes and access to relevant mental health treatments. In addition, the convergence of multiple specialties—dermatology, psychiatry, and psychology—enriches the treatment model of patients with illnesses that imply skin and mental illness. As has been mentioned in Ader et al. (2017), psychodermatology necessitates an interprofessional format, with specialists working together to address the complex interaction of skin, mind, and underlying mental illness. Not only does this multi-component model enhance the efficiency of treatments, but it also acts as a comprehensive foundation for understanding how all elements converge to form the patient's experience. By establishing a consensus treatment model, health professionals can offer integrated care considering the physical and psychological health needs, which is central to effectively treating disorders like BDD. Finally, continuing education and interprofessional training for health professionals are needed in advancing a more enlightened style in psychodermatology. As Sanchez. (2023) inferred, initiatives aimed at sensitizing individuals to body image impairment and its respective mental health risks are vital in increasing the ability of health practitioners to spot and address such issues. Through interventions in education, practitioners can enhance the manner in which they screen patients suffering from dermatological conditions for mental disorders and, by the same token, ensure enhanced mental health outcomes. This proactive action not only relieves the mental stress borne by the patients but also underscores the agency of healthcare professionals as defenders of all-inclusive care, reaffirming the significance of treating both dermatological and psychic aspects of health.

10.5.1. Importance of Interdisciplinary Collaboration

Psychodermatology emphasizes the significant benefits of interdisciplinarity, particularly in the treatment of difficult conditions like BDD. Such interdisciplinarity could involve dermatologists, psychiatrists, psychologists, and other healthcare professionals with the ability to offer specialized insight into the treatment of the patients. Dermatologists, for instance, possess experience with skin diseases that can concurrently provoke psychological symptoms, while mental health specialists can assist in making sense of the emotional and cognitive mechanisms of the disorders. Such interaction allows for a deeper understanding of the patient's condition, and this in itself leads to integrative treatment plans that are capable of addressing both the outward symptoms of the skin and psychological factors. Ultimately, such a construction of an interdisciplinary approach ensures all elements of a patient's well-being are considered, allowing for more effective and specific interventions to be provided. Moreover, the significance of interdepartmental conferences and case conferences cannot be stressed too much for the management of BDD patients and patients with concomitant conditions. Regular consultations between mental health specialists and dermatologists can facilitate the exchange of valuable observations gleaned from heterogenous clinical experiences. For example, the observations derived from dermatological examinations may provide valuable information that can contribute to the early detection of psychological distress. Conversely, psychological testing can assist in dermatologic treatment by moving the orientation to how patients themselves perceive their diseases, to additional productive treatment paths. Increasing the knowledge base not only expands the model of care but also assists in more complete understanding of the psychosocial implications of skin disorders in order to provide a higher level of care to patients in general. Interdisciplinary training and education complement the collaborative practice necessary in psychodermatology. Through educating healthcare professionals in areas of overlap between dermatology and mental health, awareness of body image concerns and associated psychological suffering can be raised significantly. As seen in Sanchez. (2023), programs that seek to raise healthcare professionals' awareness of mental health risk factors for dermatological conditions are essential. The knowledge that atopic dermatitis and other skin diseases can impair patients' mental health establishes the bond of both fields. This knowledge encourages practitioners to be more interdisciplinary in their practice, being properly prepared to identify and treat patients with issues connecting physical appearance and psychological health, eventually improving patient outcomes in BDD and other comorbidities treatment (Figure 10.10).

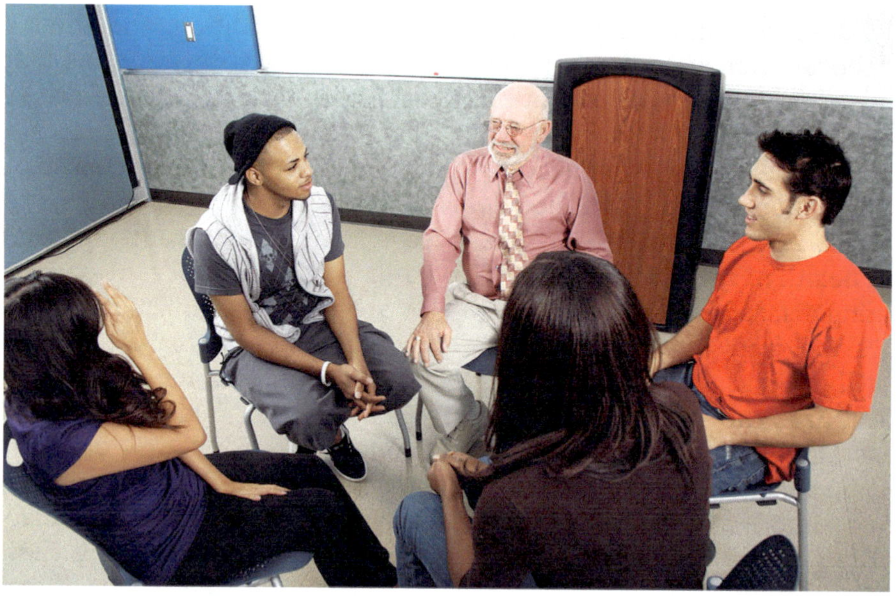

Figure 10.10. A diverse support group participates in a discussion led by a facilitator.

Source: https://bdd.iocdf.org/wp-content/uploads/sites/5/2023/04/iStock_000004966293Medium.jpg.

10.5.2. Training and Awareness for Dermatologists and Psychologists

Sensitization and training for psychologists and dermatologists are essential to successfully meet the challenges of psychodermatology, especially when treating patients diagnosed with BDD. Dermatologists being the first skin healthcare providers often have to treat patients who bring with them psychological tension in the form of skin issues. There is therefore an urgent need for extensive knowledge of the interfaces between dermatological and psychological conditions. This training equips dermatologists to recognize signs of BDD and other co-morbid conditions, with a multi-disciplinary treatment response incorporating psychological therapy. Enhanced awareness among clinicians has a direct effect on patient outcomes through the timely referral of patients to mental health professionals, which serves to greatly alleviate patient distress related to concern over their skin appearance and, as such, improving quality of life. These integrative approaches are underscored in guidelines provided during conferences, where education and inter-specialty communication are emphasized (Sanchez, 2023). Psychologists also require specialized training to address the nuances of psychodermatology, , such as how chronic skin conditions can amplify psychological distress. Familiarity with dermatology vocabulary and treatments enables psychologists to treat BDD-affected patients more successfully. An implicit knowledge of skin disease not only helps psychologists validate the patients experience but also helps in framing a detailed treatment plan. Further, training programs designed to infuse psychological insight into dermatology can make therapy more effective, curtailing the psychological effect associated with visible skin problems. Synergetic collaboration of these two fields necessitates the involvement of both psychologists and dermatologists in collaborative training, thereby improving patient care and a healthier treatment process. Integration of psychodermatology training into medical school curricula is necessary for care improvement. Having organized workshops and ongoing continuing medical education (CME) sessions on the psychosocial aspect of dermatological diseases can significantly improve practitioners' levels of understanding. These services are not merely required by psychologists and dermatologists but by other medical practitioners who deal with suffering patients. With an integrated education that unites psychological knowledge and dermatological education, healthcare professionals can better address the singular needs of patients suffering from BDD. Therefore, this new alliance of the two disciplines can lead the way to more integrative treatment approach, finally to better treatment plans and treatment outcomes for skin patients with both skin conditions and mental problems, as highlighted in recent arguments for patient-centered healthcare models (Sanchez, 2023) (Figure 10.11).

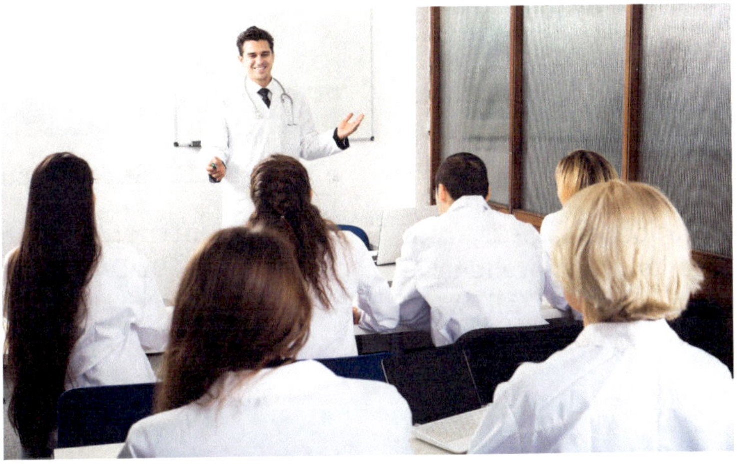

Figure 10.11. Continuing medical education (CME).

Source: https://www.nih.gov/sites/default/files/news-events/events/cme-training.jpg.

10.5.3. Strategies for Effective Patient Communication

Effective patient communication is an important factor in the management of disorders like BDD in psychodermatology. Trust forms a central prerequisite in establishing a relationship with patients, particularly as many BDD patients are bound to harbor feelings of stigma or judgment regarding their delusions of physical defects. Active listening, empathic interviewing, and patient feeling validation can also facilitate open communication. By creating a safe space for dialogue, health professionals can encourage the patient to share their worries, which, in addition to facilitating correct diagnosis, also strengthens the therapeutic relationship. This kind of practice is particularly vital, as BDD most commonly intersects with self-esteem and anxiety disorders, and thus requires sensitivity and attention towards the emotional state of the patient to develop successful outcomes (Brun et al., 2024). In addition to interpersonal skills, the presence of concise, informative materials is also vital in communicating with patients. For those with BDD, having access to correct information can eliminate false or inaccurate information and facilitate individuals to become more actively engaged with their treatment. Internet discussion groups and educational websites are valuable adjuncts to usual therapeutic intervention. They provide coping strategies, support groups, and information about their condition, which may demystify BDD. Importantly, such information may also serve to consolidate the therapeutic messages provided through direct consultations, eventually enhancing the patients' awareness of their condition, as evidenced by literature investigating the helpful impact of internet resources on mental health (Brun et al., 2024). Lastly, multidisciplinary approaches are another effective means of enhancing patient communication in psychodermatology. Multidisciplinary consultations among dermatologists, mental health professionals, and general practitioners allow an integrated treatment approach that incorporates psychological and physical treatments. During consultations, the integration of inputs from each field can offer patients a comprehensive outlook on their treatment, thus allowing informed decisions regarding it. In addition, training healthcare staff in communication skills for psychological distress can create a more responsive and compassionate healthcare environment. Such strategies emphasize the value of a coordinated model of care, which can lead to improved outcomes for patients and improved prognosis in diseases with dermatological as well as psychological components, like alopecia disorders (Figure 10.12).

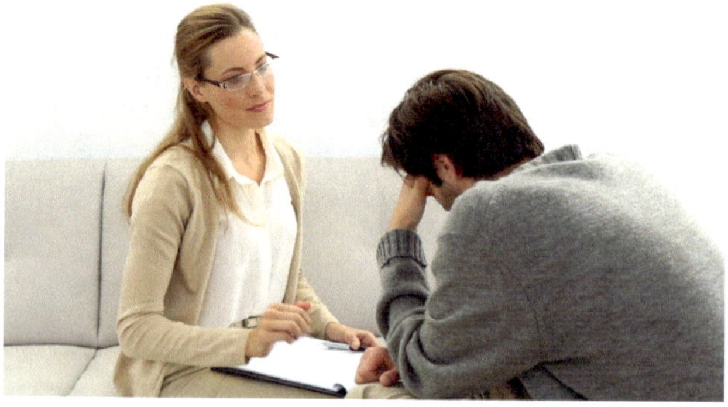

Figure 10.12. Effective patient communication.

Source: https://img.haikudeck.com/mi/D28A9FDD-69DD-4B98-AB1F-9B159693BB5B.jpg.

Test Your Knowledge

1. Why is interdisciplinary collaboration essential in the diagnosis and treatment of psychodermatological conditions like Body Dysmorphic Disorder?
2. What specific training or awareness should dermatologists receive to better recognize and manage psychodermatological disorders , such as BDD?

10.6. Current Research Trends

Learning Outcome

1. Focus on recent studies in psychodermatology
2. Understand advances in understanding BDD
3. Deal with future directions for research in the field

Recent developments in psychodermatology led researchers to explore the intersection of psychological states and dermatology, more precisely in the case of BDD. This emerging area of research investigates how psychological conditions manifest as skin issues and offers an explanation to enable conceptualizing body appearance obsession and its affective undertones. Research has increasingly indicated that BDD patients can be far more anxious and concerned with perceived defects, and this creates obsessive thinking regarding their skin. These observations imply that treatment should be interdisciplinary in nature, incorporating both psychiatric and dermatological specialists. It is supported by the emergence of diagnostic tools, , such as the Charismaphobia Scale, which tries to measure the psychological impact of social beauty standards on individuals, further emphasizing the strong relationships between body image, mental health, and dermatology (Husain, 2023). Moreover, emerging methods in psychodermatology emphasize the demand for validation and reliability when assessing psychological constructs related to dermatologic disorders. The Charismaphobia Scale is indicative of this trend through qualitative and quantitative approaches to measuring individuals' fears of unattractiveness and self-perception. By employing exploratory and confirmatory factor analyses, researchers can establish the validity of the scale in measuring charismaphobia's factors. Such attention to detail in creating instruments makes the clinical assessment and intervention planning more effective in this new area of research. Additionally, research uncovers significant intercorrelations of charismaphobia with other psychopathologies, including generalized anxiety disorder and obsessive-compulsive disorder, which demonstrate the complex interrelationship of dermatology and mental illness (Husain, 2023). Such emerging understanding requires ongoing investigation and development of therapeutic modalities to address dermatologic disorders' psychic aspects. Current studies also examine the social and cultural contexts of psychodermatology, revealing the effects of media representations of beauty on self-esteem and on the BDD conditions. Findings show that greater exposure to media use will amplify narcissistic features and exhibitionist behaviors and link them with higher charismaphobia levels. These findings reveal a social construct responsible for defining norms of attractiveness and thereby influencing the psychological life of individuals. Investigating these impacts on culture gives a better understanding of how external factors promote one's body image and subsequent psychological well-being. As scientists improve measures and methods of assessment, they will have a big impact on clinical procedures for treating the psychological and dermatologic aspects of BDD, ultimately leading to more holistic and effective patient treatment.

10.6.1. Recent Studies in Psychodermatology

Subsequent psychodermatological research has reinforced the complex relationship between psychological and dermatologic illnesses, with particular attention given to BDD. Recent evidence suggests that BDD individuals exhibit heightened sensitivity to their external appearance as a cause of aversive behavioral reactions , such as repetitive grooming and constant checking. Furthermore, studies now emphasize that neurobiological substrates significantly contribute to BDD development. For instance, neuroimaging research has revealed hyperactivity in brain regions responsible for visual processing as well as for emotional regulation and has speculated that these neurobiological deviances may be responsible for the cognitive distortions in BDD patients. This bidirectional interdependence between mental state and dermatological issues illustrates the necessity for an evenhanded understanding of psychodermatological conditions, particularly in relation to the elements of BDD that compel the suffering individuals to seek cosmetic alteration in anticipation of a healing of their imaginary imperfections. Further, collaborative treatments involving dermatologists and mental health professionals are essential to successful intervention for BDD. The clinicians have long recognized the extreme psychological impairment of dermatological symptoms, as reflected by the finding that 1–2% of the general population is afflicted with BDD, and even more so among women. They engage repeatedly in behaviors of modifying their appearance according to their profound feelings of inadequacy about perceived flaws, thus inducing severe emotional and social handicaps. The recent psychodermatologic studies emphasize that treatment must be offered in the form of combined pharmacologic treatment and specially designed cognitive-behavioral therapy aimed at resolving specific cognitive distortions of such patients. Integrated models of treatment not only address the cognitive and affective aspects of BDD but also aim to reverse the negative dermatologic consequences of maladaptive behavior. Furthermore, understanding the neurochemical mechanics of BDD has been prioritized in current psychodermatological research. Results have indicated that disturbances in neurotransmitters, chiefly serotonin and dopamine, are responsible for the primary continuation of the compulsive rituals and emotional dysregulation that follow BDD. The neurochemical mechanisms collaborate with cognitive patterns , such as catastrophic thinking and selective attention to the perceived defects to exacerbate the severity of the conditions. As observed by recent studies, women with BDD are more emotionally distressed compared to their male counterparts and resort towards maladaptive coping mechanisms, for instance, getting cosmetic surgery or applying too much makeup, to correct their imagined defect. The treatment of these interconnected biological and psychological aspects is crucial to developing effective interventions in psychodermatology. By highlighting the interdependencies among neurobiology, behavioral patterns, and cognitive distortions, future research can enhance the efficacy of therapy for BDD cases in psychodermatology clinics (Figure 10.13).

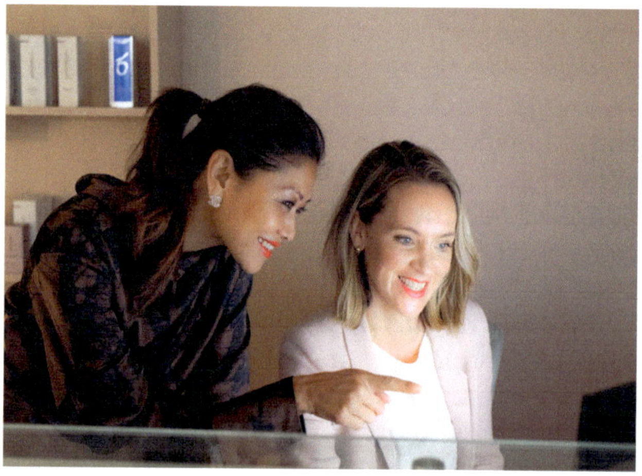

Figure 10.13. Skin Clinic collaborates while reviewing client information.

Source: https://no23skin.co.uk/wp-content/uploads/2021/12/No-23-Web-Res-18-1024x683.jpg.

10.6.2. Advances in Understanding BDD

Advances in our understanding of BDD have fostered a more empathetic response to its treatment and diagnosis, especially within the domain of psychodermatology. Recognition of BDD as an obsessive way of thinking about perceived physical flaws has facilitated interdisciplinary collaboration between dermatologists and mental health professionals. Such collaboration is necessary, as symptoms of dermatology are frequently combined with psychological distress, while underlying psychiatric conditions accompanying skin diseases are generally overlooked. As highlighted in recent literature, the complete comprehension of BDD is not merely the detection of the symptoms but also probing into inner experiences and emotional states of patients and, therefore, creating a general picture of their condition. This skin-mind interaction has become the focal point in proceeding with treatment modalities that are both useful in the management of dermatological and psychological problems (Ashwini and Kishor, 2021). The furtherance of treatment protocols with the involvement of psychodermatology principles in BDD treatment has also proven useful in providing advantages to patients. Cognitive-behavioral therapy and psychotherapeutic interventions specifically tailored to patients suffering from BDD are now being integrated by therapists. Recent studies indicate that such psychological therapies, when combined with dermatological treatment, can potentially enhance patient compliance and patient satisfaction. That a 30 to 40 percent incidence of psychiatric disorders among patients of dermatology has been reported is a reason why dermatologists should be equipped with the skills to handle such complexities. Good managerial methods not only enhance the patients' quality of life but also support a more comprehensive mode of treatment where psychological health is also respected in addition to physical health (Nguyen et al., 2015). Continuous training and education on dermatology professionals concerning the complicated interconnection of skin disease and mental illness is essential in building our own expertise in BDD. Lastly, ongoing research also teaches us much about the neurobiological correlates of BDD, which is essential to develop evidence-based focused therapeutic interventions. Investigation into the role of neurotransmitters, genetics, and brain imaging technology clarifies the pathophysiology of BDD and determines potential biomarkers that lead to earlier identification and individualized treatment regimens. Such results open the way for new pharmacological approaches that not only heal the patients' appearance problems but also their psychological torment. Furthermore, use of psychodermatology as a model for the treatment of BDD offers a multi-dimensional perspective that promotes mental health assessment in dermatology. As research continues to evolve, it may offer even greater insight into BDD, eventually leading to more effective, comprehensive care for individuals who suffer from this debilitating illness.

10.6.3. Future Directions for Research in the Field

As psychodermatology advances, future research must explore the intricate relationship between psychological and dermatological presentation, particularly for BDD. A possible future line of research is the development and assessment of internet-based interventions that offer psychological treatment for BDD patients. The growing prevalence of BDD, as seen in recent studies, necessitates new methods involving technology to expand access to treatment and education. Investigating the ways online material, , such as support groups, self-help groups, and educational papers, can improve psychological well-being, reduce anxiety, and facilitate social adaptation is key to creating effective therapeutic models. Results of these studies may not only enhance the quality of care but also provide patients with the ability to become actively involved in controlling their disorder, which might contribute to their overall quality of life (Brun et al., 2024). Another potential area for future studies is the investigation of the neuroanatomical and psychological traits underlying BDD. Recent studies indicate that BDD is more likely to present with comorbidities , such as severe depression and social dysfunction that exacerbate the disorder's effect on patients' lives (da Novaes et al., 2018). Longitudinal research tracking the development of BDD and its comorbidities enables researchers to identify key factors responsible for the disorder's onset and persistence. In addition, elucidation of the neural mechanisms behind BDD would direct the design of particular pharmacotherapies that have the goal of addressing both the psychological and physiological components of the condition. Greater understanding of these elements will not only increase diagnostic validity but also promote more individualized treatment strategies, ultimately benefiting the population afflicted with BDD. Lastly, interprofessional collaboration between psychologists, dermatologists, and other health care professionals is a key area of research for the future of psychodermatology and BDD. Multidisciplinary care models that facilitate communication and coordination will serve as an exemplar for ensuring all aspects of a patient's health are addressed comprehensively. Clinical research studies can train professionals to identify BDD symptoms, and provide a contribution towards decreasing the likelihood of patients seeking cosmetic interventions without psychiatric evaluation. In addition, studies to clarify cultural appreciation and treatment differences in BDD can determine where healthcare practice is lacking and provide the foundation for culturally responsive intervention. Through interdisciplinary collaboration, researchers are able to construct a strong base to tackle BDD effectively and with compassion (da Novaes et al., 2018).

Test Your Knowledge

1. What are the most significant findings from recent studies in psychodermatology?
2. What are the emerging research priorities in psychodermatology for patients with psychodermatological disorders?

SUMMARY

The study of psychodermatology shows important insights into the interlinked function of psychological well-being and dermatologic illness, particularly that of BDD. This disorder illustrates how an individual's perception of how they look can propel significant behavioral and psychiatric disturbances. Patients also perform damaging behaviors, , such as excessive grooming or picking at the skin, in a bid to fix supposed flaws. Recent studies bring to focus the point that such behavior is commonly linked with obsessive-compulsive disorder and other psychopathologies, so extreme therapeutic approaches are warranted. Effective therapy must combine both dermatological and psychological aspects to stop this cycle of suffering and enable holistic healing. Besides this, studies have proven that patients suffering from skin diseases like psoriasis not only have physical impacts but also have noteworthy impacts on their quality of life. The interconnectedness of the psychological well-being of a patient with dermatological health shows that treatment of the psychological aspect is crucial in the therapy of skin disease. For instance, self-esteem and anxiety exacerbate the symptoms, which create a self-perpetuating cycle of injury. Thus, a combined mode of therapy with the incorporation of therapy, lifestyle changes, and skincare can significantly benefit both psychological and dermatological symptoms within a therapeutic setting. This is in keeping with findings that integrating mental health treatment improves the prognosis for patients with psoriasis, as reaffirmed by recent studies. The association of psychodermatology with BDD merely serves to demonstrate a greater truth: body health and mind health are inseparable. Effective management strategies must thus attend not just to the visible signs of dermal ailments but, indeed, to those unconscious psychological elements that lead to their exacerbation. The biopsychosocial model is a helpful framework that advocates treatment encompassing not just bodily symptoms but also distress ensuing as an aftermath. As a specialty unfolds, a commitment to interdisciplinary consultation among dermatologists, psychologists, and psychiatrists will be imperative in making progress on patient care and optimizing overall quality of life, as evidenced by the interaction that we observe in most conditions, as outlined in the case of picking at skin and psoriasis, corroborated by outcomes of research (Benea et al., 2015; Sambura et al., 2024).

The relationship between psychological and dermatological disorders covered in the concept of psychodermatology has direct implications for the etiology of BDD. BDD is characterized by a preoccupation with physical flaws, and this may result in severe impairment of one's quality of life. Notably, patients with skin conditions, , such as atopic dermatitis, are predisposed to higher susceptibility to mental disorders. This group of people has issues that extend past physical symptoms, and hence awareness of , such associated risks is a necessity. Sadly, despite how strong the linkages between skin conditions and mental health are, physicians often do not get sufficient training on how to recognize and treat such psychological problems, with the consequence that real obstacles to effective intervention and care for persons affected are at large (Sanchez., 2023). Furthermore, treatment guidelines for BDD highlight the value of including clinical advice like that of the NICE. This would involve CBT and medication, which have been shown by research to produce substantial benefits for highly symptomatic individuals. But outcomes are variable, and evidence that, while some patients do achieve quite large decreases in BDD symptoms, others experience little or no change. This discrepancy sets the standard of individualized treatment models and the need for ongoing improvement in therapeutic protocols. Furthermore, clinician and patient feedback indicate a vital imperative for more education and training on BDD treatment methods, which indicates the evolving nature of psychodermatology as it overlaps with mental health (Govender, 2021). The findings within psychodermatology highlight not only the complexities of treating BDD but also the key importance of building effective clinician-patient relationships. Qualitative patient outcomes recognize their own perspectives, which are predominantly focused on change in quality of life and global functioning rather than symptom reduction alone. This is a distinction that emphasizes the importance of treatment models to value expansive conceptualizations of health and incorporate patient views in shaping clinical practice. Through an integrative strategy that integrates psychological and dermatological treatment, practitioners can effectively manage the interwoven nature of disorders like BDD to achieve improved treatment outcomes and enhanced patient satisfaction. All such integration not only serves the patients but also enhances the providers' knowledge base, setting the stage for future growth in the field of psychodermatology (Govender, 2021).

KEY TERMS FROM THIS CHAPTER

- Anxiety
- BDD tendencies
- BDD-type symptoms
- Charismaphobia Scale
- Continuing medical education (CME)
- Cosmetic operators
- Dermatological issues
- Interdisciplinary collaboration
- Mood disorders
- Novel alternative treatments
- BDD rates
- BDD-affected patients
- Body perception
- Cognitive behavior therapy (CBT)
- Co-occurring skin disease
- Depression
- Eczema
- Mindfulness-based interventions
- Multidisciplinary collaboration
- Obsessive-compulsive disorder

CRITICAL THINKING QUESTIONS

1. **What is the primary focus of psychodermatology?**
   a. Treatment of fungal infections of the skin
   b. Psychological impact of skin disorders and their management
   c. Surgical procedures to enhance skin appearance
   d. Study of infectious diseases affecting the skin
2. **Body dysmorphic disorder (BDD) is best characterized by:**
   a. Delusions about having a serious skin disease
   b. Fear of aging and wrinkles
   c. Obsession with a perceived flaw in appearance, often minor or not observable to others
   d. Compulsive tanning and skin bleaching
3. **Which of the following is a common behavior in individuals with body dysmorphic disorder?**
   a. Avoiding mirrors entirely
   b. Ignoring all concerns about appearance
   c. Seeking out sun exposure regularly
   d. Excessive checking of appearance in mirrors
4. **Which specialty is most likely to manage psychodermatology cases?**
   a. Dermatology and Psychiatry
   b. Orthopedics
   c. Cardiology
   d. Gastroenterology
5. **What is a common comorbid psychiatric condition in patients with body dysmorphic disorder?**
   a. Schizophrenia
   b. Obsessive-compulsive disorder (OCD)
   c. Bipolar Disorder
   d. Antisocial Personality Disorder

Short Answer Questions

1. What is psychodermatology, and how does it integrate dermatology and psychiatry?
2. What are the most common psychiatric conditions associated with dermatological disorders?
3. How can psychological stress influence or exacerbate chronic skin conditions?
4. What are the standard psychotherapeutic and pharmacological interventions used in psychodermatology?
5. How is BDD diagnosed, and what are the core features that differentiate it from normal appearance concerns?
6. What are the most common dermatological complaints or procedures sought by patients with undiagnosed BDD?
7. What role do CBT and SSRIs play in the treatment of BDD?
8. How can dermatologists and cosmetic practitioners screen for BDD before performing elective procedures?

Answer to Critical Thinking Questions

1.(b) 2.(c) 3.(d) 4.(a) 5.(b)

REFERENCES

1. Ader, R., Arck, P. C., Azambuja, R., Basavaraj, K. H., Bilbo, S. D., Botchkarev, V. A., Carmody, J., et al. (2017). The need of dermatologists, psychiatrists and psychologists joint care in psychodermatology. https://core.ac.uk/download/160475555.pdf (accessed on 11th June 2025).
2. Alhazmi, A. Y., Faqih, S. N., Alsalem, B. S., Alsalem, M., & Alnoman, H. (2024). Plastic surgeons' attitudes and understanding of body dysmorphic disorder. *Cureus, 16*. https://www.semanticscholar.org/paper/1966fa71e5ec31aac552ed28c567628d99f473f2 (accessed on 11th June 2025).
3. Al-Sarraf, Alaa (2022) Skin Lightening as An Image Enhancing Phenomenon: Investigating Risks, Motivations, and Underlying Psychological Factors. Doctoral thesis, University of Hertfordshire.(accessed on 11th June 2025).
4. Ashwini, P. K., & Kishor, M. (2021). *Essentials of Psychiatry for Dermatology and Aesthetic Practice*. https://www.mindsunited.org/_files/ugd/a5fc9c_bd2dd821b9a64b42878f5596b848074d.pdf#page=220 (accessed on 11th June 2025).
5. Bassetti, C., Sohm, F., Adamantidis, A., Schindler, K. A., Barazzoni, F., & Manconi, M. (2024). The International Master of Advanced Studies (MAS) in sleep medicine of the Universities of Bern and Svizzera Italian. *Clinical and Translational Neuroscience*. https://www.semanticscholar.org/paper/3fed730ecf08f31c4f364a912c3493fbdc3a5deb (accessed on 11th June 2025).
6. Basta-Juzbašić, A., & Bukvić Mokos, Z. (2015). Skin changes in primary psychiatric disorders. https://core.ac.uk/download/33281974.pdf (accessed on 11th June 2025).
7. Benea, V., Georgescu, S. R., Leahu, D., Raileanu, et al. (2015). Pathological skin picking: Case presentation and review of the literature. https://core.ac.uk/download/144552337.pdf (accessed on 11th June 2025).
8. Brun, E. M. (2024). Body dysmorphic disorder and internet usage: The positive impact of online resources. https://core.ac.uk/download/636341919.pdf (accessed on 11th June 2025).
9. Sambura, M., Rosołowska-Żak, S., Sas, W., Podyma, K., Ryznar, G., Rejdych, J., ... Bylica, G. (2024). Sport impact on patients with psoriasis and psychiatric problems. *Quality in Sport, 17*, 50709. https://doi.org/10.12775/QS.2024.17.001 (accessed on 11th June 2025).
10. Chiriac, A., Chiriac, A. E., Foia, L., Brzezinski, P., & Pinteala, T. (2015). Common psych cutaneous disorders in children. https://core.ac.uk/download/186770978.pdf (accessed on 11th June 2025).
11. Çınaroğlu, M. (2024). Hormonal catalysts in the addiction cycle of muscle dysmorphia: A neuroendocrine perspective. *The Journal of Neurobehavioral Sciences*. https://www.semanticscholar.org/paper/e73a17e2cd11c112bd31a27144f6e24e1c097f7d (accessed on 11th June 2025).
12. Çınaroğlu, M. (2025). A neurobehavioral perspective on body dysmorphic disorder: Understanding the brain-behavior connection. *The Journal of Neurobehavioral Sciences*. https://www.semanticscholar.org/paper/11e4bdf1b34801fef1549fe5d5d0052f170843e0 (accessed on 11th June 2025).
13. Costilla-Reyes, O., & Talbot, M. (2025). Predicting treatment response in body dysmorphic disorder with interpretable machine learning. *ArXiv, abs/2503.10741*. https://www.

semanticscholar.org/paper/c4ff2f1155af4484c646b385c54e93170ef12ee4 (accessed on 11th June 2025).

14. Czernecka, A., & Batycka-Baran, A. (2020). Acne fulminans in a patient with suspected bigorexia. *107*, 63–68. https://www.semanticscholar.org/paper/ce54c966d03988f3ec4802a37be102a933ada678 (accessed on 11th June 2025).

15. Gieler, U., Poot, F., Sampogna, F., Tomas-Aragones, L., et al. (2019). *The ESDAP Diploma in Psychodermatology*. https://core.ac.uk/download/389599286.pdf (accessed on 11th June 2025).

16. Govender A. (2021). Evaluation of a specialist service model for treating body dysmorphic disorder (BDD): application of National Institute for Health and Clinical Excellence Guidelines for BDD (NICE, 2006). *BJPsych Open*, *7*(Suppl 1), S322. https://doi.org/10.1192/bjo.2021.848 (accessed on 11th June 2025).

17. He, I. R., Gaillard, A., & Rossell, S. L. (2025). Addressing body dysmorphic disorder through mindfulness: A new therapeutic frontier. *Australian & New Zealand Journal of Psychiatry, 59*, 405–412. https://www.semanticscholar.org/paper/aa73f18102a398734a286180c02842379a5dddd1 (accessed on 11th June 2025).

18. Hocaoglu, C., & Sonmez, D. (2022). *Psychological Aspect of Alopecia*. https://core.ac.uk/download/543005590.pdf (accessed on 11th June 2025).

19. Husain, W. (2023). Charisma phobia: Diagnosis and measurement of the psych dermatological symptoms. *Journal of Skin and Stem Cell, 10*. https://doi.org/10.5812/jssc-137387 (accessed on 11th June 2025).

20. Juodikis, D., Paulauskienė, Ž., & Lukoševičiūtė, G. (2024). Understanding body dysmorphic disorder in the context of plastic surgery: A systematic review. *Chirurgia Plastyczna i Oparzenia / Plastic Surgery & Burns*. https://hdl.handle.net/20.500.12512/252027. https://www.semanticscholar.org/paper/70c3f374fd1cea609a32cede76a6665b3dc3710b (accessed on 11th June 2025).

21. Lamba, N. T. (2025). Self-esteem, body image, and the tendency of body dysmorphic disorder (BDD) in Generation Z. *Observasi: Jurnal Publikasi Ilmu Psikologi*. https://www.semanticscholar.org/paper/3c5667d9aac02d4d17a56eb70242297dd03ee76a (accessed on 11th June 2025).

22. Li, V., Frasier, K., Fritts, H., Daly, K., Christoforides, S., Harpine, C. E., Stec, K., et al. (2024). Exploring the intersection of body dysmorphic disorder (BDD) and dermatological conditions. *Clinical Dermatology and Surgery*. https://www.semanticscholar.org/paper/a889854f47c5e6dbab609534545c6e9dcbc671c9 (accessed on 11th June 2025).

23. Li, V., Frasier, K., Woolhiser, E., Daly, K., Christoforides, S., Harpine, C. E., Stech, K., et al. (2024). Exploring the intersection of body dysmorphic disorder (BDD) and dermatological conditions: A narrative review. *Dermatology and Therapy, 14*, 2693–2708. https://www.semanticscholar.org/paper/3fe728e88e4852555fa945130b1dbeb58b8ddcdf (accessed on 11th June 2025).

24. Mar, K., & Rivers, J. K. (2023). The mind body connection in dermatologic conditions: A literature review. *Journal of Cutaneous Medicine and Surgery, 27*, 628–640. https://www.semanticscholar.org/paper/6b4f4ebf6d56f85fc9ca43a3314738b96c298aea (accessed on 11th June 2025).

25. Massoud, S. (2022). *Behavioral Health Clinics in The Treatment of Psychosocial Comorbidities of Pediatric Acne*. https://open.bu.edu/bitstream/2144/43870/8/Massoud_bu_0017N_16577.pdf (accessed on 11th June 2025).

26. Nguyen, C. M., Danesh, M., Beroukhi, K., Sorenson, E., Leon, A., & Koo, J. (2015). Psychodermatology: A review. *Practical Dermatology*. https://assets.bmctoday.net/practicaldermatology/pdfs/pd0515_SF_PsychDerm.pdf (accessed on 11th June 2025).

27. Novaes, J. da S., Fernandes, H. M., Ferreira, C. M. H., et al. (2018). Body dysmorphic disorder: Characteristics, psychopathology, clinical associations, and influencing factors. https://core.ac.uk/download/322436695.pdf (accessed on 11th June 2025).

28. Osman, O., Souid, A., Al-Mugaddam, F., Eapen, B., & Jafferany, M. (2017). Attentiveness of dermatologists in the Middle East to psych cutaneous medicine. *The Primary Care Companion for CNS Disorders, 19*(2). https://www.semanticscholar.org/paper/959bb0b19a42a69ffe808dc9d0b4aee2d6981944 (accessed on 11th June 2025).

29. Patel, N. (2022). *Targeting Psychosocial Factors in Cardiac Rehabilitation of Young Women to Reduce Cardiovascular Events Following Myocardial Infarction*. Boston University ProQuest Dissertations & Theses, 2021. 28652979.(accessed on 11th June 2025).

30. Poot, F., Sampogna, F., & Onnis, L. (2007). Basic knowledge in psychodermatology. *Journal of the European Academy of Dermatology and Venereology : JEADV, 21*(2), 227–234. https://doi.org/10.1111/j.1468-3083.2006.01910.x(accessed on 11th June 2025).

31. Rodríguez-Cerdeira, C., Pera-Grasa, J. T., Molares, A., Isa-Isa, R., & Arenas-Guzmán, R. (2011). Psychodermatology: Past, present and future. *The Open Dermatology Journal, 5*, 21–27. https://www.semanticscholar.org/paper/a2aa0f6554208079254080292 5a277dde22a99cf (accessed on 11th June 2025).

32. Safitri, N. A., Suroso, & Pratitis, N. T. (2025). The Relationship between Body Image and Self-Esteem with the Tendency of Body Dysmorphic Disorder (BDD) Among Adolescents Using Social Media. *Journal of Scientific Research, Education, and Technology (JSRET), 4*(1), 656–664. https://doi.org/10.58526/jsret.v4i1.737(accessed on 11th June 2025).

33. Sanchez, Rebeca, "Knowledge Awareness of Body Image Impairment and Its Associated Mental Health Risk Factors in Pediatric Patients with Atopic Dermatitis Among Healthcare Providers in an Outpatient Allergy and Immunology Clinic in Miami, Florida: A Quality Improvement Project" (2023). *Nicole Wertheim College of Nursing Student Projects*. 215. https://digitalcommons.fiu.edu/cnhs-studentprojects/215(accessed on 11th June 2025).

34. Shakeel, A., & Zafar, H. (2024). Psychosocial effects and mental health issues associated with body dysmorphic disorder in women. *International Journal of Scientific Reports*. https://www.semanticscholar.org/paper/d924f17480793efd4a1c4fd06fc034005c920494 (accessed on 11th June 2025).

35. Zhu, Y., Du, X., Shen, S., Song, X., & Xiang, W. (2024). Body dysmorphic disorder symptoms in patients with melasma. *International Journal of Dermatology, 63*. https://www.semanticscholar.org/paper/3077f9a7a0c3f616b818c8f23d36b6fc3d1ab8d8 (accessed on 11th June 2025).

TATTOO REMOVAL AND SCAR MANAGEMENT

11

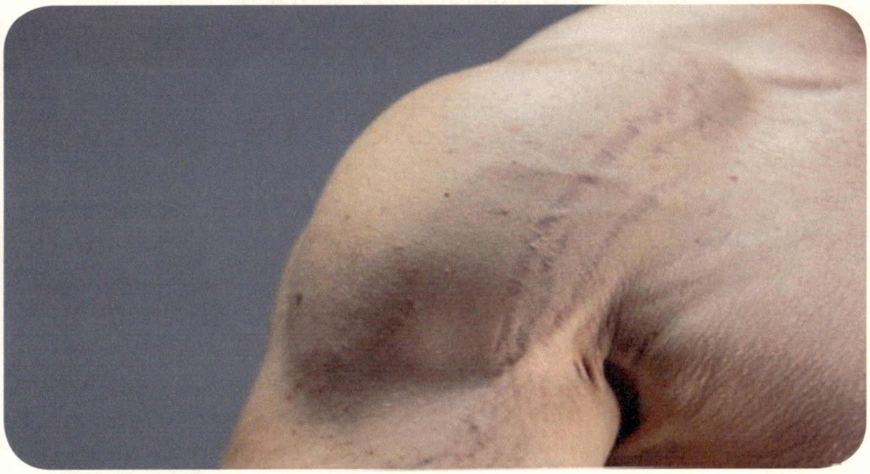

LEARNING OBJECTIVES

After studying this chapter, you will be able to:

1. Explain methods of tattoo removal
2. Explain the effectiveness of tattoo removal methods
3. Define risks and side effects of tattoo elimination
4. Control scar formation and management
5. Explain the psychological impact of tattoo removal

Introduction

The widespread popularity of tattoos among people of many different ages has made them a highly mainstream form of creativity and self-expression. Since an estimated 10–20% of European adults bear tattoos, the mainstream status that body art has achieved in modern culture also presents a myriad of health concerns. Complications from tattoos due to allergic reactions and infections have increasingly motivated individuals to have their tattoos removed. As the tattooing process is a type that is accustomed to producing a large number of dermatologic complications, understanding the same becomes a compulsion strictly while dealing with the medical and psychological aspects involved in the treatment of individuals who request unwanted tattoo removal. This context acknowledges the necessity to return not only to the tattoo removal procedures but also to skin health, particularly in terms of how scars are handled, which now becomes an integral part of follow-up and recovery (Saphale, 2017; Van et al., 2021). Tattoo removal is a multilateral process with each procedure containing different levels of effectiveness and complications. Laser treatments, tattoo removal industry leaders reveal, work at a given wavelength for the purpose of shattering tattoo ink particles so that they can be reabsorbed by the body. The treatment is not absolutely safe since there are side effects in the form of scarring, hyperpigmentation, or chronic skin irritation. Also, some skin conditions or types may yield side effects via the removal process itself, thus making the process of getting clear skin even more complicated. Therefore, thorough knowledge of all such risks is simply imperative. Proper management of scarring in the form of a result of removal of tattoos is also essential, , such as awareness about permanent care after the procedure and what ensures maximum healing and cosmetic outcome.

Technical methods of tattoo removal notwithstanding, the psychological aspect of going through the same also merits comprehensive research. A significant percentage of people think about getting their tattoos removed because of shifts in identity, a change of mind when it comes to personal beliefs, or regret, which evokes the emotional aspect of having such a bodily alteration. These are the kind of reasons for which clinician-relation becomes a necessity in clinical practice, i.e., practitioners extending their professional responsibility of dealing with the physical process of removal of tattoos to taking care of the psychological well-being of their clients. Also, due to growing demand for removal of tattoos, good practice and lucid advice in managing scars is a necessity. This combination of physical and psychological qualities emphasizes the need for an interdisciplinary approach to the treatment of scars and tattoo removal, creating avenues toward improved patient care within this new field of treatment (Saphale, 2017; Van et al., 2021).

Definition of Tattoo Removal

Treatment of tattoo removal is a course of treatments taken to eliminate the permanent color ink injected into the skin through the procedure of tattooing. One of the most popular treatments, laser therapy, applies intense beams of light to selectively kill the ink particles within the dermis. This technique has been in greater demand since it can minimize trauma to the surrounding tissue but can allow the tattoo to fade out naturally over time. As it is mixed with physical manipulation of skin and ink, success depends upon numerous factors , such as exposure to ink colors, skin type, and healing response in an individual. Recent evidence indicates that a high percentage of tattooed individuals, particularly between 26 and 40 years, regret getting tattoos and express the need for proper removal methods (Carneiro, 2023). Besides lasers, numerous other tattoo removal methods exist, each with advantages and disadvantages. Methods , such as surgical excision involve physical extraction of tattooed skin, commonly for small tattoos or cases where removal is life-critical. Chemical peels are employed to peel off or whiten the skin in less efficient and harmful methods of removal, with a high tendency to lead to scarring. Side effects of any method of tattoo removal are imminent, varying from skin infection and skin color alteration. Moreover, it is mostly oblivious to what occurs after the removal of tattoos, and more awareness of the need for informed consent and correct information in the removal process has existed (Căiță et al., 2024). Since there has also been progress in the technology of removing tattoos, applications of new technology are shifting traditional approaches and enhancing patients' outcomes. The application of artificial intelligence (AI) in treatment planning and medical imaging creates new possibilities for increased efficiency and accuracy in procedures. For instance, AI can allow monitoring and real-time optimization of laser parameters to enhance safety and minimize toxic side effects during tattoo removal. Investigations into the biochemical composition of tattoo ink pigments and their interaction with various removal methods are also being pursued as an effort to further solidify and refine treatment practices. With a focus on optimizing operational practice and information on potential complications, equally placing significance on the need for professional standards and education in tattoo removal, is the fact that both patient and practitioner wish to align beauty requirements with skin health issues (Carneiro, 2023) (Figure 11.1).

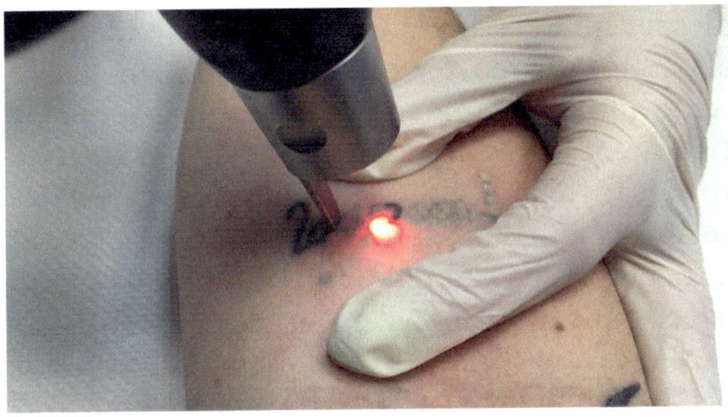

Figure 11.1. Laser treatment being performed for tattoo removal.

Source: https://dreamderma.in/wp-content/uploads/2019/04/23913068744_e827b46315_b-1024x576.jpg.

Importance of Scar Management

Proper scar management is important in the prevention of long-term physical and psychological sequelae of skin injury, particularly where tattoo removal is involved. Because more treatments for removing tattoos are being done, attention to dealing with scarring that will take place as a result of treatment increases as well. Scarring is one of the primary reasons individuals are not satisfied with the cosmetic outcome and thus will require additional treatments. Proper implementation of scar management modalities can significantly improve the healing process as well as the eventual aesthetic result. Modalities , such as laser therapy, topical therapy, and some forms of wound care are all a part of achieving the best results in healing and minimizing scar formation. Scars, if left untreated, can result in chronic scarring of pain, hyperpigmentation, or even psychological anguish, hence making anticipatory scar care not only a cosmetic concern but also a sine qua non of worldwide skin health. With the examination of mechanisms of scar development, it becomes clear that individualized care can enhance healing considerably. New technologies , such as dexpanthenol in wound healing in topical application, have been found to act as effective enhancers of scar management. Clinical trials have established that application of dexpanthenol after procedure hastens re-epithelialization and enhances skin barrier function, which is critical in scar reduction as well as promotion of the healing process overall (Baron et al., 2020). This topical treatment has also been proven to boost important genes involved in skin regeneration, making it a strong contender for inclusion in tattoo removal after-care therapies. With such evidence-based therapies, clinicians can ensure that individuals who undergo tattoo removal not only reach cosmetic objectives but also receive comprehensive care that includes addressing the patient's potential scarring. Scar management treatments are also particularly relevant in multicultural populations, where skin types become involved in the healing process. For instance, there has been a study that accepted the efficacy of Q-Switched, 1064 nm Nd: YAG laser treatment for managing Asian patients' scars, whose diverse healing responses could be determined based on their typical skin (Bennardo et al., 2022). Individualized treatments for specific skin types ensure optimal treatment and restrict unwanted side effects. This maintains the client as a focus and ensures the requirement for specialized scar management techniques stays on the agenda for tattoo removal practice. Effective scar management not only enhances the physical integrity of the skin, but it is also a key element in the construction of the emotional wellbeing of the client. With continuous developments in tattoo removal, the combination of advanced scar management techniques remains a necessity for complete patient satisfaction.

11.1. Methods of Tattoo Removal

Learning Outcome

1. Understand laser technologies in the field of tattoo removal
2. Explain how surgical excision presents a significant alternative for tattoo removal
3. Describe chemical peels and dermabrasion

Tattoo removal techniques have improved significantly over the past few years, with more focus being laid on performance as well as safety. Laser removal has become the norm now because it is a non-surgical procedure and has a relatively high success rate. Used to break down tattoo pigment particles in the skin, lasers , such as Q-switched and picosecond technology produce different wavelengths to target individual colors of the ink separately. But the treatment is administered in sessions to achieve the best possible results and often leaves the skin with varying degrees of scarring depending on individual healing processes and skin types. Knowledge of the complexities involved in scar formation can also improve management of patient expectations better, as the complete removal of scars is not always achievable, and other forms or adjuvant treatment, like a better aesthetic outcome, are desired, a view confirmed by literature reports of realistic patient expectations and surgery in scar management (Albina et al., 2024). Apart from the laser procedures, there are other methods encompassing the surgical elimination of the tattoo, dermabrasion, and chemical peels, which have some level of tattoo removal efficiency. Surgical elimination eliminates the entire dermal layer with the tattoo, resulting in instant elimination but potential scarring. Dermabrasion sands off the skin layer by layer, which can also give way to asymmetrical outcomes as far as the visibility of scars is concerned. Chemical peels utilize acid solutions to physically erase the epidermal surface and stimulate new growth. All of these modalities share certain special characteristics and limitations that need to be properly weighed regarding individual patient history and cosmetic goals. Hence, a multi-step tattoo removal process is usually followed by applying these methods along with skin hygiene and maintenance measures to prevent scarring after treatment (Albina et al., 2024). Moreover, a natural barrier in tattoo removal is the immune response triggered by treatments , such as laser. This encompasses a wide range from mild cutaneous responses to severe anaphylaxis, and elimination is thereby difficult. Understanding of the immune system is crucial since this will determine the efficacy of the tattoo removal techniques applied. For instance, hypersensitivity responses , such as irritation and redness may develop after laser treatment, which may necessitate a change in the treatment protocols. The research places great importance on careful handling of the reaction in a manner that enables medical practitioners to closely monitor patients for side effects throughout the course. Addressing patient comfort and safety is a method whereby practitioners can maximize results in tattoo removal and follow-up scar treatment.

11.1.1. Laser Removal Techniques

Laser technology has revolutionized the tattoo removal and scar management art into effective procedures for removing unwanted pigments. Laser removal techniques usually operate by concentrating high-energy light onto breaking ink fragments in the skin to enable the immune system of the body to remove them progressively. Various lasers are used, including Q-switched lasers, which produce short pulses of high-intensity light and target particular wavelengths of the ink pigments in the tattoo without damaging other tissues. Such targeting, aside from being more effective in removal, reduces healing time and complications by significant margins, setting laser removal apart from traditional methods. The ability to control laser parameters also makes it possible for practitioners to provide custom treatment to patients, thereby maximizing outcomes and patient satisfaction in aesthetic medicine. In addition to the traditional removal of tattoos, laser treatments are now viable options for treating scars from a variety of injuries or surgery (Figure 11.2).

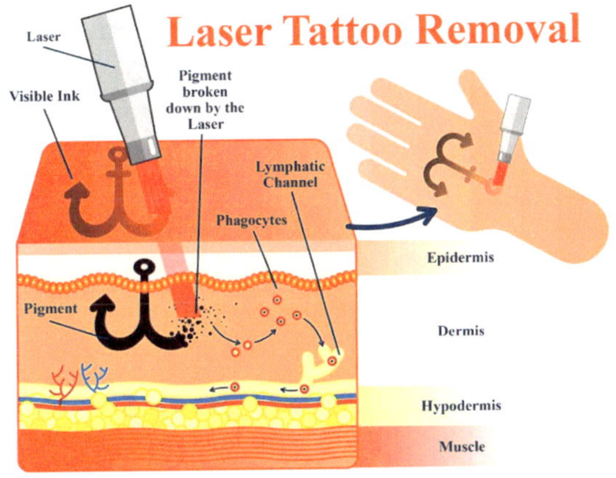

Figure 11.2. Laser tattoo removal.

Source: https://goodbyetattoos.com/wp-content/uploads/2023/01/Tattoo-removal-visual.jpg.

Fractional laser technology application is quite significant as it causes skin remodeling by delivering tiny beams of light into the dermis without damaging the surrounding tissue. It is a minimally invasive treatment that induces healing and growth of healthy tissue, which in turn decreases scars. In addition, recent studies have also explored the effectiveness of other laser wavelengths, blue (λ = 450 nm) and infrared (λ = 10.6 μm), to produce the optimum results in removing pigmented skin lesions and scar tissue. With more understanding of such treatments, practitioners can more accurately predict outcomes and reduce the risk of complications of scar treatment and thus achieve improved aesthetic outcomes. Despite the advancements in laser removal, some of the issues still remain, the most critical of which is recurrence and complication in the form of scarring. It has been estimated that approximately 6% of the patients experience severe scarring following laser treatment, which is why getting the right type of laser and optimum settings in each case matters. Also, the risk of recurrence may be as high as 41%, particularly in the case of congenital giant pigmented nevi (CGPN).

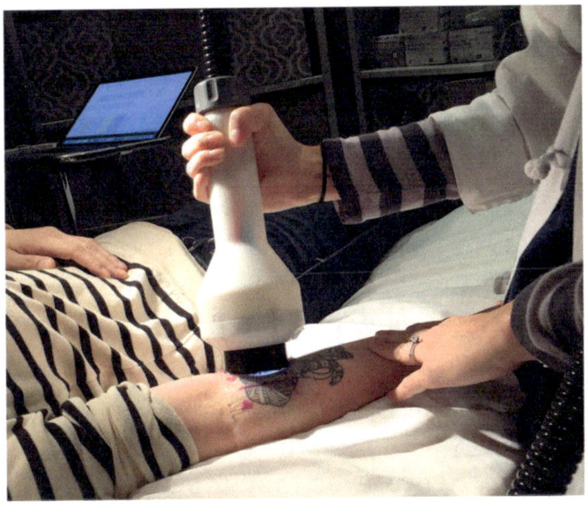

Figure 11.3. Hand Piece of Rapid Acoustic Pulse device being applied for 1 minute after a laser tattoo removal treatment to dissipate the laser whitening and allow an additional laser pass.

Source: https://www.researchgate.net/profile/David-Robertson-10/publication/335940819/figure/fig3/AS:805214445654018@1568989492508/Hand-Piece-of-Rapid-Acoustic-Pulse-device-being-applied-for-1-minute-after-a-laser-tattoo.jpg.

All this heterogeneity necessitates a planned treatment schedule, keeping in mind such details as the history of the patient, skin type, and tactile quality of the tattoo or scar. It is here that continually developing advances in advanced laser technology are significant in that current science shows greater efficacy and fewer side effects by using combinations of wavelengths. Inasmuch as technology continues to advance, clinicians are obligated to stay abreast of best practice to maximize outcomes in tattoo removal and the treatment of scars (Figure 11.3).

11.1.2. Surgical Excision

Surgical excision is a major method of tattoo removal, especially when compared with non-surgical methods like the use of lasers. The surgical procedure involves excision of the skin on which the tattoo is drawn, and thus it is a safe method for people who have unfortunate tattoos or whose tattoos are rendered disfigured after some period of time.

The procedure is straightforward; the physician uses a scalpel to excise the skin where the tattoo is and then sutures the cover of the skin. This procedure works well in the removal of small tattoos as it provides complete removal with minimal ink deposits left on the skin. The invasive surgery carries native complications , such as scarring and infection, which require meticulous planning and operation during the procedure. Hence, even though surgical removal is a final procedure, its outcome on the healing of the tissue and recovery must be properly thought out. Since patients want the best result of tattoo removal, no one should overlook the impact of surgical removal on controlling scars. The operation does create a scar whose extent is contingent upon the healing response of the patient as well as his or her genetic predisposition to develop scars. Techniques for minimizing postoperative scarring have been identified, which include meticulous suturing and topical use of silicone gel sheeting or pressure dressing. Other than that, the experts can also recommend the use of topical treatment and therapy , such as laser treatment after surgery, for better healing as well as reducing the visibility of scars. These measures must be enacted in patient management because studies have shown that proper scar care not only produces acceptable cosmetic outcomes but also results in the psychological satisfaction of patients for tattoo removal. Hence, an integrative strategy should include both surgery and post-operative therapy in an attempt to be capable of achieving satisfactory outcomes. Despite the benefits, surgery is not consideration-free and limitation-free. The procedure is more invasive than a few alternative methods of tattoo removal, like laser treatment, and this may act as a deterrent for those preferring less invasive procedures. Additionally, excision works best only on small to medium tattoos, as the process of removing the tattoo may take multiple sessions in case of a bigger tattoo or even lead to unwanted skin removal, thereby leading to a different form of scarring.

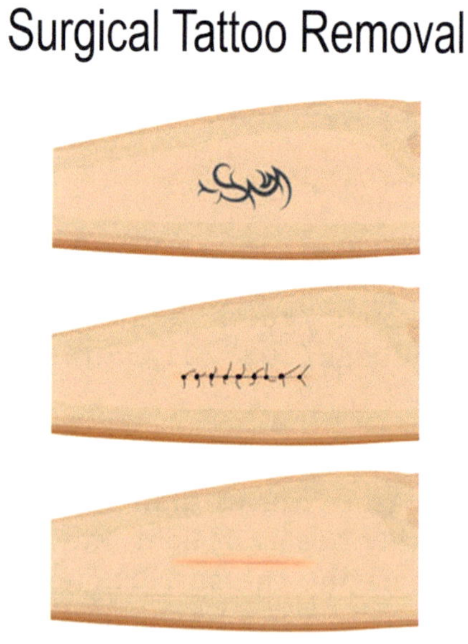

Figure 11.4. Surgical tattoo removal.

Source: https://drvinodvij.com/wp-content/uploads/2025/02/Surgical-Tattoo-Removal.png.

Also, the body site upon which the tattoo is to be performed, skin type, and composition of tattoo ink are all significant to determine. Patients should also be informed about the risk of complications arising from and after the procedure, e.g., poor cosmetic result or abnormal healing responses. Thus, surgical removal, while effective in some instances, needs to be extremely thoroughly evaluated on an individual basis to allow for a wise balance of tattoo elimination and scar reduction, as seen in the context of the entire medical scenario of such operations (Carneiro, 2023Lane et al., 2012; Carneiro, 2023) (Figure 11.4).

11.1.3. Chemical Peels and Dermabrasion

The use of dermabrasion and chemical peels for the management of scars and tattoos has been of increasing interest due to their resurfacing effect on the appearance and texture of skin. Chemical peels involve the topical deposition of chemical solutions to induce exfoliation of epidermal layers, resulting in controlled peeling. They induce stimulation of rejuvenation of skin and significantly improve the appearance of epidermal scars and tattoo-related hyperpigmentation.

Through the promotion of collagen production and cellular turnover, chemical peels effectively enhance skin texture and tone, thus becoming a desirable option for patients who would like to eliminate the visibility of tattoos or notoriety of scars. The success of the treatment warrants proper assessment of skin type and scar morphology for the provision of personalized treatment plans with optimal beneficial outcomes and minimal risk of adverse events. Dermabrasion is a mechanical exfoliant technique that involves the selective removal of superficial layers of skin. With the help of a rotating instrument, dermabrasion can quite effectively correct the abnormal surface topography so characteristically described in relation to scars, e.g., tattoo scars. Dermabrasion is particularly beneficial in atrophic scars since it acts as an agent for healing by being an agent for stimulating blood flow and collagen deposition. The depth of the dermabrasion can be adjusted according to the individualized scarring pattern of the patient and is an extremely versatile treatment modality. Keep in mind that dermabrasion does have a slower healing time than chemical peeling due to mechanical disruption of the skin and thus more trauma and more healing time. All that being said, there is value in understanding the nuances of each technique to achieve the best results for scar control.

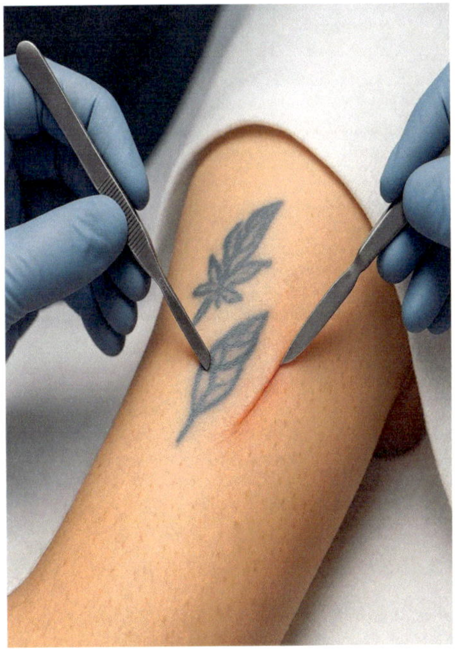

Figure 11.5. Microdermabrasion on tattoo.

Source: https://www.carewellmedicalcentre.com/wp-content/uploads/2025/05/tattoo-removal-by-surgical-excision-carewell.webp.

The incorporation of chemical peeling and dermabrasion adjunct to other treatment modalities may yield better results in the management of scars and tattoos. For instance, combination with microneedling—an established method of inducing skin repair through controlled damage—has been demonstrated to produce positive outcomes, especially for the scenario of acne scars (Sivaranjani, 2019). In addition to improving the quality of the skin, the combination also resolves pigmentation and odd tone issues at its root. In addition, as literature explains, laser treatments also have the capability to be utilized to accompany such treatments appropriately, providing individuals with other avenues to enhance the texture and look of the scars (Al-Waiz et al., 2017). Generally, the precise combination of chemical peels and dermabrasion with newer technologies provides individuals with a dual route for treating tattoos and scars, both enhancing cosmetic appearance and emotional health (Figure 11.5).

Test Your Knowledge

1. What size tattoo can be surgically removed?
2. Can chemical peels remove tattoos? Explain.

11.2. Effectiveness of Tattoo Removal Methods

Learning Outcome

1. Understand the success rates of laser treatments for tattoo removal
2. Compare surgical and non-surgical methods of tattoo removal
3. Describe factors influencing removal effectiveness

The effectiveness of tattoo removal methods is a significant area of study within dermatology and cosmetic medicine, as the increasing popularity of tattoos has led to an equal rise in demand for effective and safe removal methods. Among the various removal methods, laser treatment, particularly Q-switched lasers, has emerged as a first option due to their ability to target pigments selectively without inflicting damage to nearby tissues. The procedure operates by the release of specific wavelengths that are absorbed by the tattoo inks and then dissolved into tiny particles that can be extracted from the body. Not only does the procedure address a wide range of ink colors, but it also minimizes the risk of complications from more invasive removal techniques and is therefore preferred by those who want to eliminate unwanted tattoos. Further, the efficacy of the Q-switched, 1064 nm neodymium-doped yttrium aluminum garnet (Nd: YAG) laser is an improvement in the field of tattoo removal, particularly for darker skin tones. The literature affirms that the modality of the laser is effective for many ink colors and has a good safety profile. For instance, a study on Asian patients with Fitzpatrick skin types III–IV revealed general improvement in the appearance of scars when treated using the QSF Nd: YAG laser. The study highlighted that all volunteers experienced a significant improvement in acne scars, attesting to lasers' versatility, other than removal of tattoos, to include the solutions for treatment of scars, thereby justifying its position in current treatments of skin imperfections (Bennardo et al., 2022). Despite advancements in removal techniques, it remains crucial to control potential complications and scarring that may arise from the procedures. Control of resultant scars is typically a side issue in tattoo removal, which indicates the importance of comprehensive aftercare and management protocols. More invasive methods, , such as surgical removal or dermabrasion, may yield quicker resolution but overall carry higher potential for serious scarring and complication, , such as infection. Therefore, a general strategy for tattoo removal would have to involve honesty about outcomes along with integration of post-procedure scar correction. This combined treatment ensures that the patients not only achieve desired cosmetic results but also experience the integrity and health of their skin throughout the tattoo removal procedure (Lane et al., 2012).

11.2.1. Success Rates of Laser Treatments

The efficacy of laser therapy in tattoo removal and scar management largely depends on the nature of the laser used in addition to the nature of the tattoo or scar. For instance, Q-switched lasers are increasingly being sought after for their ability to effectively shatter ink particles in the process of tattoo removal, allowing for improved clearance through the immune system. Studies indicate that multicolored tattoos are particularly challenging, with a propensity to take several sessions for optimal results. Furthermore, patient-specific factors , such as skin type, tattoo depth, and color of ink may significantly influence outcomes. Practitioners are now integrating various laser technologies in order to achieve maximum personalized treatment efficacy and minimize side effects, foreseeing an upcoming trend in individualized treatment regimens. This technical adjustment in the area of lasers is symptomatic of an even broader knowledge of laser interactions with dermatological conditions, leading to greater success rates in tattoo removal and scar management. In keloid and hypertrophic scarring, as well as in scar management generally, laser treatment has emerged as the treatment of choice. Evidence suggests that if laser treatments are combined with adjunct therapies , such as corticosteroid injections, the success rate improves noticeably. In a systematic review, not only was the size and color of scars lessened with laser therapy, but also patient satisfaction with the aesthetic outcome. Also, when lasers are used with silicone gel or sheeting, which has been an established first-line therapy for keloids, the action becomes more pronounced. Such multimodal treatment underscores the need for clinicians to employ holistic methods that not only treat the cosmetic appearance of scars but also the underlying physiological mechanisms that result in their formation (Laura et al., 2023). Moreover, the advancements in imaging technologies and treatment protocols are moving towards imaging technologies becoming more integrated in the management of chronic wounds, which can include scarring from injuries or surgery. Chronic non-healing wounds are a certain types that require special care, and the use of wound monitoring devices in laser treatment protocols has been promising in enhancing recovery. These devices can offer physiological monitoring and diagnostic capabilities that can have the potential to increase chronic disease treatment adherence and success rates for patients. By monitoring key biomarkers and permitting real-time adjustment of the treatment protocol, laser therapy success rates are being positively affected. As is testified in recent studies, with laser therapy being used alongside new technologies to treat wounds, more effective therapy of chronic scars and tattoos is forecasted, demonstrating a shifting paradigm in dermatological treatments (Matthew et al., 2018) (Figure 11.6).

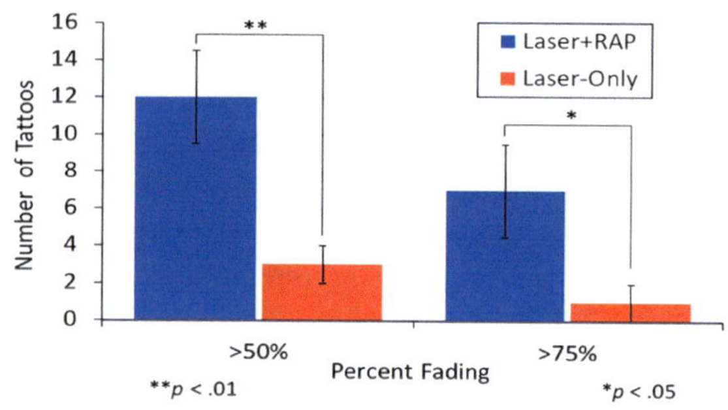

Figure 11.6. Tattoo fading distribution at 12 weeks post-treatment in a single office laser tattoo removal session. Tattoos treated with Laser + RAP achieved higher percentages of fading than Laser Only treated tattoos. RAP (Rapid Acoustic Pulse).

Source: https://www.researchgate.net/profile/David-Robertson-10/publication/335940819/figure/fig9/AS:805214445654030@1568989492852/Tattoo-fading-distribution-at-12-weeks-post-treatment-in-a-single-office-laser-tattoo.png.

11.2.2. Comparison of Surgical vs. Non-Surgical Methods

The decision to pursue tattoo removal is typically based on the available procedures, most of which are separated into surgical and non-surgical processes. Surgical processes , such as excision, involve the actual removal of the skin upon which the tattoos were done and directly provides an immediate effect. The process, however, leaves one with heavy scarring and requires careful evaluation of the healing of the removed sections. In addition, patient experience is important, since results are mostly subject to the surgeon's ability and the body's healing process. For the others opting for a more sophisticated way of doing things, technology has given rise to non-surgical means, the most common being laser therapy. Laser treatments use special wavelengths to disintegrate ink pigments, providing a less aggressive option. While laser treatment is less likely to leave scars than surgery, it involves more sessions and may not totally get rid of all of the colors, particularly tough hues , such as green or blue, so the removal is even harder. In considering the effectiveness of non-surgical methods, the new technology that could enhance the results of standard laser therapy must be taken into consideration. Current findings show that the combination of laser treatments with other modalities, , such as pulsed high intensity laser (PHIL) and pulsed high intensity focused ultrasound (PHIFU), may well yield great results in both tattoo removal and scar management. These surgery-free procedures are achieved through the application of stress waves that break down scar tissue without damaging the outer skin layer, thereby inducing a more favorable healing environment for the patient. Through the integration of these techniques into the tattoo elimination regimen, clinicians can presumably reduce the sessions required for effective ink removal without compromising on formation of new scars. This new approach demonstrates the adaptability of non-surgical technology in solving the complexities of tattoo elimination and scar treatment, paving the way for more efficient and safer patient outcomes (Hazlewood et al., 2019). Both surgical and non-surgical methods have their pros and cons, so a customized approach to tattoo removal is based on personal circumstances and desired outcome. Surgical interventions tend to be rapid and decisive in impact; the risk of scarring is an issue for all, however. Non-surgical treatment, less intrusive in most instances, also has its drawbacks, , such as longer treatment time and degrees of success. Of relevance is that practitioners must take into consideration patient tattoo history, type of skin, and personal preference when recommending a treatment regimen. The healthcare system is shifting toward a full understanding of patient care, whereby the integration of high-tech technological solutions, patient education, and tailored treatment plans works synergistically to enhance satisfaction and results in the field of tattoo removal and scar management (Carneiro, 2023) (Figure 11.7).

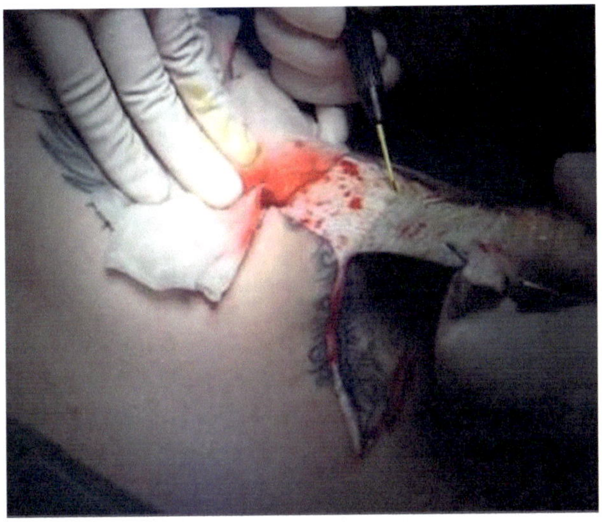

Figure 11.7. Surgical excision of skin for tattoo removal.

Source: https://www.researchgate.net/profile/Gary-Ordog/publication/372683280/figure/fig3/AS:11431281177486916@1690511009795/TATTOO-MEDICINE-PART-C-https-youtube-oCM-qmOTctE-Surgical-excision-of-skin-tattoo.png.

11.2.3. Factors Influencing Removal Effectiveness

Tattoo removal efficacy is determined by a variety of factors that can dramatically change outcomes for patients. In this regard, the composition of the ink in the tattoo is an important consideration. The composition of ink can influence the inks persistence in the skin and how it will respond to removal procedures, like laser therapy. For instance, black and other darker inks take more of the laser light than light ink shades, and hence several sessions might be required to erase them entirely. Moreover, how deeply embedded in the dermal layer the tattoo ink is decides how readily it can be targeted and dissolved by removal procedures. Clinical experience shows that increased ink pigmentation generally translates to an increased likelihood of residual tattoo marks, which are hard to remove and necessitate a particular form of treatment that considers these inherent variations like the ink. Patient-related variables are also at the center of the prediction of the success of tattoo removal treatments. Skin care differences in terms of thickness and pigmentation can influence the healing cycle as well as the efficiency of treatments. Certain patients with dark skin, for instance, can experience post-inflammatory hyperpigmentation (PIH) after laser treatment, which would camouflage the success of elimination treatments. All this is further compounded by personal healing capabilities, which also differ according to genetic constitutions and overall health. Moreover, lifestyle factors , such as sun exposure and smoking can have detrimental effects on skin regeneration and healing, leading to reduced efficacy in removal treatments. Tailoring treatment plans to include consideration of these patient-specific variables is essential to optimize results and prevent undesirable side effects, as evidenced by post-procedure recovery and satisfaction. Lastly, the tattoo removal method used may have significant influences on efficacy and patient satisfaction. Techniques , such as Q-switched lasers offer precision in the targeting of ink particles with minimal tissue destruction, enabling quicker healing and potentially better esthetic outcomes. Practitioner experience and expertise are also critical to successful outcomes. Practitioners applying careful planning and patient education on results to be expected and aftercare can ensure optimum patient satisfaction and reduce incidences of complications. Here, application of adjunct treatments , such as those that have been discussed in post-tattoo removal scar studies is very useful to improve significantly the treatment of any blemishes that ensue, thereby guaranteeing maximum success and satisfaction throughout the process of tattoo removal (Ahmed et al., 2022; Bogachev et al., 2023) (Figure 11.8).

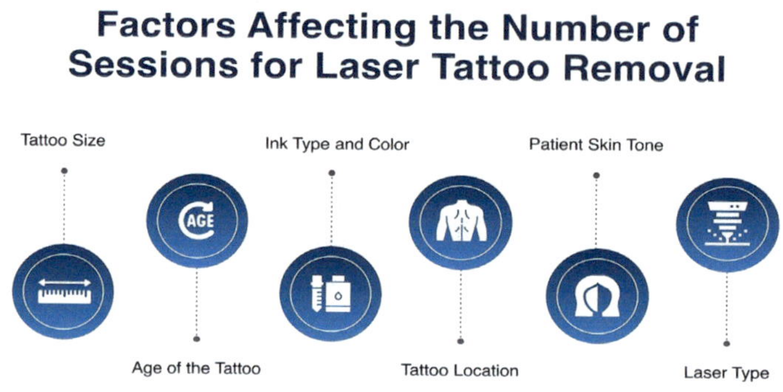

Figure 11.8. Factors affecting the number of sessions for laser tattoo removal.

Source: https://clearstonespa.com/wp-content/uploads/2024/11/image-6-1024x576.jpeg.

Test Your Knowledge

1. How effective have laser treatments been in fully or partially removing tattoos?
2. How would you compare the results, recovery time, and risks of surgical excision versus non-surgical methods like laser treatment or dermabrasion?

11.3. Risks and Side Effects of Tattoo Removal

Learning Outcome

1. Measure pain and discomfort during tattoo removal procedures
2. Understand potential for infection
3. Focus on long-term skin changes and complications

The process of tattoo removal has also grown extremely common with individuals wishing to erase or reshape their body tattoos. However, the risks and effects of such procedures are enough to warrant serious consideration. The risk of skin complications from various methods of removal, primarily laser procedures, is one , such aspect. While advanced Q-switched lasers have made the process of removal both effective and safe, they also have their share of ill effects. Studies indicate that 5–15% of the patients may develop disorders of pigmentation after laser treatment, which is defined as discoloration or darkening of tissue surrounding the treated area (Căiță et al., 2024). Additionally, improper application of laser parameters can aggravate them, leading to a permanent change in skin texture and color. Hence, awareness about the complications is essential for patients seeking tattoo removal. Apart from skin pigmentation changes, the removal of tattoos also results in infections and allergic reactions. Similar to the risks of initial tattooing, removal involves piercing of the skin surface, which could result in bacterial or other pathogen-induced infections (Cooper et al., 2023). Bacterial infection is typically temporary, but could progress to a chronic process if left untreated. Also, there are individuals who may experience allergies to the inks or the skin effects of the lasers, which can have symptoms , such as rashes or inflammation. Notably, a systematic review of tattooing and removal-related complications highlights the significance of diligent post-procedure care and monitoring in order to combat such complications and facilitate appropriate healing (Cooper et al., 2023). Individuals considering removal against their will to be free of tattoos must balance this against the risk of such complications. Lastly, the psychological effect of removal cannot be discounted, since removal can provoke intense emotional responses. Fear of pain associated with removal procedures, in addition to fears of such visible side effects as scarring, can result in fear in patients. The psychological burden of dealing with ugly scars can be staggering; while some will heal optimally, others will be left with external evidence of the removal, creating an additional burden to their body image (Căiță et al., 2024). The prevention of these scars is crucial, as this has been shown to affect the overall satisfaction with the removal procedure. To these facts, prospective patients can be instructed not only of immediate physical risk but also of psychological consequences that can arise after removal. Detailed counseling with trained staff can provide a route to informed decision and proper expectations regarding outcomes of the removal and potential scar management strategies.

11.3.1. Pain and Discomfort During Procedures

The sensation of pain and discomfort following tattoo removal procedures is a significant concern that should be addressed to promote patient comfort as well as satisfaction. The most widely applied technique in the removal of tattoos, Q-switched laser technology, has been determined to produce excellent results but comes with issues. Patients often complain that they feel as though they have been snapped with a rubber band or that they have a burning sensation in the treated area. They can create so much anxiety and discomfort that they are discouraged from having it removed, although they wish to have it removed. As per numerous studies, pain management techniques should be included in the treatment process to reduce these uncomfortable feelings and provide a better patient experience during such treatments (Căiță et al., 2024).

By managing pain through the use of topical anesthetics or injectable lidocaine, health professionals can make the environment for patients getting their tattoos removed more bearable. Furthermore, one cannot overlook the psychological considerations involved in pain perception in tattoo removal. Patients have been found to experience pain more harshly when they are not prepared well enough for the procedure or when they are deprived of adequate support from medical professionals.

This is why patient education and thorough pre-procedure consultation are very important. Through the education of patients about what to expect in terms of discomfort, anticipated side effects, and the duration of the procedure, medical personnel can alleviate anxiety and promote a feeling of calmness. These preparatory steps support patients' emotions and develop a sense of trust, therefore decreasing pain perception (Ansari et al., 2024). The role of psychological preparation in influencing pain experiences underscores the necessity for practitioners to adopt a holistic approach that incorporates physical and emotional therapy throughout the course of tattoo removal treatment. Aside from acute pain, the importance of pain during tattoo removal is also extensible to long-term management of scarring and overall patient outcomes.

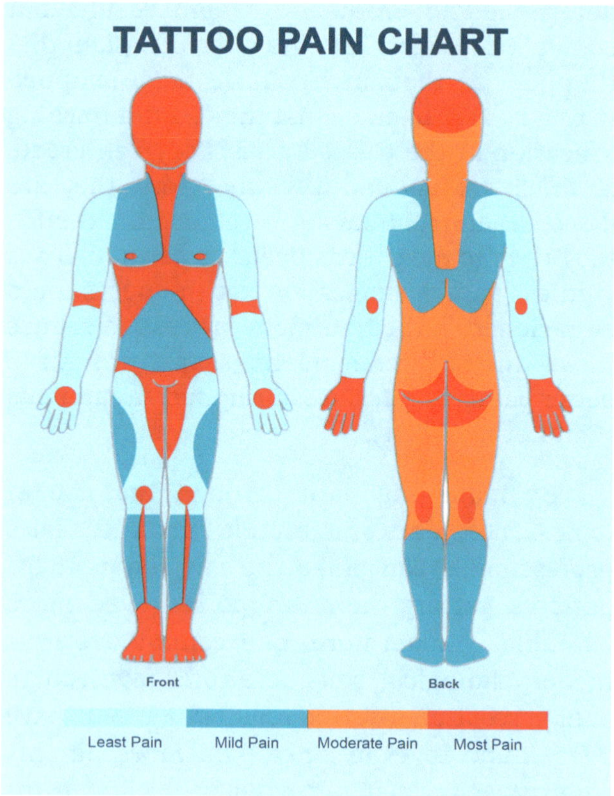

Figure 11.9. Tattoo removal pain chart.

Source: https://tatt2away.com/wp-content/uploads/2023/10/TATTOO-PAIN-CHART-Updated-800x1067.png.

The success of the Q-switched laser method relies not only on tattoo ink but also on adequate pain control during the process. Inadequate pain control can lead to increased muscle tension and stress reactions in patients, which can affect the healing process and the texture of scars. Chronic pain can create a negative feedback loop whereby patients will avoid completing the removal process, creating incomplete removal and thus suboptimal aesthetic results. Therefore, recognizing the significance of pain management during the removal process is crucial, as its impact directly relates to patient compliance and satisfaction, ultimately influencing scar management and overall success of the tattoo removal process (Căiță et al., 2024). Well-managed pain reduction techniques can significantly improve patient outcomes and create a less painful experience during and after tattoo removal (Figure 11.9).

11.3.2. Potential for Infection

Infection potential is still a significant concern in tattooing and removal, as both entail piercing the skin, which creates an opening for disease-causing agents. Bacterial and viral infections may occur if sterilization protocols are not strictly adhered to, thereby necessitating stringent hygiene standards in tattooing parlors. It is evidenced in research that short-term complications, including infection, occur days to weeks following the procedure, having a tendency to complicate the recovery process of the patients and necessitating medical intervention.

The Council of Europe has addressed the overriding necessity of safety standards in tattoo and removal procedures, advocating for improved legislation and best practice that minimizes the risk of infection (Căiță et al., 2024). Thus, awareness of the variables influencing infection prevalence is pivotal in guiding practitioners and clients about the inherent risk of tattooing. Q-switched laser removal of tattoos has been hailed as the best available, though risky. The technique may lead to complications like infection of the skin if done under relaxed conditions. Specifically, studies show that complications may occur due to improper laser parameters or lack of proper aftercare, jeopardizing the healing of the skin and potentially causing infection (Cooper et al., 2023). In spite of advancements in technology towards successful removal, the reported incidence of complications in terms of pigmentation disorder due to laser treatment has raised safety issues over the process of removal in general. With growing awareness about these risks, clients and practitioners both need to give greater importance to enhanced education in infection prevention practices and aftercare practices following tattoo removals. Public awareness of the risks associated with tattooing and removal processes is also a considerable factor influencing infection rates.

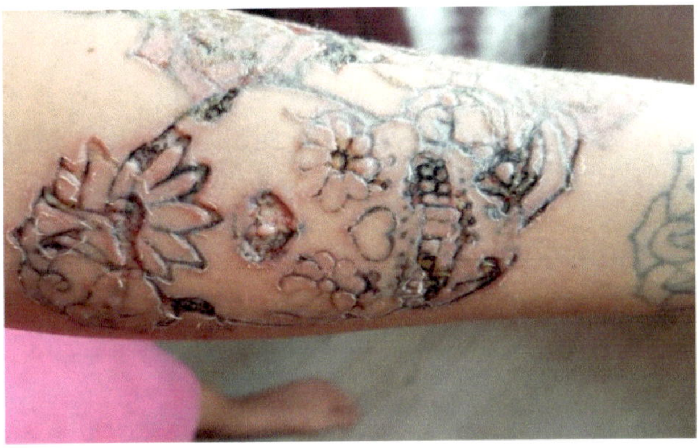

Figure 11.10. Infected tattoo after removal.

Source: https://www.reddit.com/media?url=https%3A%2F%2Fi.redd.it%2F82cu5r8k8nf81.jpg.

Research has shown that the majority of individuals may lack extensive information on possible health hazards but rely on anecdotal evidence from friends or news media rather than expert advice (Căiță et al., 2024). Interestingly, the industry has come to understand the importance of large-scale education campaigns promoting hygiene manners and risk awareness. Such programs will teach users safe practices, appropriate aftercare, as well as signs of infection that need medical attention. Addressing the knowledge gap and safety culture can greatly reduce the occurrence of tattoo and removal-related infections, enhancing patient outcomes in both environments (Cooper et al., 2023) (Figure 11.10).

11.3.3. Long-Term Skin Changes and Complications

The selection of tattoo designs and inks has grown significantly in popularity, especially among young communities, which causes several significant long-term skin changes. While individuals seek out permanent body marks, health complications with tattoos also increase. Individuals receiving tattoos usually experience immediate reactions during the healing process; however, adverse effects can happen much later than initial utilization.

Late allergic reactions and chronic inflammatory dermatoses can occur years later, complicating diagnosis and control of complications from tattoos. The risk of bacterial infections that has been estimated to be as high as 5% once more emphasizes the importance of careful observation of tattooing and removal procedures to minimize long-term skin damage (Căiță et al., 2024). With the rising prevalence of tattoo removal procedures, particularly with the newer Q-switched laser technology, the risk of long-term skin complications is an area of high concern. While efficacy and safety have been upgraded through advancements, hyper- or hypopigmentation can still occur in 5–15% of the patients undergoing treatment with these lasers (Căiță et al., 2024).

The effectiveness of such removal techniques also fluctuates according to skin type, color of the ink, and treatment variables, which must be properly adjusted to prevent unwanted side effects. Moreover, the complex mechanism of healing of the skin may trigger undesirable textural changes, thus impacting the aesthetic and functional properties of the skin. It becomes indispensable that patients who are seeking tattoo removal are informed of such potential long-term consequences. In addition, the phenomenon of tattoo regret is a new cultural nuance to body art that necessitates an exact examination of the long-term effects of tattoo permanence. Most individuals indicate they try to have them eliminated due to dissatisfaction with their tattoos, particularly those who had them as adolescents, which become regrets over time. The psychosocial component of tattoo regret includes not only dissatisfaction with aesthetic outcomes but also the effect of public opinion and shifting personal identities. This mutual makeup of tattoo regret indicates that thoughtful deliberation before inking and after-removal therapy are essential in treating skin and emotional consequences. Hence, augmenting awareness regarding the potential long-term changes associated with tattoo removal can equip a person to navigate choices with greater information and caution (Figure 11.11).

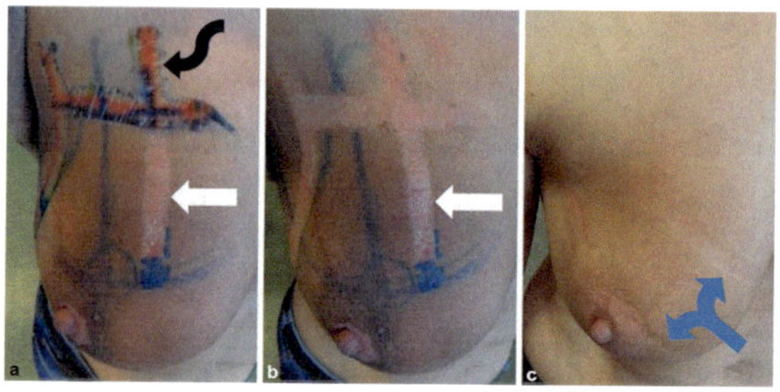

Figure 11.11. (a, b) Skin under the stripes upon removed on the final day of treatment. Black curved arrow polyurethane film stripe, white standard arrows skin beneath the stripes immediately after removal. (c) Homogeneous hyperpigmentation almost 10 weeks after completion of treatment. Blue double-arrow marks of the brassiere, revealing mild edema after radiotherapy.

Source: https://www.researchgate.net/publication/374230868/figure/fig1/AS:11431281219527141@1706064664673/a-bSkin-under-the-stripes-upon-removal-on-the-final-day-of-treatment-Black-curved.png.

Test Your Knowledge

1. How would you rate the level of pain or discomfort experienced during the tattoo removal process compared to when the tattoo was originally applied?
2. Have you noticed any lasting changes to your skin after tattoo removal?

11.4. Scar Formation and Management

Learning Outcome

1. Explain the types of scars resulting from tattoo removal
2. Describe factors affecting scar healing
3. Deal with treatments for scar management

Formation of scars is a multifaceted biological process that could be a consequence of multiple factors of injury to the skin, including those caused by tattoos. When the skin is damaged, the body's reaction includes an inflammatory, proliferative, and remodeling phase of healing. The severity of every scar type, whether hypertrophic, keloid, or atrophic, is largely dependent on individual genetic profile, tension of the skin, and the severity of the initial injury. The relationship between variables dictates the maturation and growth of the scar with time. It is vital to know about the nature of scar development, particularly in relation to tattoo removal and post-skin care, since this will significantly influence therapeutic outcomes as well as potential for scarring in individuals seeking removal of unsightly tattoos from the skin (Bennardo et al., 2022). Optimal management of scarring is required to achieve maximum cosmetic results from tattoo removal because scarring risk is a significant concern for all patients. Many different treatments are used to reduce the appearance of scarring, ranging from topical therapy to advanced laser therapy. Amongst the latter, use of the Q-Switched Nd:YAG laser with a fractionated beam pattern has proven to be promising for scar treatment, particularly in ethnic populations that may be prone to special healing challenges. Clinical studies demonstrate how this laser modality can significantly improve the cosmetic appearance of scars with minimal side effects described, , such as transient erythema (Bennardo et al., 2022). All this creativity with scar therapy also goes hand in hand with the achievement of individualized and effective solutions for addressing the aftermath of tattoos and indeed other types of dermal injury. As technology and science continue to advance, the availability of preventative measures in addition to therapeutic ones is a more holistic approach to managing scars. Preventative interventions include good wound care during healing, minimizing sun exposure, and silicone-based products in managing the development of a scar before it occurs. Besides, recent studies emphasize the recognition of scar pathology as a rationale to select treatment based on the specific needs of each patient. By acknowledging the multifactorial nature of scarring and integrating newer treatment modalities, health care providers can enhance quality of life and patient satisfaction following tattoo removal. Ultimately, a comprehensive approach that considers the complexity associated with the process of scarring and the treatment will lead to better outcomes for those who desire tattoo removal (Adamiec et al., 2024).

11.4.1. Types of Scars Resulting from Tattoo Removal

The process of tattoo removal, while often performed for various personal or professional reasons, can leave a variety of various scars based on the approach taken, skin type of the patient, and the healing process in general. More traditional forms of tattoo removal, , such as excision and dermabrasion, tend to leave more scarring because they are more invasive techniques. On the other hand, modern laser technology, for example, that by Q-switched lasers, offers higher accuracy and fewer chances of scarring. However, even by the latest technology, patients may still develop unwanted effects like PIH or scarring, particularly in individuals with darker skin. Specific data reveal that side effects from laser removal can be seen in up to 15% of patients, suggesting careful consideration of the removal procedure and post-removal measures for scar management (Căiță et al., 2024). Of the scars seen following tattoo removal, atrophic scars are most common, as evidenced by a depressed appearance resulting from collagen depletion within the skin. These are scars that may occur following improper healing or excessive damage in laser treatments. Hypertrophic, or thickened and raised, scars may also occur and are usually seen with the formation of keloids in predisposed patients.

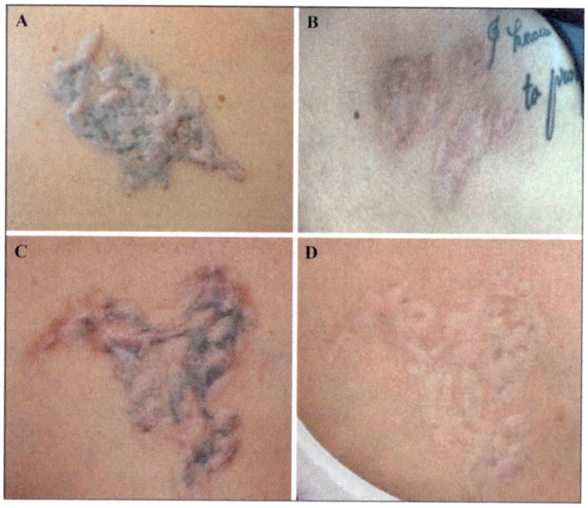

Figure 11.12. Scarring induced by chemical tattoo removal. (A) Hypertrophic scar; (B) Atrophic scar; (C) Hypertrophic scar with remnants of pigment; and before laser treatment; (D) Same scar as in (C) after two sessions of fractional ablative laser and Q-switched 1064-nm laser.

Source: https://www.researchgate.net/profile/Thierry-Passeron/publication/358672346/figure/fig1/AS:11431281091782264@1666613783644/Scarring-induced-by-chemical-tattoo-removal-A-Hypertrophic-scar-B-Atrophic-scar-C.png.

Research has shown that Asian patients, especially Fitzpatrick skin types III and IV, require personalized treatment approaches, e.g., the use of fractional Q-switched Nd:YAG lasers, which are reported to reduce scar development at the expense of effective removal (Bennardo et al., 2022). Knowledge of the special types of scars that are prone to develop is important for practitioners because it assists in the identification of treatment procedures and anticipates the potential of complications in healing. Post-removal scar care is very critical in optimizing the cosmetic outcome for those who wish to remove their tattoos. The patients are typically advised to follow some post-treatment care practices to minimize scarring, , such as keeping the area well moisturized and protected from the sun. In addition, modalities , such as silicone gel sheets, pressure dressings, and laser scar treatments can be useful during the healing process. An ongoing dialogue between patients and dermatological professionals on potential risks and preventive measures is paramount to optimal scar management. Generally, the identification of the types of scars that can result from the removal of tattoos not only directs treatment but also optimizes the chances of favorable healing results, positively contributing to the patient's overall well-being (Căiță et al., 2024) (Figure 11.12).

11.4.2. Factors Affecting Scar Healing

Scar tissue healing is a multifaceted process influenced by numerous variables, including genetic disposition, age, and prior medical conditions. Genetic disposition is a major factor in the formation of abnormal scars , such as keloids and hypertrophic scars, which form due to defective healing processes. Formation of the scars may be enhanced in individuals with such disorders running in their families, as genetic factors influence collagen formation and skin elasticity. Age also plays a role in healing scars since younger individuals will typically have better healing reactions due to improved collagen production and skin regeneration capacity. Medical conditions like diabetes or autoimmune disease can also interfere with scar healing since they may impair circulation and disrupt inflammatory response, making recovery even more problematic. Understanding these fundamental factors is crucial to the creation of effective scar management methods after tattoo removal treatments in order to obtain optimal healing outcomes for patients. Environmental aspects play a significant part in the process of healing scars, particularly after tattoo removal. Subjecting the area of healing to irritants, humidity, or excessive sunlight may lead to detrimental healing outcomes. Ultraviolet (UV) light is particularly deleterious because it can cause further damage to the skin and exacerbate pigmentation issues in healing scars. Moreover, the application of occlusive dressings might support a wet environment for healing, but their improper application might also result in infection, slowing healing. Psychological problems, including stress and anxiety, also hinder wound healing, as these can lead to disrupted hormonal balances and immunological reactions. Therefore, informing patients regarding environmental avoidance therapies and psychosocial measures of support is essential to enhance scar healing after tattoo removal. Treatment interventions are revealed to have a considerable effect on outcomes in scarring healing, with a tendency to necessitate a multimodal treatment approach. Combination therapies are evident from the literature as being effective, with the inclusion of pharmacologic and physical modalities. Medical treatments of silicone gel sheeting, laser, and corticosteroid injection are usually applied to minimize elevated scar formation by addressing varied physiological processes that play a role in scar formation. Pharmacological treatment, particularly for disorders , such as keloids and hypertrophic scars, may be mono- or combination therapy to provide the best result. Individualized treatment plans based on the patient's specific scar behavior and healing response are essential to enhance quality of life. As scar pathology evolves, continuous exploration of new treatments will become more and more responsible for directing the best practice in treating scarring, ultimately leading to improved patient outcomes from tattoo removal procedures (Ebrahimnejad et al., 2024; Murakami et al., 2024).

11.4.3. Treatments for Scar Management

Scar management is still a significant problem in medical and cosmetic environments, particularly following procedures , such as tattoo removal. Various treatment modalities have been created to address the diversity of scars, ranging from hypertrophic to atrophic in orientation. Among the most popular treatment modalities are topically applied treatments, including silicone sheets and gels, which have been discovered to flatten and soften scars by creating a barrier that maintains moisture. Furthermore, corticosteroid injections can reduce inflammation and minimize elevated scars, thereby producing symptomatic and cosmetic improvement. The optimal therapy often becomes evident depending on the site, type, and age of the scars, necessitating individualized treatment for optimal outcome. Of note is that understanding of the biologic mechanisms of scar development will direct treatment planning to permit selective application of those maneuvers that will promote healing while restricting aesthetic compromise. More intense scar treatment methods include more invasive treatments , such as laser treatments and chemical peels. Laser treatments, particularly fractional laser resurfacing, treat the deeper layers of the skin, making it possible to remodel collagen and have less tissue damage to the surrounding areas. It can greatly improve the texture and appearance of scars and is widely used as a treatment for post-tattoo removal procedures. Chemical peels, on the other hand, use acids to strip the outermost layers of skin, enhance cellular turnover, and promote healthy, unharmed growth of skin. Selection of a specific laser or chemical agent is often associated with the nature of the scars, professional ratings, and patient expectations. As these technologies continue to progress, there remains a need for ongoing research and clinical trials to determine best practices and enhance techniques, ultimately leading to more effective strategies for scar management in populations. Additionally, emerging therapies , such as microneedling and the application of platelet-rich plasma (PRP) are increasingly being debated in scar treatment. Microneedling involves the use of tiny needles to create micro-wounds in the skin, which triggers the body's healing process and stimulates collagen production. This treatment not only improves the scar but also the texture and tightness of the skin in general. Meanwhile, PRP therapy leverages the body's own growth factors to promote healing processes, providing a biological boost to mending damaged tissues. Research has yielded positive results with such techniques, particularly when it is combined with traditional therapies. The combination of various modalities functions to develop an integrative method of scar management that ultimately leads to an improvement in cosmetic results for individuals undergoing tattoo removal and other skin treatments (Baumgartner et al., 2020; Kaltenbach et al., 2020) (Figure 11.13).

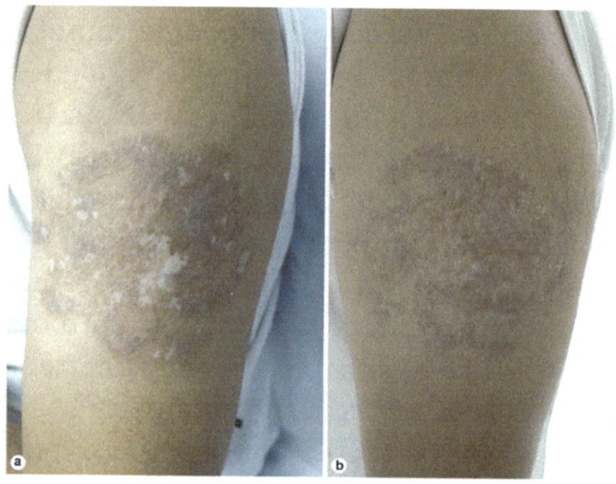

Figure 11.13. Achromic laser tattoo scars. A baseline achromic scars in the left deltoid region after 18 laser tattoo removal treatment sessions.

Source: https://www.researchgate.net/publication/333335396/figure/fig1/AS:761898052096001@1558662059396/Achromic-laser-tattoo-scars-a-Baseline-achromic-scars-in-left-deltoid-region-after-18.png.

Test Your Knowledge

1. How common is scarring from tattoo removal?
2. What are treatments for scar management?

11.5. Psychological Impact of Tattoo Removal

Learning Outcome

1. Understand emotional responses to tattoo removal
2. Focus on body image and self-esteem considerations
3. Describe support systems and counseling options for individuals seeking tattoo removal and scar management

The psychological impact of tattoo removal is often profound, a complex dynamic of self, identity, and anguish. A high proportion of participants who seek the procedure have reported regret associated with their tattoos, particularly those acquired in early adulthood. As observed in studies, such regret usually stems from the cumulative effects of several factors, , such as changes to individual lives or beauty ideals, which do not align with the initial motive for tattooing (Carneiro, 2023). This state of cognitive dissonance between present identity and the permanence of the marking can cause immense emotional anguish, leading individuals to pursue removal as a means of regaining control over their body and to create a new self. Thus, the psychological process of tattoo removal is not merely a response to remorse but a significant step toward self-coherence and psychological well-being. In addition to this, the process of removal has its psychological issues, which provide a layer to the emotional process. Although laser treatment is a common method of removal, it is susceptible to defects and requires multiple visits, which can prolong the misery of the tattoo. Research has discovered that physical pain resulting from the procedure can also enhance feelings of regret and anxiety, so a self-reinforcing cycle can ensue in which distress heightens pain (Carneiro, 2023). Fear of pain and uncertainty of outcome can increase anxiety, thus making it even more challenging to choose to remove a tattoo. Thus, the medical professionals must remain cognizant of these psychological nuances, administering overall care as well as the medical treatments to combat these unwanted effects. Finally, successful removal of tattoos can have positive psychological outcomes by significantly boosting an individual's self-esteem and psychological health. Once they have undergone the removal process, most individuals have reported feeling a heavy sense of liberation and relief as they no longer carry the unwanted tattoo around with them. The elimination of the tattoo generally enables individuals to regain their identity and better reflect their new values and experiences in life (Esparza et al., 2020). Moreover, participants undergoing successful elimination are usually observed to be reporting a higher degree of body and choice control, resulting in higher self-esteem. These, thus, are the psychological ramifications of tattoo removal that transcend aesthetics and could play a decisive role in one's quest for acceptance and emotional stability. The multifaceted psychological landscape raises the call to integrate mental health concerns into the process of removing tattoos, giving one sufficient provision in the process.

11.5.1. Emotional Responses to Tattoo Removal

The emotional climate of tattoo removal is often complex and multifactorial. Removal seekers are individuals with a strong, usually remorseful feeling regarding their tattoos, particularly those obtained in more irresponsible and less mature phases of life. Remorse is usually caused by many factors like personality growth, relationship changes, or identity shift and the quest for physical congruence in accordance with current life circumstances. The findings of the most current studies highlight that the emotional suffering of tattoo regret is not merely about looks; it is also about feelings of vulnerability and betrayal as they struggle with the consequences of their past actions (Esparza et al., 2020). Thus, the individuals who undergo tattoo removal report a range of emotions ranging from fear for the removal surgery itself to a general need to have their bodies and themselves back. In addition, the psychological weight attached to removing tattoos can present in a very real manner. Numerous people feel embarrassed or shamed by their tattoos, an outcome compounded further by the way that people view those who are tattooed. This outside judgment can be part of why someone will get their tattoos removed, a factor showing how social stigma can play a role in one's decisions.

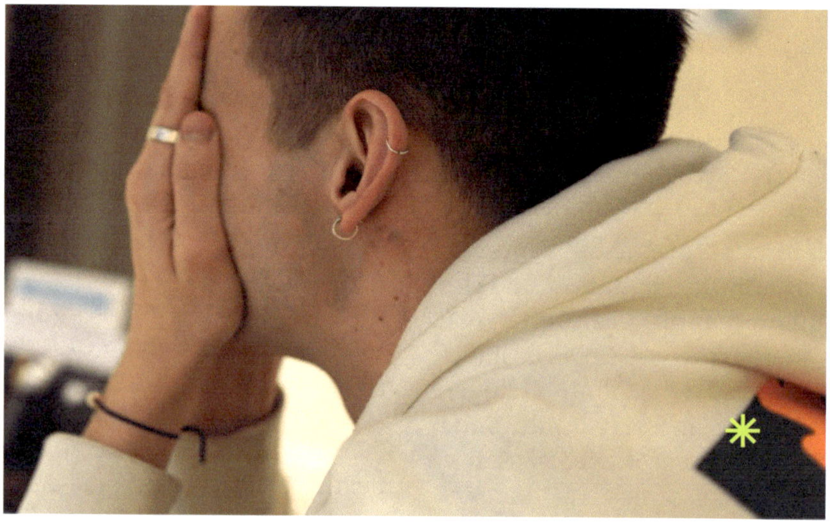

Figure 11.14. A person experiences discomfort, possibly related to tattoo removal.

Source: https://cdn.prod.website-files.com/61dedc5b29acbd6f8e108582/669ac8b69321e212d26f375a_Feeling%20Sick%20Tattoo%20Removal.png.

As the subjects have their tattoos removed, they will often wrestle with anticipating pain and the mental weight of dealing with what they regret, complicating their experiences along the way (Arora et al., 2018). Resolving these emotional responses is crucial since they play a key role in influencing the individual's overall satisfaction with the removal process and subsequent scar care. The psycho-emotional impacts of tattoo removal extend past the removal process. Individuals tend to go through numerous emotional responses to their journey towards healing. The instant gratification of physical discomfort during the laser removal process may be followed by distress and anxiety, but it will also evoke feelings of empowerment as they regain control over the story of their body. Effective removal can result in emotional liberation; yet, it might also introduce ongoing self-reflection about decisions in the past and their meaning (Esparza et al., 2020). In addition, closure might be pursued as individuals incorporate these experiences into their developing identities. In general, the emotional responses to tattoo removal constitute a spectrum of responses varying from regret and embarrassment to relief and empowerment, pointing to the relevance of these processes in the broader scar management context (Figure 11.14).

11.5.2. Body Image and Self-Esteem Considerations

The relationship between self-esteem and body image becomes especially complicated when tattoo removal and scar management are in play. People normally want to change their body art, either for removal or modification, on the basis of something more than looks, , such as underlying psychological motivations. For some, tattoos perhaps originally meant significant life stories or individual statements; however, with the passage of time and growing older, the significance attributed to them might also shift. This attitude shift will certainly result in regret, as seen in the widespread phenomenon of adults, around 19%, getting their tattoos removed once they realize that their tattoos no longer suit their new self-image or lifestyle (Carneiro, 2023). This conflict between one's internal self and socially constructed self may be the origin of low self-esteem and feelings of inadequacy, so that interventions are not only physical but also those that expand psychological health. Tattoos can be an expression of more abstract body image and self-esteem influences from society through the process of peer disapproval, cultural messages, and alteration of personal identity. Tattooed individuals are socially stigmatized, and thus, there is elevated distress towards body modification. Tattoo adversity experiences , such as regret and health problems, demonstrate the need for interventions for psychological distress caused by tattoos (Esparza et al., 2020). The majority of individuals, especially those who acquired the tattoos during initial phases of life, may end up in incongruity between the older version of oneself and who one is now. This dissonance between body image has profound mental health implications, and therefore, it is imperative to create body image safe spaces. Finally, handling body image with informed decision-making interventions, tattoo removal interventions, and self-compassion interventions can culminate in high levels of positive self-esteem and self-acceptance. Further, processes for tattoo removal and scar revision must not only be clinically efficient, but should also consider the emotional context of patients seeking to remove or alter their tattoos. The advancements in technology with lasers, promising as they are on a clinical level, must also factor in the psychology of the procedure. Those looking to get tattoos removed also suffer from emotional distress in regards to their tattoos and recalling past choices (Carneiro, 2023). Scarring, the most probable outcome of tattoo removal, also renders body image challenging, perhaps leading to loss and inadequacy. Thus, mental health practitioners and dermatologists must work together, with services delivered taking into account the overall nature of body modification in terms of the extreme impact body image assumptions have on society and the part played by individual self-esteem in the development of personal satisfaction. By ensuring an integrated approach to treatment, the practitioners can enhance the general experience for clients who are forced to deal with the problems involved in the removal of body art.

11.5.3. Support Systems and Counseling Options

Support systems are also a major player in the process of individuals seeking tattoo removal and scar treatment. Having suffered tattoo hardship, individuals are also likely to suffer from high psychological distress , such as regret and body dissatisfaction. These could be compounded by societal concerns as well as self-expectations. Good support systems, both family and friends and online support groups, are available to provide the emotional support needed for individuals to get through these kinds of problems. These systems allow for experience sharing, which can decrease feelings of loneliness and enhance emotional strength. The importance of peer support in this case cannot be overemphasized because it provides a feeling of belonging and empathy among participants with shared experiences of tattoo remorse and removal. In addition to casual support networks, there are also professional counseling services that have an important role to play in coping with the mental health issues that accompany tattoo removal. Experienced therapists and counselors who work with body image concerns can offer targeted interventions addressing the causes of tattoo regret. Narrative therapy and cognitive-behavioral therapy are two of the treatments used because these enable patients to reinterpret their experience and erase the distress of tattoos. Furthermore, art therapy is a very effective form of counseling that assists clients in expressing their feelings about their tattoos and the accompanying scars. Healing through art therapy heals and ensures personal development, where clients can gain a healthier relationship with their bodies. Pairing counseling with tattoo removal underscores the multidisciplinary care mode optimally applied to scar management. In addition, collaboration between personal choice and professional guidance is critical in refining the process of tattoo removal. When individuals attempt to remove tattoos, they will most likely be forced to deal with a complex of emotional reactions tied to historical decisions and contemporary identity. Leads professionals can empower clients by highlighting a compassionate approach that encourages self-discovery and recovery. Conditions , such as the development of sensory empathy, as used in art-based research, can encourage sensitivity to the feelings of self-cutting and tattoo removal. Emotional life therapy of tattoo remorse facilitates not just the accommodation of scar tissue but also the restoration of individual identity. This sort of holistic framework generates hope and encourages individuals to rediscover their body relationship, thus assisting them to heal and become self-accepting (Wyss, 2018; Esparza et al., 2020).

Test Your Knowledge

1. What emotions did you experience before, during, and after the tattoo removal process (e.g., relief, sadness, anxiety)?
2. How has removing your tattoo affected your body image or the way you feel about your appearance?

SUMMARY

As the consideration of scar treatment and tattoo removal winds down, the intersection of advancing medical technologies and effective treatment modalities certainly holds the greatest significance in improving patient care. The development of tattoo removal techniques has significantly lowered risks compared to traditional methods. This development has opened access to individuals who wish to eliminate unwanted ink, thereby enhancing physical appearance as well as psychological well-being. The employment of new technology, , such as laser treatment, also indicates increased understanding of the method towards cosmetic concern and the physiological impact of skin change. Awareness of and reaction to what scarring results from is also required. Awareness towards the multidisciplinary arena of tattoo removal and scar treatment will therefore become essential to provide integrative care. Of paramount importance is the value of tailored treatment protocols, particularly in the case of scar management after tattoo removal. Each patient's unique skin type, tattoo attributes, and healing patterns must be accounted for while formulating plans for best outcomes. The provision of individualized protocols makes it simpler to select appropriate technologies and methods, ranging from laser therapy to topical treatment. The integration of advanced monitoring systems, which were discussed in recent literature, enhances clinicians ability to assess healing of tattoo removal and respond appropriately to any complications during and following treatment. As observation technologies , such as the physiological monitoring methods highlighted in recent research increase widespread use, the quality of care provided to patients undergoing tattoos removed will significantly enhance. Finally, the future of scar management and tattoo removal depends on acting proactively by giving extreme importance to patient education and evidence-based practice. Accurate identification of concerns regarding risk of scarring and proper information concerning probable outcomes following removal allows for well-informed decision-making. In addition, accepting an array of treatment modalities, like lasers and non-surgical methodologies, allows practitioners to customize treatments in an effort to reduce side effects while maximizing aesthetic outcomes. New technologies, , such as the application of advanced lasers and wearable monitoring devices, promise to create safer and more effective models of treatment. Overall, establishing a culture of continued learning and adaptability in the industry will enable patients to receive the optimum care possible while they contend with the challenges of tattoo removal and scar management.

In analyzing the removal of tattoos, the necessity of learning about the several methods used and their level of effectiveness comes more into play. Most often used is the method of laser therapy, where powerful beams of light are used to break down fragments of ink in the skin. How effective the process is depends on the skill and experience of the practitioner, and therefore the need for precision when it comes to factors like laser distance and angle from skin. As mentioned, the majority who seek removal are driven by remorse, with approximately 19% of tattooed adults deciding on this option due to not enjoying their tattoos (Carneiro, 2023). Practitioners need to address such emotions because the emotional and psychological impact of tattoo regret can influence not only the removal process but also the patient experience. Due to advances in laser technology and alongside, there is a greater interest in applying AI in enhancing the process of tattoo removal. AI has been extremely promising in clinical use, especially in image processing and procedural accuracy. Applying algorithms to real-time tattoo segmenting, practitioners could theoretically optimize laser therapy by outlining the pathways of removal with pinpoint accuracy.

This kind of advance, and even improved patient outcomes, holds the promise of overall higher treatment safety and efficacy. The move towards AI solutions is only part of a broader trend in medicine, where technology incessantly attempts to plug the loopholes in the traditional methods, thereby bringing a more dynamic element into the process of scar healing and tattoo elimination (Carneiro, 2023). Furthermore, with scarring management becoming an important factor, knowledge of the healing process following tattoo elimination is of extreme significance. Scarring is a possible undesired side effect of tattoo removal, particularly laser treatments, causing inequalities in grades of skin damage. Worldwide means of scar management, including topical treatment and newer techniques , such as microneedling or laser resurfacing, leave patients with acceptable options for the return of the skin. These techniques can greatly improve aesthetic outcomes, thus eliminating after aftereffects of tattoo removal. Thus, the harmony of effective tattoo removal and expert scar management plays a vital role in the pursuit of optimal patient care through emphasis on a holistic approach involving removal and subsequent rehabilitation of the skin.

KEY TERMS FROM THIS CHAPTER

- Acne scars
- Body modification
- Chronic scars
- Congenital giant pigmented nevi (CGPN)
- Dermabrasion
- Dexpanthenol
- First-line therapy
- Health concerns
- Keloids
- Laser removal
- Allergic reactions
- Chemical peels
- Cognitive dissonance
- Cosmetic outcome
- Dermatological treatments
- Diagnostic capabilities
- Fitzpatrick skin types
- Inasmuch
- Laser parameters
- Mechanical disruption

CRITICAL THINKING QUESTIONS

1. **Which laser type is most commonly used for tattoo removal?**
   a. CO_2 laser
   b. Pulsed dye laser
   c. Q-switched Nd:YAG laser
   d. Alexandrite laser
2. **What is the primary mechanism of action in laser tattoo removal?**
   a. Thermal ablation
   b. Photochemical reaction
   c. Mechanical debridement
   d. Selective photothermolysis
3. **Which of the following is a common side effect of laser tattoo removal?**
   a. Acne
   b. Hyperpigmentation
   c. Psoriasis
   d. Rosacea
4. **What is the best initial approach to managing hypertrophic scars?**
   a. Surgical excision
   b. Silicone gel sheets or topical silicone
   c. Cryotherapy
   d. Intralesional steroids
5. **Which factor most significantly influences the success of tattoo removal?**
   a. Age of the tattoo
   b. Tattoo location
   c. Type of ink used
   d. Skin hydration level

Short Answer Questions

1. What are the most effective methods of tattoo removal available today?
2. How many sessions are typically required for complete tattoo removal, and what factors influence this?
3. Is tattoo removal painful, and what kind of aftercare is recommended post-treatment?
4. Are there any risks or side effects associated with tattoo removal procedures?
5. What types of scars can result from tattoo removal, and how common are they?
6. What are the best current treatments for managing or reducing scars after tattoo removal?
7. How soon after tattoo removal can scar treatment begin, and what are the best practices for prevention?
8. Can people with a history of keloid scarring safely undergo tattoo removal, and what precautions should they take?

Answer to Critical Thinking Questions

1.(c) 2.(d) 3.(b) 4.(b) 5.(a)

REFERENCES

1. Adamiec, D. K., Czach, M., Dąbrowska, A., et al. (2024). Scar formation, healing stages, and advanced treatment strategies–Review. https://core.ac.uk/download/620863277.pdf (accessed on 11th June 2025).
2. Ahmed, Y., Abd El Maksoud, W. M., & Sultan, M. H. (2022). A new oncoplastic technique for removal of centrally located malignant tumors and reconstruction by a local dermo-glandular flap in conservative breast surgery. *Breast Disease, 41*(1), 175–185. https://www.semanticscholar.org/paper/2902068732b5aaaeeb5dc1710b3ae8bf2c4db07c (accessed on 11th June 2025).
3. Al-Waiz, M. M., Alster, T. S., Batra, R. S., Bhalla, M., Bowes, L. E., Fife, D., Gailloud-Mathieu, M., et al. (2017). Lasers and ancillary treatments for scar management Part 2: Keloid, hypertrophic, pigmented and acne scars. https://core.ac.uk/download/187088394.pdf (accessed on 11th June 2025).
4. Ansari, A., Li, F. M., Nguyen, H. T., et al. (2024). Single-incision combined laparoscopic right hemicolectomy and cholecystectomy: A case report. https://core.ac.uk/download/652334170.pdf (accessed on 11th June 2025).
5. Arora, A. (2018). *Ink as Armor: An Examination into The Relationship Between Tattooing and The Ability to Cope with Negative Life Events*. https://core.ac.uk/download/217368298.pdf (accessed on 11th June 2025).
6. Baron, J. M., Gorski, J., Proksch, E., et al. (2020). Dex panthenol in wound healing after medical and cosmetic interventions (post procedure wound healing). https://core.ac.uk/download/358467328.pdf (accessed on 11th June 2025).
7. Baumgartner, H., De Backer, J., Babu-Narayan, S. V., Budts, W., Chessa, M., Diller, G. P., Lung, B., et al. (2020). 2020 ESC guidelines for the management of adult congenital heart disease. *European Heart Journal, 42*, 563–645. https://doi.org/10.1093/eurheartj/ehaa554 (accessed on 11th June 2025).
8. Bennardo, L., Cannarozzo, G., Fasano, G., Marigliano, M., Negosanti, F., Nistico, S. P., & Sannino, M. (2022). Fractional Q-switched 1064 nm laser for treatment of atrophic scars in Asian skin. https://core.ac.uk/download/592023342.pdf (accessed on 11th June 2025).
9. Bianchi, I., Contor, L., Pakalin, S., & Piccinini, P. (2015). Safety of tattoos and permanent make-up. *Adverse health effects and experience with the Council of Europe Resolution (2008)1*. https://core.ac.uk/download/81685083.pdf (accessed on 11th June 2025)
10. Bistarelli, S., Frassi, S., & Santini, F. (2025). Biometric standards survey. https://core.ac.uk/download/pdf/37832140.pdf (accessed on 11th June 2025).
11. Bogachev, V., Boldin, B., Alukhanyan, O. A., Turkin, P., & Lobanov, V. N. (2023). Hyperpigmentation after sclerotherapy: Modern possibilities for prevention and treatment. *Ambulatornaya khirurgiya = Ambulatory Surgery (Russia)*. https://www.semanticscholar.org/paper/1e4486537ac77a38cadfa0c9ff12866edb113b8a (accessed on 11th June 2025).
12. Brar, A., & Behera, U. C. (2025). Stuck in the posterior ocular coats! *Indian Journal of Ophthalmology–Case Reports*. https://www.semanticscholar.org/paper/a27cb5552551b2a42c592cf0e2acb634e85b7934 (accessed on 11th June 2025).

13. Brown, M. S., Ashley, B. K., & Koh, A. (2018). Wearable technology for chronic wound monitoring: Current dressings, advancements, and future prospects. *Frontiers in Bioengineering and Biotechnology, 6*. https://doi.org/10.3389/fbioe.2018.00047 (accessed on 11th June 2025).

14. Căiţă, G. A., Lascu, C. F., Bodog, F., Buhas, C., Voiţă-Mekereş, F., & Voiţă, G. F. (2024). Surgical scar management–an evaluation of surgical techniques. *Medicine and Pharmacy Reports, 97*, 149–153. https://www.semanticscholar.org/paper/41266ecdb5ae6fc9533958d92ab3ee9a1de51fcd (accessed on 11th June 2025).

15. Carneiro, J. C. R. (2023). Artificial intelligence for tattoo removal treatment planning. Dissertação de mestrado em Engenharia Eletrónica Industrial e Computadores Controlo, Automação e Robótica https://hdl.handle.net/1822/91424 (accessed on 11th June 2025).

16. Cooper, A., Csontos, J., Edwards, A., et al. (2023). A rapid review of physical health risks associated with special procedures (tattooing, body piercing, acupuncture, electrolysis). https://core.ac.uk/download/595560412.pdf (accessed on 11th June 2025).

17. Ebrahimnejad, N., Jaafar, D., & Goodarzi, H. (2024). The past, present, future: Pathophysiology, diagnosis, and treatment of human skin diseases. *Physiologic, 4*, 81–99. https://doi.org/10.3390/physiologia4010005 (accessed on 11th June 2025).

18. Esparza, L. R. (2020). *Tattoo Adversity, Regret, And Removal: Constructivist Grounded Theory*. https://core.ac.uk/download/327191839.pdf (accessed on 11th June 2025).

19. Hazlewood, D. M. (2019). *Therapeutic Applications for Pulsed Laser and Ultrasound*. https://core.ac.uk/download/250306578.pdf (accessed on 11th June 2025).

20. Kaltenbach, T., Anderson, J. C., Burke, C. A., Dominitz, J. A., Gupta, S., Lieberman, D. A., Robertson, D. J., et al. (2020). Endoscopic removal of colorectal lesions: Recommendations by the US Multi-Society Task Force on Colorectal Cancer. *The American Journal of Gastroenterology, 115*, 435–464. https://doi.org/10.14309/ajg.0000000000000555 (accessed on 11th June 2025).

21. Lane, J. C. E., & O'Toole, G. (2012). Complications of ear rings. https://core.ac.uk/download/34075664.pdf (accessed on 11th June 2025).

22. Murakami, T., & Shigeki, S. (2024). Pharmacotherapy for keloids and hypertrophic scars. *International Journal of Molecular Sciences, 25*, 4674–4674. https://doi.org/10.3390/ijms25094674 (accessed on 11th June 2025).

23. Salphale, Pankaj. (2017). Tattooed Skin and Health. (accessed on 11th June 2025).

24. Podurar, S. A., Gorbatova, N., Bryantsev, A. V., Duvansky, V. A., Tertychny, A., Varev, G. A., Nikiforov, S. M., et al. (2024). Effects of "blue" (λ = 450 nm) and pulsed periodic CO_2 (λ = 10.6 μm) laser light at the skin of laboratory animals: A comparative experimental study. *Laser Medicine*. https://www.semanticscholar.org/paper/abe695c6a990ac82a3e7f0941ba2a2036ba00bb1 (accessed on 11th June 2025).

25. Sivaranjani, J. (2019). *Percutaneous Collagen Induction in the Treatment of Atrophic Acne Scars using an Automated Microneedling Device: A Novel Approach* (Doctoral dissertation, Stanley Medical College, Chennai).(accessed on 11th June 2025).

26. Tjipta, A., Ramadhan, H., & Lubis, R. (2023). Immune response in laser tattoo removal: A systematic review. *Journal of Lasers in Medical Sciences, 14*, e66. https://www.semanticscholar.org/paper/e64e8444058da0715729e64f8771071809011476 (accessed on 11th June 2025).

27. Trivedi, M., Yang, F. C., & Cho, B. K. (2017). A review of laser and light therapy in melasma. *International Journal of Women's Dermatology, 3*, 11–20. https://doi.org/10.1016/j.ijwd.2017.01.004 (accessed on 11th June 2025).

28. van der Bent, S. A. S. (2021). *Tattoo Complications: Diagnosis and Treatment.* https://core.ac.uk/download/387937144.pdf (accessed on 11th June 2025).

29. Walsh, L. A., Wu, E. Y., Pontes, D., Kwan, K., Poondru, S., Miller, C. H., & Kundu, R. V. (2023). Keloid treatments: An evidence-based systematic review of recent advances. *Systematic Reviews, 12*. https://doi.org/10.1186/s13643-023-02192-7 (accessed on 11th June 2025).

30. Wyss, Dana, "Exploring Self-Injury: An Art-Based Approach to Cultivating Empathy and Understanding in Mental Health Professionals" (2018). *Expressive Therapies Dissertations.* 55. https://digitalcommons.lesley.edu/expressive_dissertations/55(accessed on 11th June 2025).

COSMETIC SCLEROTHERAPY

12

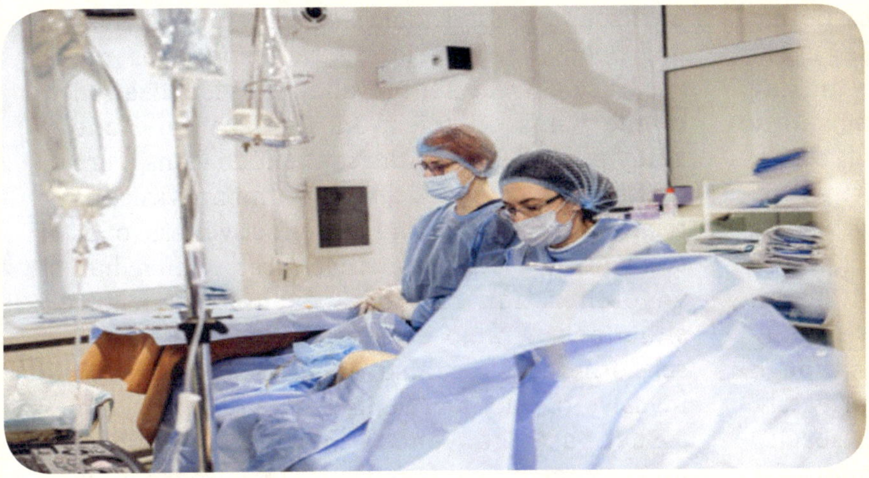

LEARNING OBJECTIVES

After studying this chapter, you will be able to:

1. Understand the science of sclerotherapy
2. Discuss cosmetic indications for sclerotherapy
3. Describe the procedure for sclerotherapy
4. Explain complications and risks of cosmetic sclerotherapy
5. Highlight the effectiveness and outcomes of cosmetic sclerotherapy
6. Assess the cost and availability of cosmetic sclerotherapy

Introduction

Cosmetic sclerotherapy is now a sought-after and successful therapy for individuals desiring relief from varicose veins and aesthetic flaws associated with them. It is a quick, minimally invasive method in which a sclerosing agent is injected into the affected veins, which will close down over time and get absorbed into the body. Increased demand for non-surgical methods is itself largely the result of enhanced awareness of aesthetics and the psychosocial implications of exposed vein flaws. With medical systems evolving to accommodate these preferences, cosmetic sclerotherapy is at the crossroads of patient satisfaction and medical effectiveness. The crossroads of aesthetic and health continue to influence interest and research in the specialty, making it obligatory to discuss its safety profiles, efficacy, as well as the implications of varied patient experiences. One of the most important elements in understanding cosmetic sclerotherapy involves its use in clinical practice. According to recent studies, the efficacy and safety of foam sclerotherapy are evinced by evidence of favorable outcomes among groups with diverse demographics. For instance, some studies point to a high rate of complications among age groups, indicating that patients over the age of 50 years have differing responses and outcomes after undergoing the procedure (Mahitha and Punitha, 2021). This means that the selection of the patient is essential in obtaining the best results, particularly in understanding how each parameter could affect tolerance and recovery. The intersection of patient age, coexisting medical conditions, and type of sclerosing agent used necessitates thorough evaluation, making available to healthcare professionals the ability to deliver the optimum interventions and results. Lastly, the setting of treatment availability within the scope of cosmetic sclerotherapy must also be investigated. Most prominently in the UK, there are discrepancies between the national health service and private clinics that create a rationing of treatments (Campbell et al., 2006). Although foam sclerotherapy is more prevalent privately, access barriers in the national health service can make initial intervention problematic for most individuals. These gaps underscore the need for health systems to design clear and equitable rules of care under which all patients are able to receive effective care regardless of fiscal or systemic limits. In furthering the discipline, the narrowing of these gaps will be essential in driving a more equitable practice for cosmetic vein treatments toward improved patient outcomes and satisfaction.

Definition of Cosmetic Sclerotherapy

Cosmetic sclerotherapy is a less invasive process that is often applied to treat small varicose veins and spider veins. The procedure involves the direct injection of a sclerosing solution into the targeted veins, which causes irritation and inflammation of the endothelium, thus causing the vein to shut down. This will cause the veins to be absorbed by the body and decrease their visibility to a large degree. As cosmetic defects significantly affect an individual's self-esteem, this treatment has gained more popularity with patients who wish to improve their cosmetic outcomes without opting for more invasive surgical treatments. Cosmetic sclerotherapy has been shown to be safe and effective through many clinical trials. Research has demonstrated that patients typically rate considerable reductions in symptoms , such as pain, swelling, and inflammation, along with a dramatic reduction in the appearance of varicose veins. Notably, ultrasound-guided foam sclerotherapy (UGFS) has been a top variation that enhances the accuracy of treatment by allowing visualization of the veins on injection. For example, one study proved 90% of the saphenous veins were obliterated 180 days after treatment with this technique, highlighting its effectiveness over conventional surgical procedures, which had an obliteration rate of 78% in comparable situations (Araujo et al., 2009). Cosmetically, sclerotherapy is compared to other minimally invasive methods of venous disease treatment , such as endovenous heat ablation and mechanochemical ablation. Each method is beneficial in its own way, but sclerotherapy is particularly in vogue due to its versatility to treat various venous pathologies, ranging from telangiectasia and small reticular veins to medium-sized varicose veins. The procedure may be paired with newer procedures , such as CLaCS (Cryo-Laser & Cryo-Sclerotherapy), to enhance outcomes, particularly for cosmetic phlebology. Practice guidelines issued by national professional vascular societies support sclerotherapy as an effective second-line management, especially for patients who present with recurrent or residual varicose veins after initial management (Antonova et al., 2022). This emphasizes the significance of sclerotherapy in aesthetic vascular therapy and its use for improving the quality of life of the patient (Figure 12.1).

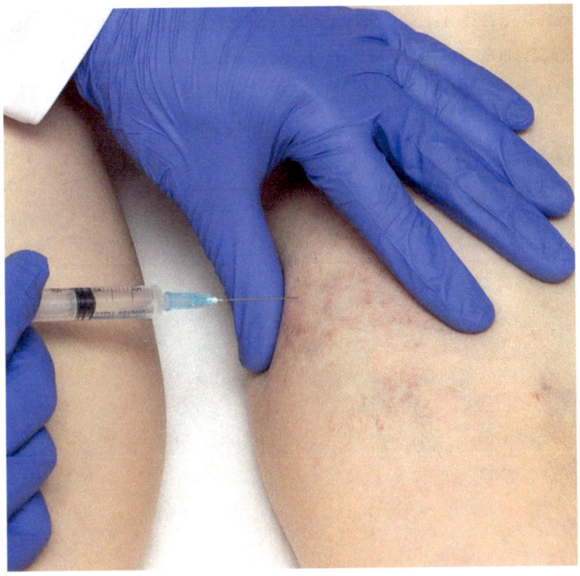

Figure 12.1. Sclerotherapy procedure being performed to treat varicose or spider veins.

Source: https://www.mplsvein.com/wp-content/uploads/2023/11/sclerotherapy.webp.

Historical Background and Development

The evolution of sclerotherapy as a treatment for venous malformations traces back to both ancient medical interventions and technological developments. Sclerotherapy was initially developed in the early 20th century, where it involved injecting agents used to cause localized inflammation and fibrosis in affected veins. The earlier therapies predominantly used chemicals, such as alcohol and iodine. These methods, however primitive, were sometimes risky, with infection and scarring, and therefore created a need for safer, more efficient alternatives. The introduction of less irritating sclerosants, , such as most importantly sodium tetradecyl sulfate (STS), was a significant turning point in the history of cosmetic sclerotherapy, emphasizing the relevance of efficacy and patient safety in the management of venous disease (Lamba, 2010). Over the years, sclerotherapy protocols and methods have been extensively refined to yield optimal outcomes and minimize side effects. The 1990s witnessed a paradigm shift with the development of ultrasound-guided sclerotherapy, which improved sclerosant delivery accuracy with a reduction in blind injections. This allowed precise mapping of venous structures and sustenance of cure by employing targeted vessel closure of offending vessels. Furthermore, increased attention to patient comfort during procedures resulted in improvements , such as the application of local anesthesia and the engineering of needle sizes to minimize pain, further increasing the acceptance of sclerotherapy as a safe outpatient therapeutic procedure for cosmetic conditions (Mohamed et al., 2021). The contemporary landscape of cosmetic sclerotherapy is characterized by a growing array of sclerosants and combination treatment paradigms, driven by findings from recent clinical trials. For instance, the recognition of the limited success of older agents has led to research into using more effective alternatives , such as ethanol, which has proved highly effective in annihilating problematic veins with minimal side effects (Lamba, 2010). The addition of adjunctive methods — , such as mechanical modalities combined with sclerotherapy, is also increasingly popular as practitioners look to continue improving outcomes and address more generalized vascular issues. With the evolution of the specialty, the emphasis on evidence-based practice likewise continues to guide treatment recommendations, ensuring continued enhanced care for patients with venous disease.

Importance of the Procedure in Modern Cosmetic Practices

In contemporary cosmetic treatments, cosmetic sclerotherapy has been an important therapy for varicose veins and superficial venous insufficiencies. Not only does this treatment address aesthetic issues surrounding unsightly veins, but it also provides the elimination of physical pain, which so often accompanies them. Clients see impressive improvements in both the quality of their life as well as their emotional states after treatment, after which the visual image of varicose veins causes patients to be self-conscious and less confident. Therefore, cosmetic sclerotherapy is done for two purposes: cosmetic enhancement and symptomatic alleviation, holding a significant position in contemporary aesthetic medicine. Moreover, the minimally invasive procedure provides faster post-treatment recovery times for patients, which is the reason behind its popularity in the context of a society that is fast-paced, where leisure time tends to be scarce. The significance of cosmetic sclerotherapy is also highlighted by its development as a key component of minimally invasive treatments, overshadowing older forms of surgery. Studies indicate that treatments like endovenous laser ablation (EVLA) have comparable efficacy to conventional surgery with reduced complications and less downtime; these benefits have led to the minimally invasive treatment becoming increasingly popular with patients seeking rapid solutions without the need for full surgery. As noted, approximately 60% of varicosities are suitable for EVLA, expanding the scope for successful treatment in a large patient population. The mounting evidence bases regarding efficacy and safety of such procedures affirm their significance in modern cosmetic treatment (Samuel et al., 2014). Within the active realm of cosmetic medicine, the integration of new techniques and technologies, such as cosmetic sclerotherapy, has larger implications for personalized care. The anticipated results of sclerotherapy align with patient expectations for effective, efficient, and aesthetically improved treatment of the issue of vein-related complications. The versatility of this procedure further allows practitioners to tailor interventions to suit individual patient requirements, enhancing patient satisfaction and results. The focus on integrating clinical effectiveness with cosmetic improvement underscores the significance of sclerotherapy in modern practices. As patients become more demanding of procedures that deliver both health benefits and cosmetic enhancement, treatments like cosmetic sclerotherapy will only continue to be characteristically part of the future of cosmetic medicines (Mekako, 2012).

12.1. The Science Behind Sclerotherapy

Learning Outcome

1. Understand the mechanism of action of sclerosing agents
2. Explain the types of veins treated with sclerotherapy
3. Compare with other vein treatment methods

The complexity of sclerotherapy stems from its inherent need to induce localized inflammation of the target veins. The minimally invasive treatment consists mainly of injecting a sclerosing agent, , such as sodium tetradecyl sulfate (STS), into offending veins. Once injected, the agent causes action by irritating the lining of the blood vessel, leading to endothelial cell injury and resulting thrombus formation. Over time, the inflammatory response causes the veins to contract and be reabsorbed by the surrounding tissue, in effect making them disappear. The mechanistic explanation for the treatment also emphasizes its advantages, including minimal downtime and less opportunity for serious complications compared to surgical procedures. Through the application of sclerotherapy in patients, they are able to experience improvements in the appearance of varicose and spider veins, thereby justifying the value of sclerotherapy as a cosmetic dermatology procedure. Though its efficacy is established, sclerotherapy is not without risk and needs to be well understood in terms of potential complications. The use of STS in the treatment of venous malformations has been a focus of many studies of its efficacy and safety. For instance, recent research demonstrated that in the application of foam sclerotherapy among head and neck venous malformation patients, several complications, although mainly tolerable, occurred. Some of these complications include localized pain, pigmentation disorders, and in some instances, more critical effects , such as allergic reaction or tissue necrosis (Gloviczki et al., 2011).

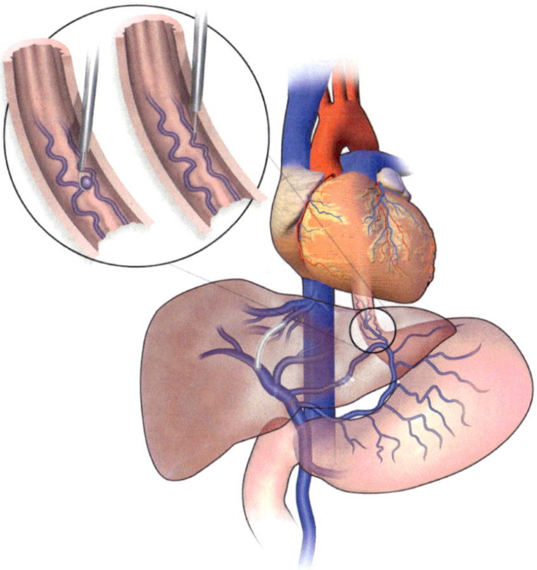

Figure 12.2. Sclerotherapy.

Source: https://upload.wikimedia.org/wikipedia/commons/thumb/c/c7/Sclerotherapy.png/800px-Sclerotherapy.png.

With these potential hazards, professionals must be vigilant in selecting patients for sclerotherapy and in conducting rigorous tests to prevent adverse outcomes during treatment. In light of ongoing scientific knowledge regarding sclerotherapy, additional research remains a priority for refining techniques and improving patient outcomes. The quest for novel sclerosing agents and new procedural methods has the potential to expand the therapeutic choices for patients with vascular conditions. As the technology improves, studies on long-term results from sclerotherapy will clarify its efficacy in various groups and disorders. In addition, existing evidence points towards the importance of patient education regarding potential side effects and likely results to facilitate informed consent and successful management of expectations (Gloviczki et al., 2011). By gaining a thorough understanding of the science behind sclerotherapy, clinicians are in a better position to control its application within cosmetic clinics and maintain patient safety and satisfaction (Figure 12.2).

12.1.1. Mechanism of Action of Sclerosing Agents

The mechanism of action of the sclerosing agents is primarily that of chemical irritation of the endothelial lining of blood vessels, leading to thrombosis and ultimately fibrosis. The process begins with the administration of the sclerosing agent into the vessel to be treated; the agent typically induces inflammation needed for the closure of the vessel. Agents , such as STS and bleomycin, which disturb endothelial cell integrity and secrete pro-inflammatory mediators, initiate a cascade of reactions that culminate in the formation of a clot. Inflammation causes a sequence of cellular interactions that enhance platelet attachment and activation of coagulation. The formation of a fibrin clot later reduces the lumen of vessels, ultimately leading to vessel obliteration and remodeling (Ahmed et al., 2016). The intrinsic process is essential for the cosmetic efficacy of sclerotherapy in the treatment of various vascular lesions. The choice of sclerosing agent also relies on its various biochemical properties and influences the results of the therapy. For instance, bleomycin functions through a novel mechanism that involves the induction of cell death and fibrosis in vascular malformations through apoptosis of cells. By direct action on endothelial cell DNA, bleomycin leads to cell death as well as activation of fibroblasts, resulting in deposition of collagen around treated vessels. This mechanism is involved in the reduction of malformation size and enhancement of skin texture and therefore results in better cosmetic results (Ahmad, 2019). The in-depth understanding of these mechanisms is critical in the selection of a treatment protocol and its outcome, particularly for cosmetic conditions like varicose veins and other vascular malformations. Lastly, the success of sclerosing agents rests not just on their biochemical action but on proper injection techniques and patient selection as well. Ultrasound has emerged as an effective tool in enhancing the precision of sclerotherapy in such a way that sclerosing agents can be injected directly into the target sites. This approach has been found to drastically improve clinical results, with heightened proportions of total resolution or significant decrease in vascular lesions (Ahmed et al., 2016). Moreover, assessment of the patient's individual factors, e.g., age, type of vascular anomaly, and previous treatment, optimizes the selection of sclerosants and modes of injection. Thus, to understand them and to implement them clinically will greatly enhance the safety and efficacy of cosmetic sclerotherapy (Figure 12.3).

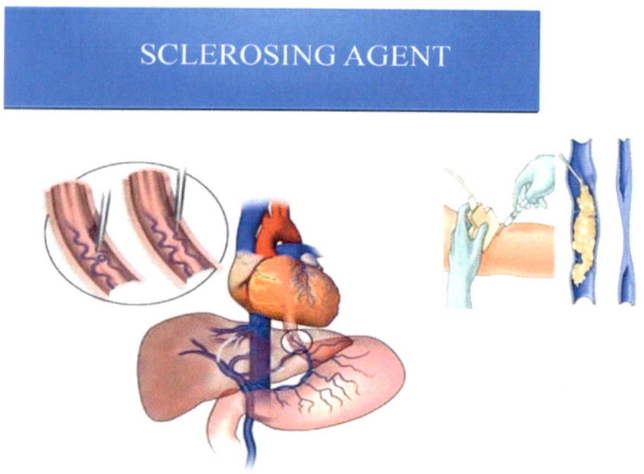

Figure 12.3. Sclerosing agents.

Source: https://cdn.slidesharecdn.com/ss_thumbnails/sclerosingagents-161217062231-thumbnail.jpg?width=640&height=640&fit=bounds.

12.1.2. Types of Veins Treated with Sclerotherapy

The efficacy of sclerotherapy extends to all superficial veins, with great focus on varicose veins and spider veins. Varicose veins, as enlarged superficial veins appearing primarily in the legs, are particularly susceptible to undergoing this treatment. Sclerotherapy not only serves aesthetic needs by reducing apparent varicosities but also corrects root functional defects, as reflected in research highlighting ultrasound-guided foam its effectiveness in treating these ailments. The treatment significantly improves signs of chronic venous disease (CVD) like heaviness, swelling, and pain and hence patients' overall condition (Darvall, 2012). Therefore, the venous groups that are targeted using sclerotherapy are both cosmetic and medical problems, hence making the treatment a widely used procedure in current vascular treatment. Besides varicose veins, spider veins, or telangiectasia, are also important targets for the intervention. They are small, narrow veins, which are normally red, blue, or purple, and appear close to the skin surface, often resulting in cosmetic problems among the patients. Sclerotherapy effectively occludes these minor veins with solutions that cause the vein to collapse and be digested by the body. Society for Vascular Surgery (SVS) and American Venous Forum (AVF) recommendations emphasize that superficial vein incompetence must be diagnosed to choose certain treatments like sclerotherapy (Gloviczki et al., 2011). Because these veins are not generally important in underlying venous disease, their treatment depends largely on individual aesthetic concerns, again highlighting the procedure's importance in cosmetic sclerotherapy and its significant impact on self-esteem. Sclerotherapy also treats incompetent tracts of the great saphenous vein (GSV) and small saphenous vein (SSV), again showing the variety of types of veins being treated. These veins are typically subjected to severe venous reflux, which exacerbates symptoms and is also the cause of varicosity and ulcers. Endovenous therapies and sclerotherapy provide reasonable alternatives in managing GSV and SSV reflux because studies show they are associated with fewer complications and improved recovery times compared to traditional surgery (Darvall, 2012). The ability to address these veins without subjecting the patient to an invasive procedure expands the indications for sclerotherapy so that practitioners have more patients to treat with fewer risks associated with more invasive treatments. The comprehensive approach is emblematic of the fusion of functional treatment and cosmetic enhancement at the core of cosmetic sclerotherapy (Figure 12.4).

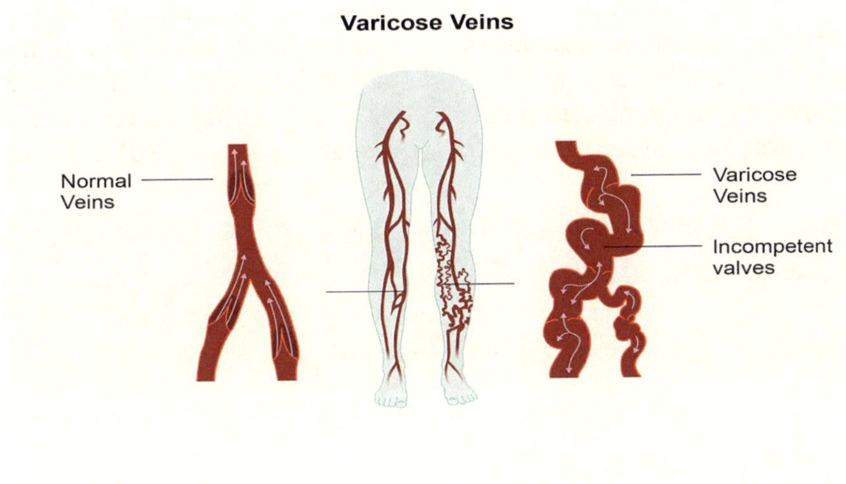

Figure 12.4. Varicose veins.

Source: https://i0.wp.com/post.healthline.com/wp-content/uploads/2021/12/1760720_Sclerotherapy-for-Varicose-and-Spider-Veins-02.jpg?w=1155&h=1837.

12.1.3. Comparison with Other Vein Treatment Methods

Among the vein treatment methodologies, there are a number, each with its own benefits and limitations. Cosmetic sclerotherapy is one of the minimally invasive procedures, and it is particularly used for spider and small varicose veins. In comparison to traditional surgery methods, like superficial venous surgery (SVS), which potentially can have more downtime and complications, sclerotherapy typically does not require much downtime. Recent studies have indicated that, compared to SVS, patients undergoing UGFS had much less bruising, pain, and a faster resumption of their normal activities. This is a compelling reason for the use of sclerotherapy as a first-line treatment, especially in those seeking cosmetic benefit alongside functional gain, e.g., reduction of the symptoms of the veins. Thus, cosmetic sclerotherapy may yield a more practical and efficient solution for the management of lower limb venous disease for the majority of patients. Cosmetic sclerotherapy is commended for its efficacy and safety, yet a comparison of its outcomes with other contemporary invasive treatments, e.g., endovenous laser treatment (EVLT) and radiofrequency ablation (RFA), is warranted. Evidence has indicated that these heat and laser treatments are approximately 90% successful at five years of follow-up, comparable to the success of sclerotherapy in cosmetic and symptom improvement. However, EVLT and RFA may be more invasive and involve the use of anesthesia, raising concerns with patient recovery and comfort. The treatments, though effective, are not necessarily what the patient would want by way of minimally invasive treatment. Sclerotherapy, especially when combined with modalities like compression therapy, reduces symptoms of CVD and enhances quality of life, well-suited for patient-centered care of vein treatment alternatives. The literature increasingly emphasizes the advantages of the utilization of sclerotherapy combined with other adjunct treatments. Current evidence has proven UGFS's efficacy to improve chronic venous ulcers when used in conjunction with compression bandaging, which shows a synergistic action that maximizes healing outcomes. Sclerotherapy's multimodal therapy further sets it apart from solitary invasive modalities, which look only at mechanical destruction of veins. Since both venous insufficiency and cosmetic aspects are addressed, sclerotherapy treats not just the functional needs of the patient but also aesthetic concerns. Therefore, just as there are different veins treatment methods, sclerotherapys efficacy, less recovery period, and more non-invasiveness make it a favorable method of treatment in venous conditions management, particularly on a cosmetic level, demonstrated by the growing patient satisfaction in recent research (Darvall, 2012; Piekarska et al., 2025).

Test Your Knowledge

1. What is the mechanism of action of sclerosing agents used in sclerotherapy?
2. Which types of veins are commonly treated with sclerotherapy?

12.2. Indications for Cosmetic Sclerotherapy

Learning Outcome

1. Understand common conditions treated by cosmetic sclerotherapy
2. Describe patient eligibility and assessment criteria
3. Deal with psychological and aesthetic motivations for treatment

The sole indications for cosmetic sclerotherapy are the treatment of spider veins and small varicose veins. These are typically a source of worry for the majority of people because they tend to significantly influence the physical outlook of an individual and his/her self-esteem. Sclerotherapy is an effective therapy for such issues through the injection of a sclerosing agent into the affected veins, subsequent collapse of the veins, and eventual disappearance. This minimally invasive procedure offers individuals a solution to their cosmetic concerns without significant downtime, thereby complying with the growing demand for effective yet non-surgical cosmetic procedures in contemporary cosmetic practice. Furthermore, the growing trend of such interventions reflects a general social interest in enhancing physical beauty, particularly among younger population groups who are concerned about avoiding the formation of vascular lesions before they appear. In addition to cosmetic use, sclerotherapy is also prescribed for some medical venous insufficiency conditions. Patients with pre-existing conditions , such as CVD, can experience pain, swelling, and discomfort, which are alleviated by this treatment. The double whammy of curing the aesthetic and functional deficit of venous health solidifies sclerotherapy's position in the medical community. With the complexities of skin aging having both environmental and genetic factors causing vascular changes and transformation, sclerotherapy steps in as a treatment option of multifaceted nature to address these complexities. The interrelationship between venous appearance and skin health is further seen with evidence pointing to the necessity of including overall aspects of skincare under treatment paradigms. Thus, combining sclerotherapy with a broad cosmetic plan highlights its effectiveness in more than mere surface treatments (Fernández-Varela-Gómez et al., 2024). Secondly, the treatment is increasingly recognized for its ability to improve outcomes when applied as an add-on to other cosmetic treatments. Combine procedures, like together as laser treatment or skin resurfacing therapies, promote not just the cosmetic result but skin health as well. With the evolving profile of cosmetic treatments, sclerotherapy remains the rage as an all-around regimen to enhance the appearance of the skin. The growing body of research on skin aging validates the effectiveness of such synergistic treatments, which address multiple signs of aging simultaneously. By understanding the relationship between vascular pathologies and overall skin well-being, aesthetic practitioners are able to provide their patients with treatment programs that are specifically tailored to individual needs, thereby maximizing satisfaction and clinical outcomes (Youngerwood, 2012).

12.2.1. Common Conditions Treated (e.g., Spider Veins, Varicose Veins)

Among the most frequent conditions that are treated with cosmetic sclerotherapy is spider veins. Spider veins are small, dilated small vessels close to the skin's surface and typically appear like spider webs or branches of a tree. Although typically benign and only cosmetically relevant, spider veins are occasionally painful and can cause itching or burning sensations. As a person gets older, the likelihood of developing spider veins increases, particularly for individuals who have a family history of venous, hormonal changes, or prolonged standing periods. Spider vein treatment typically involves injecting a sclerosing agent into the affected vessel the resulting in shrinking vessels and making them less noticeable. This mildly invasive procedure not only enhances the cosmetic appearance of the affected skin but also addresses related venous insufficiency issues, which is the reason patients love it for treating small venous conditions (Figure 12.5).

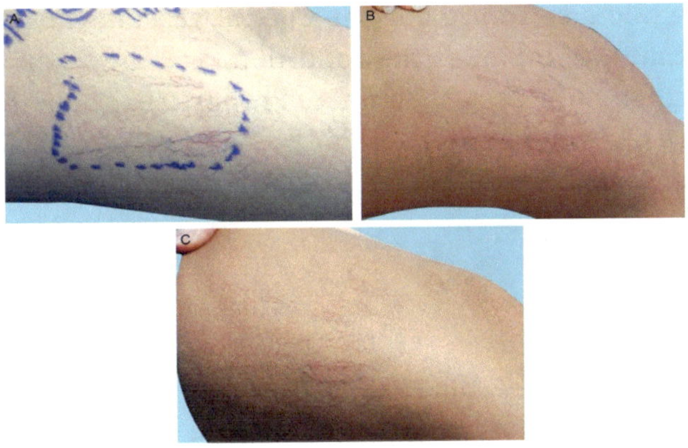

Figure 12.5. (A) This 36-year-old woman presented with untreated spider veins of the left inner knee; (B) One week after treatment; and (C) Five months after treatment.

Source: https://www.researchgate.net/profile/Edmond-Ritter/publication/280870801/figure/fig4/AS:324776733233169@1454444215910/A-This-36-year-old-woman-presented-with-untreated-spider-veins-of-the-left-inner-knee.png.

Varicose veins are a more visually obtrusive condition that is cosmetically treated by sclerotherapy, and they affect an extremely large population. Enlarged, twisted veins, which are painful and look ugly as well, varicose veins are typically a sign of CVD, a condition brought about by valvular incompetence of the venous system. Varicose veins could evolve into problems , such as superficial vein infection and deep vein thrombosis (DVT) if not given attention, which underscores the importance of curative treatment in an early stage. Sclerotherapy aims to cure by directly administering a sclerosing agent into the target veins, creating an inflammatory reaction that is managed in a way that results in vein closure. As indicated, the effectiveness of this treatment is high, with accessed studies affirming a 90% success rate after five years for varicose veins management and therefore a valid option for patients and healthcare practitioners in general (Piekarska et al., 2025). CVI is a complex condition that not only encompasses varicose and spider veins but also underlies most venous disorders. CVI is caused by an inability of the veins to pump blood back to the heart, often due to faulty valves causing increased venous pressure. CVI depends greatly on the age, genetics, and standing for extended periods of time, with catastrophic effects if left unaddressed, , such as the formation of leg ulcers or vascular complications (Micallef et al., 2011). Sclerotherapy plays a crucial role in the treatment of CVI because it targets overt symptoms while also improving the overall vascular health. The treatments alleviate the physical discomfort that accompanies the condition, and they can even help the patients psychologically by improving their physical appearance. Proper treatment of CVI through methods like sclerotherapy not only rescues the patients from the symptoms but also serves to prevent significant complications arising out of CVD (Figure 12.6).

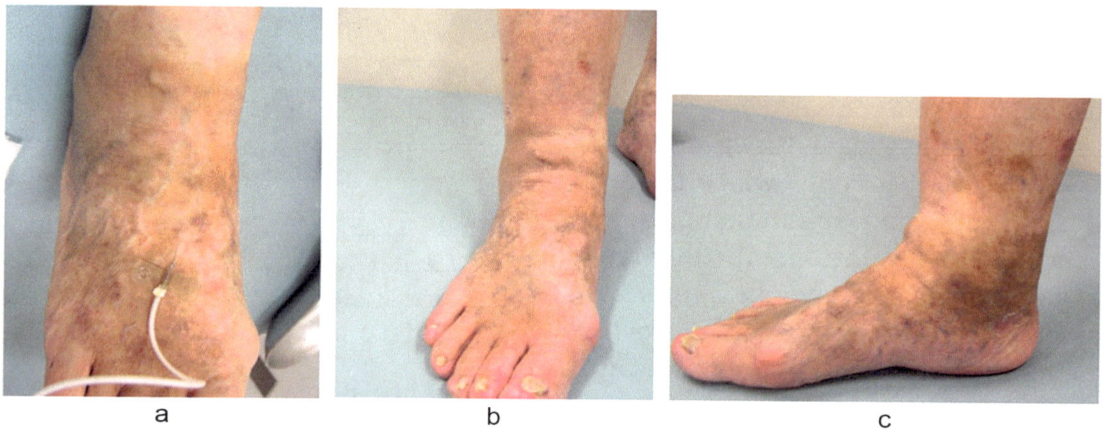

Figure 12.6. Sclerotherapy of the varicose veins of the right foot. (a) The reticular varicose vein on the dorsum of the right foot was punctured, and sclerotherapy with foam sclerosing agent (0.5% polidocanol) was performed. The sclerosing agent was manually guided into the CP around the medial condyle. (b, c) After 1 month, the reticular varicose vein on the dorsum of the foot (b) and CP on the medial aspect of the right foot (c) were relieved. CP: corona phlebectatica.

Source: https://www.researchgate.net/publication/361286267/figure/fig3/AS:11431281093798356@1667285271967/Sclerotherapy-of-the-varicose-veins-of-right-foot-a-The-reticular-varicose-vein-on-the.ppm.

12.2.2. Patient Eligibility and Assessment Criteria

In cosmetic sclerotherapy, patient selection and evaluation criteria are the most important factors that render the treatment a success. Initial assessment can involve a comprehensive review of medical history and physical examination to identify superficial venous insufficiency (SVI) or other venous diseases. Patients should be checked for comorbid disease, , such as a history of thromboembolic disease or serious cardiovascular disease, which is a contraindication for the procedure. The severity and distribution of varices are also examined because the severity and type of venous reflux might have improved outcomes after sclerotherapy. Adherence to these rigorous testing regimens enhances the efficacy and safety of the treatment and patient, and it is in adherence with principles identified in research that validates the evidence of various interventions for venous incompetence management (Mohamed et al., 2021). Apart from this, cosmetic sclerotherapy candidacy requires a clear comprehension of the patient's goal and expectation. It is crucial that the health practitioners clarify the realistic outcomes of the procedure to the patients, as patients who seek cosmetic procedures have some aesthetic expectations. The assessment typically involves determining the presence and severity of symptoms , such as pain, swelling, or cosmetic issues, to ensure that the procedure meets the expectation of benefit by the patient. Besides, health-related quality of life assessment can provide objective feedback on the way venous diseases can impact the health and daily functioning of the patient. Such evaluations can play a key role in determining whether sclerotherapy is an appropriate treatment option, particularly when it comes to addressing the psychological and emotional issues of cosmetic outcomes (El-Sheikha, 2015). Integration of patient-reported outcomes in evaluation and eligibility criteria not only strengthens the evaluation process but also supports clinical decision-making in cosmetic sclerotherapy. These outcomes can be quantified by instruments , such as the venous clinical severity score (VCSS) and the Aberdeen Varicose Vein Questionnaire (AVVQ), which assess the effect of venous disorders on patients' lives. Through the assessment of these parameters pre- and post-treatment, practitioners can assess the efficacy of sclerotherapy from both patient-centered and clinical perspectives. This dual evaluation method highlights the significance of personalized treatment, where treatment is planned according to the specific needs and conditions of individual patients. Such meticulous assessment protocols ultimately result in the optimal benefits of sclerotherapy with lesser risks of adverse effects (Mohamed et al., 2021) (Figure 12.7).

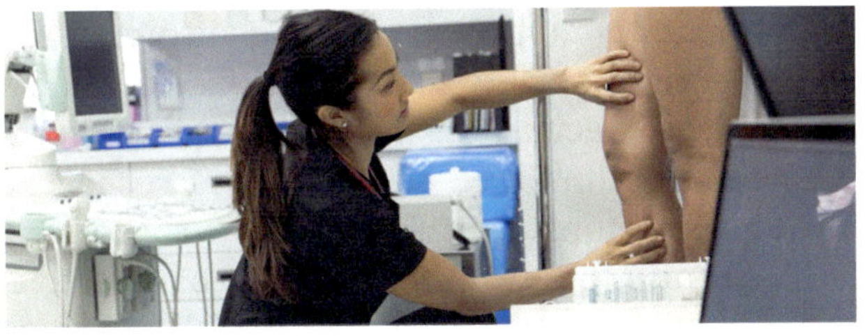

Figure 12.7. Assessing patient for the success of the treatment.

Source: https://www.ucsfhealth.org/-/media/project/ucsf/ucsf-health/treatment/hero/sclerotherapy-2x.jpg?rev=d98d3a88113045d1aa874a1dea4fdf96.

12.2.3. Psychological and Aesthetic Motivations for Treatment

Cosmetic sclerotherapy has seen widespread interest in recent times, stimulated by psychological and cosmetic motivation for treatment. Individuals who undergo the procedure have generally shown a desire to be acceptable according to a particular definition of beauty in society, as a response to a consolidation of local ideals and globalization influences. Research has demonstrated that beauty ideals are highly situational, particularly in cultures like East Asia and Latin America, where regional cultural standards dictate women's decisions regarding cosmetic procedures. Seeking aesthetic improvement is not necessarily about superficial enhancement but is highly interwoven with deep-set psychological needs, , such as the enhancement of self-esteem and empowerment through appearance. These rewards emphasize the critical role of social contexts and norms in shaping individual decision making for cosmetic treatments, illustrating a complicated interdependence among external factors and individual wants (Vorisek, 2017). Furthermore, application of nonsurgical cosmetic technologies, like sclerotherapy, provides a unique method through which to consider people's relationships with their bodies and themselves. These are actually self-presentation and impression management tactics by which individuals can negotiate society's expectations for body appearance. Because, as has been said by those who have volunteered to be part of research, undergoing nonsurgical cosmetic procedures is frequently followed by a variety of affective experiences from excitement to ambivalence, then this ambivalence may come from the pressure from society to conform to societal standards of beauty and simultaneously grapple with personal concepts of beauty. These conflicting feelings illuminate the tangled motivations behind cosmetic treatments, where individuals balance their desires for beautification in relation to cultural standards (Tyner et al., 2008). The psychological dimensions of cosmetic sclerotherapy also illuminate a broader discourse between identity and self-interpretation. When individuals undergo this treatment, they tend to have complex histories about their past, present, and future selves, showing motivations that extend beyond physical improvement. The aspiration to become an ideal self is likely to produce a dynamic relationship between personal experience and social expectations, to heighten the idea that cosmetic procedures are ways in which identity can be controlled. This implies that beyond the correction of visible imperfections, cosmetic sclerotherapy allows individuals to narrate something about who they are and who they would like to be. Thus, an understanding of these psychological and aesthetic drives provides crucial information concerning the broader implications of cosmetic surgery on self-perception and cultural values in modern society (Tyner, 2008).

Test Your Knowledge

1. What are the most common conditions treated with cosmetic sclerotherapy?
2. Who is considered eligible for cosmetic sclerotherapy, and what assessment criteria are used?

12.3. The Procedure of Sclerotherapy

Learning Outcome

1. Understand pre-procedure consultation and preparation for sclerotherapy
2. Describe a step-by-step overview of the sclerotherapy process
3. Deal with post-procedure care and recovery

Sclerotherapy is a commonly used modality for treating superficial venous pathology, particularly in cosmetic application. This extremely minimally invasive technique involves direct injection into the disease-bearing veins of a sclerosing solution, irritating and closing the vessel to be treated as a result. The procedure is routinely performed as an outpatient, with the aid of ultrasound for greater accuracy and success. The sclerosing agent employed can be variable, though the most frequent is polidocanol due to its safety profile and effectiveness. With patients wanting cures for cosmetically unappealing spider veins and varicose veins, becoming familiar with the technical aspects of the procedure becomes imperative, considering its relatively quick recovery from more invasive, traditional surgical methods. Sclerotherapy is typically a pillar of cosmetic venous treatments, both aesthetically and symptomatically. The success of sclerotherapy greatly depends on various factors, including the type of vascular malformation to be treated and the professional treating it. In a research paper on LFVMs treated with ultrasonically guided sclerotherapy with polidocanol foam, there were good results. Pain relief was noted among patients, who also had more than a 50% reduction in size after multiple sessions of therapy. The average number of sessions to obtain optimal results was approximately 2.3, and therefore, a series of well-treated sessions can result in significant improvement. This confirms the importance not only of the appropriate choice of the sclerosing agent but also of tailoring treatment regimens to the requirements of specific patients. Thus, successful sclerotherapy depends upon a deep understanding of the procedure itself and the unique properties of the vascular condition under treatment (Blaise et al., 2011). Patient evaluation and post-treatment management are part of the sclerotherapy process. Post-procedure, patients are typically counseled on managing potential side effects, , such as mild bruising or discomfort, which are commonly temporary. Compression stockings can be prescribed to optimize the effectiveness of the treatment and achieve faster recovery. Follow-up for a long period enables practitioners to see the maintenance of the result and address any developing issues regarding treated vessels. In cosmetic sclerotherapy, ongoing patient education in realistic expectations and maintenance measures also plays an important role in patient satisfaction. The incorporation of these factors into the sclerotherapy treatment serves to further solidify its status as a viable treatment method for cosmetic venous disorders, both improving physical appearance and quality of life for the afflicted (Lee et al., 2009).

12.3.1. Pre-Procedure Consultation and Preparation

The importance of pre-procedure education in cosmetic sclerotherapy cannot be overstressed. The initial meeting is a step in laying the groundwork for the patients and the healthcare providers alike to have their expectations cleared regarding the procedure. During this consultation, the clinician conducts an extensive review of the patient's medical history, including any underlying condition that might contraindicate sclerotherapy, e.g., clotting disorders or hypersensitivity to the material used in the procedure. These clinical evaluations are critical, as they not only help in the risk minimization of DVT but also decide on the choice of intervention, i.e., whether to proceed with UGFS or whether to consider other interventions like endovenous thermal ablation (ETA) or cyanoacrylate adhesive closure (Baker et al., 2019; Di Gangi et al., 2024).

An extensive pre-procedure consultation, therefore, ensures the safety of the patient and the likelihood of successful outcomes. In addition to clinical assessment, pre-procedure consultations also provide an important platform for the exchange of procedural expectations and potential side effects. Patients should be informed of what precisely the sclerotherapy entails, including information on the process, estimated duration, and follow-up care thereafter. Doctors seize this opportunity to educate patients on the possibility of temporary symptoms , such as bruising, swelling, or soreness following treatment, and to also educate them on signs that would require immediate medical attention. Research indicates that patient satisfaction is significantly influenced by how well they understand what to expect before and after the procedure (Di Gangi et al., 2024). Therefore, effective communication during the consultation can decrease anxiety, enhance patient compliance, and ultimately yield better clinical outcomes. Preparation for cosmetic sclerotherapy extends beyond the initial consultation; it is a collaborative approach that includes ensuring the provision of a safe procedural environment. Pre-procedure recommendations should be reinforced, , such as in the withdrawal of anticoagulant medication where possible and safe to do so, and requiring patients to use compression stockings post-treatment to enhance effectiveness and reduce complications (Baker et al., 2019). Moreover, instilling awareness of the patient's lifestyle, whether exercise routine or travel plan, can be a sizeable element in personalizing pre-procedure recommendation. By embracing a multi-disciplinary approach to pre-procedure preparation, healthcare professionals can significantly minimize the risk of complications of cosmetic sclerotherapy , such as DVT or allergic responses, which have been reported as severe side effects necessitating aggressive preventative measures (Baker et al., 2019; Di Gangi et al., 2024). Overall, a well-structured pre-procedure consultation and preparation process is the backbone of a successful and secure cosmetic sclerotherapy outcome (Figure 12.8).

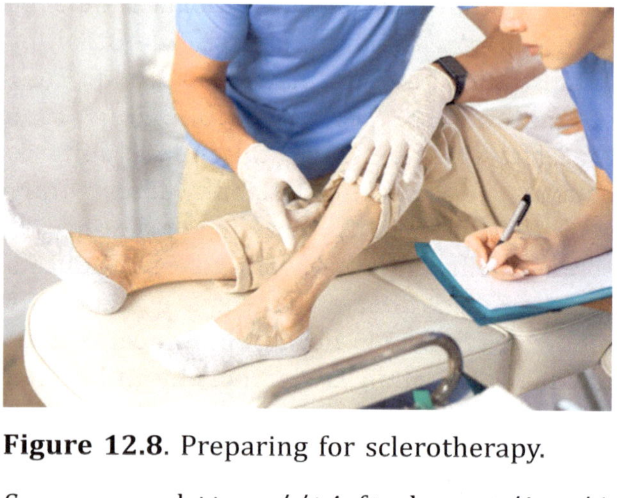

Figure 12.8. Preparing for sclerotherapy.

Source: https://t4.ftcdn.net/jpg/12/13/21/13/360_F_1213211306_sksLl3s8S1Fpw6U0hLuywjdbD8WCINYC.jpg.

12.3.2. Step-by-Step Overview of the Sclerotherapy Process

As a prelude to the sclerotherapy process, physicians initially conduct a comprehensive review of the patient's medical history and presenting symptoms. This is crucial in determining the best kind of sclerosant and identifying any underlying vascular disease that must be treated in the process. Following this assessment, the practitioner informs the patient about the procedure, its benefits and side effects, to set proper expectations before carrying on. Ultrasound guidance may also be employed, particularly when dealing with larger veins or those that are not easy to see. This initial consultation sets the foundation for a successful result of treatment since the choice of patients is a component of the effectiveness and safety of sclerotherapy as a cosmetic treatment. After preparatory actions are completed, the second phase of the sclerotherapy procedure is the injection of the sclerosant into the veins to be targeted themselves. The clinician will usually disinfect the site to reduce infection risks and may also employ a local anesthetic for enhanced patient comfort. The sclerosant is injected into the veins directly with a fine needle. This chemical irritant destroys the lining of the veins, and this causes them to seal off and eventually be reabsorbed into the body over time. Notably, there is some variation in the sclerosant chosen according to vein size and patient-dependent issues. Investigation highlights the value of attention to technique since inappropriate injection can cause unwanted effects like thrombophlebitis or hyperpigmentation and therefore puts value on the service of skilled practitioners' involvement in giving this treatment. After the sclerosant is given, the patient enters recovery, where the treated veins begin to respond to the treatment. The recovery process involves the application of compression to the involved area, most often in the form of compression stockings, which aids in the closure and absorption of the sclerosed veins. The patients are typically informed to resume light activities shortly after the procedure without heavy exercise for a specific period. Follow-up is important to monitor the success of the procedure and address any side effects or complications that may occur. Interestingly, the efficiency of sclerotherapy is realized through gradual improvements in the visual appearance of veins following treatment, enhancing patients' aesthetic satisfaction. Like any cosmetic, minimally invasive procedure, the outcome heavily relies on accurate technique and proper patient care during the entire procedure (Enespa et al., 2022; Cátia et al., 2023) (Figure 12.9).

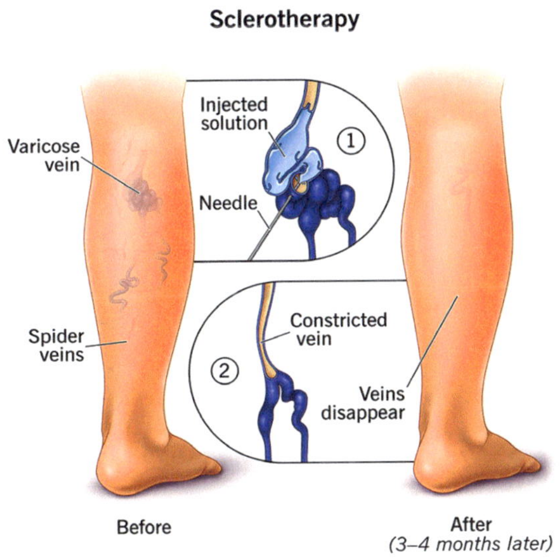

Figure 12.9. Sclerotherapy process.

Source: https://my.clevelandclinic.org/-/scassets/images/org/health/articles/6763-sclerotherapy.

12.3.3. Post-Procedure Care and Recovery

In light of the success of cosmetic sclerotherapy, post-procedure treatment can hardly be more vital. Post-procedure treatment aims to enhance recovery, minimize complications, and maximize the outcome of treatment in general. Patients are usually advised to engage in mild physical activity soon after the procedure to maximize blood flow and prevent thromboembolic complications. But avoiding heavy lifting or high-impact activities for some time is necessary, as such can interfere with the process of healing. Even the application of compression stockings can be recommended to compress the affected veins, which can add to the effectiveness of the treatment. This extensive treatment not only guarantees physical recuperation but also offers assurance to the patients about their health during this recovery process. Frequent monitoring of the treatment location for side effect evidence is a significant component of post-treatment care. Patients should be made aware of common side effects, , such as bruising, swelling, or soreness in the treated veins. They tend to fade away within a few days and are usually not a sign of serious complications. Nonetheless, patients need to be watchful and report unusual symptoms, including persistent pain, excessive swelling, or coloring, to their healthcare provider immediately. Such active monitoring helps ensure timely intervention in case there are any complications. In accordance with this patient-centered approach, the healthcare professional is assigned a key role in generating an environment that makes it safe for patients to report on their recovery status, thereby boosting their satisfaction and confidence in the cosmetic sclerotherapy treatment. Follow-up sessions become the focal point as the recovery progresses to assess the efficacy of the intervention, manage side effects, and schedule any supplemental sclerotherapy sessions as appropriate. On these visits, the doctor can assess the veins and talk with the patient about long-term results, including lifestyle changes to ensure vein health. Discussion of preventative strategies, including weight management, exercise on a regular basis, and diet changes, can also benefit patients in achieving long-term success with aesthetic outcomes after sclerotherapy. By drawing attention to ongoing care and relationship building between patients and healthcare workers, the post-procedure phase becomes an integral aspect of the total course of treatment, emphasizing the commitment to quality-of-life improvement in patients reflected in the evidence of varicose veins and their management (Haidar et al., 2023; Fayyaz et al., 2024) (Figure 12.10).

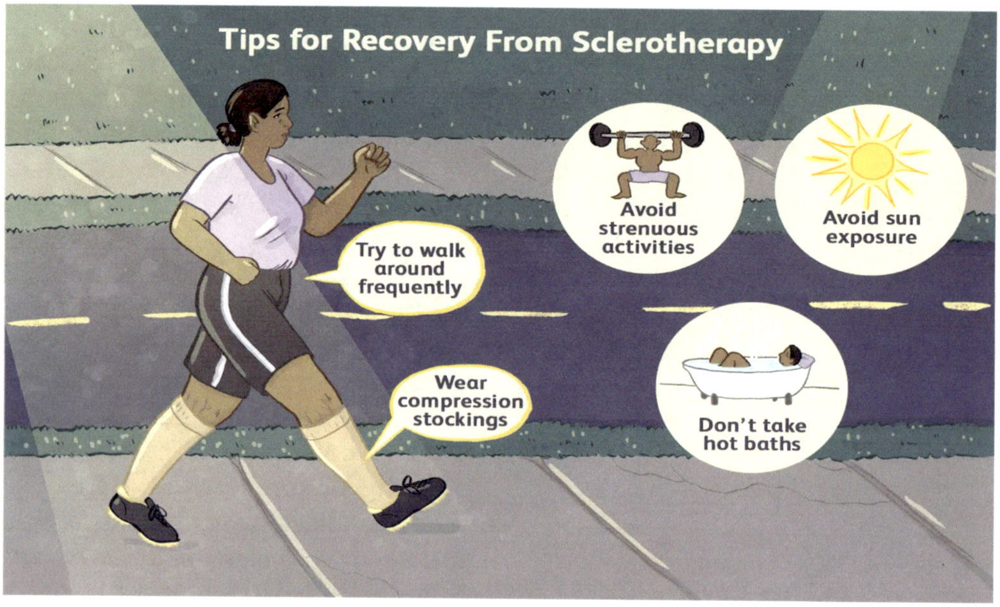
Tips for Recovery From Sclerotherapy
Avoid strenuous activities
Avoid sun exposure
Try to walk around frequently
Wear compression stockings
Don't take hot baths

Figure 12.10. Tips for recovering from sclerotherapy.

Source: https://www.verywellhealth.com/thmb/ZlNmmqUlMjywVPCHOtQUul4VT1M=/1500x0/filters:no_upscale():max_bytes(150000):strip_icc()/sclerotherapy-for-varicose-veins-4582497-5c82b264c9e77c0001f2ac45.png.

Test Your Knowledge

1. What takes place during the pre-procedure consultation and how should a patient prepare for sclerotherapy?
2. What are the step-by-step procedures involved in a typical sclerotherapy session?
3. What post-procedure care and recovery instructions are given after sclerotherapy?

12.4. Risks and Complications

Learning Outcome

1. Discuss common side effects and their management in cosmetic sclerotherapy
2. Explain rare but serious complications associated with sclerotherapy
3. Understand the importance of choosing a qualified practitioner

The cosmetic sclerotherapy treatment, which is designed to cure varicose and spider veins, is not without risks. Bruising, swelling, and reddening of the injection site are common side effects that can result from injections in patients. They tend to be temporary and resolve themselves within days, but under some conditions, they can lead to more severe complications. For instance, secondary reactions to the sclerosing agent can occur, ranging from mild irritation to anaphylactic shock, though the latter is rare. Additionally, superficial thrombophlebitis can occur with the possibility of inflammation in the veins, which results in pain and discomfort that may need further treatment. These dangers need to be familiar to patients so that they are informed about which to make decisions regarding their cosmetic therapy. In the more severe instances, sclerotherapy leads to complications that can have lasting effects on the patient's health and his/her cosmetic goals. Most worrisome is the formation of blood clots, which could migrate to organs supporting life, , such as the lungs, and produce pulmonary embolism, a lethal consequence. In addition, a few patients will develop hyperpigmentation, a condition in which dark spots on the skin at the treatment area form as a result of the interaction of sclerosing agents with the skin tissue. This is an uncomfortable complication, particularly for those undergoing the treatment for cosmetic enhancement. In addition, as CVD can complicate results, those who already have conditions would be at an increased risk for side effects. The interaction between CVD and cosmetic procedures highlights the importance of thorough pre-treatment assessments and counseling. Lastly, the psychological impacts of enduring cosmetic sclerotherapy complications cannot be overlooked. Patients undergoing treatment in pursuit of cosmetic enhancement may find themselves grappling with unforeseen outcomes or prolonged side effects, which will leave them dissatisfied and emotionally disrupted. These complications can translate into a diminished quality of life, with the initial goal of improved appearance being overshadowed by complications. As noted, CVI typically forms part of the associated conditions being treated, thus the safety and efficacy of sclerotherapy treatments becomes more complex. It is crucial that practitioner and patient share openly in the discussion of risks, agree on realistic expectations, and make arrangements for managing potential complications so that an integrated strategy for cosmetic sclerotherapy is assured.

12.4.1. Common Side Effects and Their Management

Cosmetic sclerotherapy, while successful in treating varicose and spider veins, is also far from perfect. Among the most common adverse effects that can be developed by patients are local reactions , such as redness, itchiness, and swelling at the site of treatment. These signs are typically brought about by the inflammatory reaction elicited by the sclerosing medication, as much as this might be needed to close veins, but as much as also aggravating for patients. Treatment of these side effects is primarily reassurance and education, since symptoms typically resolve spontaneously within a week. The use of cool compresses to reduce swelling and topical antihistamines for itch is also recommended by clinicians to maximize the patient's comfort during recovery. By controlling these side effects early and effectively, practitioners are able to maximize patient satisfaction and overall results in cosmetic sclerotherapy. Another significant side effect of cosmetic sclerotherapy is the potential for hyperpigmentation or brown coloration at areas of injection. This is due to blood breakdown or hematoma that is retained in the skin following the procedure. While hyperpigmentation is innocuous and will spontaneously resolve with time, it is a cosmetic concern that presents a problem to most patients. To manage this side effect, practitioners can prescribe the use of sunblock in an effort to prevent further darkening of the affected skin, as sun exposure aggravates the pigmentation changes. Furthermore, certain topical treatments like vitamin C or hydroquinone-based treatments can be used in an attempt to accelerate fading. By actively mitigating the risk of hyperpigmentation and offering choices, practitioners can potentially alleviate patient anxiety around cosmetic outcomes following treatment and enhance the overall cosmetic sclerotherapy experience. Finally, patients undergoing cosmetic sclerotherapy should be informed about the rare but perilous possible side effects, including thrombophlebitis and DVT. These difficulties can occur when the blood in the veins being treated clots and causes inflammation or swelling or worse, cardiovascular complications. Awareness of these risks is crucial for both medical personnel and patients. Prevention involves thorough screening of risk-factor patients before therapy is initiated, as well as patient education on post-procedure signs and symptoms that require immediate medical attention. Besides, the post-treatment use of compression stockings can guarantee proper blood flow and avert clot formation. The practitioners enhance patients' safety and minimize the chances of coming down with severe complications from cosmetic sclerotherapy by implementing these steps, and thereby establish a better setting for treatment as a whole (Davidson et al., 2015; Piekarska et al., 2025) (Figure 12.11).

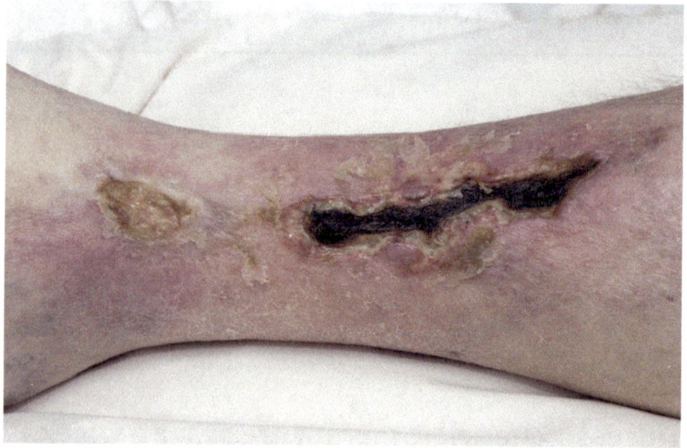

Figure 12.11. The ulcer developed 4 weeks after treatment of an incompetent short saphenous vein and lateral aspect varicosities with Aethoxysklerol ® 1% foam sclerotherapy.

Source: https://www.researchgate.net/publication/304356425/figure/fig4/AS:406968813539328@1474040334106/Patient-2-the-ulcer-developed-4-weeks-after-treatment-of-an-incompetent-short-saphenous.png.

12.4.2. Rare But Serious Complications

The cosmetic sclerotherapy treatment, while otherwise safe and effective for addressing varicose and spider veins, does carry with it the risk of rare but serious complications that must be recognized and actualized. Among these uncommon events, sensitivity reactions to the sclerosing agent do occur, varying from mild cutaneous reactions to more severe anaphylactic reactions that necessitate immediate medical attention. These allergic reactions highlight the importance of a thorough patient history before treatment, including querying for a history of previous allergic reactions or hypersensitivities. Management of these complications not only involves instant action but also reassessment of treatment to prevent risk. Awareness of these potential complications usually inspires a proactive approach in ensuring patient safety and satisfaction in cosmetic sclerotherapy procedures. The second significant problem with cosmetic sclerotherapy is thromboembolism, which may lead to complications , such as DVT or pulmonary embolism (PE). Although the development of these complications is less frequent, they are dangerous to patients' health and need to be treated with caution during and after the procedure. Thromboembolic complications result from incorrect technique, poor post-procedure care, or patient sensitivity caused by systemic disorders. Therefore, strict adherence to standards drawn by experienced authorities, , such as Gloviczki et al. (2011), is required for minimizing such risks. Through proper patient assessment, use of duplex ultrasound, and guideline compliance, professionals can considerably reduce the risk of thromboembolic complications, thus improving the overall safety of the sclerotherapy procedure. Finally, the formation of skin necrosis is a highly alarming complication of cosmetic sclerotherapy.

Table 12.1. Complications of Sclerotherapy

Complications	No. of Cases	Percentage
Bruising	19	38
Thrombophlebitis	5	10
Pigmentation	5	10
Recurrence	2	4
Deep vein thrombosis	1	2

Source: https://www.researchgate.net/publication/236338573/figure/tbl3/AS:998171492753411@1614994037318/Complications-of-sclerotherapy.png.

This complication may result when the sclerosant invades the surrounding tissues or inadvertently enters the arterial circulation instead of the treated veins. Necrosis of the skin is not only painful and potentially causes long recoveries, but also scarring or severe cosmetic deformities that undermine the original purpose of the procedure. As has been observed from clinical practice, meticulous technique at the time of injection, with the use of ultrasound guidance, plays a key role in avoiding this complication. Also, follow-up care on a regular basis is critical in the early identification and management of any side effects, contributing to the need for long care regimens to maximize the result and maintain patient safety in cosmetic sclerotherapy procedures (Table 12.1).

12.4.3. Importance of Choosing a Qualified Practitioner

Choosing a competent practitioner is of extreme importance in cosmetic sclerotherapy, primarily due to the finesse involved in the procedure and potential risks. The increasing popularity of cosmetic sclerotherapy is accompanied by an increase in the number of practitioners available, stretching from aesthetic technicians to doctors. Patients who experience this treatment must ensure that their provider possesses not only the appropriate educational background but also the appropriate clinical experience to manage the intricacies of vein anatomy and treatment technique. In the absence of proper training, there is a heightened risk of complications, including suboptimal treatment outcomes and adverse side effects. Besides, the ability to diagnose and respond to complications timely manner is crucial, underlining the necessity of a well-trained practitioner to adhere to current medical protocols and guidelines for the minimization of risks as well as protection of the patient. Furthermore, the practice of advanced techniques in cosmetic sclerotherapy necessitates continuing professional education for practitioners. As highlighted in recent research, the evolution of the aesthetic therapy environment has made it a necessity to have higher levels of education and training in somatology and aesthetics. The research respondents highlighted the need for ongoing education that addresses skill and knowledge gaps, particularly in new technology and procedure refinement (Ambrosio et al., 2018). By opting for a trained professional who keeps updating and training himself, patients are more likely to receive innovative and effective solutions most suited to their requirements. This ability enhances the possibilities of the required outcome but also creates a dependence-based relationship between the practitioner and patient, which is the top priority for a good experience. Finally, the implications of choosing an unqualified practitioner are not merely physical well-being and outcomes; they can reach as far as a patient's emotional wellness and overall satisfaction with his or her treatment process. Patients' testimonies and experts' views generally indicate that patients treated by less qualified practitioners end up more anxious and discontent due to complications or expectation mismatch (Mohamed et al., 2021). This is following the necessity of intense research and legitimacy before cosmetic sclerotherapy. Patients should prioritize practitioners with legitimate histories, patient referrals, and documented success rates of the procedure. Last but not least, patient selection of a qualified practitioner not only ensures the health of the patient but also increases confidence and satisfaction with esthetic outcomes since a significant component of the entire treatment procedure.

Test Your Knowledge

1. What are the common side effects of cosmetic sclerotherapy, and how are they typically managed?
2. What are the rare but serious complications of sclerotherapy, and how can they be recognized and addressed?

12.5. Effectiveness and Results

Learning Outcome

1. Understand expected outcomes and success rates of cosmetic sclerotherapy
2. Describe factors influencing treatment efficacy
3. Focus on long-term results and maintenance

Cosmetic sclerotherapy is also a top therapy among those who need to alleviate the discomfort of varicose veins, and it is very effective both clinically and with patient satisfaction. The effect of this minimal invasiveness of treatment is validated by clinical evidence that indicates that it can indeed eliminate symptomatology of pain and swelling and improve the cosmetic appearance of the legs. A 351-patient trial, with ultrasound-guided foam sclerotherapy, put in the foreground the point that most patients were content with the outcome of the treatment six months later. Notably, the research showed that almost all patients anticipated improvement in their symptoms in the lower limb and one-third overestimated such expectations, proving the treatment's capability to achieve more than the patient's anticipation of symptom relief and cosmetic improvement (Darvall et al., 2009). Further patient outcome evaluation reveals that cosmetic sclerotherapy not only alleviates bodily symptoms but also yields considerable psychosocial benefits. Most of the patients have experienced enhanced quality of life following treatment, particularly concerning clothing, social relationships, and lifestyle enhancement. From the above study, while two-thirds of the patients expected lifestyle improvements, the results fell a little short of expectation. However, a high percentage reported improvement in social contacts and self-esteem, with one-third indicating unexpected benefits to their social lives. This broad impact testifies to the treatment's general efficacy, and hence cosmetic sclerotherapy is a popular choice among persons suffering from the physical and psychosocial implications of varicose veins (Darvall et al., 2009). The economic viability of cosmetic sclerotherapy should be considered as well, as it is a very important factor for patients weighing their options for treatment. Recent arguments about healthcare expenditure highlight the need to balance clinical efficacy and economic viability, in particular for elective procedures. Results of studies evaluating the economic impact of cosmetic sclerotherapy suggest that, if direct medical costs and indirect gains like enhanced lifestyle and decreased work absenteeism are taken into consideration, the treatment is a valuable investment for patients. Besides, with healthcare systems becoming more clinically and economically favorable, treatment-oriented, cosmetic sclerotherapy not only comes across as a very effective treatment for varicose veins but also as cost-effective relative to the array of aesthetic medical therapies.

12.5.1. Expected Outcomes and Success Rates

The predicted outcomes of cosmetic sclerotherapy are striking and multifaceted, both physical and psychological, and point towards improvement in patients. The most commonly reported success after UGFS is the capacity to heal CVD, especially great and SSV incompetence. In research, UGFS is responsible for a significant reduction of visible varicose veins, as per duplex ultrasound scans and clinical assessment. Additionally, patients document an enhanced quality of life with maintained improvement for a period of at least twelve months following treatment. These outcomes closely reflect patient expectations as those patients undergoing cosmetic enhancement have disabling physical symptoms , such as swelling and pain, which are successfully prevented through the application of UGFS, offering an alternative to more invasive surgical treatment (Darvall, 2012). Cosmetic sclerotherapy success rates also show a hopeful trend, as shown by several studies reporting high rates of efficacy. The treatment has been especially well-received among young patients, who tend to respond more favorably to the therapy. For example, in a trial on direct percutaneous ethanol instillation for venous malformations, it was observed that a very high percentage of patients, about 73.3%, needed just one treatment session to obtain adequate outcomes.

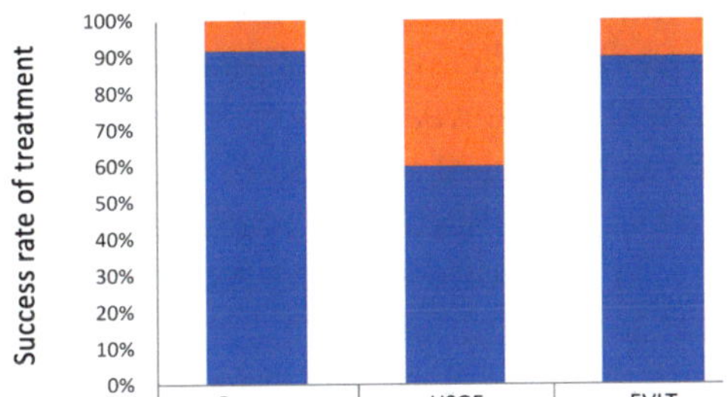

	Surgery	USGF	EVLT
fail	3	10	2
success	32	15	18

Figure 12.12. The success and failure rates of different therapeutic options. USGF: Ultrasound-guided foam sclerotherapy, EVLT: Endovenous laser therapy.

Source: https://www.researchgate.net/profile/Ahmed-Mousa-22/publication/335277128/figure/fig2/AS:794063942995968@1566331005062/The-success-and-failure-rate-between-different-therapeutic-options-USGF.png.

This is in line with the general belief that sclerotherapy is less likely to involve complications than surgical procedures, thus making it more attractive. Along with the quantitative measures of success, qualitative elements, including patient perception of body image and the significant reduction in cosmetic deformity, encouraging higher self-esteem and general wellbeing after treatment (Lamba, 2010), should also be considered. While the overall expected outcomes and success rates paint a positive picture, there may be variation in patient perceptions of cosmetic sclerotherapy. Factors , such as the severity of venous disease, age of patient, and baseline conditions can affect the effectiveness of treatment. Significantly, studies indicate that chronic venous ulcers have been found to heal better when sclerotherapy is included alongside compression treatments, thereby supporting the importance of individualization. Finally, the integration of patient expectations in pre-treatment assessments on an integrative basis can help lead to improved results and increased satisfaction. Thus, cosmetic sclerotherapy is a good bet for those looking for efficient treatments for venous disorders, with the added benefit of two-pronged aesthetic improvement and enhanced functional capacity (Darvall, 2012) (Figure 12.12).

12.5.2. Factors Influencing Treatment Efficacy

The effectiveness of cosmetic sclerotherapy is influenced by a multitude of factors, ranging from patient demographics, the inherent nature of varicosities to the sclerosant agent used. Studies have established that the age of the patient is a key factor in how responsive the patient is to the treatment, particularly for patients older than 50 years, who react differently to the treatment. For instance, studies indicated that patients below the age of 50 years experienced a widely divergent rate of complications, with a significant 57.7% of subjects in the CEAP classification C2 demonstrating decreased post-treatment complications (Mahitha and Punitha, 2021). Furthermore, the type and level of severity of the vascular condition also affect the effectiveness of sclerotherapy. Mild varicosities patients are deemed to be more appropriate candidates in general, with the capacity to facilitate easier recovery as well as better outcomes, and the importance of thorough pre-treatment evaluation to properly stratify risk and predict outcomes. The second determinant of the effectiveness of the treatment is the approach adopted during sclerotherapy. The use of ultrasound has been shown to enhance the precision of procedures and reduce opportunities for complications and hence, better patient outcomes. Where the sclerotherapy is performed using this precise method, the chance of successful treatment increases as there is better visualization of the veins and supporting tissue structures. Comparing results from various sclerosants also brings into focus that the choice of agent can significantly impact treatment results. Research has shown that the use of specific formulations, i.e., 10% STS, has less rate of complications compared to other concentrations, pointing toward the importance of individualized treatment protocols (Mahitha and Punitha, 2021). Thus, it is not just the technical method but also the type of sclerosant that plays an important role in determining the success of cosmetic sclerotherapy as a whole. Finally, patient issues , such as compliance, previous comorbidities, and expectations may play an important part in the perceived efficacy of treatment. Reactions to sclerotherapy may vary among individuals based on psychosocial traits, whereby a good attitude and awareness of the procedure result in overall satisfaction. Furthermore, patients with comorbidities may pose higher risks, which may affect post-treatment recovery. A thorough assessment using psychological evaluation coupled with the examination of a medical history will be capable of screening risk populations and facilitating individualized interventions that enhance recovery and effectiveness. Screening candidates with comorbidities before treatment, for example, allows proper preparation and planning for management, ultimately leading to improved results. Knowledge of these individual factors, coupled with clinical evaluation, forms an integrated strategy towards the optimization of the effectiveness of cosmetic sclerotherapy.

12.5.3. Long-Term Results and Maintenance

Long-term results of cosmetic sclerotherapy are a significant characteristic of its efficiency and durability as a therapeutic technique for venous malformations. Science indicates that patients undergoing this treatment will most likely experience appreciable lesion volume reduction, in most instances with good cosmetic outcomes that last in the long term. For instance, a percutaneous ethanol instillation clinical trial highlighted the fact that only 73.3% of the patients required one session for a good outcome, representing the effectiveness of a very minimally invasive method. Additionally, the follow-up period of about 7.6 months certified that the patients maintained such improvements, representing the possibility of a long-lasting effect of sclerotherapy. The recurrent statement of minimal complications is yet another consideration favoring the popularity of this mode of treatment for patients who prefer to correct superficial vascular anomalies for an extended period (Lamba, 2010). During maintenance following cosmetic sclerotherapy, one should consider factors that can influence the success as well as the duration of treatment outcomes. A key characteristic is the type of sclerosing agent used; variations in efficacy can be noted between agents like ethanol and STS, which may influence rates of recanalization and, indirectly, long-term outcomes. Reports note that although immediate results of sclerotherapy are generally positive, ongoing follow-up is essential for managing the potential for future symptoms or recurrences. Patient-specific factors for success, , such as lesion location and type, will also be important to identify in order to guide future treatment and ensure sustained results (Wallace et al., 2014). Improvements in sclerotherapy modality and technique are still important to realize enhanced long-term outcomes. Techniques that have also enhanced delivery strategies and also their complementary care pathways are also able to further enhance patient satisfaction and reduce post-operative pain, as studies have outlined enhanced endovenous laser ablation (EVLA) methods. Such clinical trials demonstrate not only enhanced clinical results compared with standard surgical methods but also notably enhanced patient quality of life. Long-term observation and research are still necessary to finding the finer points of the effectiveness of treatment and maintenance procedures. As such procedures are continually enhanced and given priority with a concentration on individualized patient care, cosmetic sclerotherapy can be an efficient and sustainable means of the treatment of venous malformations (Wallace et al., 2014) (Figure 12.13).

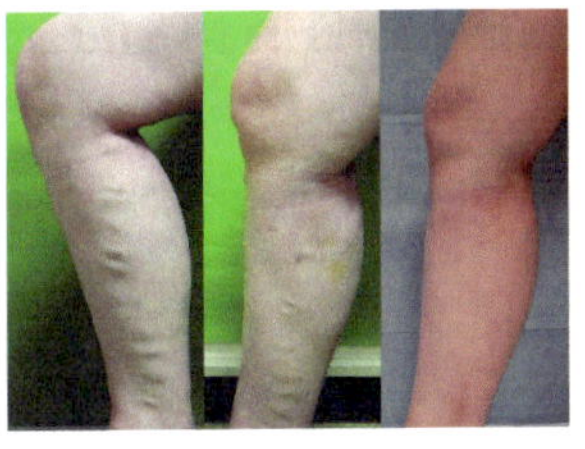

Figure 12.13. A: preoperative status, B: 1 month after EVLA (before sclerotherapy), C: 1 month after sclerotherapy.

Source: https://www.researchgate.net/publication/276830638/figure/fig3/AS:492118474006534@1494341595511/A-preoperative-status-B-1-month-after-EVLA-before-sclerotherapy-C-1-month-after.png.

Test Your Knowledge

1. What are the expected outcomes and success rates of cosmetic sclerotherapy?
2. What factors influence the effectiveness of cosmetic sclerotherapy?
3. What are the long-term results of cosmetic sclerotherapy, and is maintenance required?

12.6. Cost and Accessibility

Learning Outcome

1. Discuss about average costs associated with sclerotherapy
2. Focus on insurance coverage and financial considerations
3. Deal with the availability of services in different regions

In looking at the cost and affordability of cosmetic sclerotherapy, keep in mind that the economic impact of treatment can be dramatically influential on patient outcomes and therapy compliance. Charges associated with sclerotherapy total more than procedure fees and include ancillary-related charges , such as diagnostic imaging and postoperative garments. Various health care systems and providers have considerable variations in insurance coverage of sclerotherapy, resulting in disparate access to treatment. Some patients may face low out-of-pocket expenses, which could make them hesitant to undergo necessary treatment. Lack of homogeneity between areas as far as price and insurance coverage are concerned increases these challenges, which may leave disadvantaged patients with few options to effectively manage venous diseases. As highlighted in the updated guidelines for the treatment of CVD, cost considerations play a significant role in clinical decision-making, reflecting the extensive involvement of economic considerations in patient care plans (Maeseneer et al., 2022). Access to cosmetic sclerotherapy procedures also varies geographically, which provides an uneven situation for patients receiving interventions. Urban areas will often contain several clinics that specialize in sclerotherapy, while rural areas will often lack adequate facilities and staff. These geographical disparities are a cause of health inequities and create a situation where individuals in the less densely populated areas may forego treatment because of travel difficulties or the unavailability of competent healthcare experts. Accessibility is further undermined by the perception that sclerotherapy is elective or cosmetic, and therefore, this may result in reduced priority being given to such services within healthcare resources. It is therefore imperative that healthcare stakeholders set it as their objective to enhance access to sclerotherapy among underserved communities and make attempts to raise awareness of the medical necessity for this intervention among CVD and other related illnesses (Mimura et al., 2020). Furthermore, the integration of patient-centered care within the framework of sclerotherapy can facilitate greater access and quality in the treatment process. Patient involvement in decision-making can enable patients to weigh the pros and cons of treatment. Educational programs that explain the function of sclerotherapy in regard to aesthetic and therapeutic use are essential in maintaining an informed patient population. Fostering collaborations between health professionals and community organizations also closes the gaps in access and knowledge. These tasks can lead to increased use of sclerotherapy services, which ultimately improve patient outcomes and quality of life, along with better health and well-being. Thus, addressing costs and issues of accessibility is important so that the advantages of cosmetic sclerotherapy can reach every patient regardless of their socioeconomic status or region (Maeseneer et al., 2022).

12.6.1. Average Costs Associated with Sclerotherapy

The financial implications of sclerotherapy, particularly in cosmetic application, warrant close examination. As a cosmetic and venous insufficiency therapy with minimal invasiveness, the cost of sclerotherapy is typically in the range of $300 to $500 per session, based on location within a given region and practitioner proficiency. While the initial expense seems reasonable, potential clients must factor in the reality that multiple sessions are generally needed in order to obtain the best results. This overall cost can amount to a significant amount of money, particularly for those patients desiring to treat varicose or widespread spider veins. So, potential patients must evaluate their aesthetic and cost objectives within these budgets because over expenditure can lead to dissatisfaction if results cannot satisfy their cosmetic goals. In addition to that, when evaluating average expenses from sclerotherapy, it is also important to take other factors into account that could affect overall expenditures. For example, consultation fees, follow-up visits, and ancillary procedures could add to overall costs. Complete treatment regimens usually encompass pre-procedure evaluations, such as ultrasound exams to assess the severity of venous pathology, which could further increase costs. Further, the modality of treatment applied, , such as whether a practitioner employs traditional saline solution or newer sclerosing agents, can influence costs. Such variations imply that patients should consult multiple practitioners and inquire about complete pricing scales in order to avoid surprises in terms of extra charges. If patients are informed about the complete range of costs, they will be in a position to make good choices for their treatment methods in cosmetic sclerotherapy. Lastly, economic evaluation of sclerotherapy reveals its cost-effectiveness compared to more invasive surgery. Research shows that although initial surgery costs are more expensive, sclerotherapy has lower long-term costs, taking into account the frequency and extent of post-operative treatment required for surgical patients. For example, research finds that conventional surgical techniques may necessitate secondary interventions in the future, which tend to drive up long-term costs. By comparison, sclerotherapy entails fewer complications and less time to recover, leading to a more favorable economic status in the future. Thus, while the initial cost of sclerotherapy is outrageous, its potential to attain lesser complications and economic advantages in the future renders it an appropriate and affordable option in aesthetic treatment, according to findings of (El-Sheikha et al., 2015; Komorowski et al., 2016) (Figure 12.14).

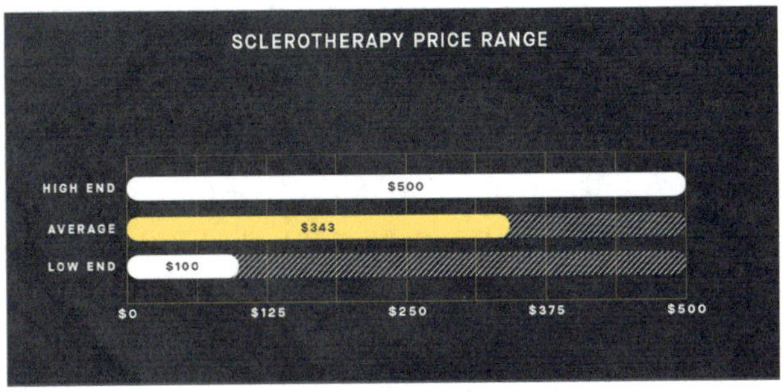

Figure 12.14. Sclerotherapy price range.

Source: https://images.ctfassets.net/zw35sfestf1t/CwzKfUAclMiH5eyeVZF8f/6784efaaef7f96d4f257704fe33c54e7/aedit-average-sclerotherapy-procedure-cost-range-chart.png.

12.6.2. Insurance Coverage and Financial Considerations

The field of cosmetic sclerotherapy also carries a unique set of insurance coverage and economic factors that patients must navigate before undergoing treatment. Most insurance policies hold sclerotherapy to be an elective cosmetic procedure, resulting in limited or no coverage at all, hence the patient assumes the total cost entirely.

Given the growing popularity of cosmetic procedures, particularly among millennials—a generation with an intense need for aesthetic treatments, therapists now have an emerging expectation to clearly describe the fees incurred by treatment. This is in line with the evidence that companies need to be able to communicate effectively with their target audience to generate understanding and appreciation of the cost of services (Kadam et al., 2015). Consequently, prospective patients need to consider not just the efficacy and safety of sclerotherapy but also whether they can afford to invest resources in what is deemed to be a luxury procedure.

Cosmetic sclerotherapy finances also involve the possibility of long-term expenses. Although the upfront cost may appear high, especially for those who need more than one treatment, knowledge of the longevity of results is important. Others may have recurring vascular issues, necessitating repeat treatments, which are cumulative in cost. Significantly, patients may also seek financing and payment plans that most clinics offer to alleviate initial costs.

The variation in pricing models across clinics also points to the need for rigorous research and comparison prior to committing to any particular provider. They must also be informed of the lack of insurance cover for such procedures, which would have lightened the financial burden, thereby highlighting the necessity of being transparent in communication by clinics (Association CM, 1988).

Lastly, the role of transparency in finances cannot be overstated. Clinics that provide clear information on the cost prospect, financing options, and lack of insurance cover engender trust and decision-making by informed clients in the future. This openness becomes ever more important in consideration of the close-up nature of cosmetic surgery; an honest understanding of cost and expense can enhance the psychological freedom which such choices so often involve. As the market for aesthetics is continually growing and changing, clinics must devise innovative ways of communicating the cost of procedures like sclerotherapy while ensuring availability to an increasing population, including the young who have an extremely high interest in such procedures (Kadam et al., 2015). Ultimately, the interaction between the cost factors and the insurance coverage is a determining force for the availability and popularity of cosmetic sclerotherapy as an efficacious mode of treatment.

12.6.3. Availability of Services in Different Regions

The rate of cosmetic sclerotherapy procedures varies significantly across different territories, depending on the standards of healthcare institutions, economic standards, and local demand for cosmetic procedures. Individuals living in large cities are offered a wide selection of clinics that offer cosmetic procedures, including sclerotherapy. The advanced machinery used in these facilities, like ultrasound-guided sclerotherapy, can be used to enhance the results of the treatment. Conversely, rural areas seldom receive specialized care, and the patients must travel long distances for treatment. Such disparity can lead to unequal access to effective care, deterring people from seeking necessary aesthetic treatment and further exacerbating existing healthcare disparities.

Furthermore, regional variation in acceptance and control of cosmetic sclerotherapy are some of the reasons why disparities exist in the delivery of services. Certain locales, particularly where cosmetic treatment is integrated into the culture, may see an influx of clinics and practitioners who offer them. Conversely, regions with stricter regulation or public reluctance toward cosmetic treatment may see a shortage. Research has shown that patients at various geographical locations have varied outcomes regarding the effectiveness and accessibility of interventions, impacting satisfaction with care. For example, studies have shown that patients who undergo treatment in areas that have adequate resources fare better compared to those in poor resource areas (Brookes et al., 2021). In addition, the evolution of cosmetic sclerotherapy practice illustrates the need for training programs with a focus on establishing the capacity of services across different areas. Training health workers in poor areas may lead to improved delivery of services such that patients receive effective and safe treatment. Following the experience of varicose vein treatments over time, adaptation into minimally invasive treatments , such as sclerotherapy, is characterized by an increased level of acceptance and demand for the treatment (Mekako, 2012). Active expansion of access to cosmetic sclerotherapy procedures through the preparation of specialists with the necessary knowledge and skills can significantly improve patient outcomes and satisfaction in a wide variety of regions, ultimately bridging this gap in this important aspect of cosmetic treatment.

Test Your Knowledge

1. What are the average costs associated with cosmetic sclerotherapy?
2. Is cosmetic sclerotherapy typically covered by insurance, and what financial considerations should patients keep in mind?
3. How accessible is cosmetic sclerotherapy in different regions or healthcare settings?

SUMMARY

The success and patient satisfaction of cosmetic sclerotherapy, particularly UGFS, underscore the value of such treatments in contemporary venous therapy. Research indicates that UGFS not only alleviates the physical complaints resulting from varicose veins but also provides excellent cosmetic improvement, a prime concern for most patients. With the large number of patients reporting that their hopes for symptom alleviation and cosmetic outcomes were achieved or exceeded, UGFS is a procedure that is clearly highly appealing to patients who desire to enhance the cosmetic appearance and function of their lower extremities. This helps to highlight the importance of correlating available therapies with patient expectations to maximize optimal therapeutic outcomes (Darvall et al., 2009). Moreover, UGFS has been found to possess great advantages when compared to traditional surgical interventions, , such as the application of SVS. The treatment is characterized by its minimally invasive approach, causing less pain, bruising, and lower analgesic demand. Furthermore, studies have shown that patients undergoing treatment using UGFS are capable of resuming work and regular activities earlier than their counterparts under traditional surgical interventions. These results not only increase the quality of care for the patients but also result in better satisfaction rates post-treatment, thus changing the treatment ambiance for CVD. The health-related quality of life improvement observed post-UGFS, particularly in physical symptoms and lifestyle, is prime evidence of its effectiveness (Darvall et al., 2012). Lastly, the long-term consequence transcends mere surface cosmetic improvement as it encompasses integral aspects of emotional and psychosocial well-being. The majority of the patients exhibit a better level of confidence and improved interpersonal relations following their procedure, which mirrors an improvement in overall quality of life. As the practitioners increasingly become dependent on patient-centered care, the comprehensive psychological benefits derived through UGFS become the most important aspect to cherish. This method of treatment not only addresses physical states but also boosts patient empowerment, which is invaluable when health and beauty are in question. Therefore, continued support for and research on cosmetic sclerotherapy is important in an attempt to enhance and refine patient outcomes within the new era of treatment for venous disease.

In the study of the field of cosmetic sclerotherapy, note is to be made of the tremendous advances and breakthroughs in treatment techniques. Of these advances, cryoablation has been particularly promising, especially in reference to venous malformations. A recent meta-analysis discussed that cryoablation had a substantial mean post-procedure decrease in lesion size by 71.7%, along with an average pain score decrease of 78.2%, with complete improvement of pain in over 63.6% of patients (Fish et al., 2022). These findings underscore the efficiency of cryoablation as a contemporary technique, as well as consolidate its role as a valid alternative in venous disease management. These reassuring outcomes point towards less aggressive methods that address both cosmetic improvement and patient comfort demands. In addition to this, developments in the management of varicose veins transformed the horizon of cosmetic sclerotherapy significantly. The trend towards minimally invasive therapies, particularly EVLA, has transformed treatment paradigms over the last two decades. Approximately 60% of varicosities are deemed suitable for EVLA, which was found to be clinically effective and significantly enhanced patients' quality of life compared to the traditional operating methods (Mekako, 2012). Furthermore, the studies illustrated that concomitant phlebectomies could enhance the result of treatments when performed along with EVLA, providing support for the effect of customized treatment approaches in optimizing patient outcomes. This evolution emphasizes the importance of tailoring treatments to unique anatomic issues to achieve the best intervention for cosmetic improvement. Lastly, cosmetic sclerotherapy discourse cannot be complete without reference to safety profiles and treatment modalities' complications. The majority of these treatments, , such as EVLA and cryoablation, carry low rates of complications; for instance, the rate of significant events in cryoablation was only 3.7% and was largely due to chronic dysesthesia (Fish et al., 2022). Protection of patient safety along with acceptable aesthetic results is paramount during sclerotherapy treatments. In addition, prophylactic antibiotic use during surgical procedures has been found to significantly decrease wound complications, further purifying clinical practice within the specialty (Mekako, 2012). Both quests for effectiveness and caution with regard to safety are at the heart of continuing to improve cosmetic sclerotherapy as well as promoting greater patient satisfaction in aesthetic procedures.

KEY TERMS FROM THIS CHAPTER

Aesthetic flaws
Ancillary procedures
Cardiovascular complications
Cosmetic improvement
Cyanoacrylate adhesive closure
Dilated small vessels
Endovenous laser ablation (EVLA)
Endovenous thermal ablation (ETA)
Health care systems
Hydroquinone-based treatments
Aesthetic vascular therapy
Ancillary-related charges
Chronic venous disease (CVD)
Cosmetic sclerotherapy
Deep vein thrombosis (DVT)
Endothelial cell DNA
Endovenous laser treatment (EVLT)
Great saphenous vein (GSV)
Healthcare systems
Invasive modalities

CRITICAL THINKING QUESTIONS

1. **What is the primary purpose of cosmetic sclerotherapy?**
   a. Treat deep vein thrombosis
   b. Remove skin tags
   c. Reduce the appearance of spider and varicose veins
   d. Increase blood circulation in major arteries
2. **Which type of agent is typically injected during a sclerotherapy procedure?**
   a. Anticoagulant
   b. Sclerosant
   c. Anesthetic
   d. Vasodilator
3. **What is a common side effect following cosmetic sclerotherapy?**
   a. Hair loss
   b. Skin tightening
   c. Increased blood pressure
   d. Bruising at the injection site
4. **Which veins are most commonly treated with cosmetic sclerotherapy?**
   a. Deep femoral veins
   b. Pulmonary veins
   c. Spider veins and small varicose veins
   d. Coronary veins
5. **Which of the following is a common complication of cosmetic sclerotherapy?**
   a. Pulmonary embolism
   b. Hyperpigmentation
   c. Myocardial infarction
   d. Stroke

Short Answer Questions

1. What is cosmetic sclerotherapy and how does it work?
2. Which types of veins are most commonly treated with sclerotherapy?
3. What are the commonly used sclerosing agents in cosmetic sclerotherapy?
4. What is the typical process of a sclerotherapy session, and how long does it take?
5. What are the contraindications to undergoing cosmetic sclerotherapy?
6. Who is considered a good candidate for cosmetic sclerotherapy?
7. What are the common side effects and risks associated with cosmetic sclerotherapy?
8. How long does it take to see results from cosmetic sclerotherapy, and are the effects permanent?

Answer to Critical Thinking Questions

1.(c) 2.(b) 3.(d) 4.(c) 5.(b)

REFERENCES

1. Darvall, K. A., Bate, G. R., Sam, R. C., Adam, D. J., Silverman, S. H., & Bradbury, A. W. (2009). Patients' expectations before and satisfaction after ultrasound guided foam sclerotherapy for varicose veins. *European journal of vascular and endovascular surgery : the official journal of the European Society for Vascular Surgery*, *38*(5), 642–647. https://doi.org/10.1016/j.ejvs.2009.07.014(accessed on 11th June 2025).
2. Ahmad, S. (2019). Efficacy of percutaneous sclerotherapy in low flow venous malformations–A single center series. https://core.ac.uk/download/442324116.pdf (accessed on 11th June 2025).
3. Ahmed, S. K., Anjum, N., Malik, N. I., et al. (2016). Ultrasound-guided intralesional bleomycin injection (IBI) for treatment of cutaneous hemangiomas and vascular malformations. https://core.ac.uk/download/56530012.pdf (accessed on 11th June 2025).
4. Ambrosio, D. V. (2018). *Incidence and Need of Advanced Aesthetic Somatology in South Africa*. https://core.ac.uk/download/222968033.pdf (accessed on 11th June 2025).
5. Antonova, S., Radev, A., & Spasov, A. (2022). Minimally invasive methods for the treatment of varicose veins of the lower extremities: Overview of the existing modern methods. https://core.ac.uk/download/599136498.pdf (accessed on 11th June 2025).
6. Di Gangi, S., Guillet, C., Anzengruber, F., Zechmann, S., & Meier, T. O. (2024). Deep vein thrombosis after sclerotherapy and endovenous laser ablation of varicose veins - an observational study. *VASA. Zeitschrift fur Gefasskrankheiten*, *53*(4), 275–285. https://doi.org/10.1024/0301-1526/a001130(accessed on 11th June 2025).
7. Araujo, S. P., Barros Junior, N. de, Figueiredo, M., et al. (2009). Results of surgical treatment compared with ultrasound-guided foam sclerotherapy in patients with varicose veins: A prospective randomized study. https://core.ac.uk/download/37735270.pdf (accessed on 11th June 2025).
8. Aronniemi, J., Castren, E., Lappalainen, K., et al. (2016). Sclerotherapy complications of peripheral venous malformations. https://core.ac.uk/download/146448263.pdf (accessed on 11th June 2025).
9. Arslan, M., Gülek, B., & Sözütok, S. (2018). Results of a long-term performance and follow-up of endogenous laser ablation procedures performed for treating great saphenous vein incompetence. https://core.ac.uk/download/227059144.pdf (accessed on 11th June 2025).
10. Baker, L., Benson, S., Berman, I., et al. (2019). Cyanoacrylate closure for peripheral veins: Consensus document of the Australasian College of Phlebology. https://core.ac.uk/download/228075109.pdf (accessed on 11th June 2025).
11. Bardazzi, A., Colletti, G., Dalmonte, P., Deganello, A., Gazzabin, L., Mattassi, R., et al. (2017). Complications after treatment of head and neck venous malformations with sodium tetradecyl sulfate foam. https://core.ac.uk/download/96519122.pdf (accessed on 11th June 2025).
12. Blaise, S., Brix, M., Carpentier, P. H., et al. (2011). Treatment of low-flow vascular malformations by ultrasound-guided sclerotherapy with polidocanol foam: 24 cases and literature review. https://core.ac.uk/download/pdf/82462051.pdf (accessed on 11th June 2025).
13. Brookes, J., Evans, N., Hamilton, G., et al. (2021). Single center experience of sirolimus therapy in head and neck low-flow vascular malformations. https://core.ac.uk/download/429123167.pdf (accessed on 11th June 2025).

14. Campbell, W. B., & Lindsey, B. (2006). Rationing of treatment for varicose veins and use of new treatment methods: A survey of practice in the United Kingdom. https://core.ac.uk/download/pdf/81135843.pdf (accessed on 11th June 2025).
15. Canadian Medical Association. (1988). Volume 31, Issue 2. https://core.ac.uk/download/215388140.pdf (accessed on 11th June 2025).
16. Gloviczki, P., Comerota, A. J., Dalsing, M. C., Eklof, B. G., Gillespie, D. L., Gloviczki, M. L., Lohr, J. M., McLafferty, R. B., Meissner, M. H., Murad, M. H., Padberg, F. T., Pappas, P. J., Passman, M. A., Raffetto, J. D., Vasquez, M. A., Wakefield, T. W., Society for Vascular Surgery, & American Venous Forum (2011). The care of patients with varicose veins and associated chronic venous diseases: clinical practice guidelines of the Society for Vascular Surgery and the American Venous Forum. *Journal of vascular surgery, 53*(5 Suppl), 2S–48S. https://doi.org/10.1016/j.jvs.2011.01.079(accessed on 11th June 2025).
17. Darvall, Katy Abigail Leigh (2012). Outcomes from ultrasound-guided foam sclerotherapy for chronic venous disease. University of Birmingham. M.D.(accessed on 11th June 2025).
18. Davidson, J., & Ford, K. (2015). *Pediatric Surgery: A Core Surgical Trainee's Guide to Vascular Malformations in Children*. https://core.ac.uk/download/336578222.pdf (accessed on 11th June 2025).
19. De Maeseneer, M., Kakkos, S. K., Aherne, T., Bækgaard, N., Black, S., Blomgren, L., Giannoukas, A., et al. (2022). Editor's choice–European Society for Vascular Surgery (ESVS) 2022 clinical practice guidelines on the management of chronic venous disease of the lower limbs. *European Journal of Vascular and Endovascular Surgery, 63*, 184–267. https://doi.org/10.1016/j.ejvs.2021.12.024 (accessed on 11th June 2025).
20. Piekarska, E., Dobrzeniecki, K., & Luter, R. (2025). Invasive Treatment of Lower Limb Varicose Veins - Comparison of Treatment Methods. *Journal of Education, Health and Sport, 77*, 56646. https://doi.org/10.12775/JEHS.2025.77.56646 (accessed on 11th June 2025).
21. El-Sheikha, J. (2015). *Long Term Outcome of Minimally Invasive Treatment for Superficial Venous Insufficiency of The Lower Limb*. https://core.ac.uk/download/556180342.pdf (accessed on 11th June 2025).
22. Enespa, P., Chandra, D., & Singh, D. (2022). Sources, purification, immobilization and industrial applications of microbial lipases: An overview. *Critical Reviews in Food Science and Nutrition, 63*, 6653–6686. https://www.semanticscholar.org/paper/36f7427b290ef70583be080a6c5d12831b0db511 (accessed on 11th June 2025).
23. Fayyaz, F., Vaghani, V., Ekhator, C., Abdullah, M., Alsubari, R. A., Daher, O. A., Bakht, D., et al. (2024). Advancements in varicose vein treatment: Anatomy, pathophysiology, minimally invasive techniques, sclerotherapy, patient satisfaction, and future directions. *Cureus*. https://doi.org/10.7759/cureus.51990 (accessed on 11th June 2025).
24. Fernández-Varela-Gómez, F., Sandoval-García, A., & Cabrera-Rios, K. V. (2024). Signs of skin aging: A review. https://core.ac.uk/download/613230159.pdf (accessed on 11th June 2025).
25. Ferreira, C., Moreira, M., Delerue-Matos, C., & Sarraguça, M. (2023). Subcritical water extraction to valorize grape biomass—A step closer to circular economy. *Molecules, 28*. https://www.semanticscholar.org/paper/a969aa75c0ea99fced9ed0045a5057634ab46758 (accessed on 11th June 2025).

26. Haidar, O., Jaques, A., McCaughran, P. W., & Metcalfe, M. (2023). AI-generated information for vascular patients: Assessing the standard of procedure-specific information provided by the ChatGPT AI-language model. *Cureus*. https://doi.org/10.7759/cureus.49764 (accessed on 11th June 2025).

27. Kadam, S. (2015). *Future Marketing and Engagement Considerations for The Non-Surgical Cosmetic Enhancement Industry for Educated and Professional Male and Female Millennial Generation Target Audiences*. https://core.ac.uk/download/ (accessed on 11th June 2025).

28. Komorowski, D., Mavropoulos, J., Slobodnik, N., et al. (2016). A randomized prospective long-term (> 1 year) clinical trial comparing the efficacy and safety of radiofrequency ablation to 980 nm laser ablation of the great saphenous vein. https://core.ac.uk/download/130355241.pdf (accessed on 11th June 2025).

29. Lamba, S. (2010). *A Prospective Non-Randomized Clinical Study to Evaluate the Role of Direct Percutaneous Ethanol Instillation in The Treatment of Venous Malformations (VMs) In the Face and Neck*. https://core.ac.uk/download/288215523.pdf (accessed on 11th June 2025).

30. Lee, I. H., Kim, K. H., Jeon, P., Byun, H. S., Kim, H. J., Kim, S. T., Kim, Y. W., et al. (2009). Ethanol sclerotherapy for the management of craniofacial venous malformations: The interim results. https://core.ac.uk/download/pdf/8280418.pdf (accessed on 11th June 2025).

31. Mahitha, M. C., & Oli, P. T. (2021). Complications, indication and tolerance of foam sclerotherapy in varicose vein management done in a tertiary care center in South India. https://core.ac.uk/download/386109622.pdf (accessed on 11th June 2025).

32. Mekako, A. Optimising outcomes in the treatment of lower limb varicose veins. (Thesis). Hull York Medical School, the University of Hull and the University of York. https://hull-repository.worktribe.com/output/4214091s (accessed on 11th June 2025).

33. Micallef, A. (2011). *Piles and More... Dealing with Incompetent Veins*. https://core.ac.uk/download/46604300.pdf (accessed on 11th June 2025).

34. Mimura, H., Akita, S., Fujino, A., Jinnin, M., Ozaki, M., Osuga, K., Nakaoka, H., et al. (2020). Japanese clinical practice guidelines for vascular anomalies 2017. *Japanese Journal of Radiology, 38*, 287–342. https://doi.org/10.1007/s11604-019-00885-5 (accessed on 11th June 2025).

35. Fish, A., Moushey, A., Chan, S. M., Staib, L., Marino, A., & Schlachter, T. (2022). Cryoablation of Venous Malformations: A Systematic Review. *Journal of vascular and interventional radiology : JVIR, 33*(8), 993–1000. https://doi.org/10.1016/j.jvir.2022.04.010(accessed on 11th June 2025).

36. Tyner, K. E. (2008). *Cosmetic Technologies of The Body: An Exploration of Self and Identity Through the Consumption of Nonsurgical Cosmetic Procedures*. https://core.ac.uk/download/38911722.pdf (accessed on 11th June 2025).

37. Vorisek, R. (2017). *Cross-Cultural Comparison of Cosmetic Procedures in Latin America and East Asia*. https://core.ac.uk/download/148696179.pdf (accessed on 11th June 2025).

38. Wallace, T., MD. (2014). *Optimizing Outcomes in The Treatment of Superficial Venous Insufficiency*. https://core.ac.uk/download/556179693.pdf (accessed on 11th June 2025).

39. Youngerwood, A. (2012). *From Creams to Lasers: Regulating the Beauty Industry in The New Millennium*. https://core.ac.uk/download/28938988.pdf (accessed on 11th June 2025).

INDEX

C

D

E

F

Q

R

S